CELLULAR
AND
MOLECULAR
IMMUNOLOGY

CELLULAR
AND
MOLECULAR
IMMUNOLOGY

ABUL K. ABBAS, M.B.B.S.
Professor of Pathology
Harvard Medical School and Brigham and Women's Hospital
Boston, Massachusetts

ANDREW H. LICHTMAN, M.D., Ph.D.
Assistant Professor of Pathology
Harvard Medical School and Brigham and Women's Hospital
Boston, Massachusetts

JORDAN S. POBER, M.D., Ph.D.
Professor of Pathology and Immunobiology
Yale University School of Medicine
New Haven, Connecticut

W.B. SAUNDERS COMPANY
Harcourt Brace Jovanovich, Inc.
Philadelphia   London   Toronto   Montreal   Sydney   Tokyo

W. B. Saunders Company
Harcourt Brace Jovanovich, Inc.

The Curtis Center
Independence Square West
Philadelphia, PA 19106

Library of Congress Cataloging-in-Publication Data

Abbas, Abul K.
    Cellular and molecular immunology / Abul K. Abbas, Andrew H.
Lichtman, Jordan S. Pober.
      p.   cm.
    ISBN 0-7216-3032-4
    1. Cellular immunity. 2. Immunity—Molecular aspects.
I. Lichtman, Andrew H. II. Pober, Jordan S. III. Title.
    [DNLM: 1. Immunity, Cellular. 2. Lymphocytes—immunology. QW
568 A122c]
QR185.5.A23 1991
616.07′9—dc20
DNLM/DLC

Editor: Martin J. Wonsiewicz
Designer: Paul M. Fry
Production Manager: Peter Faber
Manuscript Editor: Carol Robins
Illustrator: Risa Clow
Illustration Coordinator: Brett MacNaughton
Indexer: Linda Van Pelt

Cellular and Molecular Immunology   ISBN 0-7216-3032-4

Last digit is the print number: 9   8   7   6   5   4   3

To

Ann, Jonathan, Rehana

Sheila, Eben, Ariella, Amos

Barbara, Jeremy, Jonathan

PREFACE

Cellular and Molecular Immunology is intended as an introductory textbook primarily for students of medicine and related disciplines. This book evolved from a course we teach to first-year medical students at Harvard Medical School who are enrolled in the joint Harvard–MIT M.D. program in Health Sciences and Technology. The impetus for writing this book is the remarkable development of immunology as a science and the equally remarkable effect that this science has had upon clinical medicine. Over the past 20 years, the field of immunology has undergone radical changes. We can now identify the specific cells and molecules that are the essential components of the immune system, and we can predict the functions of these components based on a limited number of general principles. Students and practitioners of medicine need to be conversant with these advances in order to understand immunologic diseases and to use the rapidly emerging methods of diagnosis and therapy that are based on immunologic approaches.

Accordingly, we believe that there is a need for a new textbook that should meet two major goals. The first and foremost is to convey an accurate and up-to-date understanding of the immune system. This book emphasizes the organizing principles of immunology and is not intended to be simply a compendium of facts. The principles of immunology are derived from the shared interpretations of key experiments. To enable the student to appreciate the basis of modern immunology, these key experiments and their interpretations are described, usually in summary or schematic form. The discussion of experimental studies also serves to illustrate the evolution of immunology as a science and, we hope, to convey some of the excitement that accompanies scientific discoveries. The most important methods used in experimental analyses are described in "boxes," which are separated from the main text. As an aid to students, each chapter concludes with a list of recent review articles that may serve as a bridge to the primary scientific reports. In addition, we have listed selected research papers that present experimental studies described in the text.

The second goal is to provide students of medicine with an appreciation of how immunologic principles are being applied to understand human diseases. The importance of the immune system in clinical medicine is greatest in two broad areas — defense against infections, and diseases due to abnormal immune responses. These and other connections between immunology and medicine are highlighted throughout the book. More detailed descriptions of selected clinical disorders that illustrate important points have also been included in the boxes.

The book is organized into four sections, each focusing on different aspects of immunology. Section I presents an introduction to the cells and tissues of the immune system. Section II examines the molecular mechanisms used by the immune system to recognize antigens and the process of activation of the immune system that results from antigen recognition. Section III describes the means by which the stimulated immune system eliminates foreign molecules, cells, and organisms. Section IV is specifically devoted to clinical problems that are primarily immunologic or in which modern immunology has made a major contribution.

This book would not have been possible without the help and support of many individuals. Foremost among these were colleagues who provided invaluable constructive criticisms. Dr. Geoffrey Sunshine, of Tufts University School of Medicine, and Hal Burstein, an M.D.–Ph.D. candidate at Harvard Medical School, read the entire book and guided us through many problems of clarity and consistency. Individual chapters or topics were reviewed by the following immunologists, who are listed here in alphabetical order: Drs. Hugh Auchincloss, J. Latham Claflin, Robert Colvin, George Eisenbarth, Vic Engelhard, Frank Fitch, Steven Galli, Richard Hodes, Keith James, Stephanie James, Anne Marshak-Rothstein, Rick Mitchell, Harry Orr, David Parker, Jose Quintans, Ray Redline, Alan Sher, Richard Titus, and Janis Weis. We consider ourselves fortunate that we have been able to draw upon such a wealth of expertise. Valuable input also came from the first-year medical students on whom we first tried out the approach that is the cornerstone of this book.

We owe a great debt to many members of the staff of W.B. Saunders Company. In particular, Marty Wonsiewicz and Rosanne Hallowell, editors, and Risa Clow, illustrator, have shown extraordinary dedication and have been very much a part of the planning and writing of this book. Important contributions have also been made by Carol Robins, copy editor; Pat Morrison, Assistant Manager of Illustration and Design; Paul Fry, designer; and Pete Faber, production manager.

Many thanks are also due to Mary Jane Tawa, David Lence, and Jim Throp, who typed most of the manuscript, and to Pam Battaglino for hand-drawn illustrations.

Finally, we are grateful to the people who faithfully supported us even when we were not available for them — the members of our laboratories, who kept our research projects alive and well; Dr. Ramzi Cotran, our department chairman, whose indulgence was more than we could have asked for; and, above all, our families, who were tolerant of our many demands and awaited the completion of the book with an eagerness that matched our own.

ABUL K. ABBAS
ANDREW H. LICHTMAN
JORDAN S. POBER

CONTENTS

S E C T I O N   I V

CHAPTER FIFTEEN

CHAPTER SIXTEEN

CHAPTER SEVENTEEN

CHAPTER EIGHTEEN

CHAPTER NINETEEN

Appendix

INTRODUCTION

TO

IMMUNOLOGY

The first two chapters introduce the nomenclature of immunology and the components of the immune system. Chapter 1 describes the types of immune responses and their general properties and introduces the fundamental principles that govern all immune responses. Chapter 2 is devoted to a description of the cells and tissues of the immune system, with an emphasis on their anatomic organization and structure-function relationships. This will set the stage for a more thorough discussion of the individual cells that participate in immune responses and how the immune system recognizes and responds to antigens.

CHAPTER ONE

GENERAL PROPERTIES

OF

IMMUNE RESPONSES

Immunity is derived from the Latin word *immunitas,* which referred to the exemption from various civic duties and legal prosecution offered to Roman senators during their tenures in office. Historically, immunity meant protection from disease, and, more specifically, infectious disease. We now know that many of the mechanisms of resistance to infections are also involved in the individual's response to non-infectious foreign substances. Furthermore, mechanisms that normally protect individuals from infections and eliminate foreign substances are themselves capable of causing tissue injury and disease under some situations. Therefore, the modern definition of immunity is a reaction to foreign substances, including microbes, as well as macromolecules such as proteins and polysaccharides, without implying a physiologic or pathologic consequence of such a reaction. Immunology is the study of immunity in this broader sense and of the cellular and molecular events that occur after an organism encounters microbes and other foreign macromolecules. The cells and molecules responsible for immunity constitute the "immune system," and their collective and coordinated responses to the introduction of foreign substances comprise the "immune response."

Historians often credit Thucydides, in Athens during the fifth century B.C., as having first mentioned immunity to an infection that he called "plague" (but that was probably not the bubonic plague we recognize today). The concept of immunity may have existed long before, as suggested by the ancient Chinese custom of making children inhale powders made from the crusts of skin lesions of patients recovering from smallpox. Immunology, in its modern form, is an experimental science, in which explanations of immunologic phenomena are based on experimental observations and the conclusions drawn from them. The evolution of immunology as an experimental discipline has depended on our ability to manipulate the function of the immune system under controlled conditions. Historically, the first clear example of this, and one that remains among the most dramatic ever recorded, was Edward Jenner's successful vaccination against smallpox. Jenner, an English physician, noticed that milkmaids who had recovered from cowpox never contracted the more serious smallpox. Based on this observation, he injected the material from a cowpox pustule into the arm of an 8-year-old boy. When this boy was later intentionally inoculated with smallpox, the disease did not develop. Jenner's landmark treatise on **vaccination** (Latin *vaccus,* cow) was published in 1798. It led to the widespread acceptance of this method for inducing immunity to infectious diseases. An eloquent testament to the importance and progress of immunology was the announcement by the World Health Organization in 1980 that smallpox was the first infectious disease that had been eradicated worldwide by a program of vaccination.

In the last 20 years, there has been a remarkable transformation in our understanding of the immune system and its functions. Advances in cell culture techniques, recombinant deoxyribonucleic acid (DNA) methodology, and protein biochemistry have changed immunology from a largely descriptive science into one in which diverse immune phenomena can be tied together coherently and explained in quite precise structural and biochemical terms. This chapter outlines the general features of immune responses and introduces the concepts that form the cornerstones of modern immunology and that recur throughout the remainder of this book.

NATURAL AND ACQUIRED IMMUNITY

Healthy individuals protect themselves against microbes by means of many different mechanisms. These include physical barriers, phagocytic cells in the blood and tissues, a class of lymphocytes called natural killer (NK) cells, and various blood-borne molecules, all of which participate in defending individuals from a potentially hostile environment. Some of these defense mechanisms are present prior to exposure to infectious microbes or other foreign macromolecules, are not enhanced by such exposures, and do not discriminate among most foreign substances. These are the components of **natural (also called native** or **innate) immunity.** Other defense mechanisms are induced or stimulated by exposure to foreign substances, are exquisitely specific for distinct macromolecules, and increase in magnitude and defensive capabilities with each successive exposure to a particular macromolecule. These mechanisms constitute **acquired,** or **specific, immunity** (Table 1–1). Foreign substances that induce specific immunity are called **antigens.** By convention, immunology is the study of specific immunity and "immune responses" refer to responses that are specific for different inducing antigens.

The specific immune response is one component of an integrated system of host defense in which numerous cells and molecules function cooperatively.

TABLE 1–1. Features of Natural and Specific (Acquired) Immunity

	Natural	Specific (Acquired)
Physicochemical barriers	Skin, mucous membranes	Cutaneous and mucosal immune systems; antibody in mucosal secretions
Circulating molecules	Complement	Antibodies
Cells	Phagocytes (macrophages, neutrophils), natural killer cells	Lymphocytes
Soluble mediators active on other cells	Macrophage-derived cytokines, e.g., α and β interferons, tumor necrosis factor	Lymphocyte-derived cytokines, e.g., γ interferon

The specific immune system has retained many of the mechanisms of natural immunity that are necessary for eliminating foreign invaders and has added to them two important additional properties:

First, *the specific immune system "remembers" each encounter with a microbe or foreign antigen, so that subsequent encounters stimulate increasingly effective defense mechanisms.* This is the basis of protective vaccination against infectious diseases.

Second, *the specific immune response amplifies the protective mechanisms of natural immunity, directs or focuses these mechanisms to the sites of antigen entry, and thus makes them better able to eliminate foreign antigens.*

The concept that specific immune responses serve to enhance natural immunity is also reflected in the phylogeny of defense mechanisms (Box 1–1). Prior to the evolution of vertebrates, host defense against foreign invaders was mediated largely by the mechanisms of natural immunity, including phagocytic cells and circulating molecules that resemble components of the mammalian complement system (see Chapter 13). Specific immunity consisting of **lymphocytes** and their secreted products, such as **antibodies,** appeared in vertebrates and is clearly present in fish. Whereas phagocytes and complement cannot distinguish between distinct antigens and are not specifically enhanced by repeated exposures to the same antigen, lymphocytes and antibodies are highly specific and their production or expansion is stimulated by foreign antigens. Nevertheless, in order to carry out their function of defending the host by eliminating foreign antigens, both lymphocytes and antibodies require the participation of phagocytes and complement. Similarly, specific immune responses in the skin and mucosal surfaces serve to enhance the physical barrier functions because of which such surfaces are major components of the natural immune system. These and other examples of the cooperation between the specific immune system and the mechanisms of natural immunity are described in much more detail in subsequent chapters.

TYPES OF SPECIFIC IMMUNITY

Specific immune responses are normally stimulated when an individual is exposed to a foreign antigen. This process is called **immunization,** and the form of immunity that is induced is called **active immunity** because the immunized individual plays an active role in responding to the antigen. Specific immunity can also be conferred upon an individual by transferring cells or serum from a specifically immunized individual. The recipient of such an **adoptive transfer** becomes resistant, or immune, to the particular antigen without ever having been exposed to or having ever responded to that antigen. Therefore, this form of immunity is called **passive immunity.** Passive immunization is a useful method for conferring resistance rapidly, without having to wait for an active immune response to develop. For instance, passive immunization against snake venoms by the administration of antibodies from immunized individuals is a life-saving treatment for potentially lethal snake bites. The technique of adoptive transfer of specific immunity has also made it possible to define the various cells and molecules that are responsible for mediating immune responses.

Specific immune responses are classified into two types, based on the components of the immune system that mediate the response:

1. **Humoral immunity** can be transferred to unimmunized (also called "naive") individuals by cell-free portions of the blood, i.e., plasma or serum. Humoral immunity is mediated by molecules in the blood that are responsible for specific recognition and elimination of antigens; these are called **antibodies.**

2. **Cell-mediated immunity,** also called **cellular immunity,** can be transferred to naive individuals with cells from an immunized individual but not with plasma or serum. The cells responsible for specific antigen recognition are now known to be **lymphocytes.**

The first definitive experimental demonstration of humoral immunity was provided by Emil von Behring and Shibasabura Kitasato in 1890. They showed that if serum from animals who had recovered from diphtheria infection was transferred to naive animals, the recipients became specifically resistant to diphtheria infection. The active components of the serum were called **antitoxins** because they neutralized the pathologic effects of the bacterial toxin. In the early 1900s, Karl Landsteiner and other investigators showed that not only toxins but also other, non-microbial substances could induce humoral immunity. From such studies arose the more general term **antibodies** for the serum proteins that mediate humoral immunity. Substances that bound antibodies and generated the production of antibodies were then called **antigens.** (The properties of antibodies and antigens are described in Chapter 3.) In 1900, Paul Ehrlich provided a theoretical framework of the specificity of antigen-antibody reactions, the experimental proof for which came over the next 50 years from the work of Landsteiner and others using simple chemicals as antigens. Ehrlich's theories of the physicochemical complementarity of antigens and antibodies are remarkable for their prescience. This early emphasis on antibodies led to the general acceptance of the **humoral theory of immunity,** according to which immunity is mediated by substances present in body fluids (humors).

The **cellular theory of immunity,** which stated that host cells were the principal mediators of immunity, was championed initially by Elie Metchnikoff. His demonstration of phagocytes surrounding a thorn stuck into a translucent starfish larva, published in 1893, was perhaps the first experimental evidence that cells responded to foreign invaders. Sir Almroth Wright's observation in the early 1900s that factors in

BOX 1 – 1. EVOLUTION OF THE IMMUNE SYSTEM

Mechanisms for defending the host against foreign invaders and for healing injured self-tissues are present in some form in all members of the enormously diverse and large numbers of phyla of invertebrates. These mechanisms constitute natural immunity. The more discriminating and specialized defense mechanisms that constitute specific or acquired immunity are generally found in vertebrates only. Various cells in invertebrates respond to microbes by enclosing these infectious agents within aggregates and destroying them. These responding cells resemble phagocytes and have been called phagocytic amebocytes in acelomates, hemocytes in molluscs and arthropods, celomocytes in annelids, and blood leukocytes in tunicates. Invertebrates do not contain antigen-specific lymphocytes and do not produce immunoglobulin molecules or complement proteins. However, they contain a number of soluble molecules that bind to and lyse microbes. These molecules include lectin-like proteins, which bind to carbohydrates on microbial cell walls and agglutinate the microbes, and numerous lytic and antimicrobial factors such as lysozyme, which is also produced by neutrophils in higher organisms. Phagocytes in some invertebrates may be capable of secreting cytokines that resemble macrophage-derived cytokines in the vertebrates. Thus, *host defense in invertebrates is mediated by the cells and molecules that resemble the effector mechanisms of natural immunity in higher organisms.*

Many studies have shown that invertebrates are capable of rejecting foreign tissue transplants, or allografts. If sponges *(Porifera)* from two different colonies are parabiosed by being mechanically held together, they become necrotic in 1 to 2 weeks, whereas sponges from the same colony become fused and continue to grow. Earthworms (annelids) and starfish (echinoderms) also reject tissue grafts from other species of the phyla. These rejection reactions are mediated mainly by phagocyte-like cells. They differ from graft rejection in vertebrates in that specific memory for the grafted tissue is either not generated or is difficult to demonstrate. Nevertheless, such results indicate that even invertebrates must express cell surface molecules that distinguish self from non-self, and such molecules may be the precursors of histocompatibility molecules in vertebrates.

	Natural Immunity		Acquired (Specific) Immunity		
	Phagocytosis	*NK Cells*	*Antibodies*	*T and B Lymphocytes*	*Lymph Nodes*
Invertebrates					
Protozoa	+	−	−	−	−
Sponges	+	−	−	−	−
Annelids	+	+	−	−	−
Arthropods	+	−	−	−	−
Vertebrates					
Elasmobranchs (sharks, skates, rays)	+	+	+(IgM only)	+	−
Teleosts (common fish)	+	+	+(IgM, ? other)	+	−
Amphibians	+	+	+(2 or 3 classes)	+	−
Reptiles	+	+	+(3 classes)	+	−
Birds	+	+	+(3 classes)	+	+(some species)
Mammals	+	+	+(7 or 8 classes)	+	+

Abbreviation: NK, natural killer.
Key: +, present; −, absent.

The various components of the mammalian immune system appear to have arisen virtually together in phylogeny and have become increasingly specialized with evolution (see Table). Thus, of the cardinal features of specific immune responses, *specificity, memory, self/non-self discrimination, and a capacity for self-regulation are present in the lowest vertebrates and diversity of antigen recognition increases progressively in the higher species.* All vertebrates contain antibody molecules. Fishes have only one type of antibody, called IgM; this number increases to two types in anuran amphibians like *Xenopus,* and to seven in mammals. The diversity of antibodies is much lower in *Xenopus* than in mammals, even though the genes coding for antibodies are structurally similar. Lymphocytes that have some characteristics of both B and T cells are probably present in the earliest vertebrates, such as lampreys, and become specialized into functionally and phenotypically distinct subsets in amphibia and most clearly in birds and mammals. The **major histocompatibility complex,** which is a genetic locus that controls graft rejection and T lymphocyte antigen recognition, is present in some of the more advanced species of amphibians and fishes and in all birds and mammals. Its absence from some amphibians and fishes and all reptiles suggests that these histocompatibility genes may have evolved independently on several occasions during vertebrate phylogeny. The earliest organized lymphoid tissues detected during evolution are the gut-associated lymphoid tissues; spleen, thymus, and lymph nodes (see Chapter 2) are found in higher vertebrates.

immune serum enhanced the phagocytosis of bacteria, a process known as **opsonization,** lent support to the belief that antibodies merely prepared microbes for ingestion by phagocytes. These early "cellularists" were unable to prove that specific immunity could be mediated by cells. In 1942, Landsteiner and Merrill Chase reported that skin reactions to different chemicals could be transferred to naive animals with cells but not with serum from specifically immunized animals. The cellular theory of immunity became firmly established in the 1950s, when George Mackaness showed that resistance to an intracellular bacterium, *Listeria monocytogenes,* could also be adoptively transferred with cells but not with serum. We now know that the specificity of cell-mediated immunity is due to lymphocytes, which often function in concert with other cells such as **phagocytes** to control or eliminate microbes.

Adoptive transfer of specific immunity is one of the principal techniques for analyzing immune responses. It is now complemented by *in vitro* experiments, in which the cells of the immune system can be stimulated by defined antigens and the development of specific immune responses can be examined. As we shall discuss in subsequent chapters, such studies have shown that *humoral immunity and cell-mediated immunity are mediated by responses of distinct types of lymphocytes.* Some, called **B lymphocytes,** respond to foreign antigens by developing into antibody-producing cells, whereas others, called **T lymphocytes,** are the mediators of cellular immunity. Humoral immunity is the principal defense mechanism against extracellular microbes and their secreted toxins because antibodies can bind to these and assist in their de-

struction. In contrast, obligate intracellular microbes such as viruses and some bacteria proliferate inside host cells, where they are inaccessible to circulating antibodies. Defense against such infections is due to cell-mediated immunity, which functions by inducing and promoting the intracellular destruction of microbes or the lysis of infected cells.

CARDINAL FEATURES OF IMMUNE RESPONSES

Humoral and cell-mediated immune responses to all antigens have a number of fundamental properties. The experimental analysis of the immune response is, in fact, an attempt to provide molecular and mechanistic explanations for these cardinal features of specific immunity.

1. *Specificity.* Immune responses are specific for distinct antigens (Fig. 1–1). In fact, immune responses are specific for different structural components of most complex protein and polysaccharide antigens. The portions of such antigens that are specifically recognized by distinct lymphocytes are called **determinants,** or **epitopes.** This fine specificity exists because the B and T lymphocytes that respond to foreign antigens express membrane receptors that distinguish subtle differences between distinct antigens. Antigen-specific lymphocytes develop without antigenic stimulation, so that clones of cells with different antigen receptors and specificities are available in unimmunized individuals to recognize and respond to exposure to foreign antigens. This concept is the

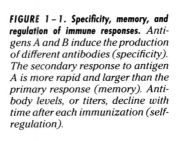

FIGURE 1–1. Specificity, memory, and regulation of immune responses. Antigens A and B induce the production of different antibodies (specificity). The secondary response to antigen A is more rapid and larger than the primary response (memory). Antibody levels, or titers, decline with time after each immunization (self-regulation).

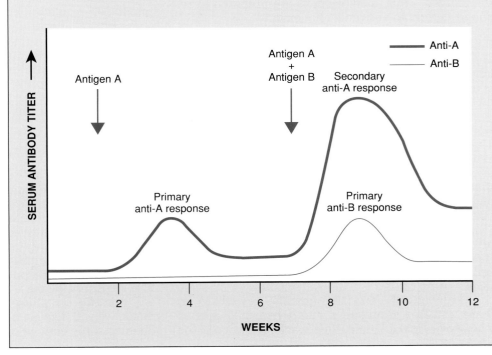

basic tenet of the **clonal selection hypothesis,** which is discussed in more detail later in this chapter.

2. *Diversity.* The total number of antigenic specificities of the lymphocytes in an individual, called the **lymphocyte repertoire,** is extremely large. It is estimated that the mammalian immune system can discriminate at least 10^9 distinct antigenic determinants. This extraordinary diversity of the repertoire is a result of variability in the structures of the antigen-binding sites of lymphocyte receptors for antigens. In other words, different clones of lymphocytes differ in the structures of their antigen receptors and, therefore, in their specificity for antigens, creating a total repertoire that is extremely diverse. One of the most important advances in immunology has been the elucidation of the molecular mechanisms that produce such structural diversity. These mechanisms are discussed in Chapters 4 and 8.

3. *Memory.* Exposure of the immune system to a foreign antigen enhances its ability to respond again to that antigen. Thus, responses to second and subsequent exposures to the same antigen, called **secondary immune responses,** are usually more rapid, larger, and often qualitatively different from the first, or primary, immune responses to that antigen (Fig. 1–1). This property of specific immunity is called **immunologic memory.** Several features of lymphocytes are responsible for memory:

a. Lymphocytes proliferate when stimulated by antigens and the progeny of a particular antigen-responsive lymphocyte has the same antigen receptors and, hence, specificity as the original cell. Therefore, each exposure to antigen expands the clone(s) of lymphocytes specific for that antigen.

b. Memory cells, which are lymphocytes that have previously responded to antigenic stimulation, survive for prolonged periods even in the absence of the antigen. Thus, memory cells are prepared to respond rapidly to antigenic challenge.

c. As we shall see in Chapters 4 and 9, memory B cells respond to lower concentrations of antigens and produce antibodies that bind antigen with higher affinity than do previously unstimulated B cells. This is only one of several qualitative differences between primary and secondary antibody responses.

4. *Self-regulation.* All normal immune responses wane with time after antigenic stimulation (Fig. 1–1). There are several reasons why immune responses are self-limited.

a. The first, and probably most important, is that immune responses are induced by antigens and function to eliminate the antigen. This results in the elimination of the stimulus for lymphocyte activation.

b. Lymphocytes perform their functions for brief periods after antigenic stimulation, after which these cells become quiescent, develop into memory cells, or differentiate into end-cells with short half-lives.

c. Antigens and the immune responses to these antigens stimulate a number of mechanisms whose principal function is feedback regulation of the response itself. These regulatory mechanisms are discussed in Chapter 10.

5. *Discrimination of self from non-self.* One of the most remarkable properties of the immune system is its ability to distinguish between foreign antigens and self antigens. Thus, the lymphocytes in each individual are able to recognize and respond to many foreign antigens but are normally unresponsive to the potentially antigenic substances present in that individual. Immunologic unresponsiveness is also called **tolerance.** Self-tolerance is an acquired process that has to be learned by the lymphocytes of each individual. It occurs in part because lymphocytes pass through a stage in their development when encounter with antigen leads to their death or inactivation. Thus, potentially self-recognizing lymphocytes come into contact with self antigens at this stage of functional immaturity and are prevented from developing to a stage at which they would be able to respond to self antigens. A great deal is now known about the selection processes that are responsible for self-tolerance, and these will be discussed in Chapters 8 and 10. Abnormalities in the induction or maintenance of self-tolerance lead to immune responses against self (autologous) antigens, and potentially fatal diseases that are called **autoimmune diseases.** The generation and pathologic consequences of autoimmunity are described in Chapter 18.

These five cardinal features of specific immunity are necessary if the immune system is to perform its normal function of host defense. Specificity and memory enable the immune system to mount heightened responses to persistent or recurring stimulation with the same antigen and thus to combat infections that are prolonged or occur repeatedly. Diversity is essential if the immune system is to defend individuals against the many potential pathogens in the environment. Self-regulation allows the system to return to a state of rest after it eliminates each foreign antigen, thus enabling it to respond optimally to other antigens that the individual encounters. Self-tolerance and the ability to distinguish between self and non-self are vital for preventing reactions against one's own cells and tissues while maintaining a diverse repertoire of lymphocytes specific for foreign antigens.

PHASES OF IMMUNE RESPONSES

All immune responses are initiated by the recognition of foreign antigens. This leads to activation of the lymphocytes that specifically recognize the antigen, and culminates in the development of mechanisms that mediate the physiologic effect of the response, namely elimination of the antigen. Thus, specific immune responses may be divided into (1) the **cognitive phase,** (2) the **activation phase,** and (3) the **effector phase** (Fig. 1–2). Throughout this book, we will discuss the mechanisms of specific immunity in the context of these three phases.

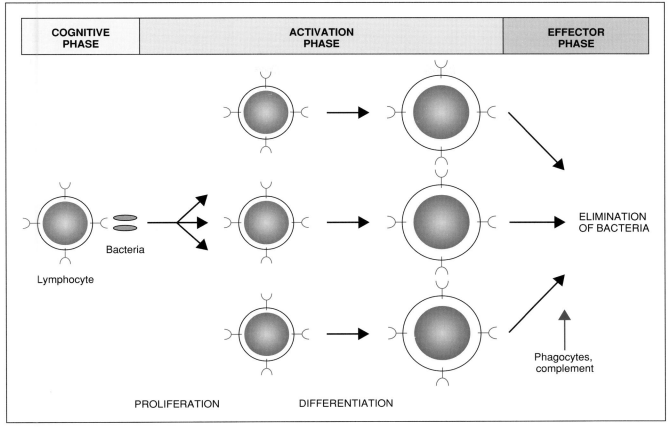

COGNITIVE PHASE	ACTIVATION PHASE	EFFECTOR PHASE

Bacteria

Lymphocyte

ELIMINATION OF BACTERIA

Phagocytes, complement

PROLIFERATION   DIFFERENTIATION

FIGURE 1 - 2. Phases of specific immune responses. *Immune responses consist of three phases:* cognitive *(antigen recognition),* activation *(proliferation and differentiation of lymphocytes), and* effector *(elimination of antigen). This example illustrates an immune response to bacteria, but the same phases are seen in all specific immune responses. Since this applies to both B and T lymphocytes, the lymphocytes shown can be of either class.*

Cognitive Phase

The cognitive phase of immune responses consists of the binding of foreign antigens to specific receptors on mature lymphocytes that exist prior to antigenic stimulation. B lymphocytes, the cells of humoral immunity, express antibody molecules on their surfaces that can bind foreign proteins, polysaccharides, or lipids in soluble form. T lymphocytes, which are responsible for cell-mediated immunity, express receptors that recognize only short peptide sequences in protein antigens. Moreover, T lymphocytes have the unique property of recognizing and responding only to peptide antigens that are present on the surfaces of other cells. The structural basis of antigen recognition by T cells and its physiologic implications are discussed in Chapter 6.

Activation Phase

The activation phase of immune responses is the sequence of events induced in lymphocytes as a consequence of specific antigen recognition. All lymphocytes undergo two major changes in response to antigens. First, they proliferate, leading to expansion of the clones of antigen-specific lymphocytes and amplification of the protective response. Second, lymphocytes differentiate from cells whose primary function is cognitive to cells that function to eliminate foreign antigens. Thus, antigen-recognizing B lymphocytes differentiate into antibody-secreting cells and the secreted antibody binds the soluble (extracellular) antigen and triggers the mechanisms that eliminate the antigen. Some T lymphocytes differentiate into cells that activate phagocytes to kill intracellular microbes, and other T lymphocytes directly lyse cells that are producing foreign antigens such as viral proteins. The ability of T cells to recognize cell-bound antigens focuses T cell responses in such a way that cell-mediated immunity is effective against intracellular microbes. A general feature of lymphocyte activation is that it usually requires two types of signals: one is provided by the antigen, and the second by other cells, which may be **"helper cells"** or **"accessory cells."** The nature of these stimuli and the sequence of T and B cell activation are discussed in Chapters 7 and 9.

Two aspects of lymphocyte activation are important in order to allow the small number of cells that respond to any one antigen to perform the many functions that lead to elimination of the antigen. First, immunization and antigen recognition trigger numerous amplification mechanisms that rapidly expand the specifically responding cells and, to a lesser extent, bystander cells as well. Second, lymphocytes preferentially migrate to sites of antigen administration and immune responses. The cellular and biochemical mechanisms of amplification and lymphocyte migration are discussed in later chapters.

Effector Phase

The effector phase of immune responses is the stage at which lymphocytes that have been specifically activated by antigens perform the functions that lead to elimination of the antigen. Lymphocytes that function in the effector phase of immune responses are called **effector cells.** Many effector functions require the participation of other, non-lymphoid cells (which are also often referred to as "effector cells") and defense mechanisms that are also operative in natural immunity. For instance, antibodies bind to foreign antigens and enhance their phagocytosis by blood neutrophils and mononuclear phagocytes. Antibodies also activate a system of plasma proteins termed **complement,** which participates in the lysis and phagocytosis of microbes (see Chapter 13). Other antibodies stimulate the degranulation of mast cells and the release of mediators, which combat infections and are responsible for the vascular components of acute inflammation (see Chapter 14). Activated T lymphocytes secrete protein hormones, called **cytokines,** which enhance the functions of phagocytes and stimulate inflammatory responses (see Chapters 11 and 12). Phagocytes, complement, mast cells, cytokines, and the leukocytes that mediate inflammation are all components of natural immunity, because they do not specifically recognize or distinguish between different foreign antigens, and they are all involved in defense against microbes, even without specific immune responses. Thus, the effector phase of specific immunity illustrates a fundamental concept that was emphasized earlier in this chapter—that specific immune responses serve to amplify and focus onto foreign antigens a variety of effector mechanisms that are also functional in the absence of lymphocyte activation.

THE CLONAL SELECTION HYPOTHESIS

From the initial demonstration that the immune system could respond specifically to a vast number of foreign antigens, the problem of explaining how such a diverse repertoire could be generated and maintained was appreciated by immunologists. Two mutually exclusive hypotheses were proposed to explain the specificity and diversity of immune responses,

even before a clear understanding of the importance of lymphocytes in antigen recognition. According to the instructional theory, immunocompetent cells and antibodies acquired their specificity after the introduction of antigen by changing the conformation of antigen-binding regions to become capable of recognizing the antigen. The alternative view, which we now know is correct, was first suggested by Niels Jerne in 1955, modified by David Talmadge and Macfarlane Burnet, and most clearly enunciated by Burnet in 1957. The key postulates of this theory, called the **clonal selection hypothesis,** have been convincingly proved by a variety of experiments, and form the cornerstone of the current concept of lymphocyte specificity and antigen recognition. In essence, the clonal selection hypothesis states the following (Fig. 1–3):

1. *Every individual contains numerous clonally derived lymphocytes, each clone having arisen from a single precursor and each clone being capable of recognizing and responding to a distinct antigenic determinant.* Thus, the development of antigen-specific clones of lymphocytes occurs prior to and independent of exposure to antigen. The cells constituting each clone have identical antigen receptors, which are different from the receptors on the cells of all other clones. Although it is difficult to place an upper limit on the number of antigenic determinants that can be recognized by the mammalian immune system, a frequently used estimate is in the order of 10^9. This is a reasonable approximation of the potential number of antigen receptor proteins that can be produced, and may, therefore, reflect the number of distinct clones of lymphocytes present in each individual.

2. *Antigen selects a specific pre-existing clone and activates it,* leading to its proliferation and its differentiation into effector and memory cells. The observation that a secondary immune response is more rapid and larger than the primary response is explained by the clonal expansion of antigen-specific lymphocytes as a result of priming (first immunization) with antigen. Because the clones that respond to any one antigen are a small fraction of the total lymphocytes in an individual, blood lymphocyte counts do not change significantly during most immune responses.

Many lines of evidence prove that both B and T lymphocytes with diverse receptors and specificities exist prior to the introduction of antigen and clones with distinct specificities are selectively activated by different antigens.

1. If lymphocytes isolated from an immunized animal are cultured at limiting dilution with antigen such that each culture well initially contains only one antibody-producing B cell, antibody of only one specificity can be detected in each well even if the lymphocytes were exposed to multiple antigens.
2. Different antigens bind to different lymphocytes, and no two structurally distinct foreign antigens bind to the same cell.
3. If an animal is injected with an antigen to which a highly radioactive tag is attached, that anti-

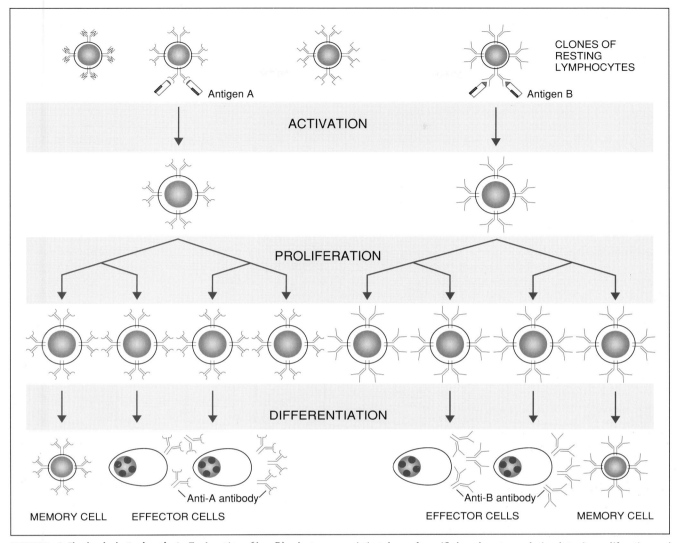

FIGURE 1 – 3. The clonal selection hypothesis. *Each antigen (A or B) selects a pre-existing clone of specific lymphocytes and stimulates its proliferation and differentiation. The diagram shows only B lymphocytes giving rise to antibody-secreting cells and memory cells, but the same principle applies to T lymphocytes as well.*

gen binds to specific lymphocytes. The lymphocytes, being radiosensitive, are killed. Injection of such an antigen makes the animal incapable of responding to that antigen (until new lymphocytes develop), but the animal responds normally to all other structurally different antigens.

4. In lymphocytes with distinct specificities, the antigen receptors have structurally different combining sites. This has been established by nucleotide and amino acid sequencing of receptors isolated from lymphocyte clones.

5. Each monoclonal lymphoid tumor contains a set of antigen receptor genes and expresses antigen receptor proteins that are unique and different from all other tumors.

The specific immune system is remarkable for its complexity and diversity. Immune responses require the coordinated and precisely regulated interplay of many different cells and secreted molecules. Perhaps the greatest achievement of modern immunology is the application of a reductionist approach to analyzing the complexity of the immune system. As we shall see throughout this book, it is now possible to separate the interacting components of the immune system and to dissect their functions individually. Such analyses have led to a clear understanding of the molecular basis of specific antigen recognition, so that the essential features of the cognitive phase of humoral and cell-mediated immune responses are known. In particular, the structure of B and T lymphocyte receptors for antigens is now understood and the molecular genetic basis of the expression of diverse antigen receptors is known. The antigenic epitopes of numerous model protein antigens that are recognized by lymphocytes have been completely defined. The selection of the lymphocyte repertoire and the mechanisms responsible for discrimination between self and non-self are being elucidated, so that approaches for analyzing autoimmune diseases are becoming feasible. We have also learned a great deal about lymphocyte surface proteins and biochemical signals involved in the proliferative and differentiative responses of these cells to foreign antigens. Among the most impressive advances is the identification of the cytokines that mediate many of the effector functions of lymphocytes and are responsible for the communications among cells of the immune system that serve to amplify and regulate immune responses. The potential use of cytokines as biological response modifiers for treating human diseases is one of the exciting applications of this basic research. Thus, immunology has progressed from a science of phenomena to one of defined genes, molecules, and cells. The challenge in the years to come is to apply our knowledge of these molecules and cells to understand how physiologic immune responses are initiated and regulated in normal individuals and how responses become deficient or aberrant, leading to pathologic tissue injury and clinical diseases.

SUMMARY

The specific immune response is initiated by the recognition of foreign antigens by specific lymphocytes, which respond by proliferating and differentiating into effector cells whose function is to eliminate the antigen. The effector phase of specific immunity requires the participation of various defense mechanisms, including the complement system, phagocytes, inflammatory cells, and cytokines, that are also operative in natural immunity. The specific immune response amplifies the mechanisms of natural immunity and enhances their function, particularly upon repeated exposures to the same foreign antigen. The immune system possesses several properties that are of fundamental importance for its normal functions. These include: specificity for distinct antigens, diversity of antigen recognition, memory for antigen exposure, capacity for self-regulation, and the ability to discriminate between self and foreign antigens.

In the remainder of this book we describe the biology of lymphocytes, in particular, the structural basis of antigen recognition by lymphocytes, their stimulation leading to the development of effector cells, their regulation, the nature of effector mechanisms, and the abnormalities that lead to diseases of deficient or excessive immunity.

SELECTED READINGS

Burnet, F. M. A modification of Jerne's theory of antibody production using the concept of clonal selection. Australian Journal of Science 20:67–69, 1957.

Jerne, N. K. The natural-selection theory of antibody formation. Proceedings of the National Academy of Sciences USA 41:849–857, 1955.

Silverstein, A. M. A History of Immunology. San Diego, Academic Press, 1989.

CHAPTER TWO

CELLS AND TISSUES OF THE IMMUNE SYSTEM

The cells of the immune system are normally present as circulating cells in the blood and lymph, as anatomically defined collections in lymphoid organs, and as scattered cells in virtually all tissues except the central nervous system. The anatomic organization of these cells and their ability to circulate and exchange among the blood, lymph, and tissues are of critical importance for the generation of immune responses. The immune system has to be able to respond to a very large number of foreign antigens introduced at any site in the body, and only a small number of lymphocytes specifically respond to any one antigen. Numerous mechanisms enable the immune system to perform its protective functions. These include:

1. The close bidirectional interactions between antigen-specific lymphocytes and other cells that are involved in the cognitive and effector phases of immune responses.
2. The ability of lymphocytes to migrate and exchange between the circulation and tissues, to home to sites of antigen exposure, and to be retained at these sites.
3. Multiple amplification loops that magnify the effects of stimulating the few lymphocytes that are specific for any one antigen.
4. The anatomic organization of cells into organs that are optimal sites for antigen-induced lymphocyte growth and differentiation.

This chapter describes the morphology of the cells and tissues of the immune system, with an emphasis on the ways in which their structural characteristics reflect or contribute to their functions.

Lymphocytes are the cells that specifically recognize and respond to foreign antigens. However, both the cognitive and activation phases of immune responses depend on non-lymphoid cells, called **accessory cells,** which are not specific for different antigens and whose functions will be described in greater detail in later chapters. Mononuclear phagocytes, dendritic cells, and several other cell populations function as accessory cells in the induction of immune responses. The activation of lymphocytes leads to the generation of numerous effector mechanisms, whose principal function is to eliminate the antigen. Many of these effector mechanisms also require the participation of **effector cells,** such as mononuclear phagocytes and other leukocytes (white blood cells). All these cell types are present in the blood, from where they can migrate to peripheral sites of antigen exposure. Lymphocytes and accessory cells are also organized in anatomically discrete lymphoid organs where they interact with one another to initiate and amplify immune responses. The cellular constituents of the blood are listed in Table 2–1. We will describe first the properties of the individual cell types and then the functional anatomy of lymphoid organs.

LYMPHOCYTES

The *specificity of immune responses is due to lymphocytes,* which are the only cells in the body capable of specifically recognizing and distinguishing different antigenic determinants. This has been established by several lines of evidence:

1. Adoptive transfer of humoral and cell-mediated immunity from immunized to naive individuals can be achieved only by lymphocytes or their secreted products.
2. Some congenital and acquired immunodeficiencies are associated with reduction of lymphocytes in the peripheral circulation and in lymphoid tissues. Furthermore, selective depletion of lymphocytes with drugs, irradiation, or cell type–specific antibodies leads to impaired immune responses.
3. Lymphocytes are often found in increased numbers at sites of immunization and/or in lymphoid tissues that drain these sites.
4. Stimulation of lymphocytes by antigens in culture leads to immune responses *in vitro* that show many of the characteristics of such responses induced under more physiologic conditions *in vivo.*
5. Most importantly, specific high-affinity receptors for antigens are produced by lymphocytes and no other cells.

TABLE 2–1. Normal Blood Cell Counts

	Number per mm³ (Mean ± S.D.)	Per Cent of Leukocytes	
		Mean	*95 Per Cent Range*
White blood cells (× 10³) (leukocytes)	7.25 ± 1.7		
Neutrophils		55	34.6 – 71.4
Eosinophils		3	0 – 7.8
Basophils		0.5	0 – 1.8
Lymphocytes		35	19.6 – 52.7
Monocytes		6.5	2.4 – 11.8
Red blood cells (× 10⁶) (erythrocytes)	5.0 ± 0.35		
Platelets (× 10³)	248 ± 50		

Abbreviation: S.D., standard deviation.

Lymphocyte Development and Heterogeneity

The **small lymphocyte** is 8 to 10 micrometers (μm) in diameter, and has a large nucleus with dense heterochromatin. There is a thin rim of cytoplasm that contains a few mitochondria, ribosomes, and lysosomes but no specialized organelles (Fig. 2-1). This bland morphologic pattern provides no clues to the remarkable functional capabilities of lymphocytes. Like all blood cells, lymphocytes originate in the bone marrow. This was first demonstrated by experiments with radiation-induced bone marrow chimeras. Lymphocytes and bone marrow stem cells are radiosensitive and are killed by high doses of γ-irradiation. If an irradiated mouse of one inbred strain is injected with bone marrow cells of another strain that can be distinguished from the host, all the lymphocytes that develop subsequently are derived from the bone marrow cells of the donor (Fig. 2-2). Such approaches have proved useful for defining the maturation of lymphocytes and other blood cells, as we shall see later in this and subsequent chapters. In the initial stages of their development, lymphocytes do not produce surface receptors for antigens and are, therefore, unresponsive to antigens. As they mature, they begin to express antigen receptors, become responsive to antigenic stimulation, and develop into different functional classes.

Lymphocytes consist of distinct subsets that are quite different in their functions and protein products, even though they all appear morphologically similar (Table 2-2). One class of lymphocytes consists of **B lymphocytes** (Fig. 2-3), so called because in birds they were first shown to mature in an organ called the bursa of Fabricius. In mammals, there is no anatomic equivalent of the bursa and the early stages of B cell maturation occur in the bone marrow. Thus, "B" lymphocyte refers to bursa- or bone marrow–derived. *B lymphocytes are the only cells capable of producing antibodies.* The antigen receptors of B lymphocytes are membrane-bound antibodies. Interaction of antigens with these membrane antibody molecules initiates the sequence of B cell activation, which culminates in the development of effector cells that actively secrete antibody molecules (see Chapter 9).

The second major class of lymphocytes consists of **T lymphocytes,** which arise in the bone marrow and then migrate to and mature in the thymus (the name "T" lymphocyte referring to thymus-derived). T lymphocytes are further subdivided into functionally distinct populations, the best defined of which are **helper T cells** and **cytolytic (or cytotoxic) T cells** (Fig. 2-3). T cells do not produce antibody molecules. Their antigen receptors are membrane molecules distinct from but structurally related to antibodies (see Chapter 7). Helper and cytolytic T lymphocytes have an unusual specificity for antigens — they recognize only peptide antigens that are attached to proteins encoded in the major histocompatibility complex (MHC) expressed on the surfaces of accessory cells. As a result, these T cells recognize and respond to cell surface–associated but not soluble antigens (see Chapter 6). In response to antigenic stimulation, helper T cells secrete protein hormones called **cytokines,** whose function is to promote the proliferation and differentiation of the T cells as well as other cells, including B cells and macrophages. Cytokines also recruit and activate inflammatory leukocytes, providing an important link between specific T cell immunity and one form of natural immunity, the inflammatory

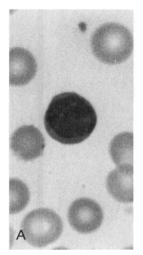
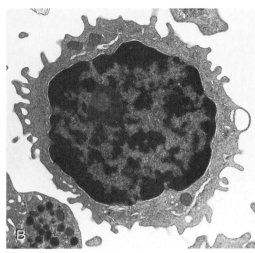
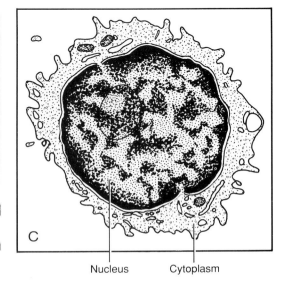

Nucleus   Cytoplasm

FIGURE 2–1. Morphology of a small lymphocyte.
A. *Light micrograph of a lymphocyte in a peripheral blood smear.*
B. *Electron micrograph of a small lymphocyte. (Courtesy of Dr. Noel Weidner, Department of Pathology, Brigham and Women's Hospital, Boston.)*
C. *Schematic diagram of the lymphocyte depicted in B illustrating the large nucleus and scant cytoplasm with few organelles.*

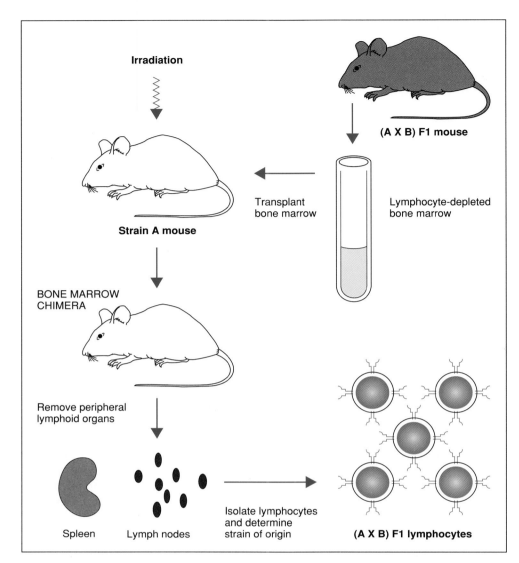

Irradiation

Transplant
bone marrow

Strain A mouse

(A X B) F1 mouse

Lymphocyte-depleted
bone marrow

BONE MARROW
CHIMERA

Remove peripheral
lymphoid organs

Spleen   Lymph nodes

Isolate lymphocytes
and determine
strain of origin

(A X B) F1 lymphocytes

FIGURE 2 – 2. Origin of lymphocytes defined in bone marrow chimeras. In an irradiated strain A mouse reconstituted with bone marrow cells from an (A × B)F1 hybrid (i.e., the offspring of a mating between a strain A and a strain B mouse), the mature lymphocytes that are recovered from peripheral lymphoid tissues are derived from the donor strain.

response. Cytolytic T lymphocytes (CTLs) lyse cells that produce foreign antigens. The mechanisms of action and physiologic functions of these T cell populations are described in detail in later chapters. In addition to providing helper and cytolytic functions, T cells may also inhibit immune responses. There is, at present, considerable controversy about the nature and physiologic roles of these so-called "suppressor T cells." In fact, it is not clear whether suppression of immune responses is mediated by a distinct T cell subset or by cells that, under various situations, can function as helper or cytolytic cells (see Chapter 10).

The most important advance in the identification and analysis of these T cell subsets has been the discovery that *functionally distinct populations express different membrane proteins.* These proteins serve as phenotypic markers of different lymphocyte populations. For instance, most helper T cells express a surface protein called CD4, and most CTLs express a different marker called CD8. Antibodies against such markers

can, therefore, be used to identify and isolate various lymphocyte populations. In addition, many of the surface proteins that were initially recognized as phenotypic markers for various lymphocytes turned out, upon further analysis, to play important roles in the biologic functions of these cells. In this book we use the unified CD nomenclature for lymphocyte markers. CD stands for "cluster of differentiation" and refers to a molecule recognized by a "cluster" of monoclonal antibodies that can be used to identify the lineage or stage of differentiation of lymphocytes and thus to distinguish one class of lymphocyte from another (Box 2 – 1). CD proteins were first used for subclassifying T cells, but different CD molecules recognized by specific antibodies now serve as useful markers of B cells and other leukocytes that participate in immune and inflammatory responses. Examples of some CD proteins are mentioned in Table 2 – 2, and the biochemistry and functions of the most important ones are described in Chapters 7 and 9. A current list of

TABLE 2–2. Lymphocyte Classes

Class	Functions	Antigen Receptor	Selected Phenotypic Markers	Per Cent of Total Lymphocytes		
				Blood	Lymph Node	Spleen
B LYMPHOCYTES						
	Antibody production (humoral immunity)	Surface antibody (immunoglobulin)	Fc and C3d receptors; class II MHC	10–15	20–25	40–45
T LYMPHOCYTES				70–75*	70–75*	40–45*
Helper	Stimuli for B cell growth and differentiation (humoral immunity) Macrophage activation by secreted cytokines (cell-mediated immunity)	$\alpha\beta$ heterodimers	CD3+ CD4+, CD8− CD2+			
Cytolytic	Lysis of antigen-bearing (e.g., virally infected) cells, allografts	$\alpha\beta$ heterodimers	CD3+ CD4−CD8+ CD2+			
Suppressor	Inhibition of immune response	?	?CD3+ Usually CD4−CD8+			
NATURAL KILLER CELLS						
	Lysis of tumor cells, antibody-dependent cellular cytotoxicity	?	Fc receptor for IgG (CD16)	~10	Rare	~10

* In most tissues, ratio of CD4+CD8− to CD8+CD4− cells is about 2:1.

known CD markers for leukocytes is provided in the Appendix, p. 398.

The third major class of lymphocytes does not express markers for either T or B cells and was, therefore, initially called the **null cell** population. It is now apparent that most null cells are large lymphocytes with numerous cytoplasmic granules and are capable of lysing a variety of tumor- and virus-infected cells without overt antigenic stimulation. As a result, these lymphocytes are called **large granular lymphocytes** or **natural killer (NK) cells,** designations that define a morphologic or functional group whose ontogeny and specificity are incompletely understood. The properties and functions of NK cells are discussed in more detail in Chapter 12.

Morphologic Changes Associated with Lymphocyte Activation

Lymphocytes undergo a well-defined pattern of changes upon activation. It is technically difficult to study the responses of lymphocytes to antigens because a very small fraction of the total population is specific for any one antigen. Immunologists have overcome this problem by using **polyclonal activators,** e.g., antibodies against antigen receptors, that stimulate many B or T lymphocytes irrespective of antigenic specificity. It is generally assumed that polyclonal activators mimic antigens; i.e., the changes induced by the former in many lymphocytes are similar to the changes induced by antigens in antigen-specific clones.

Prior to antigenic or polyclonal stimulation, small lymphocytes are in a state of rest, or in the G_0 stage of the cell cycle. If resting lymphocytes do not encounter antigen, they probably die within a few days and the population is maintained at a steady-state level by the development of new cells from precursors in the bone marrow. In response to antigenic (or polyclonal) stimulation, resting small lymphocytes enter the G_1 stage of the cell cycle. They become larger and are called large lymphocytes, or **lymphoblasts.** These cells are 10 to 15 μm in diameter and have a wider rim of cytoplasm, more organelles, and increased amounts of cytoplasmic ribonucleic acid (RNA) compared with unstimulated small lymphocytes. Progression to the S phase of the cell cycle continues, and the activated large lymphocytes divide. This sequence of events is called **blast transformation.** Mitotic division is responsible for proliferation of the antigen-responsive clones of lymphocytes. Subsequent to or in concert with proliferation, the stimulated lymphocytes differentiate from a cognitive stage at which they recognize antigen to an effector stage at which they function to eliminate the antigen. Differentiated helper T cells have essentially the same morphologic appearance as small lymphocytes. Differentiated CTLs may contain increased numbers of cytolytic granules whose contents consist of proteins that lyse target cells. Antibody-producing B cells often differentiate into specialized forms called **plasma cells.** Plasma cells are found only in lymphoid organs and at sites of immune

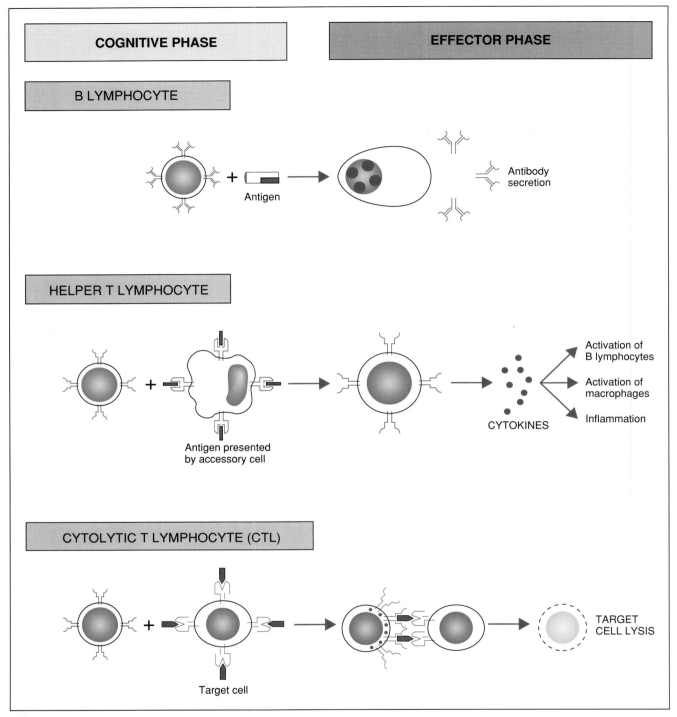

FIGURE 2 – 3. Classes of antigen-specific (B and T) lymphocytes. *B lymphocytes recognize soluble antigens and develop into antibody-secreting cells. Helper T lymphocytes recognize antigens on the surfaces of accessory cells and secrete cytokines, which stimulate different components of immunity and inflammation. Cytolytic T lymphocytes recognize antigens on target cells and lyse these targets.*

responses and normally do not circulate in blood or lymph. They have a characteristic morphology with eccentric nuclei, abundant cytoplasm, and distinct perinuclear haloes (Fig. 2 – 4). Under the electron microscope, the cytoplasm can be seen to contain dense rough endoplasmic reticulum, which is the site where antibodies (and other secreted and membrane proteins) are synthesized. There is also a large Golgi complex, which stains poorly with routinely used histologic stains and is responsible for the perinuclear halo; antibody molecules are converted to their final forms and packaged for secretion in this organelle.

From the time that functionally and developmentally distinct classes of lymphocytes were recognized, immunologists have attempted to develop methods for distinguishing them. The basic approach was to produce antibodies that would selectively recognize different subpopulations. This was initially done by raising "alloantibodies," i.e., antibodies that might recognize allelic forms of cell surface proteins, by immunizing inbred strains of mice with lymphocytes from other strains. Such techniques were remarkably successful and led to the development of antibodies that reacted with murine T cells (anti–Thy-1 antibodies) and even against functionally different subsets of T lymphocytes (anti–Lyt-1 and –Lyt-2 antibodies). The limitations of this approach, however, are obvious, since it is only useful for murine cell surface proteins that exist in allelic forms. Other approaches that met with some success but also have major limitations included searching for lymphocyte-specific autoantibodies in patients with autoimmune diseases. The advent of hybridoma technology gave such analyses a tremendous boost, and the most dramatic development was the production of monoclonal antibodies that reacted specifically and selectively with defined populations of lymphocytes, first human and subsequently in many other species. (Alloantibodies and monoclonal antibodies are described in Chapter 3.)

The cell surface molecules recognized by monoclonal antibodies are called "antigens," since antibodies can be raised against them, or "markers," since they identify and discriminate between ("mark") different cell populations. These markers can be grouped into several categories — some are specific for cells of a particular lineage or maturational pathway, and the expression of others varies according to the state of activation or differentiation of the same cells. Biochemical analyses of cell surface proteins recognized by different monoclonal antibodies in the same species or even in different species demonstrated that in many instances these antibodies were specific for the same evolutionar-

ily conserved cellular proteins. Considerable confusion was created because these surface markers were initially named according to the antibodies that reacted with them. In order to resolve this, a uniform nomenclature system was adopted, initially for human leukocytes. According to this system, a surface marker that identifies a particular lineage or differentiation stage, that has a defined structure, and that is recognized by a group ("cluster") of monoclonal antibodies, is called a member of a **cluster of differentiation.** Thus, all leukocyte surface antigens whose structures are defined are given a "CD" designation, i.e., CD1, CD2, etc. Although this nomenclature was originally used for human leukocyte antigens, it is now common practice to refer to homologous markers in other species by the same CD designation. Newly developed monoclonal antibodies are periodically exchanged among laboratories, and the antigens recognized are assigned to existing CD structures or introduced as new "workshop" candidates ("CDw").

The value of CD antigens in classifying lymphocytes is enormous. For instance, most helper T lymphocytes are $CD3^+CD4^+CD8^-$, and most CTLs are $CD3^+CD4^-CD8^+$. This has allowed immunologists to identify the cells participating in various immune responses, isolate them, and individually analyze their specificities, response patterns, and effector functions. Such antibodies have also been used to define specific alterations in particular subsets of lymphocytes that might be occurring in various diseases. Further investigations of the effects of monoclonal antibodies on lymphocyte function have shown that these surface proteins are not merely phenotypic markers but are themselves involved in a variety of lymphocyte responses. The two most frequent functions attributed to various CD antigens are (1) to promote cell-cell interactions and adhesion, and (2) to transduce signals that lead to lymphocyte activation. Examples of both types of functions are described in Chapter 7.

Plasma cells are believed to be terminally differentiated cells with little or no capacity for mitotic division, and are, in essence, factories for the synthesis and secretion of antibody molecules. It is estimated that half or more of the messenger RNA (mRNA) in plasma cells codes for antibody proteins.

Some of the progeny of antigen-stimulated B and T lymphocytes do not differentiate into effector cells. Instead, they become **memory lymphocytes,** which are capable of surviving for long periods, perhaps 20 years or more, apparently in the absence of antigenic stimulation. The development of memory cells is crucial to the success of vaccination as a method of providing long-lived immunity against infections. It is believed that memory cells are morphologically similar to small lymphocytes; this is difficult to prove, however, because memory cells are defined by their survival and until recently there were virtually no phenotypic markers to clearly distinguish them from resting or recently activated lymphocytes. It is now appreciated that naive and memory T cells express different surface proteins. Naive cells that have not been exposed to antigens express the CD45RA isoform of a surface molecule called CD45; such cells also express

high levels of the peripheral lymph node homing receptor but low levels of other surface proteins involved in cell-cell adhesion. In contrast, memory T cells express a form of CD45 called CD45RO, low levels of the peripheral lymph node homing receptor, but higher levels of other adhesion molecules. The significance of these differences will be discussed later in this chapter when we describe lymphocyte recirculation.

MONONUCLEAR PHAGOCYTES

The **mononuclear phagocyte system** constitutes the second major cell population of the immune system and consists of cells that have a common lineage whose primary function is phagocytosis. In the early 20th century, morphologists observed that certain cells took up dyes injected intravenously (called "vital dyes," since they stained live cells). Aschoff identified these cells as macrophages in connective tissues, microglia in the central nervous system, endothelial cells lining vascular sinusoids, and reticular cells of lymphoid organs and suggested that these

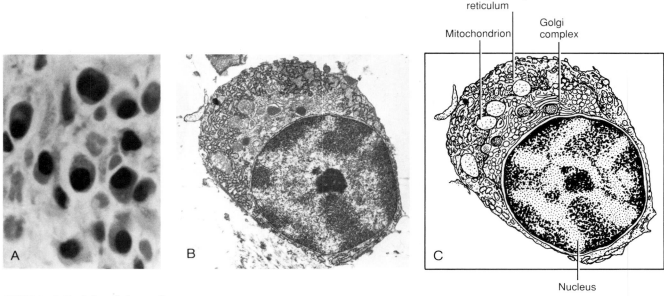

FIGURE 2 – 4. Morphology of plasma cells.
A. *Light micrograph of plasma cells in tissues.*
B. *Electron micrograph of a plasma cell. (Courtesy of Dr. Noel Weidner, Department of Pathology, Brigham and Women's Hospital, Boston.)*
C. *Schematic diagram of the plasma cell depicted in B, illustrating the eccentric nucleus with a "cartwheel" pattern of chromatin, the abundant cisternae of the rough endoplasmic reticulum, and the prominent Golgi complex.*

varied cell types functioned in host defense by phagocytosis of foreign invaders such as microbes. He grouped them collectively into the **reticuloendothelial system** (RES). It is now clear that the pinocytosis of which the endothelial and reticular cells are capable is fundamentally different from the active phagocytosis of macrophages. It is, therefore, more appropriate to classify monocytes and macrophages as members of the mononuclear phagocyte system.

Development

All the cells of the mononuclear phagocyte system originate in the bone marrow and, after maturation and subsequent activation, can achieve varied morphologic forms (Fig. 2–5). The first cell type that enters the peripheral blood after leaving the marrow is incompletely differentiated and is called the **monocyte.** Monocytes are 12 to 20 μm in diameter, and they have bean-shaped nuclei and finely granular cytoplasm containing lysosomes, phagocytic vacuoles, and cytoskeletal filaments (Fig. 2–6). Once they settle in tissues, these cells mature and become **macrophages,** which are also called "histiocytes." Macrophages can be activated by a variety of stimuli and may assume different forms. Some develop abundant cytoplasm and are called **epithelioid cells** because of their resemblance to epithelial cells of the skin. Macrophages can fuse to form polykaryons, also termed **multinucleate giant cells.** Macrophages are found in all organs and connective tissues, and have been given special names to designate specific locations.

For instance, in the central nervous system they are the "microglia"; when lining the vascular sinusoids of the liver, they are called "Kupffer cells"; and in pulmonary airways, they are the "alveolar macrophages."

Activation and Function

Mononuclear phagocytes represent the clearest example of a cell population that is critical for natural immunity, but has also become adapted to play a central role in specific acquired immunity. This illustrates a concept that was introduced in Chapter 1, namely that the immune response imparts specificity to and enhances defense mechanisms that are operative even in the absence of specific antigen recognition by lymphocytes.

The principal *functions of mononuclear phagocytes in natural immunity* include the following:

1. Macrophages phagocytose foreign particles, such as microbes, macromolecules, including antigens, and even self tissues that are injured or dead, such as senescent erythrocytes. Phagocytosed substances are degraded within macrophages by lysosomal enzymes. In addition, the cells secrete enzymes, reactive oxygen species, and lipid-derived mediators such as prostaglandins, all of which serve to kill microbes, control the spread of infections, and can injure even normal tissues in the immediate vicinity.

2. Macrophages produce cytokines, which recruit other inflammatory cells, especially neutrophils, and are responsible for many of the systemic effects of

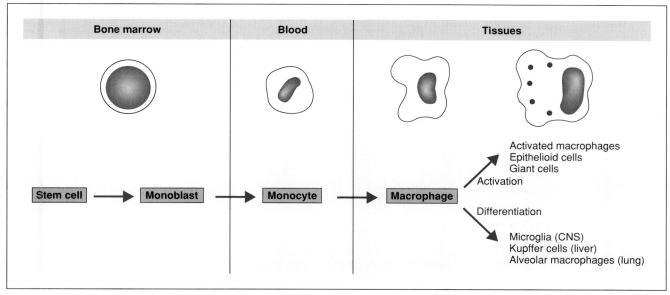

FIGURE 2 – 5. Maturation of mononuclear phagocytes.

inflammation, such as fever. Macrophages also produce growth factors for fibroblasts and vascular endothelium that promote the repair of injured tissues.

Mononuclear phagocytes play the following important roles in the cognitive, activation, and effector phases of specific immune responses.

1. Macrophages display foreign antigens on their surface in a form that can be recognized by antigen-specific T lymphocytes. This function of macrophages as **antigen-presenting cells** (APCs) is described in Chapter 6. Macrophages also express secreted and membrane proteins that promote T cell activation.

2. In the effector phase of cell-mediated immune responses, helper T cells secrete cytokines that activate macrophages. Such activated macrophages are more efficient at performing phagocytic, degradative, and cytocidal functions than are unstimulated cells. Thus, *macrophages are among the principal effector cells of cell-mediated immunity* (see Chapter 12).

3. In the effector phase of humoral immune responses, foreign antigens, such as microbes, become

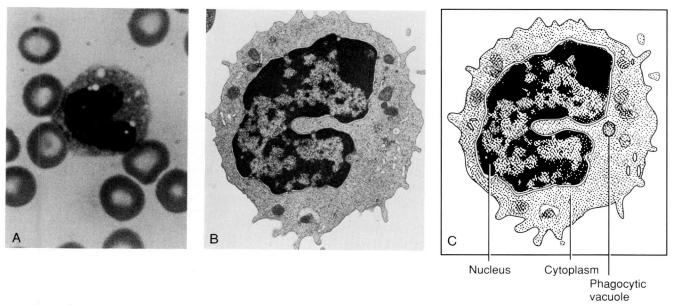

FIGURE 2 – 6. Morphology of mononuclear phagocytes.
A. *Light micrograph of a monocyte in a peripheral blood smear.*
B. *Electron micrograph of a peripheral blood monocyte. (Courtesy of Dr. Noel Weidner, Department of Pathology, Brigham and Women's Hospital, Boston.)*
C. *Schematic diagram of the monocyte depicted in B, illustrating the characteristic nucleus, scant cytoplasmic organelles, and phagocytic vacuoles.*

coated, or opsonized, by antibody molecules and complement proteins. Because macrophages express surface receptors for antibodies and for certain complement proteins, they bind and phagocytose opsonized particles much more avidly than uncoated particles. *Thus, macrophages participate in the elimination of foreign antigens by humoral immune responses.*

The ability of macrophages and lymphocytes to stimulate each other's functions provides an important amplification mechanism for specific immunity. The mechanisms and physiologic consequences of the bi-directional interactions between immunocompetent lymphocytes and non-lymphoid accessory and effector cells will be referred to in many sections of this book.

GRANULOCYTES

In addition to lymphocytes and mononuclear phagocytes, other leukocytes, which are called **granulocytes** because they contain abundant cytoplasmic granules, participate in the effector phase of specific immune responses. The details of the morphology, biochemistry, and functions of granulocytes are beyond the scope of this book. These leukocytes are often referred to as **inflammatory cells,** because they play important roles in inflammation and natural immunity, and function to eliminate microbes and dead tissues. However, like macrophages, granulocytes are stimulated by T cell–derived cytokines and phagocytose opsonized particles, so that these cells serve important effector functions in specific immune responses as well.

Peripheral blood contains three types of granulocytes, which are classified according to the staining characteristics of their predominant granules.

Neutrophils, also called **polymorphonuclear leukocytes** because of their multilobed, morphologically diverse nuclei, are the most numerous. They respond rapidly to chemotactic stimuli, perform many of the phagocytic and degradative functions of macrophages, can be activated by cytokines produced primarily by macrophages, and are the major cell population in the acute inflammatory response. Neutrophils also possess receptors for the Fc portions of antibodies and for complement proteins, and they migrate to and accumulate at sites of complement activation (see Chapter 3). Therefore, they avidly phagocytose opsonized particles and function as effector cells of humoral immunity.

Eosinophils, like neutrophils, contain numerous lysosomes and generally perform similar functions. However, presumably because they express Fc receptors specific for a class of antibodies called IgE, eosinophils are important effector cells in immune reactions to antigens that induce high levels of IgE antibody, such as parasites. Eosinophils may be particularly effective at destroying parasites such as helminths, which are often resistant to the lysosomal enzymes of neutrophils and macrophages. Eosino-phils are also abundant at sites of immediate hypersensitivity (allergic) reactions, which are due to the production of IgE antibodies. Eosinophils are also activated by other classes of antibodies, especially the secretory form of IgA (see Chapter 3). The growth and differentiation of eosinophils are stimulated by a helper T cell–derived cytokine called interleukin-5, and T cell activation may contribute to eosinophil accumulation at sites of parasitic infestation and allergic reactions.

Basophils are the circulating counterparts of tissue mast cells. Both basophils and mast cells express high-affinity receptors for IgE and, therefore, avidly bind IgE antibodies. Interaction of antigens with these IgE molecules stimulates basophils and mast cells to secrete their granule contents, which are the chemical mediators of immediate hypersensitivity (see Chapter 14). Thus, these granulocytes are effector cells of IgE-mediated immediate hypersensitivity.

FUNCTIONAL ANATOMY OF LYMPHOID TISSUES

In order to optimize cellular interactions necessary for the cognitive, activation, and effector phases of specific immune responses, the majority of lymphocytes, mononuclear phagocytes, and other accessory cells are localized and concentrated in anatomically defined tissues or organs and often in specific areas of these organs. Such anatomic compartmentalization is not fixed because, as discussed later in this chapter, many lymphocytes recirculate and constantly exchange between the circulation and tissues. Lymphoid tissues can be classified into two groups: (1) the **generative organs** are the ones in which lymphocytes arise and mature, and (2) the **peripheral organs** are the sites where mature lymphocytes respond to foreign antigens (Fig. 2–7). Included in the generative lymphoid organs of mammals are the bone marrow, where all lymphocytes arise, and the thymus, where T cells mature and reach a stage of functional competence. In birds another generative organ is the bursa of Fabricius, the site of B cell maturation; the bursal equivalent of mammals is probably the bone marrow itself. The peripheral lymphoid tissues include the lymph nodes, spleen, mucosa-associated lymphoid tissues, and the cutaneous immune system. In addition, poorly defined aggregates of lymphocytes are found in connective tissues and in virtually all organs except the central nervous system.

Bone Marrow

During fetal life, the generation of all blood cells, called **hematopoiesis,** occurs initially in the yolk sac and then in the liver and spleen. This function is gradually taken over by the bone marrow and increasingly by the marrow of the flat bones, so that by puberty hematopoiesis occurs mostly in the sternum, verte-

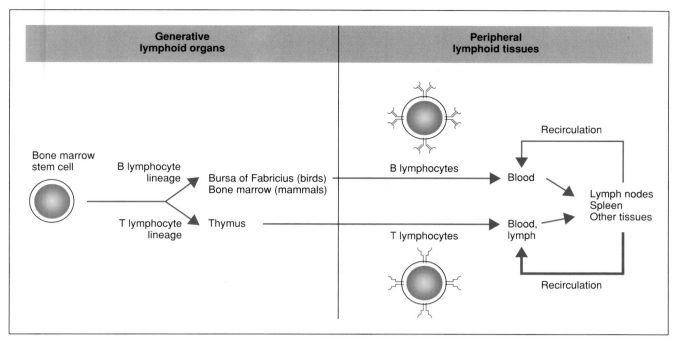

FIGURE 2 – 7. Maturation of lymphocytes. *Development of mature lymphocytes prior to antigen exposure occurs in the generative lymphoid organs, and immune responses to foreign antigens occur in the peripheral lymphoid tissues.*

brae, iliac bones, and ribs. The red marrow that is found in these bones consists of a sponge-like reticular framework located between bony trabeculae. The spaces in this framework are filled by fat cells and the precursors of blood cells, which mature and exit via the dense network of vascular sinuses to become part of the circulatory system.

All the blood cells originate from a common **stem cell** that becomes committed to differentiate along particular lineages, i.e., erythroid, megakaryocytic, granulocytic, monocytic, and lymphocytic (Fig. 2–8). Cytokines are known to stimulate the proliferation and maturation of various precursors. Since these growth factors are assayed by their ability to stimulate different types of leukocyte colonies to develop from marrow cells *in vitro,* they are called "colony-stimulating factors" (CSFs). Several of these cytokines are produced by T lymphocytes, including interleukin-3 (IL–3, also called multi-CSF), which acts on all stem cells, and granulocyte-monocyte–CSF (GM–CSF), which stimulates the formation of granulocytes and monocytes. Macrophages and marrow stromal cells produce GM–CSF and additional CSFs specific for granulocytes (G–CSF) or monocytes (M–CSF). Macrophages and stromal cells in the bone marrow produce two other cytokines, called interleukin-1 and interleukin-6, which further enhance colony formation by hematopoietic precursors in the presence of CSFs. A cytokine called interleukin-7, also produced by marrow stromal cells, has been shown to preferentially stimulate the maturation of B lymphocytes from marrow precursors. The properties and functions of these cytokines are described in Chapter 11. However, little is known about the nature of the uncommit-

ted stem cell or the mechanisms that regulate its commitment to specific lineages. In 1988, techniques for reconstituting the immune system of congenitally immunodeficient mice with human lymphohematopoietic stem cells were described. These immunodeficient mice lack T and B lymphocytes, and after the implantation of human hematopoietic tissues, mature human T and B cells develop in the animals and populate the circulation and peripheral lymphoid tissues. Such approaches hold great promise for more precise identification and characterization of stem cells and their developmental pathways.

Thymus

The thymus is a bilobed organ situated in the anterior mediastinum. Each lobe is divided into multiple lobules by fibrous septa, and each lobule consists of an outer cortex and an inner medulla (Fig. 2–9). The cortex contains a dense collection of T lymphocytes, and the lighter-staining medulla is more sparsely populated with lymphocytes. Scattered throughout the thymus are non-lymphoid epithelial cells, which have abundant cytoplasm, as well as bone marrow–derived dendritic cells and macrophages. In the medulla are structures called **Hassall's corpuscles,** which are composed of tightly packed whorls of epithelial cells that may be remnants of degenerating cells. The thymus has a rich vascular supply and efferent lymphatic vessels that drain into mediastinal lymph nodes.

The lymphocytes in the thymus, also called **thymocytes,** are T lymphocytes at various stages of matu-

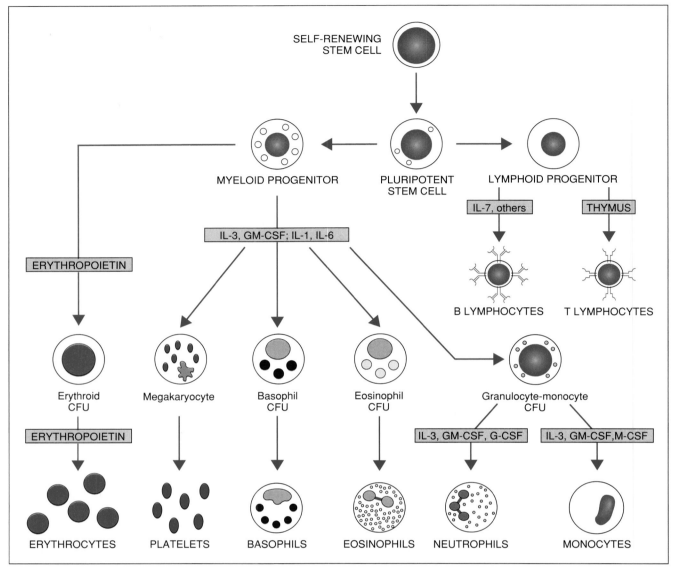

FIGURE 2 – 8. Maturation of blood cells: the hematopoietic "tree." *The maturation of different lineages of blood cells is regulated by various cytokines. Note that the maturation of T and B lymphocytes is illustrated in summary form and is discussed in detail in later chapters. CFU, colony-forming unit; IL, interleukin; GM – CSF, granulocyte-macrophage colony-stimulating factor.*

ration. Precursors that are committed to the T cell lineage enter the thymic cortex via blood vessels. It is not known whether B cell precursors enter the thymus and fail to survive or whether there are mechanisms that ensure that only cells committed to developing into T lymphocytes can enter the thymus. The most immature thymocytes do not express receptors for antigens or surface markers, including CD4 and CD8, that are characteristic of the mature phenotype. These immature cells migrate from the cortex toward the medulla and come into contact with epithelial cells, macrophages, and dendritic cells. Efficient contact may occur in lymphoepithelial complexes in which lymphocytes are found closely apposed to the invaginated plasma membranes of large epithelial cells called **"nurse cells."** En route to the medulla, thymocytes begin to express receptors for antigens

and surface markers that are present on mature, peripheral T lymphocytes. Thus, the medulla contains mostly mature T cells, and only mature CD4+ or CD8+ T cells exit the thymus and enter the blood, lymph, and peripheral lymphoid tissues.

From the large number of primitive T cells that enter the thymus, cells that might recognize self antigens do not survive, whereas cells whose receptors are specific for foreign antigens are stimulated to mature. These selection processes, which are critical for the ability of the immune system to discriminate between self and non-self, are described in considerable detail in Chapter 8. The thymus is the site of remarkable proliferation as well as elimination of lymphocytes, which presumably reflect the selection of foreign antigen-specific cells and the deletion of potentially self-reactive T cells. It is estimated that in

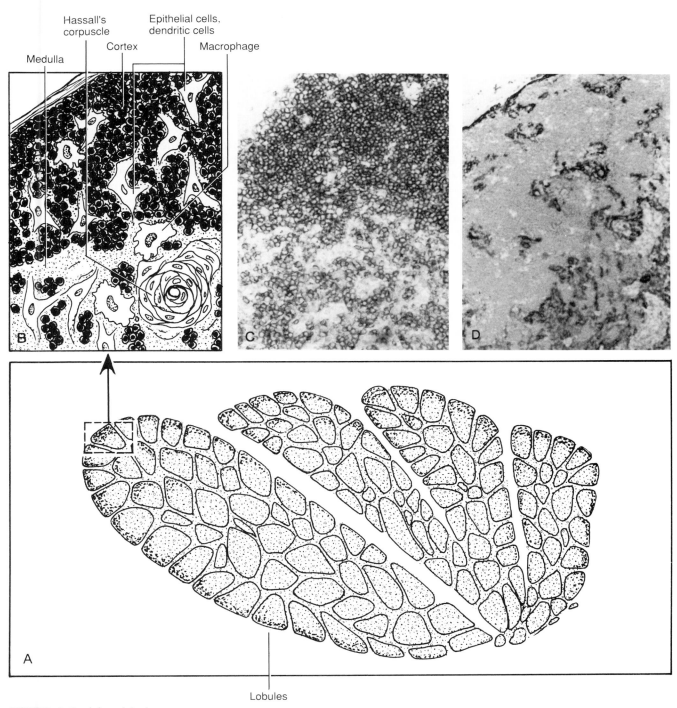

FIGURE 2–9. Morphology of the thymus.

A. *Schematic diagram of the thymus, illustrating two main lobes (the one on the right being subdivided into smaller lobes in this thymus), composed of multiple lobules.*

B. *Diagram of the edge of a lobule showing the cells of the cortex and medulla.*

C. *T lymphocytes in the cortex of the thymus, detected by an immunoperoxidase stain with an antibody specific for T cells. (Immunoperoxidase staining is described in Chapter 3; positive cells appear dark.) (Courtesy of Dr. G. S. Pinkus, Department of Pathology, Brigham and Women's Hospital, Boston.)*

D. *Epithelial cells scattered throughout the cortex and medulla, detected by an immunoperoxidase stain specific for keratin, an intracellular intermediate filament protein. (Courtesy of Dr. G. S. Pinkus, Department of Pathology, Brigham and Women's Hospital, Boston.)*

mice, about 50×10^6 immature cells enter the thymus each day and fewer than 1×10^6 mature cells leave. The thymus undergoes physiologic involution with aging, so that by puberty it is difficult to locate. Maturation and selection of T lymphocytes continue well into adult life, suggesting that either the remnants of the thymus that are present in adults are adequate for performing these functions or extrathymic T cell maturation can also occur. However, no such extrathymic sites of T cell development have been identified.

Lymph Nodes

Lymph nodes are small nodular aggregates of lymphoid tissue situated along lymphatic channels throughout the body. Epithelia, such as the skin and the mucosa of the gastrointestinal and respiratory tracts, as well as connective tissues and most organs have a lymphatic drainage. Antigens that enter through any of these portals end up in lymphatic vessels whose contents are "sampled" by lymph nodes for the presence of foreign substances. Each node is surrounded by a fibrous capsule that is pierced by numerous afferent lymphatics, which empty the lymph into a subcapsular sinus (Fig. 2–10). The node consists of an outer cortex in which there are aggregates of cells constituting the **follicles,** some of which contain central areas called **germinal centers** that stain lightly with commonly used histologic stains. The inner medulla contains less dense lymphocytes and mononuclear phagocytes scattered among lymphatic and vascular sinusoids. Lymphocytes and accessory cells are often found in close proximity but do not form intercellular junctions, which is probably important for maintaining their ability to migrate and recirculate between the lymph, blood, and tissues. The lymph that enters the subcapsular sinus percolates through the cortex and medulla and exits via a single efferent lymphatic located in the hilum of the node. In addition, each node has a vascular supply with afferent and efferent vessels at the hilum.

Different classes of lymphocytes and non-lymphoid accessory cells are sequestered in particular areas of the node. Follicles without germinal centers, which are called **primary follicles,** contain predominantly mature, resting B lymphocytes that have apparently not been stimulated recently by antigens. The germinal centers, which develop in response to antigenic stimulation, contain numerous large lymphocytes with phenotypic characteristics of activated B cells. The germinal centers are believed to be one of the sites where B lymphocytes proliferate and differentiate into antibody-secreting cells in response to antigenic stimulation. It is estimated that the cell cycle time of germinal center B cells is as short as 6 hours. Since plasma cells are rare at these sites, it is possible that the terminal differentiation of B cells occurs outside the germinal centers. It is also believed that the activation of memory B cells, the production of antibodies with increased affinities for antigens, and the

appearance of different classes of antibodies (described in Chapters 4 and 9) are three aspects of antigen-stimulated B cell differentiation that are initiated largely in germinal centers. Since these events usually require the participation of helper T lymphocytes, it is not surprising that germinal center development is T cell–dependent and is not seen in individuals congenitally deficient in T cells. In addition to lymphocytes, lymphoid follicles contain macrophages and scattered **dendritic cells** (also called interdigitating reticular cells) that function as accessory cells in immune responses. Also, in the germinal centers there are **follicular dendritic cells** that have long cytoplasmic processes, express large numbers of receptors for antibodies (Fc receptors) on their surfaces, and are different from the "dendritic cells" mentioned above. Follicular dendritic cells are believed to be important in capturing antigens complexed with preformed antibodies and, therefore, in the activation of memory B cells to generate secondary antibody responses.

The T lymphocytes are located predominantly in the interfollicular areas of the cortex and paracortical zones in the medulla (Fig. 2–10). Most of these are CD4$^+$ helper T cells, intermingled with relatively sparse CD8$^+$ cells. Some CD4$^+$ T cells are also scattered in germinal centers, where their role may be to help the proliferation and differentiation of antigen-stimulated B lymphocytes. The proximity of helper T cells and the B cells that are the recipients of T cell help is important because helper function is mediated largely by secreted cytokines, which act at short distances, close to the sites where they are produced (see Chapter 9). Dendritic (interdigitating reticular) cells are abundant in the T cell areas, which is consistent with their postulated role in presenting foreign antigens to T lymphocytes.

The medulla contains scattered lymphocytes, large numbers of macrophages and dendritic cells, and, in nodes draining sites of immunization, numerous plasma cells, all of which are interspersed with lymphatic channels.

The mechanisms responsible for the anatomic sequestration of different classes of lymphocytes in distinct areas of the node are unclear. One possibility is that compartmentalization is maintained by specific adhesions of different lymphocytes with stromal cells or extracellular matrix proteins. Although the anatomy of the immune response is poorly understood, it is likely that this cellular organization promotes interactions between the participating cell types and is critically important for the generation of immunity. Studies using labeled antigens indicate that a protein antigen that enters the lymph node in an unimmunized individual is trapped by macrophages and dendritic cells and largely degraded. Peptide fragments of the injected antigen, attached to the surfaces of accessory cells, stimulate helper T lymphocytes (see Chapter 6). The first wave of mitotic activity is seen in the T cell zones within 1 to 2 days after immunization. Proliferation of B cells follows, after which germinal centers develop and the B lympho-

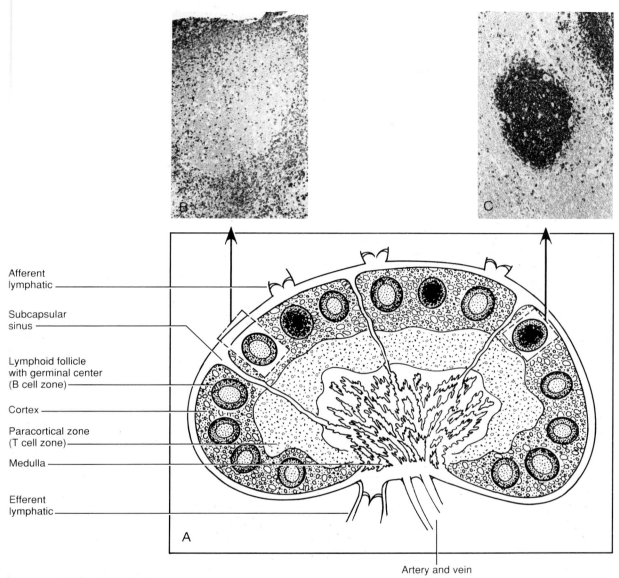

FIGURE 2 – 10. Morphology of a lymph node.
A. *Schematic diagram of a lymph node showing the distinct cortex with lymphoid follicles and dense lymphocytes and the medulla with lymphatic cords and vessels.*
B. *T lymphocytes in the parafollicular region of the cortex, detected by an immunoperoxidase stain with an antibody specific for T cells. (Courtesy of Dr. G. S. Pinkus, Department of Pathology, Brigham and Women's Hospital, Boston.)*
C. *B lymphocytes in a follicle in the cortex, detected by an immunoperoxidase stain with an antibody specific for B cells. (Courtesy of Dr. G. S. Pinkus, Department of Pathology, Brigham and Women's Hospital, Boston.)*

cytes differentiate into antibody-secreting cells. Fully differentiated plasma cells reside in the medulla, where they secrete antibodies into the circulation. Memory B cells circulate in lymphatic and blood vessels and migrate through the germinal centers of lymphoid follicles. Effector T lymphocytes that develop after immunization enter the lymphatic and vascular systems, so that they can recognize and respond to antigens at sites of immunization. In previously immunized individuals in whom circulating antibodies are already present, challenge with antigen leads to the formation of antigen-antibody complexes, which bind avidly to the surfaces of follicular dendritic cells in the germinal centers. Here the antigen remains largely undegraded and is recognized by memory B cells, which were generated by the first immunization and reside in and circulate through the germinal centers. The anatomy of lymph nodes (and other lymphoid tissues) is not fixed, but changes with antigen exposure. Thus, lymphocyte proliferation and germinal centers gradually regress after the antigenic stimulus is eliminated.

Spleen

The spleen is an organ weighing about 150 gm in adults, located in the left upper quadrant of the abdomen. It is supplied by a single splenic artery, which pierces the capsule at the hilum and divides into progressively smaller branches that remain surrounded by protective and supporting fibrous trabeculae (Fig. 2–11). Small arterioles are surrounded by cuffs of lymphocytes, called **periarteriolar lymphoid sheaths,** to which are attached the lymphoid follicles, some of which contain germinal centers. These dense lymphoid tissues constitute the **white pulp** of the spleen. The arterioles ultimately end in vascular sinusoids, scattered among which are large numbers of macrophages, dendritic cells, sparse lymphocytes, and plasma cells; these constitute the **red pulp.** The sinusoids form venules that drain into the splenic vein, which carries blood out of the spleen and into the portal circulation.

Lymphocytes and accessory cells are anatomically segregated in the spleen as they are in lymph nodes (Fig. 2–11). The periarteriolar sheaths contain mainly T lymphocytes, about two thirds of which are of the CD4+ helper class, about one third are CD8+. The follicles and germinal centers are the predominantly B cell zones, having the same anatomic features and presumed functions as in lymph nodes.

In principle, the function of the spleen and its responses to antigens are much like those of lymph nodes, the essential difference being that the spleen is the major site of immune responses to blood-borne antigens whereas lymph nodes are involved in responses to antigens in the lymph. The spleen is also an important "filter" for the blood, with its red pulp macrophages being responsible for clearing the blood of unwanted foreign substances and senescent erythrocytes even in the absence of specific immunity.

Other Peripheral Lymphoid Tissues

In addition to the lymph nodes and spleen, lymphocytes are found either scattered or in aggregates in many tissues. Some of these collections are anatomically well organized and have unique properties. The **mucosal immune system** consists of aggregates of lymphocytes, macrophages, and other accessory cells located beneath the mucosal epithelium as well as diffusely scattered intraepithelial lymphocytes. The anatomically defined aggregates of mucosa-associated lymphoid tissues include the **Peyer's patches** in the lamina propria of the small intestine, lymphoid follicles in the appendix, tonsils in the pharynx, and submucosal lymphoid follicles throughout the upper airways and bronchi.

The **cutaneous immune system** consists of intraepidermal lymphocytes and of lymphocytes and accessory cells in the dermis. It is the site of immune responses to topically applied antigens. An important antigen-presenting cell in the skin is the epidermal **Langerhans cell,** which has been postulated to be related to the dendritic cell of lymphoid organs on the basis of phenotypic markers, ontogeny, and functions.

In addition to these normal lymphoid organs, **ectopic lymphoid tissues** can develop at sites of strong immune responses. A striking example of this is the disease rheumatoid arthritis, in which an immune response in the synovium ultimately leads to destruction of the cartilage and bone in joints. In severe cases, synovial tissues contain well-developed lymphoid follicles with prominent germinal centers.

LYMPHOCYTE RECIRCULATION

Because the total population of lymphocytes in an individual can respond to many distinct antigens, it follows that only a small number of lymphocytes can specifically recognize any one antigen. Nevertheless, foreign antigens are introduced into the body by several different portals of entry, through the skin or mucosal surfaces. In order to increase the likelihood that the specific immunocompetent cells will see an antigen, the lymphocytes, especially T cells, continuously circulate throughout the body (Fig. 2–12). Blood-borne lymphocytes enter into the tissues by crawling between the endothelial cells of post-capillary venules, a process called **diapedesis.** Once in the tissues, the lymphocytes may remain in residence or may make their way through lymphatic endothelium into the lymphatic circulation. Lymphocytes in the lymphatic vessels then either enter a draining lymph node through the afferent lymphatics or return to the blood through the thoracic duct. Thus, the circulation pathway of lymphocytes allows efficient cellular communications between the blood, lymph, peripheral sites of antigen entry, and lymphoid tissues where immune responses develop. Furthermore, naive (CD45RA+) T cells and memory (CD45RO+) T cells follow somewhat different recirculation pathways. Naive T cells directly enter lymph nodes from the blood, and are thus able to "sample" nodes for the presence of foreign antigens brought via lymphatic vessels. In contrast, memory T cells preferentially migrate into sites of antigen exposure and inflammation in peripheral tissues, and to mucosal lymphoid tissues, such as Peyer's patches. Thus, memory cells home to sites of antigen accumulation (see Chapter 12).

Classical experiments in the 1950s and 1960s by James Gowans and his colleagues first demonstrated the migration of lymphocytes from the blood into the organized peripheral lymphoid organs, namely lymph nodes, spleen, and mucosal lymphoid tissues such as Peyer's patches. Some of the post-capillary venules in these organs are specialized to facilitate the transendothelial migration of circulating lymphocytes. These modified venules are lined by tall, metabolically active endothelial cells and, therefore, are called **high endothelial venules** (HEVs) (Fig. 2–13).

The HEVs develop from flat endothelial venules in

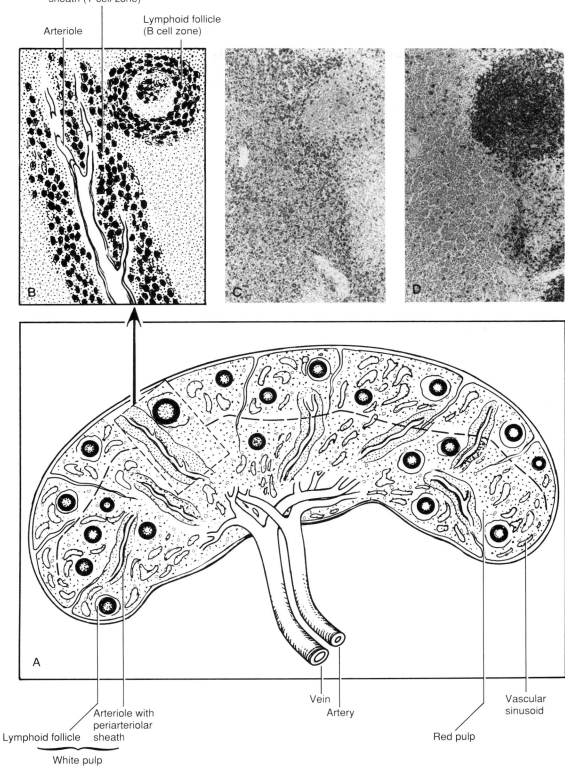

FIGURE 2–11. Morphology of the spleen.

A. *Schematic diagram of the spleen. Note that the white pulp, made up of dense lymphoid tissues in periarteriolar sheaths and follicles, is intermingled with the red pulp, composed of vascular sinusoids and scattered cells.*

B. *Diagram of an arteriole and the adjacent lymphoid tissues composing the white pulp.*

C. *T lymphocytes in the periarteriolar lymphoid sheath, detected by an immunoperoxidase stain with an antibody specific for T cells. (Courtesy of Dr. G. S. Pinkus, Department of Pathology, Brigham and Women's Hospital, Boston.)*

D. *B lymphocytes in a lymphoid follicle, detected by an immunoperoxidase stain with an antibody specific for B cells. (Courtesy of Dr. G. S. Pinkus, Department of Pathology, Brigham and Women's Hospital, Boston.)*

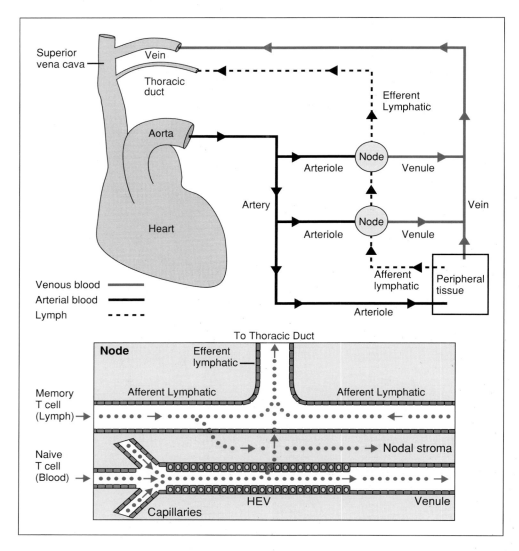

FIGURE 2–12. Pathway of lymphocyte recirculation. *Naive T cells preferentially leave the blood and enter lymph nodes across the high endothelial venules (HEVs). Memory T cells leave the blood and enter peripheral tissues through flat venules and reach the lymph nodes through afferent lymphatics. Lymphocytes return to the circulation through the efferent lymphatics and the thoracic duct, which empties into the superior vena cava.*

response to cytokines produced by antigen-stimulated T lymphocytes. This conclusion is based on several observations:

1. HEVs develop after birth only when animals are exposed to environmental antigens; HEVs fail to develop in animals raised in germ-free environments.

2. HEVs revert to flat endothelial venules when delivery of antigen to a lymph node is prevented, for instance, by surgically disrupting the afferent lymphatics.

3. HEVs are not found in animals that do not have functional T lymphocytes.

4. The endothelial cells of HEVs express surface proteins that can be induced in cultured endothelial cells only by adding cytokines, such as γ interferon, that are secreted by activated T cells (see Chapter 11).

5. High endothelial morphologic patterns can similarly be induced in cell culture or *in situ* in the skin by adding T cell–derived cytokines.

Thus, T lymphocytes, which actively recirculate between the blood and lymphoid tissues, are them-

selves responsible for inducing the development of endothelial cells that facilitate this recirculation. This is one mechanism that promotes the accumulation of lymphocytes at sites of antigenic stimulation.

Recent studies have indicated that the principal reason why lymphocytes migrate preferentially through HEVs is that the endothelial cells of HEVs are much more adhesive for lymphocytes than are the flat endothelial cells lining other venules. When circulating lymphocytes encounter a high endothelial cell, they bind and remain attached for a much longer time on average than after an encounter with a flat endothelial cell. The longer a lymphocyte remains attached to a venular endothelial cell, the greater the probability of diapedesis through the endothelial lining. It is possible that alterations in the structure of the subendothelium and surrounding cells of the HEVs may also favor diapedesis, but this is unproven. By direct comparisons using videomicroscopy on live animals, it has been found that although HEVs account for only about 2 per cent of all venules in the small intestine, about half of the lymphocytes entering the mucosa

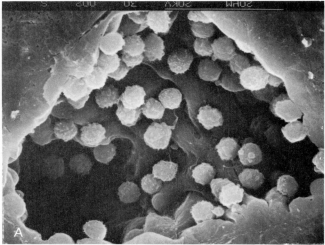

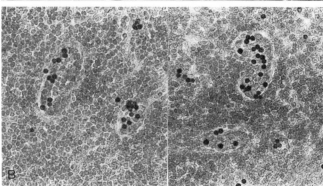

FIGURE 2 – 13. Lymphocyte adhesion to high endothelial venules.
A. *Scanning electron micrograph of a high endothelial venule with lymphocytes attached to the luminal surface of the endothelial cells. (Courtesy of J. Emerson, T. Yednock, and S. D. Rosen, University of California San Francisco School of Medicine, San Francisco. Reproduced with permission from Rosen, S. D., and L. M. Stoolman. Potential role of cell surface lectin in lymphocyte recirculation. In Olden, K., and J. Parent (eds.).* Vertebrate Lectins. *New York, Van Nostrand Reinhold, 1987.)*
B. *A frozen section binding assay showing preferential attachment of added lymphocytes (stained darkly) to high endothelial venules, which are seen in cross section. (Reproduced with permission from Rosen, S. D. Lymphocyte homing: progress and prospects. Current Opinion in Cell Biology 1:913–919, 1989.)*

exit the blood stream through HEVs and thus enter Peyer's patches, whereas the other half enter the lamina propria of the mucosa throughout the flat venules. *Thus, HEVs focus diapedesis by binding lymphocytes.*

The preferential binding of lymphocytes to HEVs *in vitro* can be observed directly and quantitated by pouring lymphocyte suspensions on frozen sections of lymphoid organs and determining the numbers of lymphocytes that bind to endothelial cells (Fig. 2–13). This frozen section binding assay led to the remarkable observation that lymphocytes of different phenotypic or functional classes, and leukemic cells derived from these lymphocytes, preferentially adhere to the HEVs of particular lymphoid organs. For example, naive T cells preferentially exit the blood stream in peripheral lymph nodes and bind avidly to lymph node HEVs. In contrast, memory T cells bind better to HEVs in mucosal lymphoid tissues, such as Peyer's patches. Such results suggest that different lymphocytes express receptors for molecules unique to HEVs of different tissues. The relative amounts of these receptors expressed by different lymphocytes may account for the relative efficiency with which lymphocytes "home" to particular lymphoid tissues. Therefore, these lymphocyte receptors for HEVs of particular organs are also called **homing receptors** (Box 2–2). In addition to the homing receptors, a number of lymphocyte surface molecules contribute

to the adhesion between lymphocytes and HEVs, irrespective of anatomic site; the most important **adhesion molecules** of these are also described in Box 2–2.

The molecules on HEVs that are the ligands for various lymphocyte homing receptors are called **vascular addressins**. Addressins have not been fully characterized yet. However, studies with antibodies reactive with these molecules have shown that the expression of addressins is related to tissue type and development but not to antigenic stimulation or cytokine production. In summary, *lymphocyte homing receptors, addressins, and adhesion molecules account for the tissue specificity of lymphocyte homing and the preferential binding of lymphocytes to HEVs compared to flat venules.*

SUMMARY

The principal cellular constituents of the immune system are lymphocytes, mononuclear phagocytes, and related accessory cells. Lymphocytes are the only immunocompetent cells capable of specific recognition of antigens. They are morphologically homogeneous but consist of distinct subsets that perform different functions and can be distinguished phenotypically. Mononuclear phagocytes are critical for

BOX 2 – 2.   LYMPHOCYTE HOMING RECEPTORS

The frozen section binding assay described in the text has allowed immunologists to elucidate the molecular basis of lymphocyte-HEV interactions by testing the ability of monoclonal antibodies against lymphocytes or against HEVs to block the binding of lymphocytes to HEVs. Once a blocking antibody is obtained, it can be used to identify the surface structures that mediate lymphocyte binding to HEVs. From such studies, it is now known that at least two separate classes of lymphocyte surface proteins are responsible for the binding of lymphocytes to HEVs:

1. *The selective homing of lymphocytes to particular lymphoid tissues is mediated by the binding of lymphocyte homing receptors to organ-specific HEV molecules.* Three candidate homing receptors have been identified:

a. The best characterized of these is recognized by a monoclonal antibody called MEL – 14, which reacts with a 90 kilodalton (kD) surface glycoprotein that is present on all murine lymphocytes that home to peripheral lymph nodes but is absent from lymphocytes that home selectively to Peyer's patches. MEL – 14 blocks lymphocyte binding to frozen sections of lymph nodes *in vitro* and inhibits homing of lymphocytes to lymph nodes *in vivo*. The protein recognized by MEL – 14, is called the "MEL – 14 antigen," or the "peripheral lymph node receptor." Recently, the MEL – 14 antigen and its human homolog have been molecularly cloned and sequenced. The extracellular portion of this homing receptor consists of an N-terminal domain that is homologous to the lectin (carbohydrate-binding) domain of the hepatocyte asialoglycoprotein receptor, a region homologous to epidermal growth factor receptor, and a series of two repeated units homologous to complement receptors (see Chapter 13). The MEL – 14 antigen may itself function as a lectin, binding to carbohydrate moieties on lymph node HEV cells. The MEL – 14 antigen is more abundant on naive than on memory T cells, and this may account for the preference of naive T cells for peripheral lymph node HEVs.

b. A second murine lymphocyte homing receptor that specifically mediates lymphocyte binding to Peyer's patch HEVs has been identified using the same approaches that were first developed with MEL – 14. This lymphocyte surface molecule, called VLA – 4, is a two-chain heterodimer and belongs to a family of membrane proteins called **integrins,** which are involved in adhesive interactions between many different cell types (see Chapter

7). This Peyer's patch homing receptor is present on many leukocytes other than lymphocytes. VLA – 4 expression is increased on memory T cells compared to naive cells, and this may contribute to the preferential binding of memory cells to Peyer's patch HEVs.

c. The third type of homing receptor is a 90 kD protein called CD44. It was identified by a panel of antibodies raised against human lymphocytes that inhibit binding to Peyer's patch but not lymph node HEVs. CD44 is present on lymphocyte cell lines that bind to both lymph node and Peyer's patch HEVs and is also expressed on many epithelial, neural, and connective tissue cells in addition to lymphocytes. The CD44 protein is structurally related to proteoglycans found on cartilage and is distinct from the MEL – 14 antigen (although the two are of similar size). Like VLA – 4, CD44 expression is increased on memory T cells.

Thus, naive T cells may enter lymph nodes mainly by binding of MEL – 14 antigen to lymph node HEVs, and memory T cells enter sites of inflammation and mucosal lymphoid tissues primarily by binding of VLA – 4 and CD44 to their respective ligands.

2. *The major lymphocyte protein involved in non-organspecific binding to HEVs is known as* **lymphocyte function – associated antigen – 1** (LFA – 1).

LFA – 1 is also an integrin, but it is distinct from the Peyer's patch homing receptor VLA – 4. LFA – 1 is a two-chain molecule that binds specifically to two target proteins on endothelial (and other) cells, called intercellular adhesion molecules (ICAM) 1 and 2, whose expression is not tissue-specific. ICAM – 1 is the main ligand for LFA – 1. As we shall discuss in Chapters 7 and 12, LFA – 1 also functions to strengthen the adhesion of lymphocytes to many other cell types and in many other circumstances besides attachment to HEVs. For instance, LFA – 1 plays an important role in antigen recognition by T cells and in the CTL – mediated lysis of target cells. In addition, the ability of lymphocytes to bind preferentially to HEVs at different anatomic sites is not attributable to lymphocyte LFA – 1. For these reasons, LFA – 1 is not classified as a "homing receptor," even though it is clearly involved in lymphocyte recirculation. Memory T cells also express more LFA – 1 than naive cells and LFA-1 contributes to the binding of memory cells to endothelium at peripheral sites of inflammation (see Chapter 12).

---

host defense in the absence of specific immunity and have also evolved into key participants in the cognitive, activation, and effector phases of specific immune responses. Lymphocytes originate in the bone marrow, mature in different generative organs, and are located in anatomically defined peripheral lymphoid tissues. The structural organization of lymphoid tissues optimizes intimate cell contact and short-range interactions between the cell populations that cooperate in the generation of immune responses. The ability of lymphocytes to circulate, to bind to endothelium by specific molecular interactions, and to migrate through vessels allows these cells to exchange between the tissues and the circulation and ensures that they can interact with foreign antigens at various sites of antigen entry.

SELECTED READINGS

Bhan, A. K., and I. Bhan. In situ characterization of human lymphoid cells using monoclonal antibodies. *In* M. Miyasaka and Z. Trnka (eds.). Differentiation Antigens in Lymphohemopoietic Tissues. M. Dekker Inc., New York and Basel, 1988, pp. 13–46.

Butcher, E. C. Cellular and molecular mechanisms that direct leukocyte traffic. American Journal of Pathology 136:1–11, 1990.

Duijvestijn, A., and A. Hamann. Mechanisms and regulation of lymphocyte migration. Immunology Today 10:23–28, 1989.

Heinen, E., N. Corwann, and C. Kinet-Denoel. The lymph follicle: a hard nut to crack. Immunology Today 9:240–243, 1988.

Hsu, S.-M., J. Cossman, and E. S. Jaffe. Lymphocyte subsets in normal human lymphoid tissues. American Journal of Clinical Pathology 80:21–30, 1983.

Kincade, P. W. Experimental models for understanding B lymphocyte formation. Advances in Immunology 41:181–267, 1987.

MacLennan, I. C. M. The evolution of B-cell clones. Current Topics in Microbiology and Immunology 159:37–63, 1990.

McCune, J. M., R. Namikawa, H. Kaneshima, L.D. Shultz, M. Lieberman, and I.L. Weissman. The SCID-hu mouse: murine model for the analysis of human hematolymphoid differentiation and function. Science 241:1632–1639, 1988.

Stoolman, L. M. Adhesion molecules controlling lymphocyte migration. Cell 56:907–910, 1989.

Szakal, A. K., M. H. Kosco, and J. G. Tew. Microanatomy of lymphoid tissue during humoral immune responses: structure function relationships. Annual Review of Immunology 7:91–109, 1989.

LYMPHOCYTE

SPECIFICITY

AND

ACTIVATION

The initial phases of specific immune responses are the specific recognition of antigen by lymphocytes and the responses of lymphocytes to antigenic stimulation. This section is devoted to a discussion of the cellular and molecular basis of antigen recognition and lymphocyte activation.

We will begin with antibodies, which are the antigen receptors and effector molecules of B lymphocytes, because the structure and production of antibodies are understood in great detail. Chapter 3 describes the molecular structure of antibodies and how these proteins recognize antigens and perform their effector functions. Chapter 4 deals with antibody genes, particularly the genetic basis of antibody production, the generation of antibody diversity, and the development of the B cell repertoire. Before continuing with a discussion of antibody production, the next four chapters will consider antigen recognition by T cells, which play a central role in all immune responses to protein antigens, including antibody responses. Because helper and cytolytic T lymphocytes (CTLs) are uniquely specific for peptide antigens bound to major histocompatibility complex (MHC) encoded cell surface molecules, in Chapter 5 we will describe the discovery, genetics, and biochemistry of the MHC. Chapter 6 discusses the association of foreign antigens with MHC molecules and the biochemistry and physiologic significance of T cell antigen recognition. Chapter 7 deals with the structure of the T cell antigen receptor, the role of other T cell surface proteins in responses to antigens, and the mechanisms of T lymphocyte activation. The expression of T cell receptor genes and the development of mature T lymphocytes are described in Chapter 8. We will return to humoral immunity in Chapter 9 and discuss the responses of B lymphocytes to antigens and to stimuli provided by helper T cells. Finally, Chapter 10 describes how these immune responses are regulated and the phenomenon of immunologic tolerance or unresponsiveness.

CHAPTER THREE

ANTIBODIES AND

ANTIGENS

One of the earliest experimental demonstrations of acquired immunity was the induction of humoral immunity to microbial toxins. The protective effects of humoral immunity are now known to be mediated by a family of structurally related glycoproteins called **antibodies** (commonly written as Ab). *Antibodies always initiate their biologic effects by binding to antigens.* Antibodies are not enzymes and, except in unusual circumstances, do not modify the covalent structure of antigens. Antibody binding to antigen, although entirely non-covalent, is nevertheless exquisitely specific for one antigen versus another and often very strong. Antibodies, along with MHC molecules (see Chapter 5) and T cell antigen receptors (see Chapter 7), comprise the three classes of molecules used by the immune system to specifically recognize antigens. Of these three, antibodies are distinguished by the widest range of antigenic structures they can recognize, by the greatest ability to distinguish between different antigens, and by the greatest strength of binding to antigen. Antibodies are also the best studied of these antigen-binding molecules. Therefore, we will begin our discussion of how the immune system specifically recognizes antigens by describing in molecular terms how antibodies perform this function.

Antibodies are produced in a membrane-bound form by B lymphocytes, and these membrane molecules function as B cell receptors for antigens. *The interaction of antigen with membrane antibodies on B cells constitutes the cognitive phase of humoral immunity.* Antibodies are also produced in a secreted form by the progeny of B cells that differentiate in response to antigenic stimulation. *These secreted antibodies bind to antigens and trigger several of the effector functions of the immune system.* The specificity of the effector phase is due to the antigen-antibody interaction, but the effector functions themselves are usually not specific for the eliciting antigen. In fact, these functions are often mediated by portions of the antibody molecule that are spatially distinct from the site of antigen binding. In this chapter, we will also describe the structural features of antibody molecules that underlie their effector functions. Finally, we will describe how antibodies can be used as laboratory reagents to analyze biologic systems, including the immune system itself.

MOLECULAR STRUCTURE OF ANTIBODIES

Structural analyses of antibody molecules involving the efforts of many laboratories have been in progress for more than 50 years. Early studies were performed with naturally occurring mixtures of antibodies present in the blood of immunized individuals. Blood contains many different antibodies, each derived from a particular clone of B cells and each having a distinct structure and specificity for antigen. Nevertheless, antibodies are sufficiently similar to each other that Michael Heidelberger and colleagues were able to purify mixtures of antibodies from blood, laying the groundwork for subsequent structural studies. Working with these mixtures, immunologists were able to deduce the overall structure of antibody molecules. However, the molecular heterogeneity of these polyclonal antibodies interfered with more detailed analysis of antibody structure, such as amino acid sequence determination. The key methodological breakthrough in this endeavor was the discovery that patients or animals with multiple myeloma, a monoclonal tumor of antibody-secreting plasma cells, often have high levels of biochemically identical antibodies or portions of antibodies in their blood or urine, providing a source of individual antibody molecules of a single (albeit usually unknown) specificity. In 1975, Georges Kohler and Cesar Milstein described a method for immortalizing individual antibody-secreting cells from an immunized animal, permitting the selection of individual **monoclonal antibodies** of predetermined specificity (Box 3–1). The availability of homogeneous populations of antibodies and antibody-producing cells permitted complete amino acid sequence determination of several individual antibody molecules and, eventually, molecular cloning and genetic analysis of antibodies. These studies have culminated in the x-ray crystallographic determinations of the three-dimensional structure of several antibody molecules and, in a few cases, of antibody with bound antigen. As a result, we now know more about the structure of antibody molecules than about any other element of the immune system. This portion of the chapter describes the purification of antibody molecules and their general structural features.

Natural Distribution and Purification of Antibody Molecules

Although antibodies were first isolated from the fluid portion of the blood, they are found in several distinct anatomic locations:

1. Antibodies are present within cytoplasmic membrane-bound compartments (endoplasmic reticulum and Golgi apparatus) and on the surface of B lymphocytes, which synthesize antibody molecules.

2. Antibodies are present in the plasma (fluid portion) of the blood and, to a lesser extent, in the interstitial fluid of the tissues where secreted antibody from B cells accumulates.

3. Antibodies are present on the surface of certain immune effector cells, such as mononuclear phagocytes, natural killer (NK) cells, and mast cells, which do not synthesize antibody but have specific receptors for binding antibody molecules.

4. Antibodies are present in secretory fluids such as mucus and milk, into which certain types of antibody molecules are specifically transported.

When blood or plasma forms a clot, antibodies remain in the residual fluid, called **serum.** A sample of

BOX 3–1. HYBRIDOMAS AND MONOCLONAL ANTIBODIES

The technique of producing virtually unlimited quantities of a single antibody specific for a particular antigenic determinant has revolutionized immunology and has had a far-reaching impact on research in diverse fields as well as in clinical medicine. This technique is based on the fact that each B lymphocyte produces antibody of a single specificity. Therefore, each monoclonal tumor derived from a B lymphocyte, called a **myeloma,** produces only one antibody. Such tumors occur spontaneously in man and can be induced experimentally by various treatments. Myeloma-derived homogeneous antibodies have proved invaluable for elucidating the structure of Ig proteins, and Ig genes were first isolated from myelomas. However, most myelomas secrete antibodies of unknown antigenic specificities, because the transformation process that gives rise to these tumors affects B lymphocytes randomly and it is not possible to predict the specificity of any randomly transformed clone of B cells. Many attempts have been made to produce homogeneous or monoclonal antibodies of known specificity. Since normal B lymphocytes cannot grow indefinitely, such attempts have focused on immortalizing B cells that produce a specific antibody. The first and now generally used technique for doing this was described by Georges Kohler and Cesar Milstein in 1975. The method involves cell fusion or **somatic cell hybridization** between a normal antibody-producing B cell and a myeloma line, and selection of fused cells that secrete antibody of the desired specificity derived from the normal B cell. Such fusion-derived immortalized antibody-producing cell lines are called **hybridomas,** and the antibodies they produce are **monoclonal antibodies.**

The success of this technique depended on the development of cultured myeloma lines that would grow in normal culture medium but would not grow in a defined "selection" medium because they lacked a functional gene(s) required for DNA synthesis in this selection medium. Fusing normal cells to these defective myeloma fusion partners would provide the necessary gene(s) from the normal cells, so that only the somatic cell hybrids would continue to grow in the selection medium. Moreover, genes from the myeloma cell make such hybrids immortal. Cell lines that can be used as fusion partners are created by inducing defects in nucleotide synthesis pathways (Fig. A). Normal animal cells synthesize purine nucleotides and thymidylate *de novo* from

phosphoribosyl pyrophosphate and uridylate, respectively, in several steps, one of which involves the transfer of a methyl or formyl group from activated tetrahydrofolate. Anti-folate drugs, such as aminopterin, block the reactivation of tetrahydrofolate, thereby inhibiting the synthesis of purine and thymidylate. Since these are necessary components of DNA, aminopterin blocks DNA synthesis via the *de novo* pathway. Aminopterin-treated cells can use a salvage pathway in which purine is synthesized from exogenously supplied hypoxanthine using the enzyme hypoxanthine-guanine phosphoribosyl transferase (HGPRT) and thymidylate from thymidine using the enzyme thymidine kinase (TK). Therefore, cells grow normally in the presence of aminopterin if the culture medium is also supplemented with hypoxanthine and thymidine (called HAT medium). Cell lines, however, can be made defective in HGPRT if they are mutagenized and selected in thioguanine or azaguinine, which are analogs of normal metabolites that function as substrates for HGPRT but give rise to nonfunctional purines. Similarly, cells can be made defective in TK by mutagenesis and selection in bromodeoxyuridine, which is metabolized by TK to form a light-sensitive, lethal product. Such HGPRT- or TK-negative cells cannot use the salvage pathway and will, therefore, die in HAT medium. If normal cells are fused to HGPRT-negative or TK-negative cells, the normal cells provide the necessary enzyme(s), so that the hybrids synthesize DNA and grow in HAT medium.

This principle was applied to the generation of antibody-producing hybridomas by first developing HGPRT-negative and/or TK-negative myeloma lines. Myeloma lines are the best fusion partners for B cells, since like cells tend to fuse and give rise to stable hybrids more efficiently than unlike cells. Kohler and Milstein fused an HGPRT-defective mouse myeloma line to normal B cells from mice immunized with a known antigen using Sendai virus, which expresses an envelope protein ("fusion protein") that fuses cells together. Hybrids were selected for growth in HAT medium; under these conditions, unfused myeloma cells die because they cannot use the salvage pathway and the B cells cannot survive for more than 1 to 2 weeks because they are not immortalized, so that only hybrids will grow (Fig. B). More recent advances in this basic technique include the use of myeloma lines that do not produce their own Ig and the use of polyethylene glycol in-

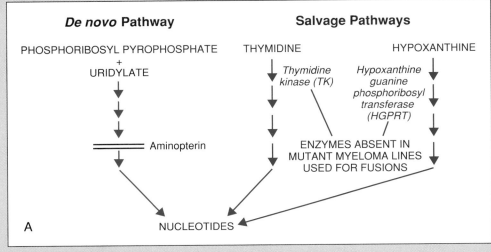

A. *Pathways of purine synthesis.*

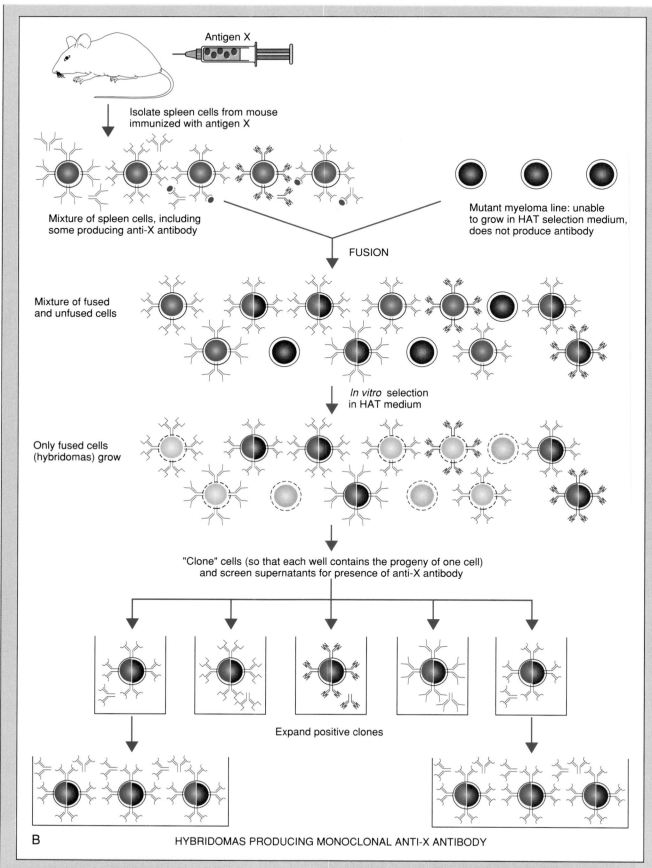

Antigen X

Isolate spleen cells from mouse immunized with antigen X

Mixture of spleen cells, including some producing anti-X antibody

Mutant myeloma line: unable to grow in HAT selection medium, does not produce antibody

FUSION

Mixture of fused and unfused cells

In vitro selection in HAT medium

Only fused cells (hybridomas) grow

"Clone" cells (so that each well contains the progeny of one cell) and screen supernatants for presence of anti-X antibody

Expand positive clones

B   HYBRIDOMAS PRODUCING MONOCLONAL ANTI-X ANTIBODY

B. *Production of hybridomas.*

Continued

stead of Sendai virus as the fusing agent because of technical ease. The fused cells are cultured at a concentration at which each culture well is expected to contain only one hybridoma cell. The culture supernatant from each well in which growing cells are detected is then tested for the presence of antibody reactive with the antigen used for immunization. The screening method depends on the antigen being used. For soluble antigens, the usual technique is RIA or ELISA, and for cell surface antigens a variety of assays for antibody binding to viable cells can be used. Once positive wells are identified, i.e., wells containing hybridomas producing the desired antibody, the cells are cloned in semisolid agar or by limiting dilution and clones producing the antibody are isolated by another round of screening. These cloned hybridomas produce monoclonal antibodies of a desired specificity. Hybridomas can be grown in large volumes or as ascitic tumors in syngeneic mice in order to produce large quantities of monoclonal antibodies.

Two features of this somatic cell hybridization make it extremely valuable. First, it is the best method for producing a monoclonal antibody against a known antigenic determinant. Second, it can be used to identify unknown antigens present in a mixture because each hybridoma is specific for only one antigenic determinant. For instance, if several hybridomas are produced that secrete antibodies that bind to the surface of a particular cell, each hybridoma clone will secrete an antibody specific for only one surface antigenic determinant. These monoclonal antibodies can then be used to purify different cell surface molecules, some of which may be known molecules and others which may not have been identified previously. Some of the commonest applications of hybridomas and monoclonal antibodies include the following:

1. *Identification of phenotypic markers unique to particular cell types.* The basis for the modern classification of lymphocytes and mononuclear phagocytes is the binding of population-specific monoclonal antibodies. These have been used to define "clusters of differentiation" for various cell types (see Chapter 2).

2. *Immunodiagnosis.* The diagnosis of many infectious and systemic diseases relies upon the detection of specific antigens and/or antibodies in the circulation or in tissues, using monoclonal antibodies in immunoassays.

3. *Tumor diagnosis and therapy.* Tumor-specific monoclonal antibodies are used for detection of tumors by imaging techniques and for immunotherapy of tumors *in vivo*.

4. *Functional analysis of cell surface and secreted molecules.* In immunologic research, monoclonal antibodies that bind to cell surface molecules and either stimulate or inhibit particular cellular functions are invaluable tools for defining the functions of surface molecules, including receptors for antigens. Antibodies that neutralize cytokines are routinely used for detecting the presence and functional roles of these protein hormones *in vitro* and *in vivo*.

At present, hybridomas are most often produced by fusing HAT-sensitive mouse myelomas with B cells from immunized mice, rats, or hamsters. Attempts are being made to generate human monoclonal antibodies, primarily for administration to patients, by developing human myeloma lines as fusion partners. (It is a general rule that the stability of hybrids is low if cells from species that are far apart in evolution are fused, and this is presumably why human B cells do not form hybridomas with mouse myeloma lines at high efficiency.) The same principle is used to generate mouse T cell hybridomas, by fusing T cells with a HAT-sensitive, T cell-derived tumor line; uses of such monoclonal T cell populations are described in Chapter 7.

serum that contains a large number of antibody molecules that bind to a particular antigen is commonly called an **antiserum**. (The study of antibodies and their reactions with antigens is therefore classically called **serology**.) The number of antibody molecules in a serum specific for a particular antigen is often measured by serially diluting the serum until binding can no longer be observed; sera with a large number of antibody molecules specific for a particular antigen are said to be "strong" or have a "high titer."

Plasma or serum glycoproteins are traditionally separated by solubility characteristics into albumins and globulins and may be further separated by migration in an electric field, a process called **electrophoresis** (Fig. 3-1). Elvin Kabat and colleagues demonstrated that most antibodies are found in the third fastest migrating group of globulins, named **gamma globulins** for the third letter of the Greek alphabet. Another common name for antibody is **immunoglobulin** (Ig), referring to the immunity-conferring portion of the gamma globulin fraction. The terms immunoglobulin and antibody are synonymous and will be used interchangeably throughout this book.

Currently, antibody molecules are generally purified from plasma or other natural fluids by a two-step procedure. The first step is to precipitate antibodies from the biologic fluid by adding a concentration of ammonium sulfate that ranges from 40 to 50 per cent of saturation. Under these conditions, albumin and most small molecules remain in solution so that par-

tially purified antibody can be collected in a pellet by centrifugation. The antibody-containing pellet is redissolved in buffer and then purified by **chromatography**. Homogeneous antibodies can be isolated from other proteins in the pellet by size *(gel filtration chromatography)*, charge *(ion exchange chromatography)*, or specific binding to an antibody-binding molecule such as staphylococcal protein A. When the antibody of interest in the biologic fluid is specific for a known antigen, the antigen can be immobilized on a column matrix and used to bind the antibody, a method called *affinity chromatography*. In all cases, antibody can be removed from the column matrix by a suitable change in buffer conditions. In the case of affinity chromatography, release often involves temporary and reversible denaturation with a salt solution such as magnesium chloride or a change in pH. Many such chromatographic procedures are routinely run under high pressure using special column matrices to achieve rapid and highly resolved separations. This technique is called *high-pressure liquid chromatography* (HPLC).

Overview of Antibody Structure

A number of the structural and functional features of antibodies were determined from the early studies of these molecules:

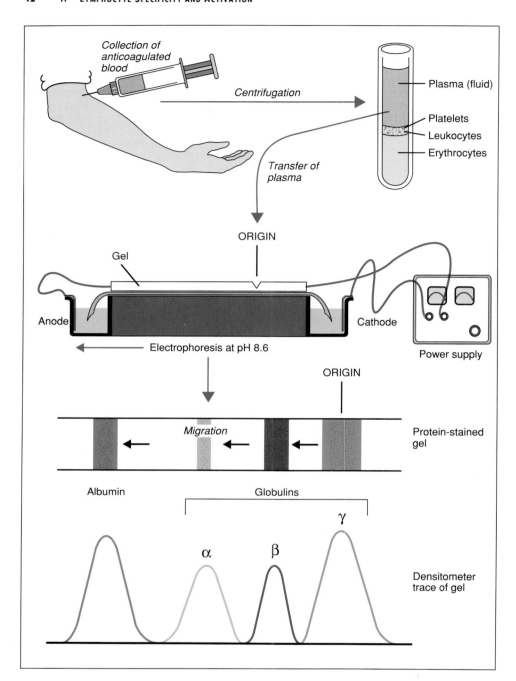

FIGURE 3 – 1. Separation of plasma proteins by electrophoresis. *Electrophoresis separates plasma proteins into albumin and globulins. Most antibodies are found in the γ globulin fraction.*

1. *All antibody molecules are similar in overall structure, accounting for certain common physiochemical features, such as charge and solubility.* These common properties may be exploited as a basis for the purification of antibody molecules from fluids such as blood. *All antibodies have a common core structure of two identical light chains (about 24 kilodaltons [kD]) and two identical heavy chains (about 55 or 70 kD)* (Fig. 3 – 2). One light chain is attached to each heavy chain, and the two heavy chains are attached to each other. Both the light chains and the heavy chains contain a

series of repeating, homologous units, each about 110 amino acid residues in length, which fold independently in a common globular motif, called an **immunoglobulin domain.** All Ig domains contain two layers of β-pleated sheet with three or four strands of antiparallel polypeptide chain. As will be discussed in Chapter 7, many other proteins of importance in the immune system contain regions that use the same folding motif and show structural relatedness to Ig amino acid sequences. All molecules that contain this motif are said to belong to the **Ig gene superfamily,**

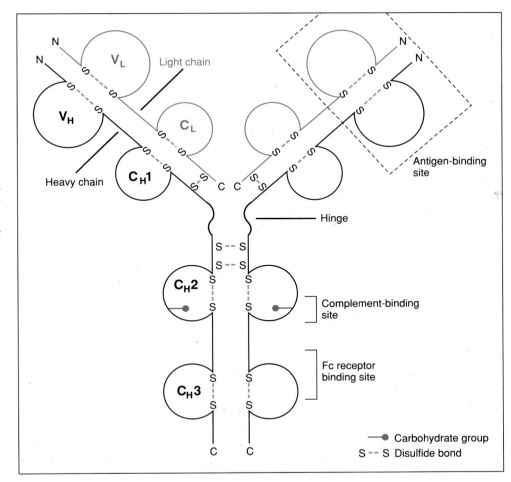

FIGURE 3–2. Schematic diagram of an immunoglobulin molecule. *In this drawing of an IgG molecule, the antigen-binding sites are formed by the juxtaposition of V_L and V_H domains. The locations of complement and Fc receptor–binding sites within the heavy chain constant regions are approximations. S--S refers to intrachain and interchain disulfide bonds; N and C refer to amino and carboxy termini of the polypeptide chains, respectively.*

and all of the gene segments encoding the Ig-like domains are believed to have evolved from the same common ancestral gene (see Chapter 7, Box 7–3).

2. Despite their overall similarity, *antibody molecules can be readily divided into a small number of distinct classes and subclasses, based on minor differences in physicochemical characteristics such as size, charge, and solubility and on their behavior as antigens* (Box 3–2). In man, the classes of antibody molecules are called IgA, IgD, IgE, IgG, and IgM, and members of each class are said to have the same **isotype** (Table 3–1). IgA and IgG isotypes can be further subdivided into closely related subclasses, or subtypes, called IgA1 and IgA2, and IgG1, IgG2, IgG3, and IgG4, respectively. In certain instances, it will be convenient to refer to studies of mouse antibody. Mice have the same general isotypes as man, but the IgG isotype is divided into the IgG1, IgG2a, IgG2b, and IgG3 subclasses. The heavy chains of all antibody molecules of an isotype or subtype share extensive regions of amino acid sequence identity but differ from antibodies belonging to other isotypes or subtypes. Heavy chains are designated by the letter of the Greek alphabet corresponding to the overall isotype of the antibody: IgA1 contains α1 heavy chains; IgA2, α2; IgD, δ; IgE, ε; IgG1, γ1; IgG2, γ2; IgG3, γ3; IgG4, γ4; and IgM, μ.

The shared regions of heavy chain amino acid sequences are responsible for both the common physicochemical properties and the common antigenic properties of antibodies of the same isotype. In addition, the shared regions of the heavy chains provide members of each isotype with common abilities to bind to certain cell surface receptors or to other macromolecules like complement and thereby activate particular immune effector functions. Thus, the separation of antibody molecules into isotypes and subtypes on the basis of common structural features also separates antibodies according to which set of effector functions they commonly activate. In other words, *isotypes and subtypes determine the effector functions of humoral immunity.* As we shall see later, there are two isotypes of antibody light chains, called κ and λ. The light chains, however, do not mediate or influence the effector functions of antibodies.

3. *There are more than 1×10^7, and perhaps as many as 10^9, different antibody molecules in every individual, each with unique amino acid sequences in their antigen-combining sites.* This extraordinary diversity of structure (whose generation is explained in Chapter 4) accounts for the extraordinary specificity of antibodies for antigens because each amino acid difference may produce a difference in antigen binding. In

BOX 3-2.   ANTI-IMMUNOGLOBULIN ANTIBODIES

Antibody molecules are proteins and therefore can be antigenic. Immunologists have exploited this fact to produce antibodies specific for Ig molecules that can be used as reagents to analyze the structure and function of other Ig molecules. In order to obtain an anti-antibody response, it is necessary that the Ig molecules used to immunize an animal be recognized in whole or in part as foreign. The simplest approach is to immunize one species, e.g., rabbit, with Ig molecules of a second species, e.g., mouse. Populations of antibodies may be generated by such cross-species immunizations and are largely specific for epitopes present in the constant regions of light or heavy chains. Such sera can be used to define the **isotype** of an antibody.

When an animal is immunized with Ig molecules derived from another animal of the same species, the immune response is confined to epitopes of the immunizing Ig which are absent or uncommon on the Ig molecules of the responder animal. Two types of determinants have been defined by this approach. First, determinants may be formed by minor structural differences (polymorphisms) in amino acid sequences located in the conserved portions of Ig molecules. Ig genes that encode such polymorphic structures are inherited as Mendelian alleles. (The concepts of **polymorphism** and **allelic genes** are discussed more fully in Chapter 5.) Determinants on Ig molecules that differ among animals which have inherited different alleles are called **allotopes.** All antibody molecules that share a particular allotope are said to belong to the same **allotype.** Most allotopes are located in the constant regions of light or heavy chains, but some are found in the framework portions of variable regions. Allotypic differences have no functional significance, but they have been important in the study of Ig genetics. For example, allotypes detected by anti-Ig antibodies were initially used to locate the position of Ig genes by linkage analysis. In addition, the remarkable observation that, in homozygous animals, all of the heavy chains of a particular isotype (e.g., IgM) share the same allotype even though the V regions of these antibodies have different amino acid sequences, provided the first evidence that the constant portions of all Ig molecules of a particular isotype are encoded by a single

gene separate from the genes encoding V regions. As will be discussed in Chapter 4, we now know that this surprising conclusion is correct.

The second type of determinant on antibody molecules that can be recognized as foreign by other animals of the same species is that formed largely or entirely by the hypervariable regions of an Ig variable domain. When a homogeneous population of antibody molecules, e.g., a myeloma protein or a monoclonal antibody, is used as an immunogen, antibodies are produced that react with the hypervariable loops. These determinants are recognized as "foreign" because they are usually present in very small quantities in any given animal, i.e., at too low a level to induce self-tolerance (see Chapter 10). Such determinants are **idiotopes,** and all antibody molecules that share an idiotope are said to belong to the same **idiotype.** As will be discussed in Chapter 4, hypervariable sequences arise both from inherited germline diversity and from somatic events. Individual idiotopes that arise from somatic events are rare and may define the products of one or a few clones of antibody-producing B cells. Idiotopes that arise from the germline are less rare and, in some cases, may be present on the majority of antibody molecules that recognize a particular antigen (**dominant idiotypes**). Unlike allotopes, idiotopes may be functionally significant because they may be involved in regulation of B cell functions. The theory of lymphocyte regulation through antibody-binding idiotopes expressed on membrane Ig molecules, called the **network hypothesis,** is discussed further in Chapter 10.

In addition to experimentally elicited anti-Ig antibodies, immunologists have also been interested in naturally occurring antibodies reactive with self Ig molecules. Small quantities of anti-idiotypic antibodies may be found in normal individuals. Anti-Ig antibodies are particularly prevalent in an autoimmune disease called rheumatoid arthritis (see Chapter 18), in which setting they are known as **rheumatoid factor.** Rheumatoid factor is usually an IgM antibody that reacts with the constant regions of self IgG. The significance of rheumatoid factor in the pathogenesis of rheumatoid arthritis is unknown.

TABLE 3-1. Human Antibody Isotypes*

Antibody	Subtypes	H Chain (Designation)	H Chain Domains (Number)	Hinge	Tail Piece	Serum Concentration (mg/ml)	Secretory Form	Molecular Weight of Secretory Form (kD)
IgA	IgA1	$\alpha 1$	4	Yes	Yes	3	Monomer, dimer, trimer	150, 300, or 400
	IgA2	$\alpha 2$	4	Yes	Yes	0.5	Monomer, dimer, trimer	150, 300, or 400
IgD	None	δ	4	Yes	Yes	Trace	—	180
IgE	None	ϵ	5	No	No	Trace	Monomer	190
IgG	IgG1	$\gamma 1$	4	Yes	No	9	Monomer	150
	IgG2	$\gamma 2$	4	Yes	No	3	Monomer	150
	IgG3	$\gamma 3$	4	Yes	No	1	Monomer	150
	IgG4	$\gamma 4$	4	Yes	No	0.5	Monomer	150
IgM	None	μ	5	No	Yes	1.5	Pentamer	950

* Multimeric forms of IgA and IgM are associated with J chain via the tail piece region of the heavy chain. IgA in mucus is also associated with secretory piece.

theory, such extensive sequence diversity poses a structural problem because the three-dimensional structure of any protein is completely determined by its amino acid sequence and certain sequences are incapable of folding into soluble, stable proteins. In an antibody molecule, this problem is solved by confining the sequence diversity to three short stretches within the amino terminal domains of the heavy and light chains. The amino acid sequences of the amino terminal domains are called **variable (V) regions,** to distinguish them from the more conserved **constant (C) regions** of the remainder of each chain. The highly divergent stretches within the V regions are called **hypervariable regions** and they are held in place by more conserved **framework regions.** In an intact immunoglobulin, the three hypervariable regions of each light chain and the three hypervariable regions of each heavy chain can be brought together in three-dimensional space to form an antigen-binding surface. Because these sequences are thought to form a surface complementary to the three-dimensional surface of a bound antigen, the hypervariable regions are also called **complementarity-determining regions** (CDRs).

With this overview of antibody structure and function in mind, we will now consider antibody structure in greater detail.

Detailed View of Antibody Structure

LIGHT CHAIN STRUCTURE

All antibody light chains fall into one of two classes or isotypes, κ and λ. Each member of a light-chain isotype shares complete amino acid sequence identity of the carboxy terminal C region with all other members of that isotype. In man, antibodies with κ and λ light chains are present in about equal number. In mice, κ-containing antibodies are about ten times more frequent than λ-containing antibodies. There are no known differences in function between κ-containing and λ-containing antibodies.

Each light chain, whether κ or λ, is folded into separate V and C domains corresponding to the amino terminal and carboxy terminal halves of the polypeptide, respectively (Fig. 3–3). Each domain is about 110 amino acids long. As noted above, most of the amino acid sequence variation among different light chains is confined to three separate locations in the V region. These three hypervariable segments, or CDRs, are each about ten amino acids long (Fig. 3–4). Proceeding from the amino terminus, these regions are the CDR1, CDR2, and CDR3, respectively. CDR3 is the most variable of the CDRs and, as will be discussed in Chapter 4, there are more genetic mechanisms for generating sequence diversity in this region than in CDR1 or CDR2. V region folding into an Ig domain is determined by the sequence of the framework regions adjacent to the CDRs. Within the framework regions, certain amino acid residues and certain structural features are very highly conserved. For example, all V region sequences contain an internal disulfide loop of about 90 amino acid residues. Other portions of the framework regions differ between κ and λ chains. When V_κ or V_λ regions fold into an Ig domain, the CDRs are present on the surface as projecting loops (Fig. 3–3). Recent studies suggest that each CDR folds similarly, regardless of the precise amino acid sequence. Sequence differences contribute to variation in the chemical surface of the loops.

The carboxy terminus of the C region of the light chain also folds into an Ig domain. Although C_κ and C_λ differ in exact amino acid sequence, they are structur-

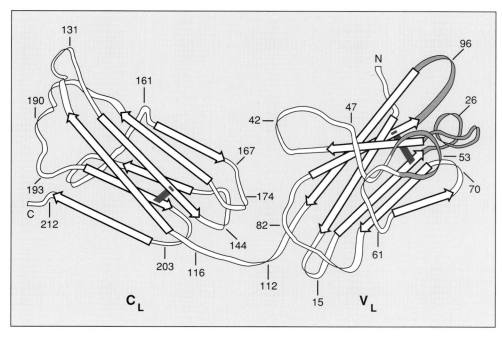

FIGURE 3–3. Polypeptide folding into Ig domains in a human antibody light chain. *The V and C regions each independently fold into Ig domains. The white arrows represent polypeptide arranged in β pleated sheets, the dark blue bars are intrachain disulfide bonds, and the numbers indicate the positions of amino acid residues counting from the amino (N) terminus. The CDR1, CDR2, and CDR3 loops of the V region, colored in light blue, are brought together to form the antigen-binding surface of the light chain. (Adapted with permission from Edmundson, A. B., K. R. Ely, E. E. Abola, M. Schiffer, and N. Panagiotopoulos. Rotational allostery and divergent evolution of domains in immunoglobulin light chains. Biochemistry 14: 3953–3961, 1975. Copyright 1975, American Chemical Society.)*

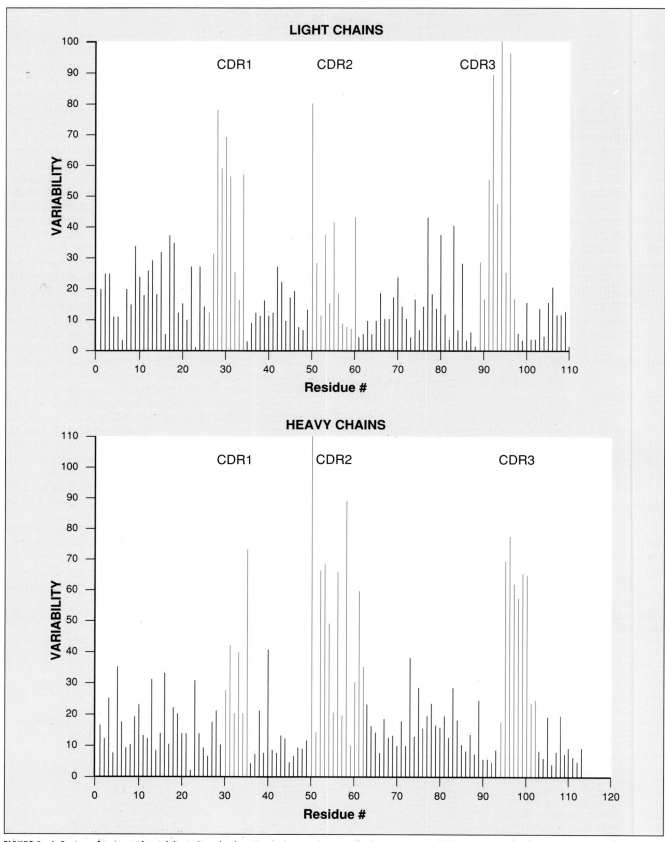

FIGURE 3 – 4. Regions of amino acid variability in Ig molecules. *The histograms depict the extent of variability, defined as the number of differences in each amino acid residue among various independently sequenced Ig heavy and light chains, plotted against amino acid residue number, measured from the amino terminus. This method of analysis, developed by Elvin Kabat and Tai Te Wu, indicates that the most variable residues are clustered in three "hypervariable" regions, colored in blue, corresponding to the three CDRs shown in Figure 3 – 3. (Courtesy of Dr. E. A. Kabat, Department of Microbiology, Columbia University College of Physicians and Surgeons, New York.)*

ally related, or homologous, to each other and, to a lesser extent, to V_κ and V_λ.

HEAVY CHAIN STRUCTURE

All heavy chain polypeptides, regardless of antibody isotype, contain a tandem series of approximately 110 amino acid residue sequences. These sequences are homologous to each other, and all undergo characteristic folding into 12 kD Ig domains. As in light chains, the amino terminal variable, or V_H, domain displays the greatest sequence variation among heavy chains and the most variable residues are concentrated into three short (up to ten amino acid residue) stretches called CDR1, CDR2, and CDR3 (Fig. 3–4). Also similar to light chains, the heavy chain CDR3 shows greater sequence variability than CDR1 or CDR2.

The remainder of the heavy chain, which forms the constant (C) region, differs among isotypes; however, it is invariant among the member antibodies within a particular isotype. In IgM and IgE antibodies, the constant region is of sufficient length to form four separate Ig domains. In IgG, IgA, and IgD antibodies, the shorter constant regions form three Ig domains. (In the mouse, the δ chain gene has undergone a deletion such that the protein product forms only two Ig domains.)

In γ, α, and δ heavy chains, there is a nonglobular region of amino acid sequence, containing from about ten (in α1, α2, γ1, γ2, and γ4) to over 60 (in γ3 or δ) residues, located between the first and second constant region domains (called C_H1 and C_H2, respectively). Although portions of this sequence form rod-like helical structures, other portions assume a random and flexible conformation, permitting molecular motion between C_H1 and C_H2. For this reason, this portion of the heavy chain is called the **hinge.** Some of the greatest differences between the constant regions of the IgG subclasses are concentrated in the hinge region. For steric reasons, antibody subtypes with flexible hinges may be better able to use more than one antigen-binding site to attach to a particular antigen; as discussed later in this chapter, binding involving more than one attachment point will increase the strength of attachment.

All heavy chains may be expressed in one of two molecular forms that differ in amino acid sequence on the carboxy terminal side of the last C_H domain. The secretory form, found in blood plasma, terminates with a sequence containing charged and hydrophilic amino acids. The membrane form, found only on the plasma membrane of the B lymphocyte that synthesized the antibody, has distinct carboxy terminal sequences that include approximately 26 uncharged, hydrophobic side chains followed by variable numbers of charged (usually basic) amino acids that form the cytoplasmic segments (Fig. 3–5). This structural motif is characteristic of transmembrane proteins. The hydrophobic residues are believed to form an α-helix, which extends across the hydrophobic portion of the membrane lipid bilayer; the basic side

chains of the cytoplasmic amino acids interact with the phospholipid head groups on the cytoplasmic surface of the membrane. In membrane IgM or IgD, the extreme carboxy terminus or cytoplasmic portion of the heavy chain is very short, only three amino acid residues; in membrane IgG or IgE, it is somewhat longer, up to about 30 amino acid residues in length.

The secretory forms of μ, α, and δ heavy chains, but not γ or ϵ, have additional extended nonglobular sequences on the carboxy-terminal side of the last C_H domain. These extensions are called **tail pieces.** In secreted IgM and IgA molecules, the tail pieces permit intermolecular interactions, resulting in multimeric Ig molecules. Specifically, IgM forms a pentamer, containing ten heavy chains and ten light chains, and IgA can form dimers containing four heavy chains and four light chains, or trimers, containing six heavy chains and six light chains (Fig. 3–6). Little is known about the usual form of circulating IgD because it is normally present in only trace amounts. Multimeric IgM and IgA also contain an additional 15 kD polypeptide, called the **joining (J) chain,** which is disulfide-bonded to the tail pieces, stabilizing the multimer. All membrane Ig molecules, regardless of isotype, are believed to be monomeric, containing two heavy and two light chains.

All heavy chains are characteristically N-glycosylated; that is, the polypeptide contains N-linked oligosaccharide groups attached to asparagine side chains. The location of oligosaccharides may vary in different Ig isotypes. The precise composition of the oligosaccharides is not fully determined by the polypeptide sequence and may also vary with the physiologic state of the host at the time of antibody synthesis.

ASSOCIATION OF LIGHT AND HEAVY CHAINS

The basic pattern of chain association in all antibody molecules is that each light chain is attached to a heavy chain and each heavy chain pairs with another heavy chain. The interactions between light and heavy chains involve both covalent and non-covalent interactions (see Fig. 3–2). Covalent interactions are in the form of disulfide bonds between the carboxy terminus of the light chain and the carboxy terminal region of the V_H domain or of the C_H1 domain of the heavy chain. The exact position of the heavy chain cysteine that participates in disulfide bond formation varies with the isotype. Non-covalent interactions arise primarily from hydrophobic interactions between the C_L domain and the C_H1 domain. This association of C_L and C_H1 brings the V_L and V_H domains into spatial apposition such that the juxtaposed V domains can each contribute to the binding of antigen (see Plate I, opposite page 52).

The pairing of heavy chains is best understood from studies of IgG molecules. As in the case of light and heavy chain association, both covalent and non-covalent interactions are involved. Heavy chains form interchain disulfide bonds in the region near the carboxy terminus of the hinge. Strong hydrophobic in-

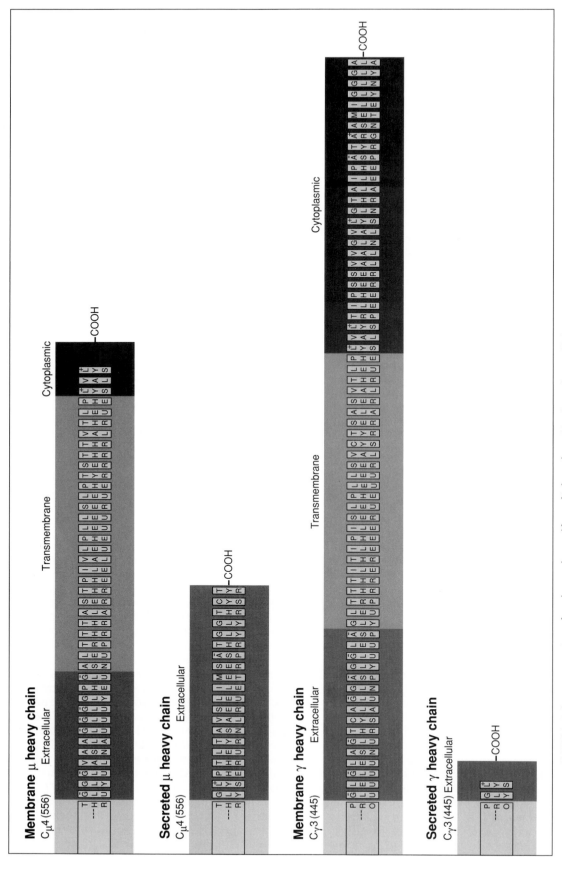

FIGURE 3–5. *Sequence comparisons of membrane and secreted forms of Ig heavy chains. Membrane forms of Ig heavy chains contain characteristic hydrophobic sequences, the transmembrane region, which span the lipid bilayer of the plasma membrane. The cytoplasmic domains of membrane heavy chains of different isotypes are significantly different: μ contains only three residues whereas γ3 contains 28. The carboxy termini of secreted forms also differ among isotypes: μ has a long tail piece involved in pentamer formation, whereas γ3 does not. Amino acids are shown in the three-letter code, and charged residues are marked + or −; the numbers in parentheses mark the amino acid residue number of the carboxy terminus of the last Ig domain (i.e., $C_\mu 4$ or $C_\gamma 3$).*

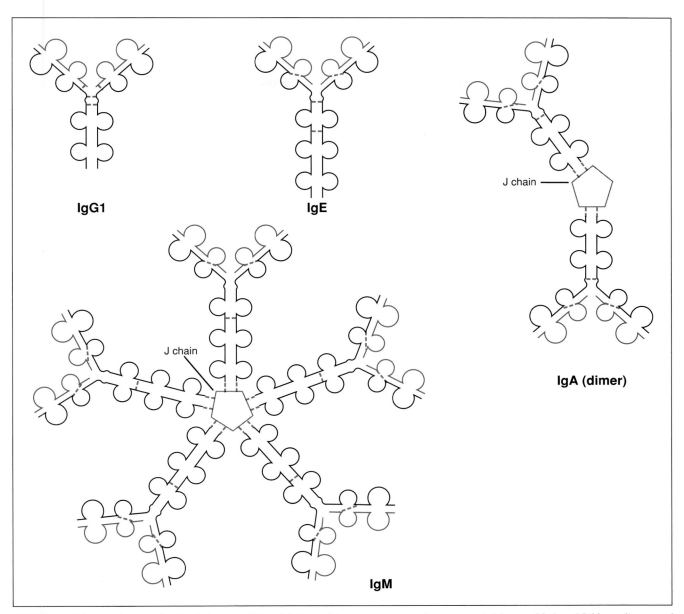

FIGURE 3–6. *Schematic diagrams of various Ig isotypes. IgG and IgE circulate as monomers, whereas secreted forms of IgA and IgM are dimers and pentamers, respectively, stabilized by the J chain. (Some IgA molecules are trimers, not shown.)*

teractions occur between the C_H3 domains. In contrast, there is little favorable interaction between C_H2 domains, and some of the N-linked oligosaccharides may actually be located in a physical gap formed between these portions of the chain. The length and flexibility of the hinge regions differ significantly among IgG subclasses because, as noted above, most of the amino acid sequence differences among the four subclasses are located in the hinge region. These sequence differences lead to very different overall shapes among the IgG subtypes, as depicted in Figure 3–7.

These structural features of chain association explain the results of the classical limited proteolysis studies of rabbit IgG conducted by Rodney Porter and

colleagues. The theory of limited proteolysis is that globular or rodlike domains of folded proteins are more resistant to the peptide-bond cleaving actions of proteolytic enzymes than are extended, flexible regions of polypeptide. In IgG molecules, the most susceptible region is therefore the hinge located between C_H1 and C_H2 of the heavy chain. The proteolytic enzyme papain preferentially cleaves rabbit IgG molecules into three separate pieces (Fig. 3–8). Two of the pieces are identical to each other and consist of an intact light chain associated with a V_H–$C\gamma1$ fragment of the heavy chain. These fragments each retain the ability to bind antigen, a function of the V_L and V_H domains, and are therefore called **Fab** (fragment, antigen-binding). The third piece contains identical

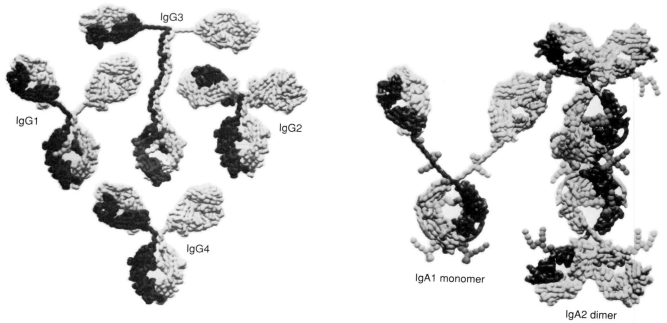

FIGURE 3–7. Three-dimensional shapes of various Ig isotypes. *These computer-generated space filling models of different Ig isotypes illustrate that the shapes of antibody molecules are quite distinct, largely due to differences in the lengths of the hinge regions. (Courtesy of Dr. R. S. H. Pumphrey, Regional Immunology Service, St. Mary's Hospital, Manchester.)*

fragments of the γ heavy chain composed of the $C\gamma2$ and $C\gamma3$ domains. This piece of IgG has a propensity to self-associate and to crystallize into a lattice. It is therefore called **Fc** (fragment, crystalline). As we shall discuss later in this chapter, many of the effector functions of immunoglobulins are mediated by the Fc portions of the molecule.

Different results are obtained when the proteolytic enzyme pepsin is used instead of papain to cleave rabbit IgG molecules (Fig. 3–8). In this case, under limiting conditions of enzyme concentration and time, proteolysis is restricted to the carboxy terminus of the hinge region near the $C\gamma2$ domain such that the antigen binding fragment of IgG retains the hinge and the interchain disulfide bonds. Fab fragments containing the heavy chain hinge are called Fab'; when the interchain disulfide bonds are intact, the two Fab' fragments remain associated in a form called **F(ab')$_2$**. The Fc fragment is often extensively degraded and does not survive proteolysis by pepsin.

These proteolysis experiments are not readily extended to other antibody isotypes such as IgM. In fact, they are often not applicable even to IgG molecules in many species other than rabbit. However, the basic organization of the Ig molecule that Porter deduced from his studies of rabbit IgG is common to all Ig molecules of all isotypes and of all species. These features may be summarized as follows:

1. Each $V_L V_H$ pairing properly positioned by C_L–C_H1 interactions forms an independent antigen-binding site. Thus, all monomeric IgG molecules have two separate antigen-binding sites and secreted pentameric IgM molecules have ten separate antigen-binding sites (see Figs. 3–2 and 3–6).

2. The structure of the hinge region (or lack of one in certain isotypes) sterically determines how many binding sites of a single antibody molecule can simultaneously interact with antigen molecules, e.g., on a cell surface.

3. The Fc portion of an antibody molecule is spatially distinct from and functions independently of the antigen-binding site formed by the Fab regions. Since Fc regions activate immune effector functions, the kinds of effector functions activated by a particular Ig molecule are largely independent of the specificity for antigen and instead depend primarily on the isotype of the antibody.

ANTIBODY BINDING OF ANTIGENS

In the preceding sections, we have developed a general description of the structure of antibody molecules. Now we will turn to a more detailed discussion of the structural basis and physicochemical characteristics of antigen binding.

Structural Aspects of Biologic Antigens

An **antigen** can be defined as any substance that may be specifically bound by an antibody molecule. This differs from the original (historical) definition of

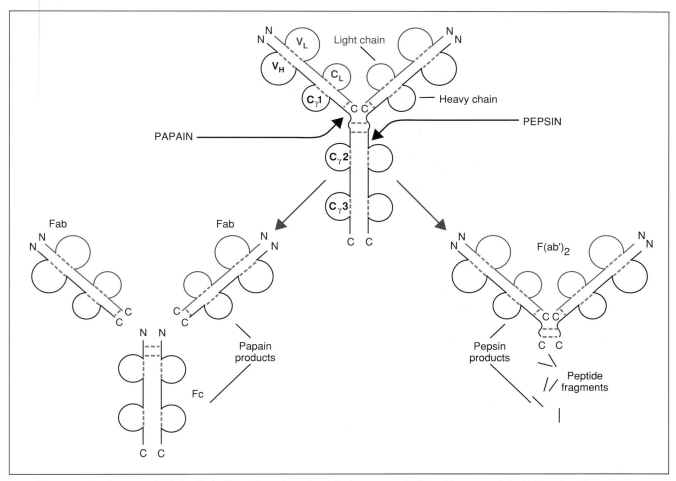

FIGURE 3 – 8. Proteolytic fragments of an IgG molecule. *Sites of papain and pepsin cleavage are indicated by arrows. Papain digestion allows separation of two antigen-binding regions (the Fab fragments) from the portion of the IgG molecule that activates complement and binds to Fc receptors (the Fc fragment). Pepsin generates a single bivalent antigen-binding fragment [F(ab')$_2$] with higher avidity for antigen than the two monovalent Fab fragments produced by papain cleavage.*

antigen as a molecule that generates an antibody. We now know that almost every kind of biologic molecule, including simple intermediary metabolites, sugars, lipids, autacoids, and hormones as well as macromolecules such as complex carbohydrates, phospholipids, nucleic acids, and proteins can serve as antigens. However, only macromolecules can initiate lymphocyte activation necessary for an antibody response. Molecules that generate immune responses are called **immunogens.** In order to generate antibodies specific for small molecules, immunologists commonly attach such small molecules to macromolecules before immunization. In this system, the small molecule is called a **hapten** and the macromolecule, usually a foreign protein, is called a **carrier.** The hapten-carrier complex, unlike free hapten, can act as an immunogen.

In general, macromolecules are much bigger than the antigen-binding region of an antibody molecule. Therefore, an antibody binds to only a specific portion of the macromolecule, called a **determinant,** or **epitope.** These two words are synonymous and are used interchangeably throughout the book. A hapten

may be thought of as an exogenous determinant that is attached to a macromolecule.

Macromolecules typically contain multiple determinants, each of which, by definition, can be bound by an antibody. In some cases, the determinants are spatially well separated and two individual antibody molecules can be bound to the same antigen molecule without influencing each other; such determinants are said to be non-overlapping. In other cases, the first antibody bound to an antigen may sterically interfere with the binding of the second and the determinants of the antigen are said to be overlapping. In rarer cases, binding of the first antibody may cause a conformational change in the structure of the antigen, influencing the binding of the second antibody by means other than steric hindrance. Such interactions are called allosteric effects.

In the case of phospholipids or of complex carbohydrates, the antigenic determinants are entirely a function of the covalent structure of the macromolecule. However, in the case of nucleic acids and even more so in the case of proteins, the non-covalent folding of the macromolecule may also contribute to the

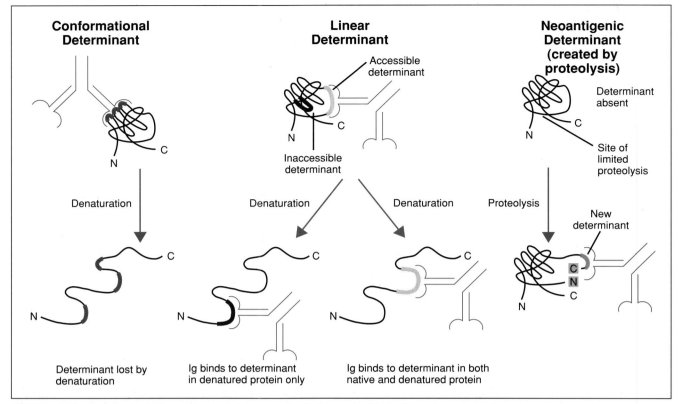

FIGURE 3 – 9. The nature of antigenic determinants. *Antigenic determinants in proteins (shown in gray) may depend upon protein folding (conformation) as well as upon covalent structure. Some linear determinants are accessible in native proteins, whereas others are exposed only upon protein unfolding. Neodeterminants arise from covalent modifications such as peptide bond cleavage.*

formation of determinants. For proteins, epitopes formed by adjacent amino acid residues in the covalent sequence are called **linear determinants** (Fig. 3–9). It is estimated that in a protein antigen the size of the linear determinant that forms contacts with specific antibody is about 6 amino acids long. Linear determinants may be accessible to antibodies in the native folded protein if they appear on the surface or in a region of extended conformation. More often, linear determinants may be inaccessible in the native conformation and appear only when the protein is denatured. In contrast, **conformational determinants** are formed by amino acid residues from separated portions of the linear amino acid sequence that are spatially juxtaposed only upon folding (Fig. 3–9). In theory, denatured proteins could transiently give rise to conformational determinants; however, such determinants are too short-lived unless they are maintained by energetically favorable interactions such as those found in native proteins. Thus, antibodies specific for certain linear determinants and antibodies specific for conformational determinants can be used to ascertain whether a protein is denatured or in its native conformation, respectively. When there is more than one stable conformation, antibodies may be specific for one or the other. The energy of antibody binding may actually alter the relative stability of the two conformations, shifting the dynamic equilibrium.

Proteins may be subjected to covalent modifica-

tions such as phosphorylation or specific proteolysis. These modifications, by altering the covalent structure, can produce new antigenic epitopes. Such epitopes, called **neoantigens,** may be recognized by specific antibodies (Fig. 3–9).

At the beginning of this chapter, we made the general assertion that antibodies are not enzymes. However, certain antigen-binding sites may coincidentally resemble the active site of enzymes and function to catalyze reactions. It should be emphasized that this is an area of intense research activity as a means of designing enzymes but is unlikely to play much of a role in normal immunity.

A final consideration about macromolecules as antigens is that proteins, nucleic acids, and complex carbohydrates may have internally repetitive structures, forming more than one identical determinant per molecule. For proteins, such structures commonly arise from polymerization of monomeric units. Molecules with repetitive structures are said to be **multivalent** and can interact with more than one binding site on an individual antibody or with more than one antibody.

Structural Basis of Antigen Binding

The limited proteolysis of antibody molecules described above indicated that the antigen-binding

PLATE I

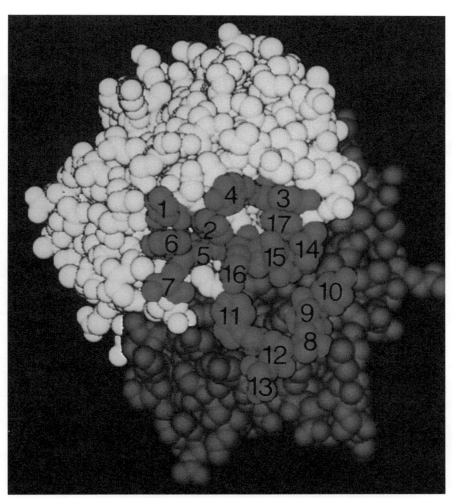

PLATE I. En face *view of the antigen-binding site of an anti-lysozyme antibody, revealed by x-ray crystallography of an antigen-antibody complex. In this space-filling model, the variable regions of the heavy and light chains are shown in yellow and blue, respectively. The numbered side chains in red indicate amino acid residues in the complementarity-determining regions (CDRs) of the light chain (1–7) and heavy chain (8–17) that contact the protein antigen on this planar surface. (Courtesy of Dr. R. J. Poljak, Pasteur Institute, Paris, France, and reproduced with permission from A. G. Amit, R. A. Mariuzza, S. E. V. Phillips, and R. J. Poljak. Three-dimensional structure of an antigen-antibody complex at 2.8 Å resolution. Science 233: 747–753, 1986. Copyright 1986 by the American Association for the Advancement of Science.)*

PLATE II

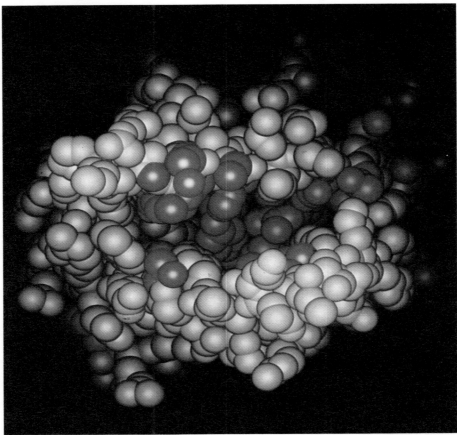

PLATE II. En face *view of the antigen-binding cleft of a class I major histocompatibility complex molecule, HLA–A2, revealed by x-ray crystallography. In this space-filling model, the conserved portions of the antigen-binding region, composed of the α1 and α2 domains of the heavy chain, are shown in light blue and the polymorphic residues, which differ among alleles, are shown in red. These polymorphic residues are located in such a way that they determine the specificity of peptide binding in the cleft. (Courtesy of Drs. Mark A. Saper and Donald C. Wiley, Department of Biochemistry and Molecular Biology and Howard Hughes Medical Institute, Harvard University, Cambridge, Mass.)*

region of antibody is contained within the Fab fragment. Several lines of evidence provide a more precise localization of this function to the hypervariable regions of V_L and V_H.

1. V_L and V_H vary among antibodies of different antigenic specificity, and most of this variation is confined to the hypervariable regions.

2. Changes in the hypervariable regions, either by spontaneous mutation or by specifically directed mutagenesis, can alter antigen-binding specificity.

3. Crystallographic analysis of many antibody structures reveals that the hypervariable regions form extended loops which are exposed on the surface of the antibody and are thus able to interact with antigen.

4. Crystallographic analysis of a limited number of antigen-antibody complexes shows that the amino acid residues of the hypervariable regions form extensive contact with bound antigen. The most extensive contact is with the third hypervariable region, the most variable of the three. (See Plate 1.)

The assignment of antigen-binding specificity to the hypervariable regions led to the alternative name for these sequences as complementarity-determining regions described earlier in the chapter. *The amino acid sequences of the CDRs are primarily responsible for the specificity of antigen binding.* However, it should be noted that antigen binding is not completely a function of the CDRs. Some framework region residues also may contact the antigen. Moreover, in binding of small antigens, one or more of the CDRs may be outside the region of contact with antigen, thus unlikely to participate in antigen binding.

The original models for antigen binding, based on analogy to enzymes, proposed that antibodies contained clefts for binding antigens. Indeed, some of the earliest characterized antibody-antigen complexes involved small carbohydrate antigens and the antibodies that were studied did have clefts lined by amino acid residues of the hypervariable regions. However, more recently analyzed antibody-antigen complexes have revealed that native protein antigens may interact with a more planar antibody-combining site. This is critical for recognition of native proteins, as globular protein antigens are unlikely to fit into clefts. As will be discussed in Chapters 5 and 6, this is a key difference between the antigen-binding site of antibody molecules and those of the other antigen-binding molecules of the immune system, namely MHC molecules and T cell receptors, which cannot bind to native globular proteins.

Affinity and Avidity of Antigen Binding

To describe the physicochemical characteristics of antigen binding to antibody, we will first consider a simplified system consisting of an antigen that has only one determinant per molecule and a population of identical antibody molecules specific for this determinant. When this antigen and antibody are mixed in solution, antigen-antibody complexes constantly form and spontaneously dissociate. After a period of time, the rate of complex formation will exactly equal the rate of complex dissociation and a state of **dynamic equilibrium** will have been reached. If antibody is present at much lower concentration than antigen, the proportion of antibody molecules that have bound antigen at equilibrium is determined by two factors: the concentration of antigen molecules and the strength of the binding interaction. (The strength of the binding interaction is also influenced by other factors such as temperature and solvent conditions, but to simplify the analysis, we will hold these constant.) Under such conditions, the concentration of antigen that allows one half of the antibodies to be in complex with antigen and leaves one half free is a measure of the strength or **affinity** of the binding interaction. This concentration of antigen, measured in molarity, is called the **dissociation constant** (K_d) of the interaction. *A smaller K_d means a greater affinity;* i.e., a lower concentration of antigen is needed to reach half maximal occupancy. It is important to note that affinity depends on both the antibody and the antigen. A given antibody molecule can have different affinities for different related antigens.

The K_d of antigen binding can be measured directly for small antigens by means of equilibrium dialysis (Fig. 3–10). In this method, a solution of antibody is confined within a "semipermeable" membrane of porous cellulose and is immersed in a solution containing the antigen. (Semipermeable in this context means that small molecules, like antigen, can pass freely through the membrane pores but that macromolecules, like antibody, cannot.) If no antibody were present within the membrane, the antigen in the bathing solution would enter the membrane-bound compartment until the concentration of antigen within the membrane-bound compartment became exactly the same as that outside. Another way to view the system is that, at dynamic equilibrium, antigen enters and leaves the membrane-bound compartment at exactly the same rate. However, when antibody is present inside the membrane, the net amount of antigen inside the membrane at equilibrium increases by the quantity that is bound to antibody. This occurs because only unbound antigen can diffuse across the membrane and, at equilibrium, it is the unbound concentration of antigen that must be identical inside and outside the membrane. The extent of the increase in antigen inside the membrane depends on the antigen concentration, on the antibody concentration, and on the K_d of the binding interaction. By measuring the antigen and antibody concentrations, by spectroscopy or by other means, the K_d can be calculated.

An alternative way to determine the K_d is by measuring the rates of antigen-antibody complex formation and dissociation. These rates depend on the concentrations of antibody and antigen, on the affinity of the interaction, and on certain geometric parameters that equally influence the rate in both directions. All parameters except the concentrations can be summarized as rate constants, and both the **on rate constant**

A

ANTIGEN ALONE

B

ANTIGEN + ANTIBODY

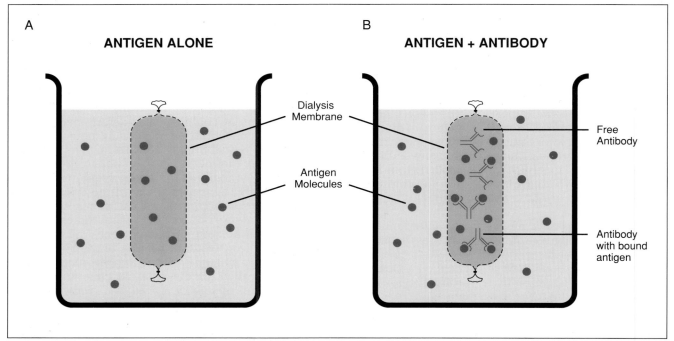

Dialysis Membrane

Antigen Molecules

Free Antibody

Antibody with bound antigen

FIGURE 3–10. *Analysis of antigen-antibody binding by equilibrium dialysis. In the presence of antibody (B), the amount of antigen within the dialysis membrane is increased compared with the absence of antibody (A). As described in the text, this difference, caused by antibody binding of antigen, can be used to measure the affinity of the antibody for the antigen.*

(k_{on}) and the **off rate constant** (k_{off}) can be calculated experimentally by determining the concentrations and the actual rates of association or dissociation, respectively. The ratio of k_{off}/k_{on} allows one to cancel out all of the parameters not related to affinity and is exactly equal to the dissociation constant K_d. Thus, one can measure K_d at equilibrium by equilibrium dialysis or calculate K_d from rate constants measured under non-equilibrium conditions.

So far we have considered only the situation in which the antigen contains a single determinant and thus can interact with a single antibody-combining site. For antibodies specific for an antigen of interest, the K_d usually varies from about 10^{-7} M to 10^{-11} M. In a natural serum, there will be a mixture of such antibodies with different affinities for the specific antigen, depending primarily upon the precise amino acid sequences of the CDRs. (The average affinity of the antibody molecules in a population will increase with repeated immunization, a phenomenon called **affinity maturation;** this is discussed in Chapter 4.) Natural antigens often contain more than one determinant and therefore bind more than one antibody molecule. Moreover, multivalent antigens will have more than one copy of a particular determinant. (Multivalency may arise because a macromolecule may be multimeric or may have an internal repeating structure.) A cell surface will also be multivalent by virtue of having multiple copies of a particular surface antigen. Unless inhibited by steric constraints, a single antibody may be able to attach to a single multivalent antigen by more than one binding site. For IgG or IgE, this attachment can involve, at most, two binding sites because there are only two combining regions per antibody molecule, one on each Fab. For IgM, however, a single antibody may bind at up to ten different sites! Although the affinities of any one site will be unchanged, the overall strength of attachment must take into account binding at all of the sites. This overall strength of attachment is called the **avidity** and will be much stronger than the affinity of any given site. Mathematically, the strength of the avidity increases almost geometrically (rather than additively) for each occupied site. Thus, a low-affinity IgM molecule can still bind very tightly to a multivalent antigen because many low-affinity interactions can produce a single high-avidity interaction.

Multivalent interactions between antigen and antibody are of biologic significance. If a multivalent antigen is mixed with a specific antibody in a test tube, the two will associate to form **immune complexes** (Fig. 3–11). At the correct concentrations, called a "zone of equivalence," antibody and antigen form an extensively cross-linked network of non-covalently attached molecules such that most or all of the antigen and antibody molecules are complexed into large masses. Although the primary non-covalent interactions involve the Fab portions of the antibody and antigen, Fc-Fc associations between antibody molecules may also contribute. (Recall that Fc was named for its propensity to self-associate, leading to crystal formation.) Thus, intact IgG molecules form larger complexes than F(ab')₂, despite similar specific antigen-binding properties.

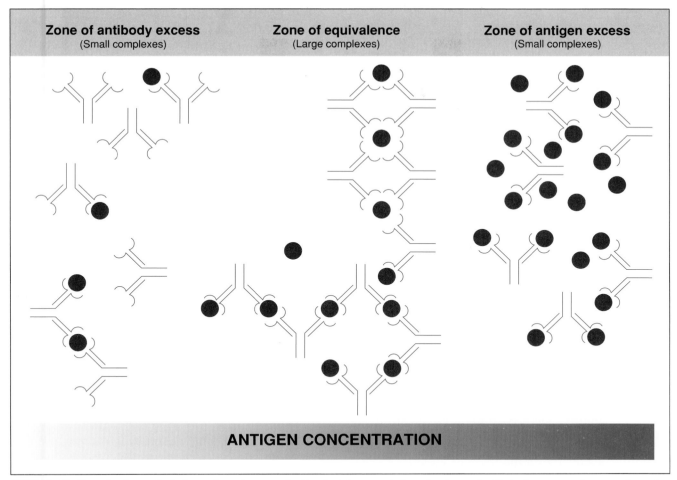

Zone of antibody excess
(Small complexes)

Zone of equivalence
(Large complexes)

Zone of antigen excess
(Small complexes)

ANTIGEN CONCENTRATION

FIGURE 3–11. Sizes of antigen-antibody (immune) complexes as a function of relative concentrations of antigen and antibody. *Large complexes are formed at concentrations of multivalent antigens and antibodies that are termed the "zone of equivalence"; the complexes are smaller in relative antigen or antibody excess.*

Immune complexes can be dissociated into smaller aggregates either by increasing the concentration of antigen so that free antigen molecules will displace cross-linked antigen from antibody-combining sites ("zone of antigen excess") or by increasing antibody so that free antibody molecules will displace cross-linked antibody from antigen determinants ("zone of antibody excess"). If a "zone of equivalence" is reached *in vivo,* large immune complexes can form in the circulation. If such complexes are trapped in tissue (or form in tissue), they can initiate an inflammatory reaction (see Chapter 18).

EFFECTOR FUNCTIONS OF ANTIBODIES

The effector function of an antibody is triggered by binding of antigen. Once antigen is bound, different consequences may ensue, depending on the structure, anatomic location, and isotype of the antibody. The following sections consider the various biologic effects of antibody binding to antigen.

Membrane Antibody As the B Cell Antigen Receptor

Resting B cells are activated to proliferate and secrete antibody by encounter with specific antigen. The specificity and recognition are provided by the membrane forms of antibody expressed on the B cell surface. At different points in the history of a B cell, different heavy chain isotypes may be expressed. For example, immature B cells may express IgM, previously unstimulated mature B cells may express IgM and IgD, and previously stimulated memory B cells may express any isotype or subtype. As noted earlier, membrane Ig differs structurally from secreted Ig of the same isotype, in that membrane Ig contains an extra hydrophobic sequence of about 26 amino acids near the carboxy terminus (see Fig. 3–5). This sequence spans the hydrophobic region of the plasma membrane lipid bilayer so that the extreme carboxy terminal amino acids are located in the cytoplasm. At the present time, it is not known whether these cytoplasmic segments interact with other cytoplasmic or membrane proteins or how the information that antigen is bound to membrane Ig is communicated to the inside of the B cell. However, much evidence suggests that cross-linking of cell surface antibody by multivalent antigen may be an important signal that contributes to B cell activation (see Chapter 9).

As discussed in Box 3–2, the Ig molecules produced by any one B cell contain hypervariable regions that are different from those in Ig molecules produced by most or all other B cells. The unique determinants of Ig hypervariable regions are the **idiotopes,** and the collection of idiotopes on a particular antibody molecule constitutes its **idiotype.** It has been postulated that during immune responses to antigens, anti-idiotypic antibodies specific for the responding lymphocytes are also produced. These anti-idiotypes bind to the surface Ig of the responding B cells and may regulate the magnitude of the immune response (see Chapter 10).

Neutralization of Antigen by Secreted Antibody

The initial discovery of antibodies arose by analyzing the humoral factors that protect immunized hosts against microbial toxins. Many injurious agents, such as toxins, drugs, viruses, bacteria, and other parasites, initiate cell injury by binding to specific cell surface receptors. Secreted antibodies can sterically hinder this interaction by binding to antigenic determinants on the agent (or, less commonly, on the cell receptor), **neutralizing** the toxic or infectious process. This action may be mediated by antibodies of any isotype and experimentally can also be mediated by Fab or $F(ab')_2$ fragments. However, whole antibody molecules usually form more stable complexes because of the propensity of Fc regions to self-associate.

Isotype-Specific Functions of Antibodies

Many functions of antibody molecules are mediated by their Fc portions and are, therefore, specific for particular isotypes or subtypes. As will be seen in Chapter 4, B cells may undergo **heavy chain isotype switching,** allowing the same antigen-binding specificity to be expressed at different times as part of Ig molecules of different isotypes. As a consequence, the same antibody specificity for antigen can be utilized to activate different effector functions. Although the V regions of antibodies are responsible for the specificity and diversity of humoral immunity, the availability of multiple C regions in different isotypes provides an additional measure of adaptability. The production of various heavy chain isotypes serves to direct the humoral immune response along different functional and anatomic pathways, involving diverse interactions with the body's mechanisms of natural immunity and inflammation.

ACTIVATION OF COMPLEMENT BY IgG AND IgM

The **complement system** consists of a family of serum proteins that can be activated by a proteolytic cascade to generate effector molecules. The name complement refers to a heat-labile serum component that was needed to "complement" the function of heat-stable antibody in order to produce lysis of certain target cells. The complement system mediates many of the cytolytic and inflammatory effects of humoral immunity (Chapter 13). Here we will focus upon the ability of antibody to activate the complement system.

One sequence of complement activation, called the **classical complement pathway,** is triggered when a complement protein binds to the Fc region of antigen-complexed IgG or IgM. Neither free IgG nor IgM binds the first protein involved in complement activation, called C1q, so that complement is not activated by circulating free antibody. In the case of IgG, it is believed that the affinity of C1q is insufficient to bind to a single Fcγ region. However, C1q can bind to aggregated Fcγ present in immune complexes or to the clusters of Fcγ regions formed when multiple IgG molecules bind to a cell surface. The interaction of C1q occurs through the $C_\gamma 2$ domain of the IgG molecule. Different IgG subtypes are variously able to initiate this reaction. For example, IgG3 efficiently activates complement, IgG1 somewhat less so, IgG2 poorly, and IgG4 not at all. (In mice, IgG2a, IgG2b, and IgG3 all activate complement but IgG1 does not.)

Activation of complement by IgM differs from activation by IgG. Secreted IgM is already pentameric in its native form in the circulation. However, C1q is sterically hindered from binding by the three-dimensional structure of circulating IgM. The binding of IgM to a planar (e.g., cell) surface is postulated to change the conformation of the antibody, allowing access of C1q to the Fc regions. C1q binding may then occur to the $C_\mu 3$ domain (the one that most resembles $C_\gamma 2$).

OPSONIZATION BY IgG FOR ENHANCED PHAGOCYTOSIS

Both mononuclear phagocytes and granulocytes have the ability to ingest particulate matter as a prelude to intracellular killing and degradation. The ingestion process of particulate matter, called **phagocytosis,** involves attachment of surface membrane to the foreign material and then "zipping up" of membrane around it. The efficiency of the process is markedly improved if the membrane of the phagocytic cell can attach itself with specificity to the object undergoing phagocytosis (Fig. 3–12).

Both mononuclear phagocytes and neutrophils express receptors for the Fc portions of IgG molecules. In fact, at least three distinct types of Fcγ receptors are expressed, each with different affinities and selectivities for different IgG subtypes (Table 3–2). Recent studies have revealed that each of the three types of IgG Fc receptor molecules is actually a family of several structurally related proteins encoded by different genes. It is interesting that all three classes of IgG receptors on leukocytes (written FcγR) contain

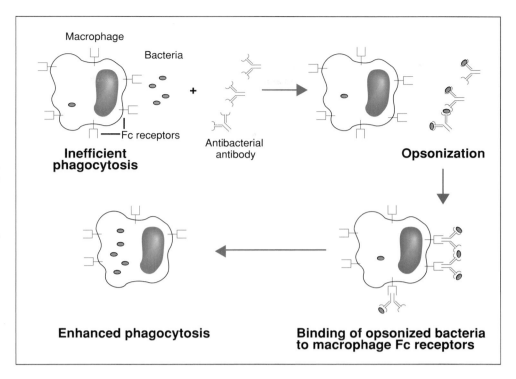

FIGURE 3–12. Antibody-dependent opsonization and phagocytosis of bacteria. *Antibody binding to particles such as bacteria can markedly enhance the efficiency of phagocytosis. The enhancement of phagocytosis in macrophages involves both increased attachment to the cell surface and activation of the phagocyte, both mediated through occupancy of Fcγ receptors.*

Ig-like domains and are thus members of the Ig gene superfamily. By means of these receptors, when IgG molecules bind to and coat antigenic particles, a process called **opsonization,** the bound IgG serves to enhance the efficiency of phagocytosis. The higher-affinity receptors (called FcRI and FcRII) are most important for phagocytosis, and the IgG subtypes that bind best to these receptors (IgG1 and IgG3) are most efficient for promoting phagocytosis.

It should be noted that a fragment derived from the third component of complement (C3b) can also opsonize particles for phagocytosis through binding to a leukocyte receptor for C3b. Since C3b can be generated and attached to cells as a consequence of the classical pathway of complement activation, IgM binding can indirectly lead to opsonization and enhanced phagocytosis.

Opsonization may lead to more than merely increasing the binding of the particulate matter to phagocytes. FcRI and FcRII also appear to be involved in metabolic activation of phagocytes, increasing the efficiency of the subsequent intracellular degradation of ingested particles.

ANTIBODY-DEPENDENT CELL-MEDIATED CYTOTOXICITY TARGETED BY IgG, IgE, AND IgA

Several different leukocyte populations other than cytolytic T lymphocytes (CTLs), including neutrophils, eosinophils, mononuclear phagocytes, and especially NK cells, are capable of lysing various target cell types. In many cases, killing of target cells requires that the target cell be precoated with specific IgG, and the lytic process is called **antibody-dependent cell-mediated cytotoxicity** (ADCC) (Fig. 3–13A). Recognition of bound antibody occurs

TABLE 3–2. Human Leukocyte Fcγ Receptors

Common Nomenclature	CD Designation*	Size*	Affinity (K_d)†	Distribution
FcRI	64	75 kD	1×10^{-8} M (IgG1 > IgG3 > IgG4 > > IgG2)	Mononuclear phagocytes, cytokine-activated neutrophils
FcRII	32	40 kD	5×10^{-7} M (IgG1 > IgG3 = IgG4 > > IgG2)	Mononuclear phagocytes, neutrophils, eosinophils, platelets
FcRIII	16	50–70 kD	2×10^{-6} M (IgG1 = IgG3; not IgG2, IgG4)	Natural killer cells, neutrophils, eosinophils, macrophages, but not monocytes

* The size and CD designation apply to the IgG–binding component; each receptor may be associated with other polypeptides. The IgG–binding domains of each receptor may exist in several isoforms.

† Indicated K_d refers to affinity for IgG1. The selectivity for IgG isotypes is still tentatively assigned.

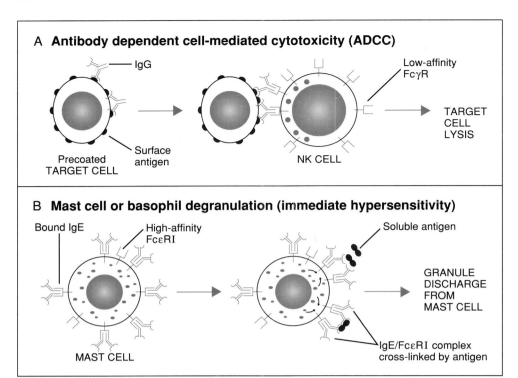

FIGURE 3–13. Functions of antibodies in natural killer (NK) cell–mediated cytolysis (A) and in degranulation of mast cells (B).
A. *NK cells express low-affinity Fcγ receptors that recognize clustered IgG molecules prebound to antigens on the surface of a target cell.*
B. *Monomeric IgE antibodies attach to high-affinity Fcε receptors on mast cells or basophils in the absence of antigen; subsequent exposure to antigen causes cross-linking of the IgE/FcεRI complex leading to mast cell or basophil degranulation.*

through low-affinity receptors for Fcγ on the leukocyte, called FcRIII or CD16. In the case of NK cells, the predominant cellular mediators of ADCC, it is now appreciated that IgG serves two distinct functions. First, it provides cognitive function; i.e., those target cells that have bound IgG will be preferentially killed compared with those not displaying IgG. Second, the occupancy (and perhaps aggregation) of FcRIII serves to activate the NK cell to synthesize and secrete cytokines such as tumor necrosis factor and interferon-γ as well as to discharge their granules. These released cytokines and granule proteins probably mediate the cytolytic functions of this cell type (see Chapter 12).

Since CD16 is a low-affinity receptor and more efficiently binds aggregated IgG than monomeric IgG, monomeric IgG in plasma neither activates NK cells nor competes effectively with cell-bound IgG for recognition. *Thus, ADCC is most efficient when the target cell is precoated with antibody.* Interestingly, a form of FcRIII is also expressed on neutrophils, but on this cell type it does not mediate ADCC. Neutrophil FcRIII is encoded by a different gene from the FcRIII of NK cells. Furthermore, neutrophil FcRIII is attached to the cell surface by a phosphatidylinositol anchor, whereas on NK cells FcRIII is a transmembrane protein.

Eosinophils mediate a special type of ADCC directed against parasites such as helminths. Helminths are relatively resistant to lysis by neutrophils and mononuclear phagocytes, but they can be killed by a basic protein present in the granules of eosinophils. In this case, IgE or IgA rather than IgG serves as the principal isotype that provides cognitive recognition and effector cell activation because eosinophils express Fc receptors for IgE and IgA antibodies.

IMMEDIATE HYPERSENSITIVITY TRIGGERED BY IgE

Mast cells and basophils express high-affinity receptors for the Fc portion of IgE molecules. The structure and function of this IgE receptor, called FcεRI, are described in Chapter 14. Because of their high affinity, FcεRI receptors are occupied by IgE monomer in the absence of antigen, a key difference from FcRIII involved in ADCC (Fig. 3–13B). The introduction of specific antigen causes aggregation of the IgE molecule and its receptor. This clustering, in turn, causes the mast cell or basophil to release inflammatory and vasoactive mediators (e.g., histamine) from preformed storage granules and to synthesize lipid-derived mediators (e.g., leukotrienes, prostaglandins, and platelet activating factor) and cytokines *de novo*. The consequence of the release of these mediators is a response called **immediate hypersensitivity,** which is discussed in Chapter 14.

MUCOSAL IMMUNITY MEDIATED BY IgA

Although IgA is a relatively unimportant component of systemic humoral immunity, it plays a key role in mucosal immunity. This is because IgA alone of the various isotypes can be selectively transported across mucosal barriers into the lumens of mucosa-lined organs. Epithelial cells of organs such as the intestine express specific Fc receptors for dimeric IgA molecules. This FcαR receptor is also called **secretory,** or

S, protein. Initially, S protein binds the antibody on the basal surface of the epithelial cell that is facing the blood. Bound IgA is passaged through the cell to the mucosal surface by vesicular transport. Surprisingly, IgA is not simply released from its receptor. Rather, the S protein itself is specifically cleaved, leaving a bound secretory-component peptide (called **secretory piece**) attached to the dimeric IgA molecule. Once in mucosal secretions, IgA functions to neutralize injurious agents.

Neonatal Immunity Mediated by Maternal IgG

Neonatal mammals often lack the ability to mount an effective immune response against microbes. However, maternally produced IgG can provide a protective action. Such IgG is secreted by the mother into breast milk and taken up from the gut lumen into the blood of the neonate, the opposite direction of IgA secretion. A distinct receptor for IgG has been identified that mediates this transport function. Interestingly, this receptor is unique among Fc receptors in that it structurally resembles a class I MHC molecule (see Chapter 5).

Feedback Inhibition of Immune Responses Mediated by IgG

Various lymphocyte populations express Fc receptors for different Ig isotypes. These receptors are believed to modulate lymphocyte function independent of antigenic specificity. The best example of this phenomenon is the binding of aggregated IgG or IgG-containing antibody-antigen complexes to Fcγ receptors on B cells, which may inhibit activation of these B cells, a process called **antibody feedback** (see Chapter 10).

Laboratory Uses of Antibodies

This portion of the chapter describes how antibodies may be used as tools in research and in clinical diagnosis. Historically, many of the uses of antibody depended upon the ability of antibody and specific antigen to form large immune complexes. Immunochemists could detect antigen by observing the formation of such complexes in solution by light scattering. In addition, specific antigens could be purified from solutions containing mixtures of molecules by collecting the specific immune complexes by centrifugation or by precipitation of antibody with chemical agents. The presence of antigen could be detected by allowing antibody-antigen precipitates to form in gels. In the classic "double-diffusion" method of Ouchterlony, antigen and antibody were allowed to diffuse into gels from separate but nearby wells and a "precipitin line" of insoluble immune complexes would form at the point where the concentrations of diffusing antibody and antigen reached a zone of equivalence (Fig. 3–14). The position of the precipitin line provided information about antigen concentration and comparisons of the precipitin lines formed by different antigen solutions allowed structural inferences about antigenic similarities or differences to be made. However, very little direct structural information could be learned about the antigens by these methods. In a later technique, the antigen solution could first be separated by electrophoresis under non-denaturing conditions and then allowed to diffuse into an antibody-containing gel. The extent of migration during electrophoresis provided additional information about the structure of the antigen. These methods were of great importance in early studies, but now have been almost entirely replaced by simpler methods based on immobilized antibodies or antigens. In the remainder of this chapter, we describe four common applications of antibodies in widespread current use.

Quantitation of Antigen

Immunologic methods of quantifying antigen concentration provide exquisite sensitivity and specificity and have become standard techniques for both research and clinical applications. All modern immunochemical methods of quantitation are based upon having a simple and accurate method for measuring the quantity of indicator molecules. When the indicator molecule is labeled with a radioisotope, as first introduced by Rosalyn Yallow and colleagues, it may be quantified by counting radioactive decay events in a scintillation counter; the assay is called a **radioimmunoassay** (RIA). When the indicator molecule is covalently coupled to an enzyme, it may be quantified by determining with a spectrophotometer the initial rate at which the enzyme converts a clear substrate to a colored product; the assay is called an **enzyme-linked immunosorbent assay** (ELISA). Several variations of RIA and ELISA are in common use.

Direct RIA (Fig. 3–15)

A fixed quantity of antibody is attached to a solid support. The immobilized antibody will bind a finite portion of added radiolabeled indicator antigen. How much antigen binds depends on the antigen concentration and on the affinity of the antibody for the antigen. In the assay, the test solution of unknown antigen concentration is compared with a series of standard solutions containing known concentrations of unlabeled antigen for their ability to inhibit competitively the binding of the radiolabeled indicator antigen to the immobilized antibody. The greater the content of competing antigen in the test or standard solution, the less radiolabeled indicator antigen is bound. The results for the standard solutions of known antigen con-

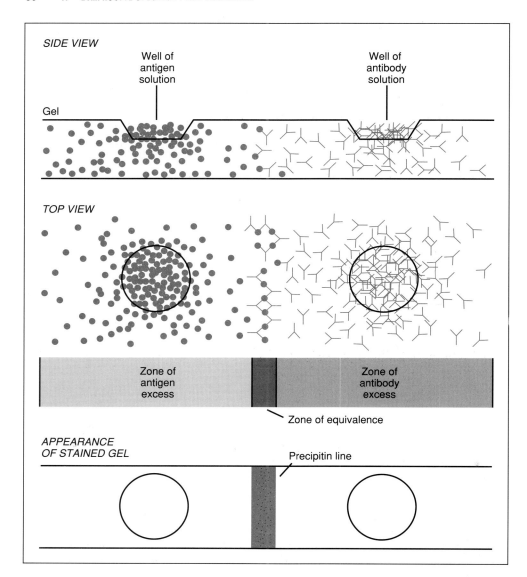

SIDE VIEW

Well of antigen solution

Well of antibody solution

Gel

TOP VIEW

Zone of antigen excess

Zone of antibody excess

Zone of equivalence

APPEARANCE OF STAINED GEL

Precipitin line

FIGURE 3–14. Analysis of the binding of antigen and antibody by agar gel diffusion (Ouchterlony technique). Diffusion of antibody and antigen leads to a zone of equivalence, where large insoluble immune complexes form and can be detected as a precipitin line.

centration are used to derive an inhibition curve as a function of antigen concentration, from which the concentration in the test sample can be inferred.

Inhibition ELISA or RIA (Fig. 3–16)

A fixed quantity of antigen is attached to a solid support, and a fixed quantity of indicator antibody in solution is allowed to bind. The amount of bound indicator antibody is measured by a linked enzyme or by an attached radioisotope label. The test solution of unknown antigen concentrations is compared with a series of standard solutions of known concentrations of antigen to inhibit competitively the binding of the antibody. The greater the content of antigen in the test or standard solution, the less antibody is bound. The results from the standard solutions of known antigen concentration are used to derive an inhibition curve

as a function of antigen concentration, from which the concentration in the test sample can be inferred.

Sandwich ELISA or RIA (Fig. 3–17)

A fixed quantity of one antibody is attached to a solid support. A test solution of unknown antigen concentration or a series of standard solutions of known concentrations of antigen is allowed to bind. Unbound antigen is removed, and a second population of enzyme-linked or radiolabeled indicator antibodies is allowed to bind. The more antigen in the test or standard solutions, the more enzyme-linked or radiolabeled second antibody will bind. The results from the standard solutions are used to construct a binding curve for second antibody as a function of antigen concentration, from which the quantity of antigen in the test solution may be inferred. When this test is performed with two antibodies, it is essential that

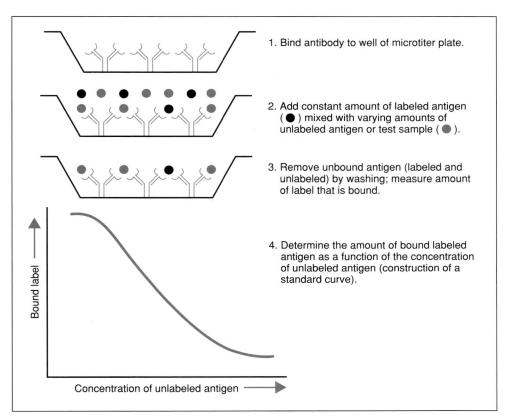

FIGURE 3 – 15. Direct radioimmunoassay (RIA). *With a fixed amount of immobilized antibody, the amount of labeled antigen bound decreases as the concentration of competing unlabeled antigen is increased, allowing quantification of unlabeled antigen.*

1. Bind antibody to well of microtiter plate.

2. Add constant amount of labeled antigen (●) mixed with varying amounts of unlabeled antigen or test sample (●).

3. Remove unbound antigen (labeled and unlabeled) by washing; measure amount of label that is bound.

4. Determine the amount of bound labeled antigen as a function of the concentration of unlabeled antigen (construction of a standard curve).

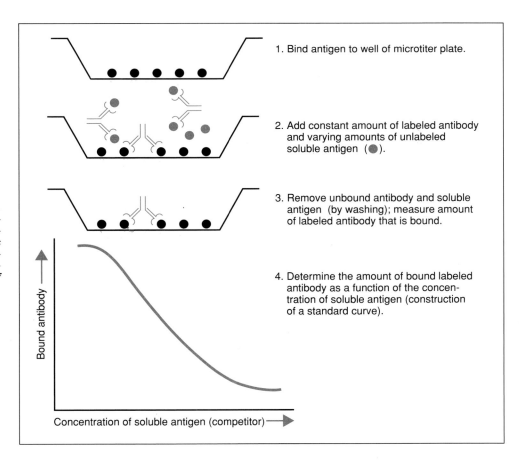

FIGURE 3 – 16. Competitive ELISA or RIA. *With a fixed amount of immobilized antigen, the amount of labeled antibody bound decreases as the concentration of unlabeled antigen (competitive inhibitor) is increased, allowing quantification of unlabeled antigen.*

1. Bind antigen to well of microtiter plate.

2. Add constant amount of labeled antibody and varying amounts of unlabeled soluble antigen (●).

3. Remove unbound antibody and soluble antigen (by washing); measure amount of labeled antibody that is bound.

4. Determine the amount of bound labeled antibody as a function of the concentration of soluble antigen (construction of a standard curve).

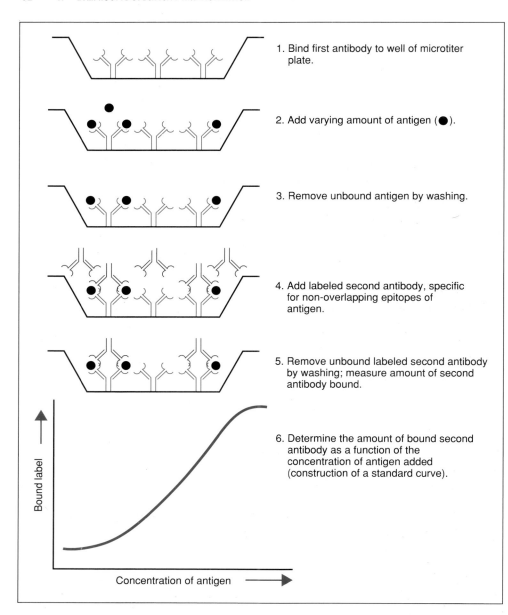

1. Bind first antibody to well of microtiter plate.

2. Add varying amount of antigen (●).

3. Remove unbound antigen by washing.

4. Add labeled second antibody, specific for non-overlapping epitopes of antigen.

5. Remove unbound labeled second antibody by washing; measure amount of second antibody bound.

6. Determine the amount of bound second antibody as a function of the concentration of antigen added (construction of a standard curve).

FIGURE 3–17. Sandwich ELISA or RIA. *With a fixed amount of one immobilized antibody, the binding of a second, labeled antibody increases as the concentration of antigen increases, allowing quantification of antigen.*

these antibodies see non-overlapping determinants on the antigen; otherwise, the second antibody cannot bind.

Identification and Characterization of Protein Antigens

The two major approaches used by immunochemists to identify and characterize protein antigens are immunoprecipitation and Western blotting.

IMMUNOPRECIPITATION (Fig. 3 – 18)

An antibody directed against one protein antigen in a mixture of proteins is used to isolate the specific antigen from the mixture. In most modern proce-dures, the antibody is attached to a solid phase parti-cle (e.g., an agarose bead), either by direct chemical coupling or indirectly. Indirect coupling may be achieved by means of an attached "second antibody" such as rabbit anti-mouse Ig antibody or by means of some other protein with specific affinity for the Fc portion of Ig molecules, such as protein A or protein G from staphylococcal bacteria. After the antibody-coated beads are incubated with the solution of antigen, unbound molecules are separated from the bead-antibody-antigen complex by washing. Specific antigen is then released (eluted) from the antibody by changing pH or by other solvent conditions that re-duce the affinity of binding. Large quantities of anti-gen can be purified by this procedure of affinity chro-matography. (Recall that affinity chromatography is also used as a method for purifying antibody mole-cules; see p. 41.) The purified antigen can then be analyzed by conventional protein chemical tech-

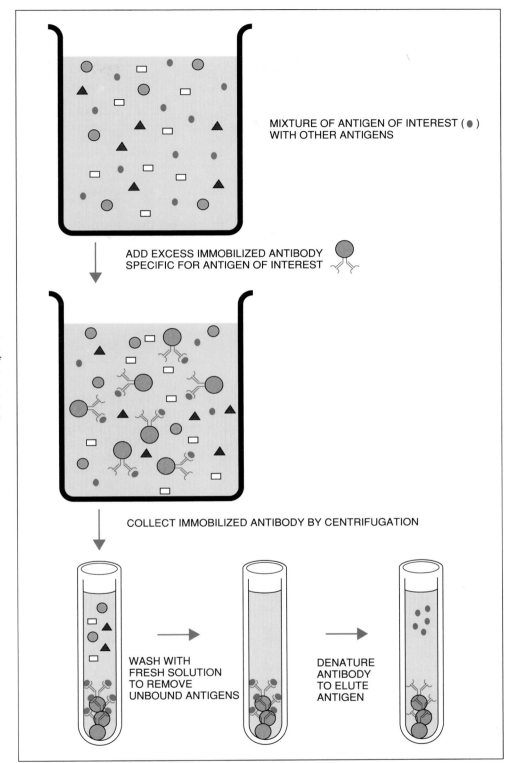

FIGURE 3–18. Isolation of an antigen by immunoprecipitation. *Immunoprecipitation can be used as a means of purification, as a means of quantification, or as a means of identification of an antigen. Antigens purified by immunoprecipitation are often analyzed by polyacrylamide gel electrophoresis (see Box 3–3).*

MIXTURE OF ANTIGEN OF INTEREST (●) WITH OTHER ANTIGENS

ADD EXCESS IMMOBILIZED ANTIBODY SPECIFIC FOR ANTIGEN OF INTEREST

COLLECT IMMOBILIZED ANTIBODY BY CENTRIFUGATION

WASH WITH FRESH SOLUTION TO REMOVE UNBOUND ANTIGENS

DENATURE ANTIBODY TO ELUTE ANTIGEN

niques. Alternatively, a small amount of radiolabeled protein can be purified and the characteristics of the macromolecule can be inferred from the behavior of the radioactive label in analytical separation techniques such as polyacrylamide gel electrophoresis or isoelectric focusing (Box 3–3).

WESTERN BLOTTING (Fig. 3–19)

If the protein antigen to be characterized is in a mixture with other antigens it may be first subjected to analytical separation, typically by sodium dodecyl sulfate (SDS)–polyacrylamide gel electrophoresis, so

Analytical separation of proteins by size is routinely accomplished by electrophoresis through cross-linked polyacrylamide gels in the presence of SDS, an ionic detergent. Dodecyl sulfate binds to proteins in proportion to their molecular size, and the net negative charge of the bound detergent overwhelms the intrinsic charge of the protein. The bound dodecyl sulfate also causes refolding of the protein into semirigid rods of length proportional to molecular size. As a result, both hydrodynamic resistance and net charge become entirely functions of molecular size, and consequently migration to the anode in an applied electric field is also a function only of size. *Stated simply, smaller proteins migrate faster.* The size of an unknown protein can be determined by comparing the distance migrated in an SDS–polyacrylamide gel with the migration of known size standards electrophoresed in parallel lanes of the same gel. In general, the gel porosity is made sufficiently large to prevent sieving effects but size resolution can be further enhanced by using gradients of cross-linked polyacrylamide concentration to introduce a small sieving effect. By this technique, one can accurately determine the size of any protein from about 5000 to 250,000 or more daltons.

An alternative analytical separation strategy is based upon isoelectric point. When proteins are electrophoresed through a pre-formed or self-generating pH gradient, they will migrate until they reach their isoelectric point, i.e., the condition of zero net charge. This separation technique is called **isoelectric focusing** and is also conveniently performed in polyacrylamide gels.

An optimal analytical separation scheme has been developed that combines these techniques. One first separates proteins by isoelectric focusing in one dimension and then subjects the initially separated array of proteins to SDS–polyacrylamide gel electrophoresis in the second, orthogonal direction. Such two-dimensional (2-D) gels can resolve over one thousand separate proteins from a typical cell!

Once separated, the positions of the proteins in the gel are localized by staining. A common technique is to fix the proteins in place by denaturing solvents and then to stain them with a dye such as Coomassie blue or to use the fixed protein as a nidus for *in situ* reduction of silver ("silver staining"). Alternatively, radiolabeled proteins can be detected by dehydrating fixed gels and using the dried gel to expose photographic x-ray film (autoradiography). Finally, as discussed in the text, proteins separated by electrophoresis may be transferred by capillary action (blotting) or electrophoresis from the gel to a membrane where they can be stained by immunochemical procedures ("Western blotting").

that the positions of different proteins in the gel are a function of their molecular sizes. The array of separated proteins is then transferred from the separating gel to a support membrane by capillary action (blotting) or by electrophoresis, such that the membrane acquires a replica of the array of separated macromolecules present in the gel. SDS is displaced from the protein during the transfer process, and native antigenic determinants are often regained as the protein refolds. The position of the antigen on the membrane can then be detected by binding of labeled antibody, thus providing information about antigen size. Both enzyme-linked and radiolabeled antibodies are commonly used.

The technique of transferring proteins from a gel to a membrane is called Western blotting as a biochemist's joke. Southern is the last name of the scientist who first blotted deoxyribonucleic acid (DNA) from a separating gel to a membrane, a technique since called Southern blotting. By analogy, "Northern blotting" was applied to the technique of transferring ribonucleic acid (RNA) from a gel to a membrane and "Western blotting" was applied to protein transfer. A more detailed description of both Southern and Northern blotting will be presented in Box 4–1, Chapter 4.

Cell Surface Labeling and Separation

Antibodies are commonly used to characterize, identify, or separate cell populations. In these methods, the antibody can be radiolabeled, enzyme linked, or, most commonly, fluorescently labeled. In the case of fluorescent labels, the amount of bound antibody on every individual cell in a population is measured by passing suspended cells one at a time through a fluorimeter. This ability to analyze individual cells more than compensates for the fact that fluorescence intensity is always an arbitrary quantity and, unlike radioactivity or absorbance, cannot be related to an absolute number of molecules except by comparison to known standards. The flowing cells can also be differentially deflected by electromagnetic fields whose strength and direction are varied according to the measured intensity of the fluorescence signal, thereby allowing one to separate cell populations according to surface antibody binding (Fig. 3–20). The instrument that performs this task is called a **fluorescence activated cell sorter** (FACS). Modern FACS instruments routinely allow simultaneous detection of three or more different fluorescent signals, each attached to a different antibody, permitting analysis or separation of cells according to any specified combination of surface antibody-binding patterns. A less sophisticated separation can be accomplished by allowing cells to attach to antibodies bound to plates ("panning").

Localization of Antigen Within Tissues or Cells

Antibodies can be used to identify the anatomic distribution of an antigen within a tissue or within compartments of a cell. The common principle behind these techniques is that a label is attached to the spe-

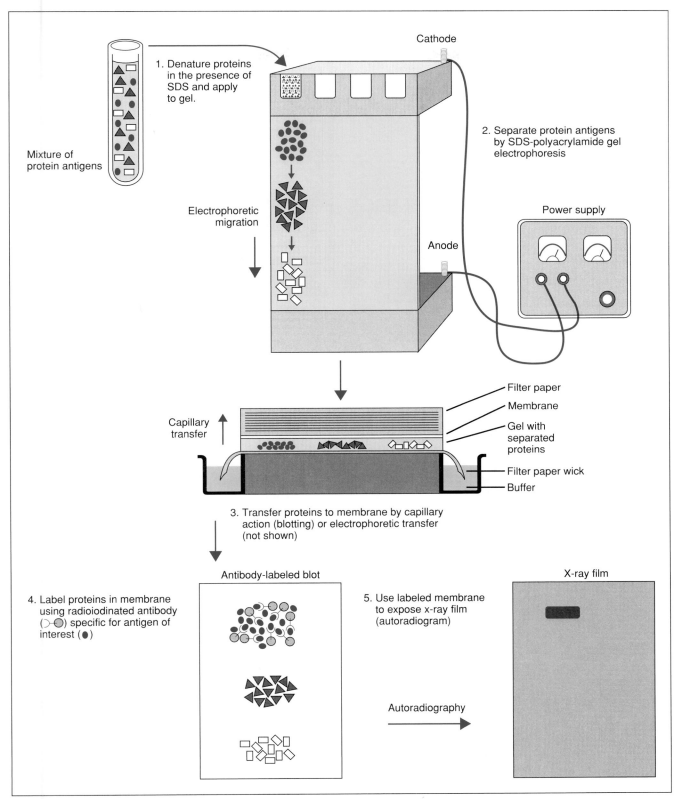

FIGURE 3–19. Characterization of antigens by Western blotting. *Protein antigens, separated by polyacrylamide gel electrophoresis and transferred to a membrane, can be labeled with radioactive or (not shown) enzyme-coupled antibodies. Analysis of an antigen by Western blotting provides information similar to that obtained from immunoprecipitation followed by polyacrylamide gel electrophoresis. Some antibodies work only in one or the other technique.*

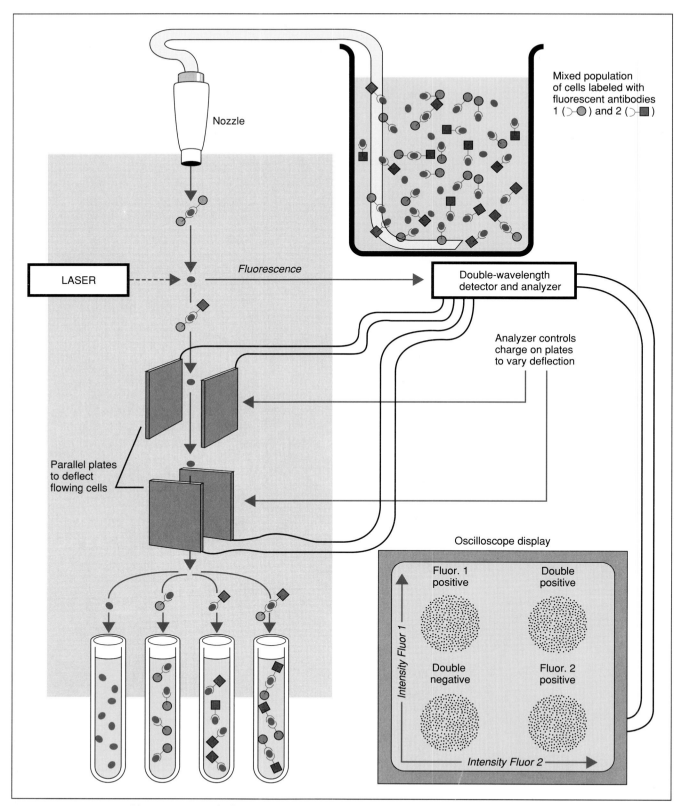

FIGURE 3 – 20. The principle of fluorescence-activated cell sorting. *The separation depicted here is based upon two antigenic markers ("two-color sorting"). Modern instruments can routinely separate cell populations based upon three or more markers.*

cific antibody and that the position of the label in the tissue or cell, determined with a suitable microscope, is used to infer the position of the antigen. In the earliest version of this method, called **immunofluorescence,** the antibody was labeled with a fluorescent group and allowed to bind to a monolayer of cells or to a frozen section of a tissue. The stained cells or tissues were examined with a fluorescence microscope to locate the antibody. Although extremely sensitive, the fluorescent microscope is not an ideal tool for identifying the normal unstained structures of the cell or tissue. Thus, it is often difficult to interpret precisely where the label has been located. More recently, antibodies have been coupled to enzymes that convert colorless substrates to colored insoluble substances that precipitate at the position of the enzyme. A conventional light microscope may then be used to localize the antibody in a stained cell or tissue. The most common variant of this method utilizes the enzyme horseradish peroxidase, and the method is commonly referred to as the **immunoperoxidase technique.** Examples of this method have been shown in Chapter 2. In other variations, antibody can be coupled to an electron-dense probe, such as colloidal gold, and the location of antibody can be determined subcellularly by means of an electron microscope, a technique called **immunoelectron microscopy.**

In all immunomicroscopic methods, signals may be enhanced by using "sandwich" techniques. For example, instead of attaching horseradish peroxidase to a specific mouse antibody directed against the antigen of interest, it can be attached to a second antibody (e.g., rabbit anti-mouse Ig antibody) that is used to bind to the first, unlabeled antibody. When the label is attached directly to the specific, primary antibody, the method is referred to as **direct;** when the label is attached to a secondary or even tertiary antibody, the method is **indirect.** In some cases, molecules other than antibody can be used in indirect methods. For example, staphylococcal protein A, which binds to IgG, or avidin, which binds to primary antibodies labeled with biotin, can be coupled to enzymes.

SUMMARY

Antibodies, or immunoglobulins, are a family of structurally related glycoproteins produced by B lymphocytes that function as the mediators of specific humoral immunity. All antibodies have a common core structure of two identical light chains and two identical heavy chains. Each chain consists of multiple independently folded domains of about 110 amino acids containing conserved intrachain disulfide bonds. The N-terminal domains of heavy and light chains form the variable regions of antibody molecules, which differ among antibodies of different specificities. The variable (V) regions of heavy and light chains each contain three separate hypervariable regions of about ten amino acids that are spatially assembled to form the antigen-combining site of the antibody molecule. Light chains contain one C region domain, and heavy chains contain three or four, which are similar in antibodies of the same class (isotype) and subclass but differ among antibodies of different classes and subclasses. Most of the effector functions of antibodies are mediated by the constant regions of the heavy chains, but these functions are triggered by binding of antigens to the spatially distant combining site in the variable region.

Macromolecular antigens contain multiple epitopes, or determinants, each of which may be recognized by an antibody. The affinity of the interaction between the combining site of a single antibody molecule and a single epitope is measured as a dissociation constant (K_d). Multivalent antigens contain multiple identical epitopes to which identical antibody molecules can bind. When multivalent antigens react with antibodies, a zone of equivalence may be reached, where the relative concentrations of antigen and antibody favor the formation of large immune complexes. In zones of antigen excess or antibody excess, these extensively cross-linked aggregates dissociate into smaller complexes.

Antibodies are produced in membrane-associated and secreted forms. Membrane Ig, on the surface of a B cell, is the B cell receptor for antigen. Secreted antibody molecules neutralize antigens, activate the complement system, and opsonize antigens and enhance their phagocytosis by various cells. In addition, different antibody isotypes bind to Fc receptors on eosinophils, mast cells, and natural killer cells and stimulate the functions of these cells as a consequence of antigen binding. Other Fc receptors on epithelial cells mediate transepithelial transport of IgA and IgG antibodies.

Antibodies are also invaluable tools in the laboratory. Radioimmunoassay and enzyme-linked immunosorbent assay are used to quantify antigens in solution. Immunoprecipitation and Western blotting are used for the purification and structural analysis of protein antigens. Fluorescence-activated cell sorting is used to identify, characterize, and purify cell populations that express particular surface antigens. Immunomicroscopic techniques such as immunofluorescence and immunoperoxidase are used to identify and localize antigens in cells and tissues.

SELECTED READINGS

Alzari, P. M., M. Lascombe, and R. J. Poljak. Three-dimensional structure of antibodies. Annual Review of Immunology 6:555–580, 1988.

Amit, A. G., R. A. Mariuzza, S. E. V. Phillips, and R. J. Poljak. Three-dimensional structure of an antigen-antibody complex at 2.8 Å resolution. Science 233:747–753, 1986.

Burton, D. R. Structure and function of antibodies. *In* F. Calabi and M. S. Neuberger (eds.). Molecular Genetics of Immunoglobulins. Amsterdam, Elsevier Science Publishers, 1987.

Davies, D. R., and H. Metzger. Structural basis of antibody function. Annual Review of Immunology 1:87–117, 1983.

Johnstone, A., and R. Thorpe. Immunochemistry in Practice, 2nd ed. Oxford, Blackwell Scientific Publishers, 1987.

Kohler, G., and C. Milstein. Continuous cultures of fused cells secreting antibody of predefined specificity. Nature 256:495–497, 1975.

Porter, R. R. The hydrolysis of rabbit γ-globulin and antibodies by crystalline papain. Biochemical Journal 73:119, 1959.

Unkeless, J. C. Function and heterogeneity of human Fc receptors of human immunoglobulin G. Journal of Clinical Investigation 83:355–361, 1989.

Wu, T. T., and E. A. Kabat. An analysis of the sequences of the variable regions of Bence-Jones proteins and myeloma light chains and their implications for antibody complementarity. Journal of Experimental Medicine 132:211–250, 1970.

CHAPTER FOUR

MATURATION OF

B LYMPHOCYTES

AND EXPRESSION OF

IMMUNOGLOBULIN

GENES

Antibodies, or immunoglobulins (Igs), are synthesized exclusively by B lymphocytes. Therefore, the humoral immune response to a foreign antigen reflects the types of Ig produced by the B cells which are stimulated by that antigen. At different stages of their maturation, B cells provide both cognitive and effector functions in the humoral immune response. Membrane Ig–expressing B cells are the cognitive cells, since they specifically recognize and respond to antigens. Following antigenic stimulation, they differentiate into effector cells that secrete Ig. Elucidation of the mechanisms of antibody synthesis has been one of the major advances in immunology during the last decade. This chapter describes the molecular genetic basis of humoral immune responses, with particular reference to the organization and expression of Ig genes, the differentiation of B lymphocytes, and the mechanisms by which antibody diversity is generated. The cellular interactions and extrinsic stimuli that lead to B cell proliferation and differentiation, including the functions of helper T cells in specific antibody responses, will be discussed in Chapter 9.

GENERAL FEATURES OF ANTIBODY PRODUCTION

The first analyses of specific antibody responses to foreign antigens were initiated in the early 1900s and focused on the types of antibodies produced in a person or experimental animal exposed to bacteria or microbial toxins. The total population of antibody specificities that an individual can produce is called the **antibody repertoire** and is a reflection of all the B cell clones capable of Ig synthesis and secretion in response to antigenic stimulation. During its life, each B lymphocyte and its clonal progeny go through a series of well-defined maturational or differentiative stages, each of which has a characteristic pattern of Ig production. Attempts to understand the development of B lymphocytes ultimately led to the isolation of Ig genes and to analyses of their expression and regulation.

Diversity of the Antibody Repertoire

The **primary antibody repertoire** consists of all the antibodies that an individual can produce in response to the first (primary) immunization with different antigens. It is ($\sim 10^9$ or more) determined by the number of B cell clones that exist prior to immunization and express membrane Ig molecules with distinct specificities for antigens. Since lymphocytes specific for different antigens develop before the introduction of these antigens, it follows that *the information needed to generate the enormously diverse repertoire of antibodies is present in the DNA of each individual.* If, however, each Ig heavy and light chain were produced by an individual gene, more than half

the genome that can code for functional proteins would be required to generate 10^9 antibody specificities. This is clearly not the case, and as we shall see later in this chapter, each Ig heavy chain and light chain polypeptide is not encoded by a discrete DNA sequence in the germline. Instead, B lymphocytes have developed remarkably effective genetic mechanisms for generating a highly diverse repertoire from a pool of Ig genes that is of more limited size.

Maturation of B Lymphocytes

All B lymphocytes arise in the bone marrow from a stem cell that does not produce Ig (Fig. 4–1). The earliest cell type that synthesizes a detectable Ig gene product contains cytoplasmic μ heavy chains composed of variable (V) and constant (C) regions. This cell is called the **pre-B lymphocyte** and is found only in hematopoietic tissues, such as the bone marrow and fetal liver. It does not express membrane IgM, since surface expression requires synthesis of both heavy and light chains. Therefore, pre-B cells cannot recognize or respond to antigen. In pre-B cells, the μ heavy chains may associate with other, non-Ig proteins whose major function may be to prevent the degradation of newly synthesized heavy chains and promote the expression of Ig molecules on the cell surface.

At the next identifiable stage in B cell maturation, κ or λ light chains are also produced. These associate with μ heavy chains and then the assembled IgM molecules are expressed on the cell surface, where they function as specific receptors for antigens. IgM-bearing B cells that are recently derived from marrow precursors are called **immature B lymphocytes** because they do not proliferate and differentiate in response to antigens. In fact, their encounter with antigens such as self antigens may lead to unresponsiveness (tolerance) rather than activation. Once a B cell expresses a complete heavy or light chain, it cannot produce another heavy or light chain containing a different V region.

Having acquired a complete Ig and, therefore, a specificity, B cells migrate out of the bone marrow and can be found in the peripheral circulation and lymphoid tissues. They continue to mature, even in the absence of antigenic stimulation. **Mature B cells** co-express μ and δ heavy chains in association with the original κ or λ light chain and, therefore, produce both membrane IgM and IgD. Both classes of membrane Ig have the same V region and hence the same antigen specificity. Such cells are responsive to antigens. It is possible that some B cells may acquire functional responsiveness to antigenic stimulation without expressing IgD. Although maturation to this stage does not require overt exposure to antigen, it is believed that unless these B lymphocytes encounter antigen, they die with a half-life of about 3 or 4 days. Once the mature B cells are stimulated by antigen (and other signals that will be described in Chapter 9), they are called **activated B lymphocytes.** Activated B cells

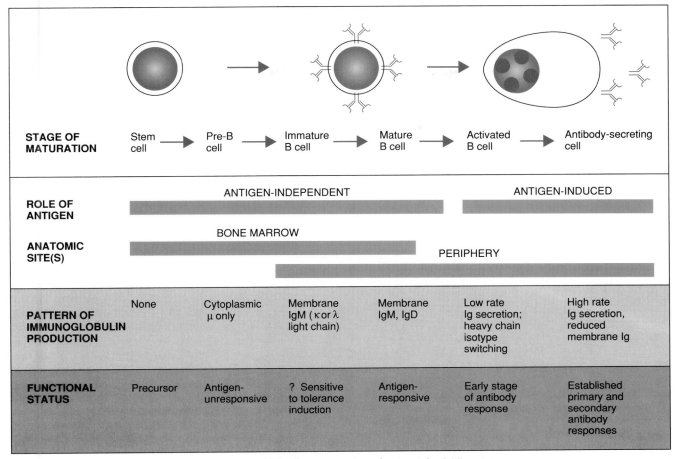

STAGE OF MATURATION	Stem cell →	Pre-B cell →	Immature B cell →	Mature B cell →	Activated B cell →	Antibody-secreting cell

	ANTIGEN-INDEPENDENT				ANTIGEN-INDUCED	
ROLE OF ANTIGEN	▬▬▬▬▬▬▬▬▬				▬▬▬▬▬▬▬▬▬	
	BONE MARROW					
ANATOMIC SITE(S)	▬▬▬▬▬▬▬		PERIPHERY			

PATTERN OF IMMUNOGLOBULIN PRODUCTION	None	Cytoplasmic μ only	Membrane IgM (κ or λ light chain)	Membrane IgM, IgD	Low rate Ig secretion; heavy chain isotype switching	High rate Ig secretion, reduced membrane Ig
FUNCTIONAL STATUS	Precursor	Antigen-unresponsive	? Sensitive to tolerance induction	Antigen-responsive	Early stage of antibody response	Established primary and secondary antibody responses

FIGURE 4–1. Sequence of B lymphocyte maturation and antigen-induced differentiation.

proliferate and differentiate, producing an increasing proportion of their Ig in a secreted form and progressively less in a membrane-bound form. Some of the progeny of activated B cells undergo **heavy chain class (isotype) switching** and begin to express Ig heavy chain classes other than μ and δ, e.g., γ, α, or ε. Other activated B lymphocytes may not secrete antibody but instead persist as membrane Ig–expressing **memory cells.** Memory cells survive for weeks or months without further antigenic stimulation and actively recirculate between the blood, lymph, and lymphoid organs. The stimulation of memory B cells by antigen leads to the secondary antibody response. Memory B cells generally express Ig molecules whose affinities for antigens are higher than those of their unstimulated clonal precursors. Antigen-induced differentiation of mature or memory B lymphocytes culminates in the development of **antibody-secreting cells,** some of which can be morphologically identified as plasma cells. In the blood or lymphoid tissues of normal individuals, the majority of B cells are IgM+ or IgM+IgD+. (For the sake of convenience, we will refer to the changes that occur in lymphocytes prior to antigen exposure as "maturation" and to antigen-induced alterations as "differentiation." These terms, however, are often used interchangeably in the immunology literature.)

Every lymphocyte that is committed to become a B cell specific for a foreign antigen is capable of maturing and differentiating through all these stages, with their distinct patterns of Ig production. Although the members of each B cell clone express the same V region and maintain essentially the same antigen specificity, subtle changes do occur. In particular, the average affinity of the secreted antibody and of membrane Ig on antigen-specific B cells increases after antigenic stimulation and is substantially higher in secondary than in primary antibody responses. This is called **affinity maturation** and is a property of humoral immune responses to protein antigens. Affinity maturation is measured at the population level, i.e., at the level of the entire antibody response. It arises from small mutations in the DNA coding for Ig V regions in individual, antigen-stimulated B lymphocytes, leading to an increase in the affinity of Ig produced by these cells. The mechanisms and consequences of somatic mutations in Ig genes are discussed later in this chapter.

Two other features of Ig production by B cells are noteworthy. First, each B cell clone and its progeny are specific for only one antigenic determinant. It is, therefore, necessary for each B cell to express only one set of Ig heavy and light chain V genes throughout its life, even though all heterozygous individuals inherit two sets of Ig genes, one from each parent. A single specificity is maintained because only one of the two parental alleles of Ig is expressed by every B cell clone from its earliest maturational stage. This phenomenon is called **allelic exclusion** and is characteristic of both B and T lymphocyte receptors for antigens. Second, each B cell clone produces either a κ or a λ light chain (but not both), and although heavy chain class switching occurs following activation, switches from one light chain class to the other do not occur throughout the life of each clone. This is called **light chain isotype exclusion.**

The pattern of Ig expression is a particularly useful marker for the stages of B cell maturation. There are two main reasons for this. First, at each stage of maturation there is an excellent correlation between the function of a B cell and the type of Ig it produces. Second, Ig is unique to B cells and is the protein primarily involved in their cognitive and effector functions. Much of our current understanding of B cell ontogeny, especially the regulation of Ig gene expression, is based on analyses of B cells during fetal life and of tumors that correspond to distinct maturational stages of B lymphocytes. Such tumors appear spontaneously in man and in experimental animals and can also be induced by oncogenic viruses *in vivo* and *in vitro*. Recently, methods have been developed for culturing mouse bone marrow stem cells on monolayers of marrow stromal cells and matrices. Pre-B cells as well as surface IgM-expressing B lymphocytes arise in these cultures, and such techniques should prove useful for defining the ontogeny of normal untransformed B cells.

In summary, analyses of the antibody repertoire and B lymphocyte maturation and differentiation have led to the following general conclusions.

1. Each clone of B cells produces one set of Ig heavy chain and light chain V regions, and different clones produce Igs with different V regions.

2. During the life history of each clone, the same heavy chain V region is expressed in association with membrane or secreted forms of C regions and with C regions of different isotypes. In contrast, the light chain C region remains the same.

3. The specificities of V regions in each B cell and its progeny remain essentially unaltered but are "fine-tuned" after antigenic stimulation, leading to affinity maturation.

Molecular biologic analyses have proved invaluable for elucidating the mechanisms of antibody production, including the generation of diversity, allelic exclusion, Ig secretion, heavy chain isotype switching, and affinity maturation. It is now clear that these processes are regulated by changes in the organization of Ig genes and by the transcription and translation of these genes. In the remainder of this chapter, we will focus on the expression of Ig genes, beginning with the earliest events in committed B lymphocytes and proceeding through the various stages of B cell maturation and differentiation.

Rearrangement of Immunoglobulin Genes
Discovery of Ig Gene Rearrangement

The first hypothesis about the organization of the genes that coded for different portions of Ig molecules was proposed even before B lymphocytes were recognized as antibody-producing cells. It was known in the 1950s that each chain of antibody molecules consisted of highly diverse V regions, which conferred upon them specificity for antigens, and relatively invariant C regions. Moreover, each C region had to be the product of a single allelic gene locus because in any individual the C regions present on all the antibodies of a particular isotype, irrespective of their antigenic specificities, contained sequences that were inherited in mendelian fashion. (These sequences constitute the allotypes of antibodies and have been described in Box 3–2, Chapter 3.) This apparent diversity of V regions and constancy of C regions of antibody molecules created a paradox, since the V and C regions made up one polypeptide chain and it was believed at that time that one protein was always encoded by one gene. Therefore one would have to propose that only the variable portion of this putative gene was subject to extensive alterations or mutations. Realizing this paradox, Dreyer and Bennett postulated in 1965 that each antibody chain was actually encoded by at least two genes, one variable and the other constant, and the two became joined at the level of the DNA or messenger RNA (mRNA) to give rise to functional Ig proteins.

Formal proof of this hypothesis came over a decade later. In a landmark study, Susumu Tonegawa and his colleagues demonstrated that the structure of Ig genes in the cells of an antibody-producing tumor, called a myeloma or plasmacytoma, is different from that in embryonic tissues not committed to Ig production (which would be the same as all adult non-lymphoid cells, as we now know). This observation is best demonstrated by a technique called Southern blot hybridization, which is used to examine the sizes of DNA fragments produced by enzymatic digestion of genomic DNA (Box 4–1). By this method it has been shown that *the sizes of DNA fragments containing Ig genes are different in cells that do and do not make antibody* (Fig. 4–2). The explanation for these different sizes is that V and C regions for any Ig light (L) or heavy (H) chain are encoded by different gene segments that are located far apart in embryonic cells and are brought close together in cells committed to antibody synthesis, i.e., B lymphocytes. *Thus, Ig genes undergo a process of somatic DNA recombination or rearrangement during B cell ontogeny.* These findings provided the first clear molecular explanation for the production of antibodies. The current concepts are best understood by describing the unrearranged, or germline, configuration of Ig genes, and then the pat-

B O X   4 – 1.   SOUTHERN BLOT HYBRIDIZATION

This technique, introduced by E. M. Southern, is used to characterize the organization of DNA surrounding a specific nucleic acid sequence, e.g., a particular gene. In a typical experiment, genomic DNA is chemically extracted from the nuclei of isolated cells or from whole tissues. At this point, the DNA will be present in extremely long segments and must be broken down into smaller fragments for analysis. This is accomplished by enzymatic

cleavage with **restriction endonucleases.** (These bacterial enzymes are so named because they function to restrict the survival of foreign bacterial DNA in a host strain by cleaving DNA at specific internal sites as opposed to digesting DNA from the ends as an exonuclease would.) Restriction endonucleases cleave double-stranded DNA only at positions of particular symmetric nucleotide sequences, usually about 6 bp in length. Such sequences

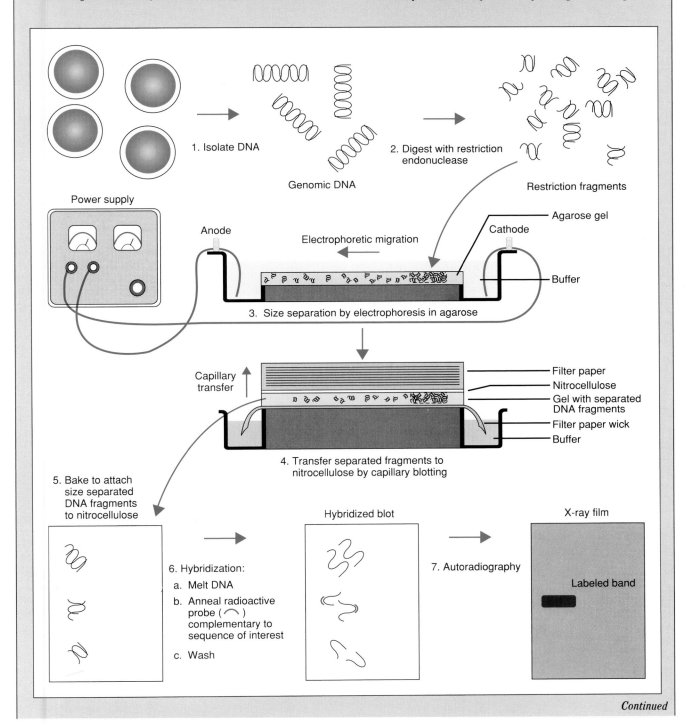

1. Isolate DNA

Genomic DNA

2. Digest with restriction endonuclease

Restriction fragments

Power supply

Anode

Electrophoretic migration

Cathode

Agarose gel

Buffer

3. Size separation by electrophoresis in agarose

Capillary transfer

Filter paper
Nitrocellulose
Gel with separated DNA fragments
Filter paper wick
Buffer

4. Transfer separated fragments to nitrocellulose by capillary blotting

5. Bake to attach size separated DNA fragments to nitrocellulose

6. Hybridization:
   a. Melt DNA
   b. Anneal radioactive probe (⌒) complementary to sequence of interest
   c. Wash

Hybridized blot

7. Autoradiography

X-ray film

Labeled band

Continued

are called **restriction sites,** and each site is uniquely recognized by a particular restriction endonuclease. Within the genome of an individual, restriction sites are present at the same positions in every cell, barring somatic mutation or DNA rearrangement. Complete digestion with a particular enzyme leads to cleavage of the genomic DNA, giving rise to an array of DNA fragments ranging from about 0.5 to 10 kb in size. Different restriction endonucleases produce different arrays of **restriction fragments,** but each enzyme generally produces the same fragments from the DNA of every cell from an individual. This, of course, is not the case when one examines genes that rearrange in different ways in different clones of cells, such as Ig and T cell receptor genes.

To analyze the fragments, the digested DNA is separated according to size by electrophoresis in an agarose gel. The separated fragments are transferred by capillary action (blotting) from the gel to a membrane of nitrocellulose or nylon. Each fragment is then attached in place to the membrane by heating or ultraviolet irradiation. The net result is that the array of fragments is arranged by size on the membrane. Any particular nucleic acid sequence, such as a gene of interest, will be present on one or two unique-sized fragments, depending only on the choice of restriction endonuclease and the distances between the relevant restriction sites that flank the gene or are located within the gene.

The analysis is completed by ascertaining the size of the restriction fragment(s) that contains the gene of interest. This is accomplished by nucleic acid **hybridization.** Double-stranded DNA can be "melted" into single-stranded DNA by changing temperature and solvent conditions. When the temperature is lowered, single-stranded DNA will reanneal to form double-stranded DNA. The rate at which reannealing of a sequence occurs is determined by the concentration of DNA containing complementary nucleic acid sequences present in the system. In the Southern blot hybridization technique, the DNA on the membrane is melted and then allowed to reanneal ("hybridize") in the presence of a solution containing a large excess of single-stranded DNA (probe) with a sequence complementary to the gene of interest. The probe, which is called a "complementary DNA" (cDNA) probe, is labeled

with radioactive phosphorus. It preferentially anneals to the melted DNA on the membrane only at the position of the restriction fragment that contains the complementary sequence. After excess probe is removed by washing, the location of the bound probe is determined by autoradiography and compared with the positions of DNA fragments of known size. By varying the conditions of the hybridizations and of the subsequent washing steps, one can control the quantity of probe that remains bound as a function of sequence complementarity. Practically, this means that at "high stringency" the probe may need to be an exact complement of the gene of interest, whereas at "low stringency" one can identify related but non-identical sequences.

Restriction sites are generally located at the same positions in the genomes of all individuals of a species. Occasionally, this is not true and a particular restriction site is present only in or near some allelic forms of a gene. This variability in the presence of a particular restriction site leads to variability in the length of the restriction fragment that is detected by Southern blot hybridization using a probe that hybridizes near the variable restriction site. The length of the fragment is inherited as a mendelian allele, and its variation among individuals is described as a **restriction fragment length polymorphism** (RFLP). Southern blotting for RFLPs is now commonly used to study the inheritance of nearby ("linked") genes.

Nucleic acid electrophoresis, blotting, and hybridization with cDNA probes have also been used to analyze mRNA molecules. In this case, mRNA is isolated from the cell of interest and subjected to electrophoresis without digestion; mRNA is already single-stranded, but the gel electrophoresis is run under denaturing conditions to prevent internal hybridization. The position of probe binding can indicate the size of the mRNA (rather than of a restriction fragment of DNA), and the extent of probe binding correlates with the abundance of mRNA present in the cell. This technique for RNA analysis is now universally referred to as **Northern blotting,** a biochemist's joke alluding to the DNA blotting technique introduced by Southern that now bears his name.

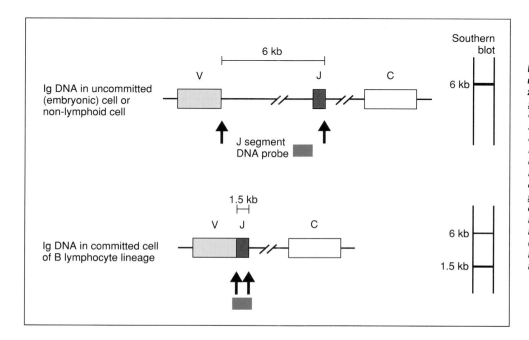

FIGURE 4–2. Detection of Ig gene rearrangement by Southern blot hybridization. In this hypothetical example, genomic DNA from an embryonic or non-lymphoid cell is cut by a restriction enzyme at sites shown by bold arrows, producing a 6 kb fragment that is detected by Southern blot hybridization using a J segment–specific DNA probe. In a clone of B cells, the same enzyme generates a 1.5 kb fragment, because VJ rearrangement has led to the deletion of the DNA between the rearranged gene segments. (Note that a 6 kb band persists in the B cells; this band is derived from the unrearranged allelic locus.)

tern and mechanisms of their rearrangement during B cell development.

Genomic Organization of Immunoglobulin Genes

The organization of Ig genes* in the germline is fundamentally similar in all species studied. Genes encoding the two light chains, κ and λ, and the single locus containing the various heavy chain genes are located on different chromosomes. Each set has a similar basic organization, which is illustrated for mouse and human Ig genes in Figs. 4–3 and 4–4, respectively.

The Ig heavy and light chain loci are composed of multiple genes that give rise to the V and C regions of the proteins, separated by stretches of non-coding DNA. At the 5' end of each Ig locus are the **V region exons,** each about 300 base-pairs (bp) long, separated from one another by non-coding DNA of varying lengths. About 90 bp 5' of each V region exon is a small (60 to 90 bp long) exon that encodes the translation initiation signal and 20 to 30 amino terminal residues of the translated protein. These residues are moderately hydrophobic and make up the **signal** or **leader peptides.** Leader sequences are found in secretory and transmembrane proteins, and are involved in guiding the emerging polypeptides during their synthesis on ribosomes into the lumen of the endoplasmic reticulum. Here, the leader sequences are rapidly cleaved and lost from the mature proteins, probably before translation is complete. The numbers of V genes (used here synonymously with V region exons) in the mouse vary from two for λ chains to about 1000 for heavy chains and can be found over large stretches of genomic DNA, at least 1000 to 2000 kilobases (kb) long (Figs. 4–3 and 4–4). The numbers of V genes in other species are not as well defined. In all species examined to date, V genes are organized into multiple **families.** The members of each family are identical at more than 80 per cent of their nucleotide sequences and usually share less than 70 per cent homology with other families. Each family is thought to have originated by duplication of a single V gene. The "com-

plexity" of a family is defined by the number of genes in that family. In the mouse H chain, for instance, there are at least nine V gene (V_H) families, each consisting of two to 60 members. The sizes and complexities of V gene families in other Ig loci and other species are not fully known yet.

At varying distances 3' of the V genes are the **C region genes.** In both mouse and man, the κ light chain locus has a single C gene, λ has three to six, and the genes for heavy chain C regions (C_H) of different isotypes are arranged in a tandem array whose order is characteristic for each species. Each heavy chain C region gene actually consists of three to four exons (each similar in size to a V region exon) that make up the complete C region, and smaller exons that code for the carboxy terminal transmembrane and cytoplasmic domains of the heavy chains. Between the V and C genes, and separated by introns of varying lengths, are additional coding sequences, 30 to 50 bp long, which make up the **joining (J) segments** and, in the H chain locus only, the **diversity (D) segments.** The J and D gene segments code for the carboxy terminal ends of the V regions, including the third hypervariable (complementarity-determining) regions of antibody molecules. Thus, in an Ig light chain protein (κ or λ), the variable region is encoded by the V and J exons and the constant region by a C exon (which does not have transmembrane or cytoplasmic segments). In the heavy chain protein, the variable region is encoded by the V, D, and J exons. The constant region of the protein is derived from the multiple C exons and, for membrane-associated heavy chains, the exons encoding the transmembrane and cytoplasmic domains (Fig. 4–5).

Based on the tandem organization of V and C genes in each Ig locus and on the structural homologies between them, it is likely that these genes evolved from repeated duplication of a primordial gene. Each V and C exon codes for an individual domain of an antibody molecule. Other proteins that contain Ig-like disulfide-bonded domains are considered to be members of the Ig gene superfamily (see Box 7–3, Chapter 7) and are encoded by genes that are homologous to Ig V and C genes.

Although the introns and the non-coding DNA sequences between exons are not expressed in mature mRNA, they play an important role in the production of antibodies. As we shall see later, recognition sequences that dictate rearrangement of various exons are present in the non-coding DNA and nucleotide sequences that regulate transcription and RNA splicing are located in the introns.

Sequence of Immunoglobulin Gene Rearrangement

All cells except B lymphocytes contain Ig genes in the germline configuration, and only B lymphocytes express these genes in functionally rearranged forms, capable of giving rise to functional proteins. The stim-

---

* In the Ig loci, the term "gene" refers either to the DNA encoding an entire heavy or light chain polypeptide, or to segments of DNA encoding only the V or C regions. In the germline, the V and C region "genes" are separated from one another by large stretches of DNA that are never transcribed. Each V and C region "gene" may actually be composed of segments of DNA that encode sequences present in the mature mRNA; these DNA segments are called **exons.** For instance, each C_H gene that gives rise to a heavy chain C region is composed of five to six exons. Exons are separated by pieces of DNA, called **introns,** that are transcribed and present in the primay (nuclear) RNA but are absent from the mRNA. The removal of introns from the primary transcript is the process of RNA **splicing.** Sometimes, the terms "gene" and "exon" are used interchangeably. For instance, "V gene" might refer to the gene coding for the complete V region of an Ig heavy or light chain, which actually consists of a V region exon and additional segments (J and D, as we shall see later), or "V gene" might refer to a V region exon only (as in "V gene families," discussed in this chapter).

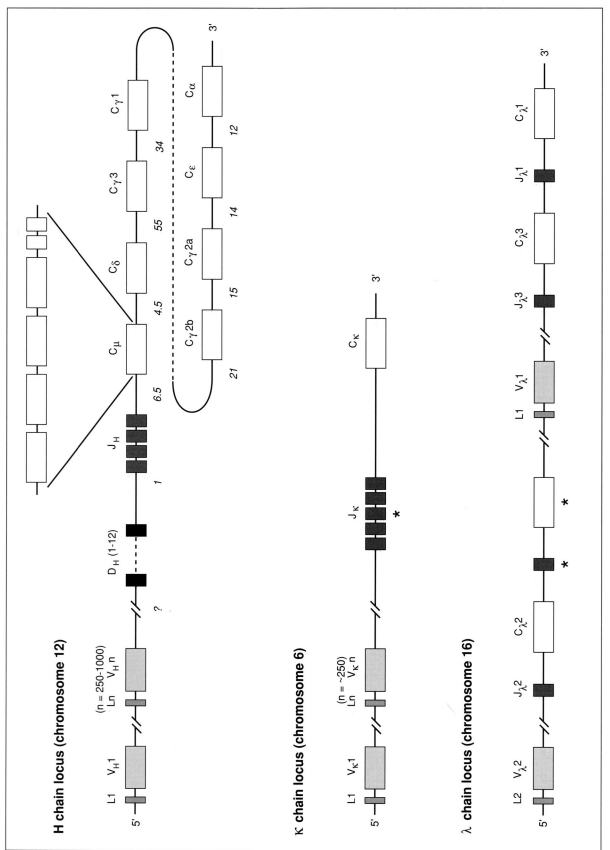

H chain locus (chromosome 12)

κ chain locus (chromosome 6)

λ chain locus (chromosome 16)

FIGURE 4–3. Organization of mouse Ig genes in the germline. *Sizes of exons and intervening DNA segments are not to scale. Numbers in italics refer to approximate lengths of DNA segments in kilobases (kb). Asterisks indicate nonfunctional pseudogenes. Each C_H gene is shown as a single box but is composed of several exons; the actual exon composition of C_H genes is shown for μ only. Gene segments are indicated as follows: L, leader; V, variable; D, diversity; J, joining; C, constant.*

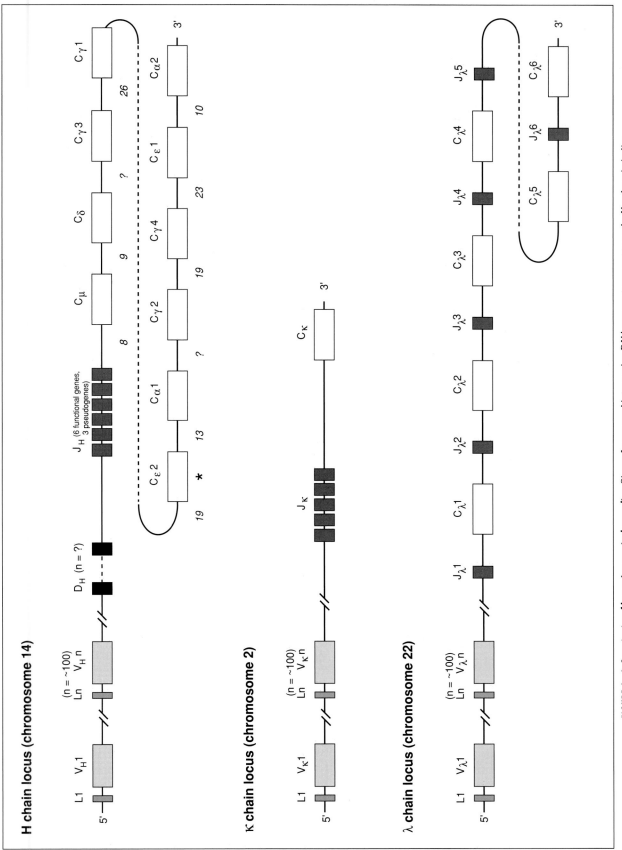

FIGURE 4 – 4. Organization of human Ig genes in the germline. *Sizes of exons and intervening DNA segments are not to scale. Numbers in italics refer to approximate lengths of DNA segments in kilobases (kb). Asterisks indicate nonfunctional pseudogenes. Each C_H gene is shown as a single box but is composed of several exons. Gene segments are indicated as follows: L, leader; V, variable; D, diversity; J, joining; C, constant.*

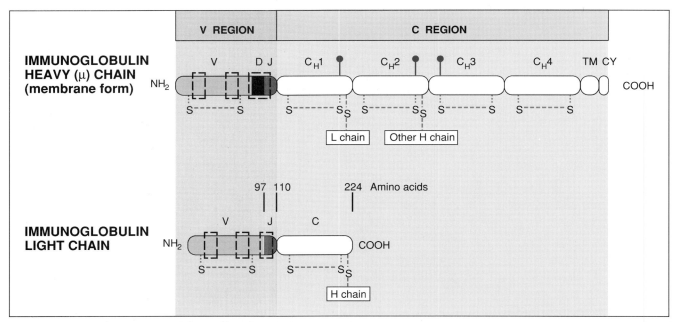

FIGURE 4 – 5. Relation of Ig gene segments to domains of Ig polypeptide chains. *The V and C regions of Ig polypeptides are encoded by different gene segments. The locations of intrachain and interchain disulfide bonds (S—S) and of carbohydrates (♦) as shown are approximate. Areas in dashed boxes indicate hypervariable (complementarity determining) regions. In the μ chain, transmembrane (TM) and cytoplasmic (CY) domains are encoded by separate exons. In the light chain, numbers refer to positions of amino acids; see Figure 3–3 for the locations of these residues in the three-dimensional structure.*

uli that determine the commitment of a bone marrow stem cell to mature along the B lymphocyte lineage are largely unknown. Such commitment, however, leads to somatic recombination or rearrangement of Ig genes. *DNA rearrangements in Ig gene loci occur in a precise order;* this explains the pattern of B cell maturation described earlier (see Fig. 4–1). The first rearrangement involves the heavy chain locus and leads to the joining of one D and one J segment with deletion of the intervening DNA (Fig. 4–6). The D segments 5′ of the rearranged D and the J segments 3′ of the rearranged J are not affected by this recombination (D1 and J2–4 in Fig. 4–6). DJ rearrangement may actually occur prior to commitment of a lymphoid precursor to the B cell lineage, because about 20 per cent of T cell–derived tumors contain DJ rearrangements in Ig heavy chain loci. Following the DJ rearrangement, one of the many V genes is joined to the DJ complex, giving rise to a rearranged VDJ gene. At this stage, all D segments 5′ of the rearranged D are also deleted. This VDJ recombination occurs only in cells committed to become B lymphocytes and is a critical control point in Ig expression because only the rearranged V gene is subsequently transcribed. The C region genes remain separated from this VDJ complex by an intron (presumably containing the unrearranged J segments), and the primary (nuclear) RNA transcript has the same organization. It is not known whether all the C regions are expressed in the primary transcript. Subsequent processing of the RNA leads to splicing out of the intron between the VDJ complex and the most proximal C region gene, which is C_μ, giving rise to a functional mRNA for the μ heavy chain. Multiple adenine nucleotides, called poly-A

tails, are added to one of several consensus polyadenylation sites located 3′ of the C_μ RNA. Genes coding for other C_H classes also have 3′ polyadenylation sites, which are utilized when these C regions are expressed (see below). It is thought that cleavage of the primary RNA transcript and splicing are tightly coupled to polyadenylation, since most functional, complete mRNAs have poly-A tails. How these events are coordinately regulated is not known. Translation of the μ heavy chain mRNA leads to production of the μ protein, giving rise to the "cytoplasmic μ only" phenotype of the pre-B lymphocyte.

The next somatic DNA recombination involves a light chain locus (κ and then λ; see below) and follows an essentially similar sequence (Fig. 4–7). One V segment is joined to one J segment, forming a VJ complex, which remains separated from the C region by an intron, and this gives rise to the primary RNA transcript. Splicing of the intron from the primary transcript joins the C gene to the VJ complex, forming an mRNA that is translated to produce the κ or λ protein. The light chain assembles with the previously synthesized μ in the endoplasmic reticulum to form the complete membrane IgM molecule, which is expressed on the cell surface, and the cell is now the immature B lymphocyte.

Rearrangements of Ig genes are the essential first steps in the production of antibodies. *In addition, the μ heavy chain protein that is synthesized in a developing B cell itself regulates the somatic recombination of Ig genes in two ways (Fig. 4–8):*

1. First, it irreversibly inhibits rearrangement on the other chromosome, accounting for *allelic exclusion*

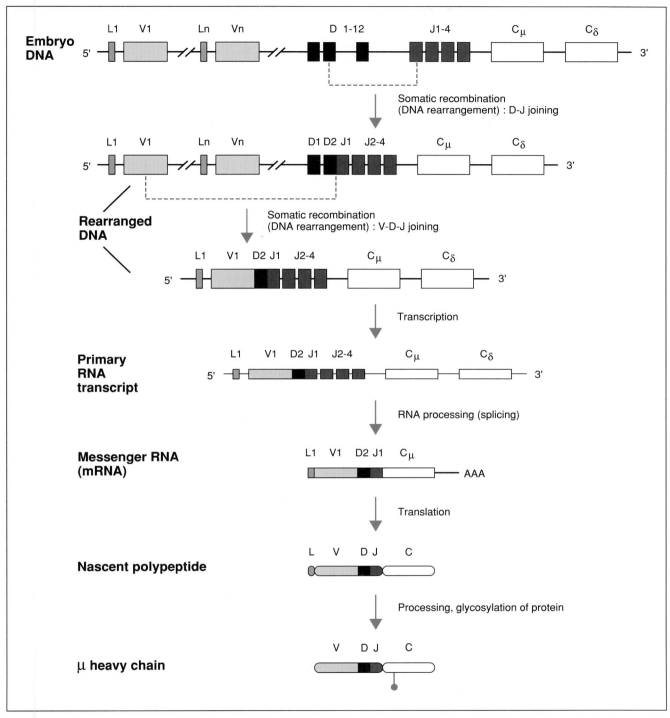

FIGURE 4 – 6. Sequence of gene rearrangement, transcription, and synthesis of the mouse Ig μ heavy chain. In this example, the V region is encoded by the exons V1, D2, and J1. V genes are indicated as V1 to Vn; C_H genes 3' of Cδ are not shown; the location of carbohydrates (●) is schematic; and gene segments and distances between them are not shown to scale.

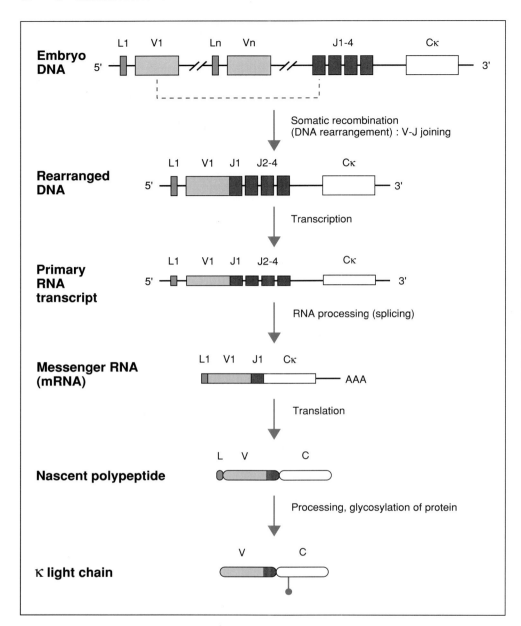

FIGURE 4–7. Sequence of gene rearrangement, transcription, and synthesis of mouse Igκ light chain. In this example, the V region is encoded by the exons V1 and J1. V genes are indicated as V1 to Vn; the location of carbohydrates (♦) is schematic; and gene segments and distances between them are not shown to scale.

of Ig heavy chains. Heavy chain genes on the second allelic chromosome will rearrange only if the first is nonproductive. Such nonproductive DNA rearrangements may be due to deletions, mutations, or frameshifts during recombination that generate stop codons. Thus, in any B cell, one heavy chain allele is productively rearranged and expressed and the other is in the germline configuration or is aberrantly rearranged. If both alleles undergo nonproductive recombinations, the cell cannot produce Ig, will be unable to recognize and respond to antigens, and presumably dies. Recently, transgenic mice have been constructed (Box 4–2) in which a rearranged membrane or secretory form of a μ gene is expressed as a transgene. Most B cells contain this transgene and

produce the encoded protein. B cells with the membrane μ transgene do not rearrange their endogenous Ig heavy chain genes, whereas the secretory μ has no effect on endogenous Ig gene rearrangement. This indicates that the membrane but not the secreted form of the μ protein suppresses heavy chain gene rearrangement and is responsible for allelic exclusion; however, the precise mechanism of this suppression is unknown.

2. The second effect of the production of a μ protein in a pre-B cell is *stimulation of light chain gene rearrangement*. This has been suggested by analyses of pre-B tumor lines in which VJ_κ rearrangements spontaneously occur in culture. Such light chain DNA recombinations are seen only in daughter cells of the

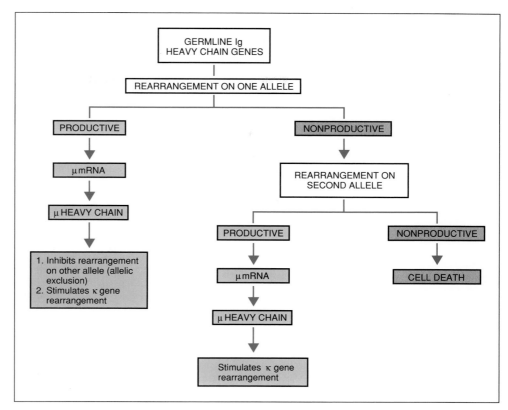

FIGURE 4–8. Order of rearrangement and expression of Ig heavy chain (μ) genes. *The consequences of productive (functional) and nonproductive (aberrant) rearrangements of Ig heavy chain genes on the two allelic chromosomes are shown. The μ chain is the first Ig protein produced in a developing B lymphocyte.*

original clone that synthesize μ protein. Again, the molecular signals by which the μ protein stimulates light chain gene rearrangement are not known.

Rearrangement of light chain genes occurs first in the κ locus (Fig. 4–9). If the κ rearrangement is productive, giving rise to a κ protein, subsequent rearrangement of the λ light chain is blocked. Rearrangement of the λ locus occurs only if the rearranged κ genes on both parental chromosomes are unable to code for a functional protein. This explains why an individual B cell clone can produce only one of the two types of light chains during its life (light chain isotype exclusion). It also accounts for the observation that in κ-producing B cells, the λ genes are in a germline or unrearranged configuration, whereas in λ-producing B cells, the κ genes on both chromosomes are either deleted or aberrantly recombined. As in the heavy chain locus, functional rearrangement involving either light chain locus on one of the two parental chromosomes actively prevents rearrangement at the other allele, accounting for allelic exclusion of light chains in individual B cells. Also, as for heavy chains, if one allele undergoes nonfunctional rearrangement, DNA recombination can occur on the other allele; however, if both alleles of both κ and λ chains are nonfunctional, that cell presumably dies.

Mechanisms of Immunoglobulin Gene Rearrangement

Rearrangement of Ig (and, as we shall discuss in Chapter 8, T cell receptor) genes occurs principally by a mechanism of excision (looping out) of the DNA between various gene segments followed by ligation of these segments. Rarely, it is possible that inversion may occur such that one gene segment is inverted and attached to another and the non-coding DNA is excised. Ig gene rearrangements represent a special kind of recombination involving non-homologous gene segments that is mediated by a system of enzymes collectively called **recombinases.** Some features of these enzymes have been deduced by transfecting fragments of germline Ig genes into various tumors or cell lines and following the spontaneous rearrangement of these genes:

1. Recombinases are cell type–specific. They are active in lymphocytes but not in non-lymphoid cells such as fibroblasts. This may explain why Ig gene rearrangement is observed only in B lymphocytes. It is, however, unlikely to be the complete answer, because the same or similar recombinases appear to act on Ig and T cell receptor genes *in vitro* and yet *in vivo*

BOX 4 – 2.   TRANSGENIC MICE

Techniques for introducing foreign genes into intact organisms are being increasingly used in many areas of mammalian biology. Much of this work has been done with mice, although the same principles are applicable to other species, such as sheep, pigs, and rabbits. Mice bearing a foreign gene introduced into their germline are called **transgenic,** and the introduced genes are called **transgenes.** In essence, this method involves microinjecting linearized DNA into the pronuclei of recently fertilized eggs, transferring the eggs into the oviducts of pseudopregnant females, and allowing development to proceed. Usually, if a few hundred copies of a gene are injected into pronuclei, about 25 per cent of the mice that are born are transgenic. The transgene integrates into a random site of breakage in a mouse chromosome. Typically, one to 50 copies of the gene integrate in a tandem, head-to-tail array at a single chromosomal site and are subsequently inherited together as a simple mendelian trait. Because integration usually occurs before DNA replication, about 70 per cent of the transgenic pups carry the transgene in all their cells, including the germ cells. The remaining 30 per cent are mosaics, indicating that integration occurred after one round of DNA replication. Such mosaicism is usually present equally in somatic and germ cells, so that lines of mice capable of transmitting the transgene can be established by breeding. In addition, the transgene inserts into one chromosome, so that the founder mouse is heterozygous. Homozygous lines can be bred if the integration of the transgene does not disrupt normal development. In most cases, the transgene is stably transmitted for many generations without detectable rearrangement.

The great value of transgenic animals derives from the observation that in most cases transgenes are expressed appropriately. Thus, if a gene is injected with its tissue-specific regulatory elements, such as promoters and enhancers (see p. 92), it will be expressed in the tissues where these regulatory elements are normally active. The level and tissue distribution of gene expression can, however, vary, depending on how many copies of the integrated transgene are expressed in different mice, the site of chromosomal integration, and other factors that remain poorly understood. Nevertheless, qualitatively the expression of a transgene seems to depend more on the presence of *cis*-acting regulatory nucleotide sequences than on chromosomal location or copy number.

Transgenic mice have been used for many different kinds of studies, some examples of which are the following:

1. To examine the effects of genes not present normally *in vivo*. Viral oncogenes can be expressed in mice in particular tissues by attaching tissue-specific promoters and enhancers to the oncogenes. Such mice may develop tumors in these tissues.

2. To study alterations in developmentally regulated genes. By introducing rearranged Ig or T cell receptor genes, transgenic mice can be created in which the rearrangement and expression of endogenous Ig and T cell receptor genes are blocked and most or all B or T cells express the transgenic Ig or T cell receptor, respectively.

3. To express normal genes in cells that do not express these genes normally, by using cell type–specific regulatory elements.

4. To delete specific cell populations with transgenes encoding toxic proteins, such as diphtheria toxin, attached to promoters and enhancers that are active only in these cells. More recently, it has become possible to specifically delete particular genes in transgenic mice using a technique called homologous recombination.

Thus, transgenic mice provide a potentially powerful approach for expressing genes in vivo that can be specifically "targeted" to particular cell or tissue types, for altering developmentally regulated gene expression, and for creating animals in which many or all cells of a particular type express a gene of interest or are deleted. As we shall see in this book, transgenic mice have already demonstrated their potential in the field of immunology.

---

complete, functional rearrangements of Ig genes occur in B cells and of T cell receptor genes in T lymphocytes.

2. Recombinases function only at the early developmental stages of B cells. They are active in immature B cells such as pre-B cell lines and tumors, but not in antibody-secreting cells like myelomas. Therefore, cells already producing functional antibodies cannot rearrange additional Ig genes and cannot alter their specificity.

The recombination mechanism appears to recognize specific DNA **recognition sequences** located in the intervening DNA 3′ of each V exon and 5′ of each J segment and flanking both sides of each D segment (Fig. 4–10). The recognition sequences are highly conserved stretches of seven or nine nucleotides separated by non-conserved 12 or 23 nucleotide spacers. In a light chain gene, each heptamer or nonamer adjacent to a V exon recognizes a complementary stretch adjacent to a J exon. This allows recombinases to bring the two exons into apposition, forming a loop of intervening DNA. Enzymes then excise the intervening DNA in this loop and anneal the ends of the V and J exons. This same basic mechanism is responsible for DJ and VDJ recombinations in the H chain locus. The term "recombinase" is used for the functional activity that mediates somatic recombination of Ig (and T cell receptor) genes. This may actually consist of multiple enzymatic activities that bring together the DNA segments of Ig and T cell receptors. Other enzymes may not be lymphocyte-specific and function like exonucleases and ligases. Recently, two genes that stimulate Ig gene recombination, called recombination activating genes 1 and 2 (RAG–1 and RAG–2), have been identified in pre-B cells. It is not known whether these two genes code for the recombinases themselves or for proteins that regulate gene rearrangement. Abnormalities in the function of recombinases lead to a failure to produce both Ig and T cell receptor proteins. This is the postulated genetic defect in a strain of mice that develop a hereditary syndrome called "severe

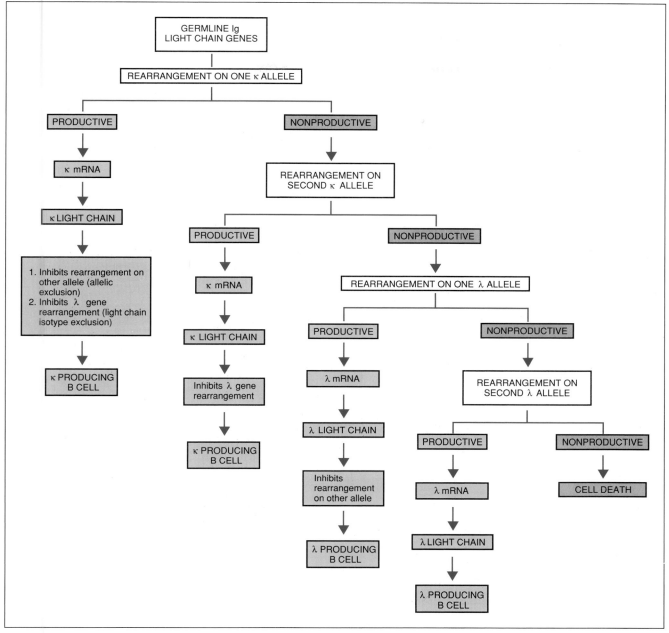

FIGURE 4 – 9. Order of rearrangement and expression of Ig light chain (κ and λ) genes. *The consequences of productive and nonproductive rearrangements of Ig κ and λ chain genes on the two allelic chromosomes are shown.*

combined immunodeficiency" (SCID), which is characterized by an almost complete absence of mature B and T lymphocytes (see Chapter 19).

Rearrangement of Ig genes during B cell development is also controlled by accessibility of the DNA to recombinases. In eukaryotic cells, most regions of DNA are covered by proteins, condensed into a structure called chromatin, which prevent the uncontrolled expression of the DNA. Early in B cell maturation the chromatin structure of Ig genes opens, so that the genes become accessible to the recombinases that mediate DNA recombination. This allows the func-

tional rearrangement and subsequent transcription of complete Ig genes.

There may also be constraints on the DNA rearrangement process such that some V genes rearrange preferentially, especially early in B cell development. For instance, if one examines large numbers of cell lines derived from pre-B cells, which have not recognized and responded to antigens, the V_H gene families that are closest to the D and J_H segments are overrepresented in proportion to their complexity relative to other, more 5' V_H families. This suggests that the recombination machinery may work by scanning

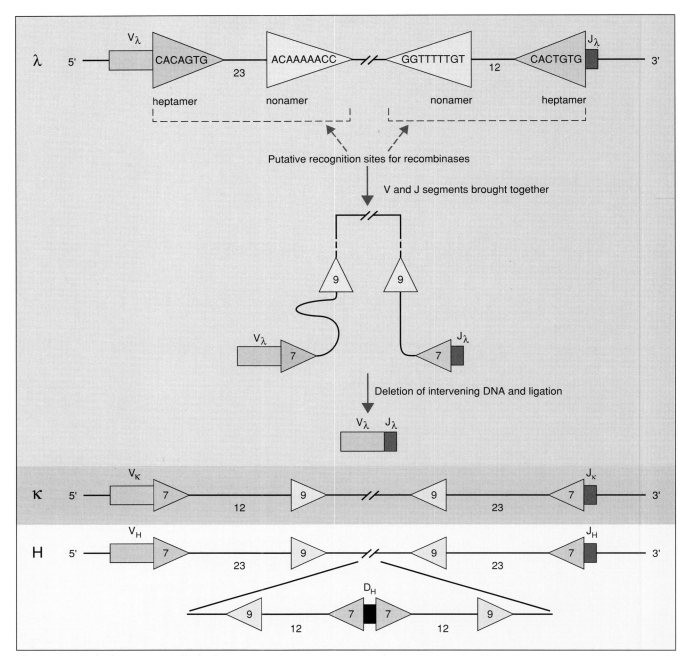

FIGURE 4 – 10. DNA recognition sequences for recombinases that mediate Ig gene rearrangement. *Heptamer and nonamer sequences, separated by 12 or 23 base pair spacers, are located adjacent to V and J exons (for κ and λ loci), or V, D, and J exons (in the H chain locus). Recombinases presumably recognize these regions and bring the exons together, forming loops of non-coding intervening DNA that are excised and the exons are joined. Alternatively, the exons can be joined by a process of inversion, followed by excision and ligation. (Adapted with permission from Tonegawa, S. Somatic generation of antibody diversity. Nature 302:575 – 581, 1983. Copyright © 1983, Macmillan Magazines Ltd.)*

upstream from the rearranged DJ_H complex and, as a result, the proximal V_H genes that are encountered early are more frequently recombined to form the VDJ_H complex. However, mature B cells in peripheral lymphoid organs do not reveal the bias in expression of V_H gene families that is seen in pre-B lines. Thus, if cell lines derived from mature B cells are examined, the frequency of different V_H families present reflects their relative size and complexity. This "correction" in V gene usage that occurs during maturation may be due to programmed changes in the development of the B cell repertoire or selection pressures imposed by environmental antigens.

Somatic Mutations in Immunoglobulin Genes

Somatic DNA recombinations involving Ig genes occur in the absence of antigenic stimulation and lead to the appearance of clones of B cells committed to recognizing different antigenic determinants. We shall summarize the mechanisms by which such rearrangements generate antibody diversity later in this chapter. After antigenic stimulation, the Ig heavy and light chain genes undergo another type of structural alteration, namely somatic mutations. *Somatic mutations in Ig genes involve primarily V genes and are principally responsible for the affinity maturation of antibodies.* In addition, mutations that alter antigen-binding specificities of Ig molecules can contribute to the generation of even more diversity of the B cell repertoire.

Comparison of V region amino acid and nucleotide sequences of IgM and IgG antibodies specific for the same antigen first revealed the existence of large numbers of point mutations in the IgG antibodies. Several features of the somatic mutations that occur in Ig genes have been established:

1. In any clone of B cells responding to a protein antigen or a hapten, the numbers of mutations in heavy and light chain V genes are higher in IgG than in IgM antibodies, increase with time after the first immunization, and are even more frequent after secondary and tertiary immunizations (Fig. 4–11). These

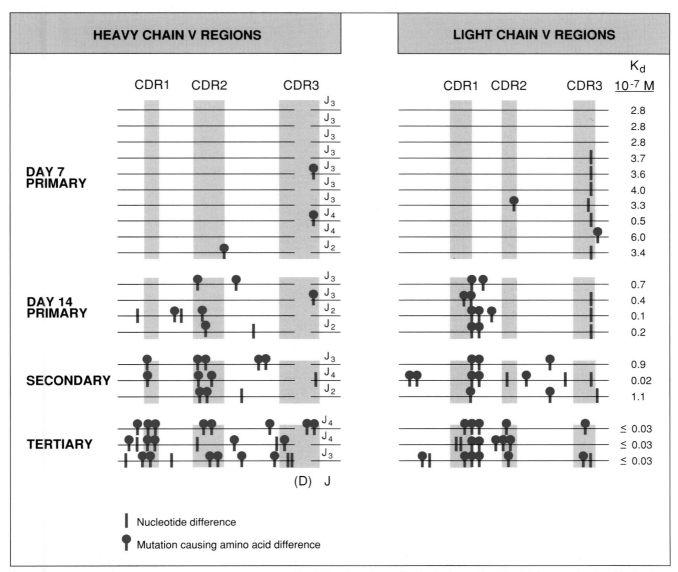

FIGURE 4 – 11. *Somatic mutations in Ig V genes. Hybridomas were produced from the spleen cells of mice immunized 7 or 14 days previously with a hapten, oxazolone, coupled to a protein, or from spleen cells obtained after secondary and tertiary immunizations with the same antigen. Hybridomas producing oxazolone-specific monoclonal antibodies were isolated, and the nucleotide sequences of the V genes encoding the Ig H and L chains were determined. Mutations in V genes increase with time after immunization and with repeated immunizations, and are clustered in the complementarity determining regions (CDRs). The location of CDR3 in the heavy chains is approximate. The affinities of the antibodies also tend to increase with more mutations, as indicated by the lower dissociation constants (K_d) for hapten binding. Note that the use of different J segments also contributes to variability of antibodies. (Adapted with permission from Berek, C., and C. Milstein. Mutation drift and repertoire shift in the maturation of the immune response. Immunological Reviews 96:23–41, 1987. Munksgaard International Publishers Ltd, Copenhagen, Denmark.)*

conclusions are based largely on comparisons of IgM- and IgG-producing antigen-specific hybridomas derived from B cells at different times after immunizations with the antigen.

2. Point mutations tend to be clustered in V region exons and adjacent flanking sequences of both H and L chains and are most numerous in the hypervariable regions (Fig. 4–11). One possible explanation for this localization of somatic mutations is that particular areas of the gene are mutation-sensitive. Alternatively, and more probably, mutations may occur randomly throughout V genes, but only the ones involving antigen-combining sites lead to increased affinities of antibodies. B cells that produce antibodies of higher affinities are positively selected by antigen. This is because as the immune response develops, more antibody is produced and the concentration of available antigen decreases. Under these conditions, B cells that bind the antigen with higher affinity are preferentially stimulated. Such high-affinity B cells also dominate secondary (IgG) antibody responses, which are stimulated by lower concentrations of antigens than primary responses; this explains the increased frequency of somatic mutations in IgG antibodies. *Thus, affinity maturation of antibody responses is due to somatic mutations in Ig V genes and subsequent selection of high-affinity clones of antigen-specific B cells.*

3. Mutations may lead to loss of antigen-binding activity, so that B cells in which this happens become antigen-unresponsive and may die. Alternatively, as a result of somatic mutations, the Ig produced by a particular B cell may no longer be specific for the immunizing antigen but may acquire a new specificity for a different antigen. This is a potential mechanism for increasing the diversity of antibodies.

4. The somatic mutation rate is estimated to be 10^{-3} per V gene base-pair per cell division, which is 10^3 to 10^4 times higher than the spontaneous rate of mutation in other mammalian genes. Because the V genes of expressed heavy and light chains in each B cell contain a total of about 700 nucleotides, this implies that mutations will accumulate in expressed V regions at an average rate of almost one per cell division. It is estimated that as a result of somatic mutations, IgG antibodies derived from one clone of B cells can diverge 1 to 5 per cent from the original germline sequence. This usually translates to less than ten amino acid substitutions because mutations located in flanking sequences or involving third-base positions may not change the V region amino acid sequence.

5. Affinity maturation is observed mostly in antibody responses to helper T cell–dependent protein antigens. Therefore, it is likely that T cells or their products are involved in stimulating mutational mechanisms or in selecting and stimulating B cells whose expressed V genes contain mutations that lead to increased antibody affinities (see Chapter 9).

The precise mechanisms of somatic mutations in Ig genes are poorly understood. Immunologists are actively searching for cell lines in which mutations can be induced *in vitro* by antigens and helper T cells or by T cell–derived cytokines. Such models should prove valuable for analyzing the extrinsic signals, enzymes, and regulatory mechanisms responsible for the extraordinarily high mutation rate in Ig V genes.

Generation of Antibody Diversity

Several different genetic mechanisms contribute to the diversity of membrane-bound and secreted antibodies in each individual. The estimated contribution of each of these mechanisms to the total repertoire of antibodies is summarized in Table 4–1.

1. *Multiple germline genes.* Both heavy chains and light chains may be encoded by multiple germline V genes, which have different sequences and produce Ig molecules with different specificities. Because D genes and J genes also encode portions of the antigen-binding regions of Ig molecules, the utilization of different germline D and J genes also contributes to diversity. The amount of diversity generated at a particular Ig locus correlates with the number of gene segments at that locus. For instance, in mice 90 to 95 per cent of antibodies produced contain κ light chains and the λ-containing antibodies recognize a quite restricted set of antigens. In mice, the λ locus contains only two functional V genes. In humans, on the other hand, the κ and λ loci contain roughly equal numbers of V genes, are equally represented in antibodies produced, and are similar in their diversity.

2. *Combinatorial diversity.* The somatic recombination of Ig DNA participates in the generation of antibody diversity in several ways. The combinatorial associations of different V, D, and J gene segments lead to a large potential for generating different antibody specificities. The maximum possible number of combinations is the product of the number of V, D (if present), and J exons at each locus. Every clone of B

TABLE 4–1. Mechanisms Contributing to the Generation of Antibody Diversity in the Mouse*

	H	κ	λ
Germline genes*			
V gene segments	250–1000	250	2
J segments	4	4	3
D segments	12	0	0
Combinatorial joining			
V × J (×D)	10,000–40,000	1000	6
H-L chain associations			
H × κ	1–4 × 10^7		
H × λ	5–10 × 10^4		
Total potential repertoire with junctional diversity	10^9–10^{11}		

* Numbers of gene segments are estimates. The mouse is unusual among all species examined because of the low number of V_λ genes and the limited diversity in antibodies with λ light chains. Apart from this, other mammalian species (including humans) are essentially similar.

BOX 4-3. IMMUNOGLOBULIN GENES IN B LYMPHOCYTE –DERIVED TUMORS

Since the presence of functionally rearranged Ig heavy and light chain genes is the *sine qua non* of a B lymphocyte, examination of tumors for the presence of such rearrangements has proved to be a useful diagnostic and analytical method. Perhaps the earliest significant result of such studies was that tumors that did not express phenotypic markers characteristic of a particular cell lineage could be classified unambiguously. For instance, the cell of origin of hairy cell leukemias was an issue of great debate until the demonstration that virtually all these tumors contained rearranged Ig genes, establishing their derivation from B lymphocytes. The expression of Ig proteins can also be used as a marker for the clonality of B cell tumors. This was initially done by analyzing the frequency of cells producing κ or λ light chains within a proliferative lesion of B lymphocytes. In humans, approximately half of all antibody molecules contain κ and half contain λ light chains. Therefore, if all the B cells in a lesion express either κ or λ, it is likely that this lesion is a monoclonal tumor. Conversely, if equal numbers of cells express κ and λ, the lesion is a polyclonal or non-neoplastic proliferation. This approach has been refined and tremendously improved by our ability to analyze Ig gene rearrangements by Southern blot hybridization, because every clone of B lymphocytes contains unique rearranged VJ and

VDJ complexes in light chain and heavy chain loci, respectively. Thus, if genomic DNA from B cell tumors is isolated and digested with a panel of restriction enzymes, and then Southern blots are probed with cDNA probes for J or C regions, the pattern of restriction fragments containing these genes is unique for each clonally derived tumor. This pattern is reflected in the bands detected by Southern blot hybridization. Provided that a sufficiently large panel of restriction enzymes is used, no two tumors will exhibit identical bands. If the lesion being studied is not a tumor but a polyclonal hyperplasia of B lymphocytes, no one rearrangement is present in enough cells to give a discernible band and a smear of DNA fragments will be visible in Southern blots. Such a distinction between hyperplastic and neoplastic lesions has important therapeutic implications. Moreover, the identification of a unique restriction fragment pattern of a B cell tumor is useful for determining if recurrences in patients are due to new tumors or to growth of tumor cells that resisted treatment. Similarly, if circulating tumor cells develop in the blood of patients with lymphoma initially confined to lymphoid organs, Southern blot analysis can establish whether or not this reflects conversion of the original lymphoma to a leukemic growth phase.

---

cells and its progeny express a unique combination of V, D, and J genes. One corollary of this observation is that every monoclonal tumor derived from a B cell is also different from all other tumors. Therefore, the pattern of Ig gene rearrangement is a useful marker for assessing the clonality of B cell–derived lymphomas and leukemias (Box 4–3). Because of combinatorial diversity, *antibody molecules show the greatest diversity at the junctions of V and C regions* in both heavy and light chains. These junctions form the third hypervariable region, or CDR3, which is the most important portion of the Ig molecule for binding antigen (see Chapter 3). The CDR3 of heavy and light chains is actually encoded in a large part by J and/or D gene segments.

3. *Junctional diversity.* Even the same set of germline V, D, and J gene segments can generate different amino acid sequences at the junctions. This additional junctional diversity arises from two mechanisms:

a. The first is inaccurate or **imprecise DNA rearrangement,** which occurs because nucleotide sequences at the 3' end of a V gene and the 5' end of a J segment in a light chain, or at the ends of V, J, and D gene segments in a heavy chain, can each recombine at any of several nucleotides in the germline sequence. As long as the recombination does not generate nonfunctional DNA, different nucleotide and, subsequently, amino acid sequences can arise (Fig. 4–12). Imprecise joining can also lead to nonfunctional recombinations that are out of frame so that the DNA cannot be transcribed, and this may be a price that is paid for generating diversity. B cells occasionally compensate for out-of-frame joining

events by deleting one or two nucleotides upstream of the joint.

b. The second mechanism for junctional diversity is **N region diversification.** Nucleotides, called N sequences, which are not present in the germline, can be added to the junctions of rearranged VJ or VDJ genes. This addition of new nucleotides is a random process probably mediated by an enzyme called terminal deoxyribonucleotidyl transferase (TdT). Because of junctional diversity, the number of different amino acid sequences that are present in the third hypervariable regions of antibody molecules is actually greater than the number of germline J and D segments present in the genome. As we shall see in Chapter 8, both junctional inaccuracies and N region addition are even more important for generating diversity in T cell antigen receptor genes than in Ig genes. In fact, T cell receptor loci contain fewer V genes and yet the potential for diversity is greater in T cell antigen receptors than in antibody molecules.

4. *Somatic mutations.* Changes in antigen-binding specificity as a result of somatic mutations in V genes can lead to a vast potential for generating additional diversity.

5. *Combinations of H and L chain proteins.* In addition to these mechanisms operative at the level of Ig genes, the combination of different H and L chain proteins also contributes to diversity because the V region of each chain participates in antigen recognition.

The expression of different germline V, D, and J genes, combinatorial VJ and VDJ associations, junctional diversity, and H–L chain associations all occur

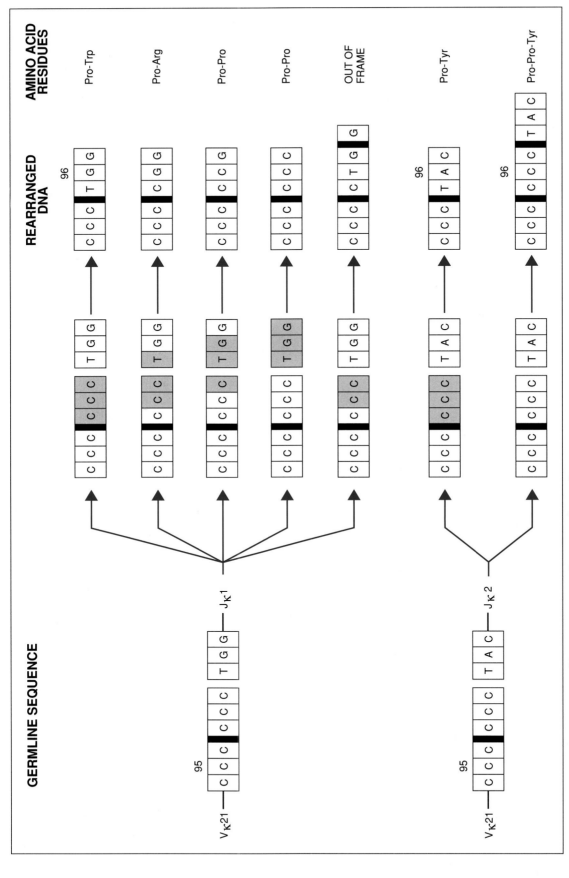

FIGURE 4–12. Generation of diversity at VJ junctions by imprecise DNA recombination. *During the joining of different V and J exons, deletion of nucleotides (indicated as shaded boxes) may lead to the generation of novel nucleotide and amino acid sequences or to out-of-frame nonfunctional recombinations. All the indicated amino acid sequences have been detected in different $V_\kappa 21$ containing mouse antibodies. Two examples are shown, one in which $J_\kappa 1$ was used and another in which $J_\kappa 2$ was used. (Adapted with permission from Weigert, M., R. Perry, D. Kelley, T. Hunkapiller, J. Schilling, and L. Hood. The joining of V and J gene segments creates antibody diversity. Nature 283:497–499, 1980. Copyright© 1980, Macmillan Magazines Ltd.)*

prior to antigenic stimulation. These are the mechanisms responsible for the diversity of the primary, or naive, B cell repertoire. Therefore, in primary antibody responses to multideterminant antigens, multiple antigen-reactive B cell clones expressing different V genes and VJ_L and VDJ_H combinations may be stimulated. This may give rise to specific antibodies with a wide range of affinities for the antigen. In contrast, the secondary antibody response to the same antigen is dominated by only a few of the clones that were stimulated by the first immunization. These clones contain numerous somatic mutations in their Ig V genes, and the cells producing Ig with the highest affinities for antigen are preferentially activated. As a result, the secondary response often consists of a more restricted population of antibodies with a higher average affinity for the antigen.

It is also interesting that in the naive repertoire of B cells in an individual, clones specific for particular antigens may arise or mature to functional competence in a defined sequence. For instance, in inbred mice, responsiveness to the hapten 2,4,6-trinitrophenyl appears earlier in neonatal life than responsiveness to antigens on sheep erythrocytes, and other antigens can be ranked in a similar manner. This is not solely attributable to the order of V genes in the germline; i.e., the first specificities expressed, as B cells mature, are not necessarily encoded by the most 3' V genes.

EXPRESSION OF DIFFERENT CLASSES AND TYPES OF IMMUNOGLOBULINS

The molecular genetic events in the early life of a B cell, which we have described in the previous portion of the chapter, lead to the appearance of cells which express a membrane-associated IgM molecule. This IgM consists of μ heavy chains derived from one of the two parental chromosomes, complexed with κ or λ light chains also derived from one allele. The subsequent changes in Ig gene expression, other than mutations, occur only in the constant regions of heavy chains and result in the production of membrane or secreted forms of heavy chains of various isotypes. Many of these changes lead to alterations in the functions of the antibody produced by the B cell, but the antigenic specificity of each Ig-producing B cell clone is retained. For instance, the switch in Ig production from a membrane to a secreted form converts the B cell from a cognitive to an effector cell. Because different Ig heavy chain isotypes perform distinct functions, heavy chain class switching is important for the elimination of microbes that are susceptible to different effector mechanisms (see Chapter 3). We now know in considerable detail how the clonal progeny of a membrane IgM-producing B cell can express different types of Ig molecules with the same antigen-binding regions as the original, or parent, cell.

Co-expression of IgM and IgD

The mature B lymphocyte is the functionally responsive stage in B cell maturation at which membrane-associated μ and δ heavy chains are co-expressed on the surface of each cell in association with κ or λ light chains. Both classes of Ig heavy chains on each cell have the same V region and, therefore, the same antigen specificity. Simultaneous expression of a single V_H with both C_μ and C_δ to form the two heavy chains is thought to occur by alternative RNA splicing. A long primary RNA transcript is produced containing the rearranged VDJ complex as well as sequences encoded by both C_μ and C_δ genes (Fig. 4–13). If the introns are spliced out such that the VDJ complex is attached to the C_μ RNA, it gives rise to a μ mRNA. If however, the C_μ RNA is spliced out as well so that the

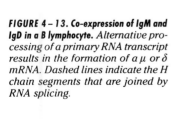

FIGURE 4–13. Co-expression of IgM and IgD in a B lymphocyte. Alternative processing of a primary RNA transcript results in the formation of a μ or δ mRNA. Dashed lines indicate the H chain segments that are joined by RNA splicing.

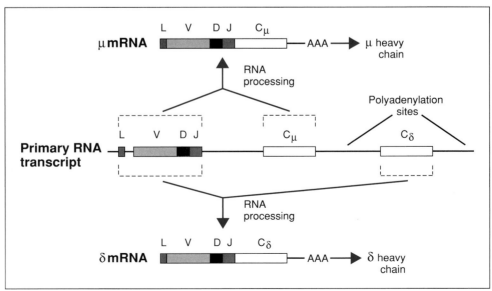

VDJ complex becomes contiguous with C_δ, a δ mRNA is produced. Subsequent translation results in the synthesis of a complete μ or δ heavy chain protein. *Thus, alternative splicing allows a B cell to simultaneously produce mature mRNAs of two different heavy chain isotypes.* The precise mechanisms that regulate the choice of polyadenylation and/or splice acceptor sites by which the rearranged VDJ is joined to C_μ or C_δ are not known, nor are the signals that determine when and why a B cell expresses both IgM and IgD rather than IgM alone.

Secretion of Immunoglobulin

Activation of a membrane Ig-expressing mature B lymphocyte by antigen leads to its proliferation and the induction of Ig secretion. Membrane and secreted Ig molecules differ at their carboxy termini (see Fig. 3–5). For instance, in secreted μ, the $C_\mu 4$ domain is followed by a tail piece containing charged amino acids. In membrane μ, on the other hand, $C_\mu 4$ is followed by a short spacer, 26 hydrophobic transmembrane residues, and a cytoplasmic tail of three amino acids (lysine, valine, and lysine). *The transition from membrane to secreted heavy chain occurs at the level of mRNA processing.* This was first suggested by the observation that in tumors with membrane IgM the size of the μ mRNA is about 2.7 kb and in tumors with secreted IgM it is about 2.4 kb. It is now believed that the primary RNA transcript in all IgM-producing B cells contains the rearranged VDJ, the four C_μ exons coding for the C region domains, a small exon immediately 3' of the fourth C_μ exon encoding the tail piece, and the two exons encoding the transmembrane and cytoplasmic domains. Alternative processing of this transcript, which is regulated by RNA cleavage and the choice of polyadenylation sites, determines whether or not the transmembrane and cytoplasmic exons are included in the mature mRNA (Fig. 4–14). If they are, the μ chain produced contains the hydrophobic amino acids that make up the transmembrane

segment and is, therefore, anchored in the lipid bilayer of the plasma membrane. If, on the other hand, the transmembrane segment is excluded from the μ chain, the carboxy terminus consists of about 20 amino acids constituting the tail piece. Since this protein does not have a stretch of hydrophobic amino acids or a positively charged cytoplasmic domain, it cannot remain anchored in the cell membrane and is secreted. Thus, each B cell can synthesize both membrane and secreted Ig. As differentiation proceeds, more and more of the Ig is secreted. All other C_H genes contain similar membrane exons, and all heavy chains can apparently be expressed in membrane-bound and secreted forms, although IgD is rarely secreted.

Heavy Chain Class (Isotype) Switching

After antigenic stimulation, mature IgM- and IgD-expressing B cells also undergo the process of heavy chain class (isotype) switching, allowing their progeny to produce antibodies with heavy chains of different classes, such as γ, α, and ϵ. Two molecular mechanisms can cause isotype switching. The first involves a linear *orderly deletion of H chain genes* and was suggested by the finding that myelomas producing one Ig isotype have deleted all rearranged C_H genes 5' of this isotype. Thus, if the C_μ and C_δ exons are deleted, the rearranged VDJ will be attached to the next C_H complex, which is $C_\gamma 3$ in the mouse, giving rise to $\gamma 3$ heavy chains; subsequent deletion of all γ subclass–encoding genes will result (in the mouse) in the production of ϵ heavy chains; and so on (Fig. 4–15A). These DNA recombination events are believed to occur at or near nucleotide sequences called **switch regions,** which are located in the introns at the 5' end of each C_H locus. Switch regions occupy distances of 1 to 10 kb and contain numerous tandem repeats of highly conserved DNA sequences, each of which is up to 52 bp long. Their precise function is not known. The

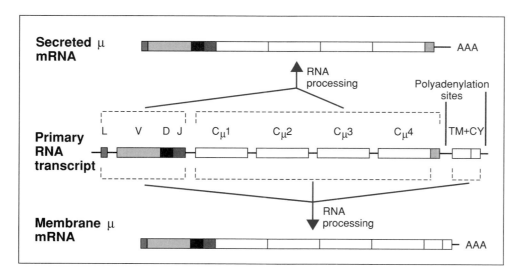

FIGURE 4–14. Expression of membrane and secreted μ chains by B lymphocytes. Alternative processing of a primary RNA transcript results in the formation of a membrane or secreted μ mRNA. Dashed lines indicate the μ chain segments that are joined by RNA splicing. TM and CY refer to transmembrane and cytoplasmic segments, respectively. $C_\mu 1$, $C_\mu 2$, $C_\mu 3$, and $C_\mu 4$ are four exons of the C_μ gene.

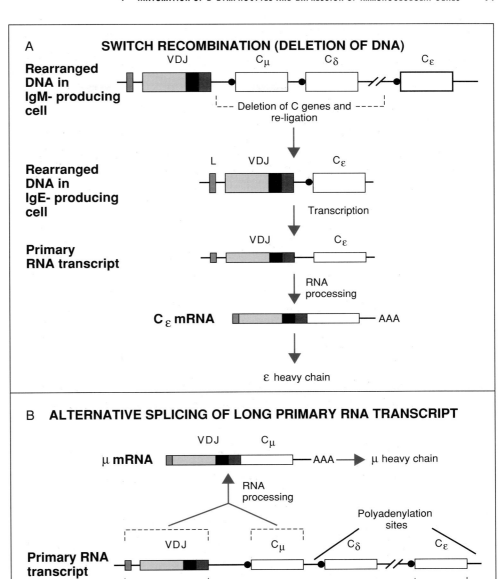

FIGURE 4–15. *Mechanisms of heavy chain class (isotype) switching.*
Heavy chain class (isotype) switching may be due to two mechanisms:
A. Switch recombination: Deletion of C_H genes, of which only C_μ and C_δ are shown, leads to recombination of the VDJ complex with the next, i.e., 3' C_H gene and expression of this gene, which is C_ϵ in the example shown. Switch regions are indicated by dark circles. (Note that the C_γ genes are located between C_δ and C_ϵ but are not shown.)
B. Alternative processing of a primary RNA transcript may lead to co-expression of multiple C_H genes, e.g., C_μ and C_ϵ.

model of linear orderly deletion of C_H genes during B cell differentiation is supported by the observation that if mouse B cells are stimulated to differentiate in culture, the temporal sequence in which different Ig isotypes are secreted often corresponds to the sequence of C_H genes in the heavy chain locus, i.e., IgM, then IgG3 and IgG1, and so on.

This model, however, does not explain the frequently observed co-expression of multiple heavy chain isotypes by single B cells in immunized animals or in antigen-stimulated cultures. Another mechanism for isotype switching is the production of a long

primary transcript containing many or all C_H genes, followed by **alternative RNA splicing** and production of different mRNAs, much like the process that leads to co-expression of μ and δ or membrane and secreted Ig (Fig. 4–15B). It is possible that early during isotype switching in each B cell clone, alternative RNA splicing leads to co-expression of multiple heavy chain classes in individual cells. As differentiation proceeds, switch recombination at the level of DNA results in the appearance of cells that produce only the more 3' heavy chain C regions. Throughout these differentiative events, the expressed VDJ complex and, therefore, the specificity of the Ig heavy chain remain unaltered (except, of course, for somatic mutations). Also, each B cell clone continues to produce only one light chain isotype, either κ or λ.

Heavy chain class switching is not a random process but is regulated by helper T cells and their secreted cytokines (see Chapter 9). For instance, the production of IgE is stimulated by a T cell–derived cytokine called interleukin-4 (IL–4), which is a necessary and sufficient "IgE switch factor." Similarly, the cytokine γ-interferon (IFN-γ) selectively induces switching to IgG2a in mice. It has been postulated that such cytokines specifically alter the structure of chromatin and/or DNA, making switch regions located 5' of particular C_H genes as well as the C_H genes accessible to factors that regulate DNA recombination and transcription. This hypothesis is supported by studies with B cell lines that normally produce IgM and can be induced to synthesize IgE by culture with IL-4, or produce IgG2a by culture with IFN–γ. In such lines, 1 to 3 days after exposure to IL-4, short "sterile" C_ϵ transcripts containing the C region but not the VDJ complex can be detected. A few days later, the complete ϵ mRNA, consisting of VDJ and C_ϵ, is produced. These findings suggest that cytokine-induced increased accessibility of the switch sites first leads to transcription detected by the presence of sterile C region transcripts, followed by DNA recombination and the production of full-length mature mRNA. T lymphocytes may not be the only regulators of heavy chain class switching. There is a strong genetic predisposition for the development of allergies, which are due to the production of IgE antibodies. IgA is synthesized mostly in mucosal lymphoid tissues, suggesting that the lymphoid microenvironment may also regulate heavy chain isotype switching. The role of cytokines in these situations is being actively investigated at present (see Chapter 9).

TRANSCRIPTIONAL AND TRANSLATIONAL CONTROL OF ANTIBODY PRODUCTION

The elucidation of the structure and expression of Ig genes during B cell maturation has been a remarkable milestone in the progress of immunology. More recently, attention has been devoted to a better understanding of the regulation of Ig gene expression. There are several reasons why this is an important area of scientific investigation. First, the production of Ig is an excellent example of the expression of cell type–specific, developmentally regulated genes. Second, changes in the pattern of Ig biosynthesis and secretion can be induced by well-defined external stimuli such as antigens, polyclonal activators, and helper T cells or T cell–derived cytokines (see Chapter 9). Finally, abnormalities in antibody production contribute to the pathogenesis of many diseases associated with deficient or excessive immune responses.

The general principles of transcriptional regulation of Ig genes are probably similar to those for other genes. Transcription is controlled primarily by *cis*-acting nucleotide sequences and by proteins that bind to these sequences. The synthesis of antibodies is also influenced by the rate of turnover of mRNAs, their translation, and the post-translational modification and assembly of heavy and light chains.

Cell Type–Specific Regulation of Immunoglobulin Gene Transcription

The transcription of most eukaryotic genes, including Ig genes, is regulated by two types of DNA sequences, called **promoters** and **enhancers.** The functions of these regulatory sequences have been defined by attaching the sequences to synthetic "reporter" genes, transfecting the constructs into cell lines, and monitoring the expression of the "reporter" mRNA and proteins. By mutating or deleting nucleotides within the regulatory sequences, it is possible to identify segments that function to varying degrees to control gene transcription.

Promoters are located immediately 5' of the site where transcription is initiated, and their principal function is to ensure accurate and efficient transcription. The basic organization of Ig promoters is similar to promoters for other genes. Ig promoters contain AT–rich sequences, called TATA boxes, located immediately 5' of each V gene segment, which function to determine where transcription is initiated by RNA polymerase II. Most Ig promoters also contain numerous DNA sequences, including a conserved octanucleotide (which is also found in other genes), that stimulate transcription of adjacent genes preferentially in lymphoid cells and are believed to be the targets of nuclear DNA–binding proteins. Such proteins are derived from other distant genes and are, therefore, said to be *trans*-acting. They are postulated to play a prominent role in regulating transcription (Box 4–4).

Enhancer elements are DNA sequences whose major function is to increase the rate of transcription of linked genes. Enhancers function in an orientation-independent manner and, unlike promoters, are capable of enhancing transcription when situated at substantial distances upstream or downstream from the gene being transcribed. Enhancers are typically tissue-specific; i.e., they function best in particular cell types and are maximally active in concert with the appropriate promoters. Such enhancer elements have been identified in mouse and human heavy and light (κ) chain loci. One mouse heavy chain enhancer is located 3' of the J_H segments, and it is believed that a consequence of VDJ recombination is to bring the promoter located 5' of a V gene closer to this enhancer, permitting more efficient initiation of transcription (Fig. 4–16). Nuclear factors that are activated by external stimuli and bind to Ig heavy and κ chain en-

BOX 4 – 4. NUCLEAR FACTORS AND THE REGULATION OF Ig GENE TRANSCRIPTION

The transcriptional activity of Ig genes, like that of other genes, is regulated by two *cis*-acting elements, promoters and enhancers. Deletion and mutational analyses have revealed the existence of several critical nucleotide sequences in Ig promoters and enhancers that are necessary for their function. Some of these sequences are active preferentially in B cells, whereas others stimulate transcription of a wide variety of genes in addition to Ig in diverse cell types. In general, the Ig heavy chain enhancer functions maximally in concert with the heavy chain promoter in B cells and serves to facilitate the formation of stable transcription-initiation complexes.

The functions of promoters and enhancers are controlled by **trans-acting nuclear factors.** These factors are also called **DNA – binding proteins** because they bind to specific nucleotide sequences in promoters and enhancers and are capable of inhibiting or stimulating the activities of these regulatory DNA elements. In many cell types, particular DNA – binding proteins are induced or activated by stimuli that elicit biologic responses. Therefore, DNA – binding proteins may provide an important link between external stimulation of a cell and the subsequent response, which leads to specific changes in gene expression.

Several *assays* for DNA – binding proteins have been described:

1. *DNA footprinting.* If a segment of DNA has a protein bound to it, that segment will be resistant to digestion by deoxyribonuclease (DNase). If a radioactively labeled DNA fragment (probe) is incubated with a putative DNA-binding protein, digested, and electrophoresed to separate fragments of different sizes, the protected fragments that contain bound proteins will resist enzymatic degradation and, therefore, will not be detected as digested pieces. Thus, each protected DNA sequence with associated protein will exhibit a characteristic "footprint."

2. *Methylation interference.* The same principle is used in an assay in which specific nucleotides are methylated, and attached methyl groups detected by cleavage at methylated G residues and electrophoresis. Bound proteins interfere with methylation and, therefore, create detectable "gaps" in the pattern of methylation.

3. *Gel retardation.* If a putative DNA – binding protein contained in a cell extract is incubated with a radioactively labeled target nucleotide sequence *in vitro* and then electrophoresed, the complex that is formed will migrate slowly in comparison to the nucleotide sequence alone. Thus, retardation of the target nucleotide indicates an increase in size as a consequence of the binding of a protein.

Using such assays, nuclear factors have been described that bind to several sites in the promoters and enhancers of Ig genes. Ig heavy chain promoters contain a conserved octanucleotide (ATGCAAAT) that is also present in the κ chain promoter, in reverse orientation in the Ig heavy chain enhancer, and in many non-Ig promoters as well. Transcription of Ig genes in B cells is critically dependent on the presence of an intact octamer motif in promoters. At least three proteins that specifically bind to the octamer have been isolated from nuclear extracts of mammalian cells. One, called Oct1 (or OTF1, for Octamer Transcription Factor 1), is a ubiquitous mammalian transcription activator. Two others, Oct2 (OTF2A) and OTF2B, are lymphoid-specific and activate transcription of Ig genes. Oct2 has recently been molecularly cloned and has been shown to contain a domain homologous to a homeobox motif, which was originally identified as a component of *Drosophila* genes involved in morphogenesis. Expression of Oct2 cDNA in non-lymphoid cell lines strongly activates co-transfected "reporter" genes if these genes are linked to octamer-containing Ig promoter sequences. Such experiments provide formal proof of the specificity and transcriptional activity of DNA – binding proteins like Oct2. The mouse κ chain enhancer contains a 10 bp sequence that is the target of a DNA – binding protein called NF – κB (NF = nuclear factor). The NF – κB site is present in many other genes, such as the gene encoding the cytokine interleukin-2 (see Chapter 7). NF – κB has some particularly interesting properties. It is inactive in pre-B cell lines, which do not transcribe κ genes constitutively. Treatment of such cell lines with lipopolysaccharide (LPS) induces functional NF – κB and coordinately stimulates κ gene transcription. Recent experiments suggest that NF – κB is present in the cytoplasm of unstimulated cells bound to an inhibitor. Activation of the cellular enzyme protein kinase C phosphorylates and then releases this inhibitor and presumably allows NF – κB to migrate to the nucleus, bind to the κ enhancer, and stimulate transcription. Interestingly, as we shall see in Chapter 9, stimulation of B cells by antigens that bind to membrane Ig generates a number of intracellular "second messengers," one of which is active protein kinase C, and LPS may also activate this enzyme. Moreover, NF – κB is inactive or absent in myeloma cells that do actively synthesize κ chains, suggesting that this nuclear factor and, by implication, the κ enhancer may be required early in B cell differentiation to initiate κ gene transcription but are not needed to maintain transcription later in development.

Research in *trans*-acting transcription factors and the regulation of cell type – specific gene expression is still in its infancy. Nevertheless, it is possible to come to some basic, albeit tentative, conclusions about the *general properties* of DNA – binding proteins.

1. Many DNA – binding proteins are widely distributed among different cell types and are not specific for particular genes.

2. Their activity may be inducible by external stimuli and may be related to the maturational stage of the cell.

3. They have positive and negative effects whose interplay determines the net level of gene transcription.

4. Although DNA – binding proteins are widely distributed, some of them do have effects that are cell type – specific and/or developmentally regulated. This may be because the binding sites on promoters and enhancers are unique and regulated or because of endogenous inhibitors whose activity is specifically altered by cellular maturation or stimulation.

---

hancers have also been identified. The interactions of these protein factors with one another and with regulatory DNA sequences may be critical for stimulating cell type – specific Ig gene transcription in response to external signals and spontaneously during B cell maturation (Box 4 – 4).

Since Ig genes are transcriptionally active in B cells and are sites for multiple DNA recombinational

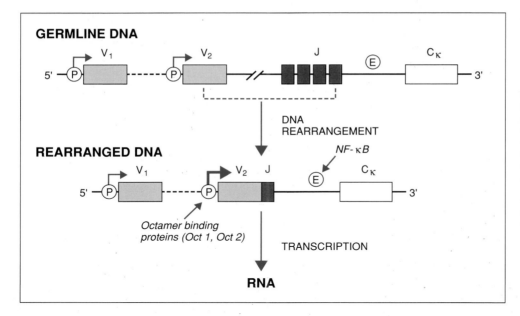

GERMLINE DNA

REARRANGED DNA

DNA REARRANGEMENT

TRANSCRIPTION

RNA

Octamer binding proteins (Oct 1, Oct 2)

NF-κB

FIGURE 4–16. Transcriptional regulation of immunoglobulin genes. *VDJ rearrangement brings promoter sequences (shown as (P)) close to the enhancer (E) located between the J and C loci, resulting in increased transcription of the rearranged V gene (V2, whose active promoter is indicated by a bold arrow). Also shown are the sites of binding of the nuclear factors Oct1, Oct2 and NF–κB.*

events, foreign genes can be abnormally translocated to Ig loci and, as a result, may become transcriptionally active. For instance, in certain tumors of B cells, oncogenes are translocated to switch sites located 5' of heavy or light chain C region genes. Such chromosomal translocations are frequently accompanied by enhanced transcription of the oncogenes and are believed to be one of the factors causing the development of tumors of B lymphocytes (Box 4–5).

Regulation of Messenger RNA Turnover and Translation

The turnover rate of Ig mRNA changes during B cell differentiation and correlates with the quantity of Ig synthesized. For instance, the half-life of Ig mRNA in myelomas, which actively secrete large amounts of antibodies, is as long as 20 to 40 hours; in B cell lymphomas, which produce much lower quantities of Ig only in the membrane-bound form, the half-life is less than 6 hours. This may be one of the reasons why plasma cells contain 100 to 500 times more cytoplasmic Ig mRNA than do nonsecreting B lymphocytes. Moreover, if B lymphoma cell lines are stimulated to secrete more Ig, the level of steady-state Ig mRNA increases five to ten times more than the transcription rate, as measured by nuclear run-off assays. This implies that Ig mRNA is stabilized after stimulation and its half-life is prolonged. The mechanisms that control turnover of mRNA are largely unknown.

The importance of translational control in regulating Ig production is suggested by several observations. Mature B cells, despite containing about ten times more μ mRNA (for the membrane form) than δ mRNA, express more membrane IgD than IgM. Antibody-secreting cells often contain mRNAs for the membrane forms of heavy chains even when they do not express detectable membrane Ig. Such observations indicate that translation of Ig mRNA is a regulated process that varies according to the stage of B lymphocyte maturation and differentiation, but the control mechanisms are not yet identified.

Synthesis, Glycosylation, and Assembly of Immunoglobulin Molecules

Immunoglobulin heavy and light chains, like most secreted and membrane proteins, are synthesized on membrane-bound ribosomes in the rough endoplasmic reticulum. The 5' leader peptides are cleaved co-translationally in the endoplasmic reticulum. The covalent association of heavy and light chains, created by the formation of disulfide bonds, probably occurs in the endoplasmic reticulum as well, where high-mannose oliosaccharides may be added to asparagine residues (N-linked glycosylation). Following synthesis, the polypeptide chains are directed into the cisternae of the Golgi complex, where the high-mannose carbohydrates are converted to their mature forms by the trimming of terminal mannose and the addition of other sugar side chains. Assembled antibody molecules are transported to the plasma membrane in vesicles, where they become anchored into the cell membrane or are secreted by a process of reverse pinocytosis. Moreover, other proteins that bind to Ig are coordinately regulated. For instance, the "J chains" attached to IgA and IgM (see Chapter 3) are believed to be important for the polymerization of the secreted forms of these antibodies (and are not related to J gene segments in Ig loci). In cells producing such antibodies, transcriptional activation of Ig heavy and light chains is accompanied by

BOX 4 – 5.   CHROMOSOMAL TRANSLOCATIONS IN TUMORS OF B LYMPHOCYTES

Reciprocal chromosomal translocations in many tumors, including lymphomas and leukemias, were first noted by cytogeneticists in the 1960s, but their significance remained unknown until almost 20 years later. At this time, sequencing of switch regions 5' of C_H genes in B cell tumors revealed the presence of DNA segments that were not derived from Ig genes. This was first observed in two tumors derived from B lymphocytes, human Burkitt's lymphoma and murine myelomas. The "foreign" DNA was identified as a portion of the *c-myc* proto-oncogene, which is normally present on chromosome 8 in man. Proto-oncogenes are normal cellular genes that often code for proteins involved in cell growth and regulation, such as growth factors, receptors for growth factors, or transcription-activating factors. In normal cells, their expression is tightly regulated. When these genes are altered by mutations, inappropriately expressed, or incorporated into and reintroduced in cells by RNA retroviruses, they can become transcriptionally active and function as oncogenes. Such deregulation is postulated to be one of the mechanisms that lead to enhanced cellular growth and, ultimately, neoplastic transformation.

The most common translocation in Burkitt's lymphoma is t(8;14), involving the Ig heavy chain locus on chromosome 14; less commonly, t(2;8) or t(8;22) translocations are found, involving the κ or λ light chain loci, respectively. In all cases of Burkitt's lymphoma, *c-myc* is translocated to one of the Ig loci, which explains the reciprocal 8;14, 2;8, or 8;22 chromosomal translocations detectable in these tumors. Because the Ig loci normally undergo several genetic rearrangements during B cell differentiation, they are likely sites for accidental translocations of distant genes. Detailed molecular analysis has revealed differences in the architecture of the translocations in different Burkitt's lymphomas, suggesting that rearrangements are sometimes catalyzed by isotype-switching enzymes and sometimes catalyzed by VDJ recombinase enzymes.

The product of the *myc* gene most likely acts as a nuclear regulatory factor controlling the transcription of genes required for cellular proliferation. Aberrant *myc* expression can lead to the development of malignant tumors, presumably by interfering with the normal control of cell growth. Other examples of the association of aberrant *myc* expression and tumors include the oncogenic potential of the avian myelocytomatosis virus, which carries a viral homolog of *myc*, the presence of multiple (amplified) copies of the *myc* gene in the genomes of many human tumors, and the development of B cell lymphomas in mice carrying a *myc* transgene linked to an Ig promoter.

An attractive hypothesis for the etiology of Burkitt's lymphomas is that translocations of *myc* into the Ig loci transcriptionally activate the cellular oncogene, leading to malignant transformation. In fact, these translocated *myc* genes are continually transcribed in Burkitt's lymphoma cell lines but the unrearranged *myc* alleles in the same cells are not. Just how the *myc* gene becomes transcriptionally deregulated after translocation remains unknown. One possibility is that when *myc* is translocated to a site of active gene transcription, adjacent to Ig loci, the result is enhanced transcription of *myc* itself, and this leads to tumor development in the cells in which Ig genes are active, i.e., B lymphocytes. Although the regulatory components (promoters, enhancers) of the Ig genes can be very active, it is unknown whether they influence transcription of translocated *myc* genes. Several observations suggest that this is not the case. First, translocated *myc*

genes may be in the opposite transcriptional orientation (i.e., 3' to 5') to the Ig genes. Second, the 5' IgH enhancer is often lost from the site of translocation. Third, the *myc* gene may end up quite distant from the Ig gene, out of the presumed range of influence of Ig regulatory sequences. Fourth, the *myc* gene is often translocated to the excluded allele, i.e., the functionally unrearranged, transcriptionally inactive Ig locus. It is also possible that translocation removes the *myc* gene from regulatory influences of genomic sequences that are left behind on chromosome 8. As a result, the *myc* gene becomes abnormally active. Although the precise mechanisms of *myc* deregulation are not yet known, these B cell tumors may illustrate a general concept that activation of cellular oncogenes, coupled with their location next to normal genes that are functional in particular cells, may be one of the mechanisms causing neoplastic transformation of these cells.

Other oncogenes and normal cellular genes are also involved in reciprocal chromosomal translocations in lymphomas and leukemias derived from cells other than B lymphocytes. Some examples are listed in the table. Clearly, T lymphocyte–derived tumors may be analogous to B cell lymphomas, since chromosomal translocations in the former often involve loci coding for antigen receptors on T cells.

Type of Tumor	Chromosomal Translocations
B Cell – Derived	
Burkitt's lymphoma	t(8;**14**) (q24.1; **q32.3**) Less frequently, t(8;**22**) (q24.1; **q11.2**) or t(2;8) (**p12**; q24.1)
Chronic lymphocytic leukemia	t(11;**14**) (q13.3; **q32.3**)
Follicular lymphoma	t(**14**;18) (**q32.3**; q21.3)
T Cell – Derived	
Chronic lymphocytic leukemia	t(**14**;14) (**q11.2**; q32.1)
Acute lymphoblastic leukemia	t(8;**14**) (q24.1; **q11.2**) t(7;9) (**q34**; q32) Numerous others reported

The above are illustrative examples of chromosomal translocations that have been characterized in human lymphomas and leukemias. Each translocation is indicated by the letter t. The first pair of numbers refers to the chromosomes involved, e.g., (8;**14**), and the second pair to the bands of each chromosome, e.g., (q24.1; **q32.3**). The normal chromosomal locations of antigen receptor genes (indicated in bold) are as follows: IgH 14q32.3; Igκ 2p12; Igλ 22q11.2; T cell receptor α 14q11.2; T cell receptor β 7q34; T cell receptor γ 7p15; and T cell receptor δ 14q11.

The normal location of the *c-myc* oncogene is 8q24.1, and of the *bcl-2* gene is 18q21.3. The *bcl-2* gene is a human gene identified from a translocation, and recently shown to have an oncogenic effect in transgenic mice.

Courtesy of Dr. Jeffrey Sklar, Department of Pathology, Harvard Medical School and Brigham and Women's Hospital, Boston.

coordinate stimulation of J chain gene transcription and biosynthesis.

SUMMARY

The maturation of B lymphocytes is accompanied by specific changes in Ig gene structure and mRNA expression, which correspond to changes in the production of Ig molecules in different forms (Fig. 4–17). The earliest detectable change in Ig genes during B cell ontogeny is a somatic recombination of variable (V), joining (J), and, for heavy chains, diversity (D) gene segments so that one of each is assembled together on one chromosome. The recombination of Ig genes itself occurs in a precise sequence, with H chains being first, followed by κ and then λ. Functional rearrangement at each heavy or light chain locus inhibits rearrangement on the other allele (allelic exclusion). The constant (C) region heavy or light chain gene is attached to the VDJ or VJ complex by RNA splicing to generate a mature mRNA that is translated into heavy or light chain protein. The diverse repertoire of antibody specificities is generated by the presence of multiple germline V, D, and J genes; their combinatorial associations; junctional diversity; and, particularly in secondary antibody responses to protein antigens, by somatic mutations in V genes. Coexpression of μ and δ heavy chains on the same B cell

and the change from membrane to secreted Ig are mediated by alternative splicing of primary heavy chain RNA transcripts. Heavy chain class (isotype) switching results either from a sequential and ordered deletion of C_H genes or from alternative splicing of long primary transcripts containing several or all of the C_H genes. Somatic mutations in V genes give rise to affinity maturation in antibody responses. Transcription and translation of Ig are controlled by numerous processes that are incompletely elucidated; however, many of these processes are believed to be specific for B lymphocytes.

Analysis of these molecular events has provided a clear picture of the differentiation of B lymphocytes and the molecular basis of Ig expression. In addition, such studies form the basis of our rapidly increasing understanding of related fields, such as the evolution of B cell tumors, and are providing increasingly sophisticated tools for the diagnosis of diseases of B lymphocytes.

SELECTED READINGS

Alt, F. W., T. K. Blackwell, and G. D. Yancopoulos. Development of the primary antibody repertoire. Science 238:1079–1087, 1987.
Berek, C., and C. Milstein. Mutation drift and repertoire shift in the maturation of the immune response. Immunological Reviews 96:23–41, 1987.

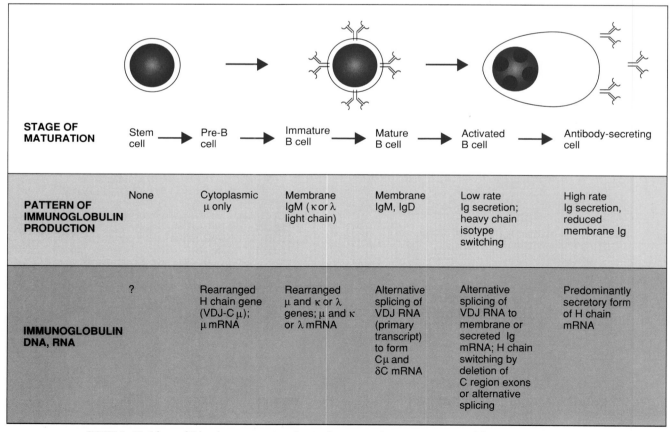

FIGURE 4–17. Scheme of B lymphocyte maturation, showing the patterns of Ig gene expression at different stages of maturation.

Calabi, F., and M. S. Neuberger (eds.). Molecular Genetics of Immunoglobulin. Elsevier Science Publishers, Amsterdam, 1987.

Calame, K., and S. Eaton. Transcriptional controlling elements in the immunoglobulin and T cell receptor loci. Advances in Immunology 43:235–275, 1988.

Esser, C., and A. Radbruch. Immunoglobulin class switching: molecular and cellular analysis. Annual Review of Immunology 8:717–735, 1990.

French, D. L., R. Laskov, and M. D. Scharff. The role of somatic hypermutation in the generation of antibody diversity. Science 244:1152–1157, 1989.

Hanahan, D. Transgenic mice as probes into complex systems. Science 246:1265–1275, 1989.

Klein, G., and E. Klein. Myc/Ig juxtaposition by chromosomal translocations: some new insights, puzzles and paradoxes. Immunology Today 6:208–215, 1985.

Lai, E., R. K. Wilson, and L. E. Hood. Physical maps of the mouse and human immunoglobulin-like loci. Advances in Immunology 46:1–60, 1989.

Oettinger, M. A., D. G. Schatz, C. Gorka, and D. Baltimore. RAG–1 and RAG–2, adjacent genes that synergistically activate V(D)J recombination. Science 248:1517–1523, 1990.

Rajewsky, K., I. Forster, and A. Cumano. Evolutionary and somatic selection of the antibody repertoire in the mouse. Science 283:1088–1094, 1987.

Sen, R., and D. Baltimore. Factors regulating immunoglobulin gene transcription. In F. W. Alt, T. Honjo, and T. H. Rabbitts (eds.). Immunoglobulin Genes. Academic Press, New York, 1989, pp. 327–342.

Showe, L. C., and C. M. Croce. The role of chromosomal translocations in B- and T-cell neoplasia. Annual Review of Immunology 5:253–277, 1987.

Storb, U. Transgenic mice with immunoglobulin genes. Annual Review of Immunology 5:151–174, 1987.

Tonegawa, S. Somatic generation of antibody diversity. Nature 302:575–581, 1983.

Waldmann, T. A. The arrangement of immunoglobulin and T cell receptor genes in human lymphoproliferative disorders. Advances in Immunology 40:247–321, 1987.

CHAPTER FIVE

THE MAJOR

HISTOCOMPATIBILITY

COMPLEX

The **major histocompatibility complex** (MHC) is a region of highly polymorphic genes whose products are expressed on the surfaces of a variety of cells. This locus was discovered in the 1940s in the artificial situation of transplantation of tissues from one individual to another. MHC–encoded proteins, which are commonly referred to as "MHC molecules" or "MHC antigens," are the principal determinants of graft rejection. Thus, individuals who express the same MHC molecules accept tissue grafts from one another, and individuals who differ at their MHC loci vigorously reject such grafts. Although the role of MHC molecules as the targets for immunologic rejection of transplants raised considerable interest, the importance of the MHC in physiologic immune responses was established almost 20 years after the discovery of these genetic loci. Baruj Benacerraf, Hugh McDevitt, and their colleagues showed in the 1960s that different inbred strains of guinea pigs and mice did or did not produce antibodies in response to immunization with simple polypeptide antigens and that this immune responsiveness was an autosomal dominant trait that mapped to the MHC region. The genes that controlled such immune responses were called **immune response (Ir) genes.** It was later shown that Ir genes controlled the activation of helper T lymphocytes, which were necessary for antibody responses to protein antigens. The central role of MHC genes in immune responses to protein antigens was explained in the late 1970s, with the demonstration that *antigen-specific T lymphocytes do not recognize antigens in free or soluble form but recognize portions of protein antigens that are non-covalently bound to MHC gene products.* There are two different types of MHC gene products, called **class I** and **class II MHC molecules,** and any given T cell recognizes foreign antigen bound to only one specific class I or class II MHC molecule. Furthermore, as we shall discuss in Chapter 6, in each individual the antigen receptors of mature T cells are specific for complexes of foreign protein antigens and self MHC molecules. Thus, MHC molecules are integral components of the ligands that T cells recognize.

Before we discuss the discovery and structure of MHC molecules, it is useful to summarize the principal physiologic importance of the specificity of T lymphocytes for self MHC–associated antigens.

1. Because MHC molecules are membrane-associated and not secreted, T lymphocytes can recognize foreign antigens only when bound to the surfaces of other cells. This limits T cell activation such that *T cells interact most effectively with other cells that bear MHC–associated antigens and not with soluble antigens.* The cell that bears the MHC molecule is said to *present* the antigen to the T lymphocyte. The recognition of antigen on a cell surface also serves to localize the effector functions of the activated T cell to the anatomic site of antigen presentation. In contrast, antibodies can function in the circulation by binding to and neutralizing soluble antigens.

2. *The patterns of antigen association with class I or class II MHC molecules determine the kinds of T cells that are stimulated by different forms of antigens.* Peptide fragments derived from extracellular proteins usually bind to class II MHC molecules, whereas endogenously synthesized peptides generally associate with class I molecules. As a consequence, exogenously and endogenously synthesized proteins are, for the most part, recognized by functionally distinct T cell populations.

3. The immune response to a foreign protein is determined by the presence or absence of MHC molecules that can bind and present fragments of that protein to T cells. MHC genes are very polymorphic; i.e., many different alleles exist within the population, and these alleles differ in their ability to bind and present different antigenic determinants of proteins. This is one way in which *MHC genes control immune responses to protein antigens.*

4. Mature T cells in any individual recognize and respond to foreign antigens but are unresponsive to self proteins. This repertoire of antigen recognition is shaped by the selection of foreign antigen-specific T cells from developing lymphocytes, based on their recognition of self MHC molecules with or without bound peptide antigens. Therefore, *a second means by which MHC genes can influence immune responses to particular antigens is through the role of MHC molecules in shaping the repertoire of mature T cells.*

The functions of MHC gene products in T cell antigen recognition and in the development of the T cell repertoire are described in much more detail in Chapters 6 to 8. However, these functional considerations make clear why our discussion of T cells must begin with a discussion of MHC molecules. The terminology and genetics of the MHC are best understood from a historical perspective, and we will begin our discussion with a description of how the MHC was discovered.

DISCOVERY OF THE MAJOR HISTOCOMPATIBILITY COMPLEX
Transplantation in Mice

The initial discovery of the murine MHC was made by George Snell and his colleagues, using classical genetic techniques to analyze the rejection of transplanted tumors and other tissues. In their simplest form, these experiments examined the outcome of skin grafts between individual animals. The key to the analysis was the use of inbred strains of laboratory mice.

In an animal population, some genes are represented by only one normal nucleic acid sequence; every variant nucleic acid sequence is an uncommon mutation and may result in a disease state. Such genes are said to be nonpolymorphic, and the normal, or wild type, gene sequence will usually be present on both chromosomes of a pair in each individual member of the species. (Recall that all chromosomes, except sex chromosomes in the male, are present in pairs in a normal diploid animal.) In other genes, the nucleic acid sequences may vary at a relatively high frequency among normal individuals in the population; i.e., at least 1 per cent of individuals may express a gene that differs from the homologous gene in remaining members of the population. Such genes are said to be **polymorphic.** Each common variant of a polymorphic gene present in the population is called an **allele.** For polymorphic genes, any individual animal can have the same allele at a genetic locus on both chromosomes of the pair (i.e., can be homozygous) or two different alleles, one on each chromosome (i.e., can be heterozygous).

Inbred mouse strains are produced by repetitive matings of siblings (Fig. 5–1). After about 20 generations, every individual animal of a given inbred mouse strain will have identical nucleic acid sequences at all locations on both members of each pair of chromosomes. In other words, *inbred mice are completely ho-*

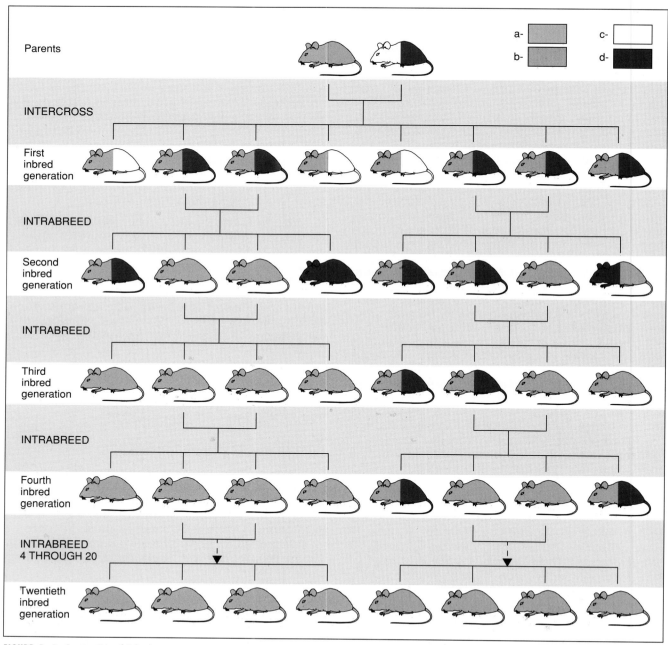

FIGURE 5–1. Construction of inbred mouse strains. *In this hypothetical breeding scheme, a particular genetic locus is represented in the outbred heterozygous parent animals by four different alleles: a, b, c, and d. Repetitive inbreeding leads to development of animal strains in which every individual is homozygous at this locus and expresses the same allele. Without selective pressure, which of the original parental alleles will be present in the inbred animals is random. In this example, two strains that preserve alleles a and b are generated; other strains that are homozygous for c or d could be derived from the same parents. Although only one locus is depicted, every other genetic locus in each inbred strain will also be homozygous and identical among all animals in the same strain.*

mozygous at every genetic locus. In addition, every mouse of an inbred strain is genetically completely identical **(syngeneic)** *to every other mouse of the same strain.* In the case of polymorphic genes, each inbred strain, because it is completely homozygous, can express only one allele from the original population. However, the determination of which of four possible alleles (one on each member of the chromosome pairs in each of the two original parents) is preserved by inbreeding is random for any particular gene; different inbred strains derived from the same two parents may preserve different alleles (Fig. 5–1). Strains or individuals that express different alleles are said to be **allogeneic** to one another.

When a tissue or an organ, such as a patch of skin, is grafted from one animal to another, two possible outcomes may ensue. In some cases, the grafted skin survives and functions as normal skin. In others, the immune system destroys the graft, a process called **rejection.** By determining whether or not grafts exchanged among various inbred strains of mice were rejected, several key observations were made about the genetic basis of graft rejection.

1. Grafts of skin from one animal to itself (isogeneic grafts or isografts) or grafts between animals of the same inbred strain (syngeneic grafts or syngrafts) are usually not rejected.
2. Grafts between animals of different inbred strains or between outbred mice (allogeneic grafts or allografts) are almost always rejected.

We will return to these experiments in Chapter 16, when we discuss transplantation. Suffice it to say here that the different outcomes for grafts between syngeneic animals and grafts between allogeneic animals established that there is a genetic basis for recognizing a graft as foreign. The genes responsible for causing a grafted tissue to be perceived as similar to one's own tissues or as foreign were called **histocompatibility genes,** and the differences between foreign and self were attributed to genetic polymorphisms among different histocompatibility alleles.

The tools of classical genetics, namely breeding and analysis of the offspring, were then applied to identify the relevant genes. The critical strategy in this effort was the breeding of **congenic mouse strains** (Box 5–1) that differed only by genes responsible for causing graft rejection. These studies indicated that although several different genes could contribute to rejection, *a single genetic region is responsible for most rejection phenomena.* The particular region identified in mice by Snell's group was linked to a gene encoding a polymorphic blood group antigen called Antigen II, and this region was subsequently called histocompatibility-2 or, simply, H-2. Initially, MHC congenic strains were thought to differ at a single gene locus. However, occasional recombination events occurred within the MHC during interbreeding of different strains, suggesting that the MHC actually contained several different but closely linked genes, each involved in graft rejection. The H-2 region in mice is now known to be homologous to genes that determine the fate of grafted tissues in other species, and all of these are grouped under the generic name, the "major histocompatibility complex."

The genetics of graft rejection indicated that the

BOX 5–1. CONGENIC MOUSE STRAINS

A key development in defining the genes responsible for causing graft rejection was the development of congenic mouse strains that differ only by the relevant genes, now known as the MHC. The strategy for such breeding depends upon two circumstances. First, there must already exist a homozygous inbred mouse strain that will reproducibly reject transplanted grafts of another strain. Second, there must be a simple assay for graft rejection. Both of these conditions are met by transplanting skin between inbred strains that differ in alleles of MHC genes. The procedure is outlined in the accompanying figure.

We begin by breeding a mouse of one inbred strain A with a mouse from a second strain B. We will refer to the MHC of a strain A mouse as being *aa* homozygous (with italics representing alleles) and that of a strain B mouse as being *bb* homozygous. All of the first filial (F1) generation will be *ab* heterozygotes. Next we will mate an F1 mouse with a strain A mouse. This is called a backcross. Half of the offspring will be *aa* and half will be *ab*. Those mice which are *ab* can be identified by the fact that their skin will be rapidly rejected by strain A mice; in contrast, the skin of *aa* offspring will not be rapidly rejected by strain A mice. Step three is again to backcross one of the heterozygous *ab* mice with a strain A mouse. Once again, half of the offspring will be *aa* and half will be *ab*, and the heterozygous ab mice can be identified by

the fact that strain A mice will rapidly reject their skin. By continuing to carry out such backcrosses for multiple generations, two things occur. First, the *b* allele of the MHC will be indefinitely maintained in the offspring because its expression is necessary for skin graft rejection and this is the positive selection being imposed by the experimenter. Second, all other genetic loci from the strain B mice will disappear as a result of random backcrosses into strain A mice. This second effect can be thought of as serial dilution. The F1 mice will contain 50 per cent strain B genes; the offspring of the first backcross will contain, on average, 25 per cent; the offspring of the next backcross, on average, 12.5 per cent and so on, until by about 20 backcrosses no strain B genes except the MHC alleles will persist. At this point, we have produced a mouse strain identical to the strain A except that the MHC is heterozygous *ab*. If we allow the new strain to interbreed, 25 per cent of the first generation offspring will be *aa* homozygous, 50 per cent will be *ab* heterozygous, and 25 per cent will be *bb* homozygous at the MHC. We can identify the *bb* MHC homozygotes as being the only mice that will rapidly reject strain A skin grafts. If we allow the *bb* mice to interbreed, we arrive at a strain that is identical to strain A at every locus except the MHC and is identical to strain B only at the MHC. These mice are congenic to strain A and are said to have the B MHC on an A background.

Continued

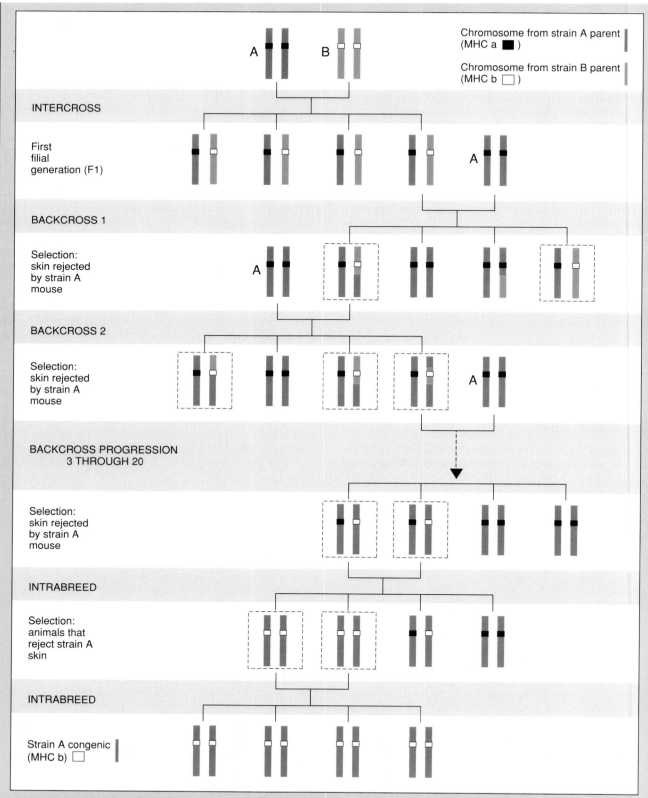

Derivation of congenic mice. *In this hypothetical breeding scheme, selection for skin graft rejection is used to derive mice congenic for MHC loci. To simplify the diagram, each animal is depicted as one chromosome pair and the MHC is represented as a single locus on this chromosome. Animals that are positively selected are indicated by dashed blue boxes around the chromosome pair. As described in the box, all non-MHC strain B genes are lost during progressive backcrosses with strain A animals; MHC b genes are preserved by selection, eventually allowing the breeding of a congenic strain that differs only at the MHC from parental strain A.*

products of MHC genes are co-dominantly expressed; i.e., the alleles on both chromosomes of a pair are expressed. As a consequence, each parent of a genetic cross between two different strains can reject a graft from the offspring by recognizing MHC alleles inherited from the other parent.

In mice, the MHC alleles of particular inbred strains are designated by lower case letters (e.g., a, b, c). The individual genes within the MHC are named for the MHC type of the mouse strain in which they were first identified. The two independent MHC loci known to be most important for graft rejection in mice are called H-2K and H-2D. The K gene was first discovered in a strain whose MHC had been designated k, and the D gene was first discovered in a strain whose MHC had been designated d. In the parlance of mouse geneticists, the allele of the K gene in a strain with the k-type MHC is called K^k (pronounced K of k) whereas the allele of the K gene in a strain of MHC d is called K^d (pronounced K of d). A third locus similar to K and D was discovered later and called L.

Several other genes were subsequently mapped to the region between the K and D genes responsible for skin rejection. For example, S genes that code for polymorphic serum proteins, now known to be components of the complement system, were identified. Most importantly, *the polymorphic Ir genes mentioned earlier in the chapter were assigned to a region within the MHC called I* (the letter, not the Roman numeral). The I region, in turn, was further subdivided into I-A and I-E subregions on the basis of recombination events during breeding between congenic strains. The I region was also found to code for certain cell surface antigens against which antibodies could be produced by interstrain immunizations. These antigens were called I region-associated or **Ia molecules.** As we shall discuss in Chapters 6 and 8, we now know that the I-A and I-E Ir genes are the structural genes that code for Ia antigens, which are called I-A and I-E molecules, respectively. The I-A molecule found in the inbred

mouse strain with the K^k and D^k alleles is called I-A^k (pronounced I big A of k). Similar terminology is used for I-E molecules. The culmination of genetic analysis was the construction of a classical genetic map of the murine MHC, schematized in Figure 5-2.

MHC genes were initially identified by graft rejection and Ir gene phenomena, which are T cell–mediated immune responses. This is not unexpected because, as stated earlier and discussed in detail in Chapter 6, MHC molecules are crucial for T cell recognition of foreign antigens. Nevertheless, immunization of one congenic mouse strain with cells of another can be used to produce antibodies (i.e., B cell products) specific for MHC gene products. Such antibodies were important in the biochemical analysis of murine MHC molecules and played a central role in the discovery of the MHC in man.

Serologic Studies in Humans

The kinds of experiments used to discover and define MHC genes in mice, namely intentional inbreeding and skin graft rejection, obviously cannot be performed in humans. However, the development of allogeneic blood transfusion and especially allogeneic organ transplantation as methods of treatment in clinical medicine provided a strong impetus to detect and define genes that control rejection reactions in humans. Jean Dausset and others noted that patients who rejected kidneys or had transfusion reactions to white blood cells often developed circulating antibodies reactive with antigens on the white blood cells of the blood or organ donor. In the presence of complement, the recipient's serum would lyse lymphocytes from the donor and also lyse lymphocytes obtained from some, but not all, third parties (i.e., individuals other than the blood or organ donor or the recipient). These sera, which react against the cells of allogeneic individuals, are called **alloantisera** (or allosera for

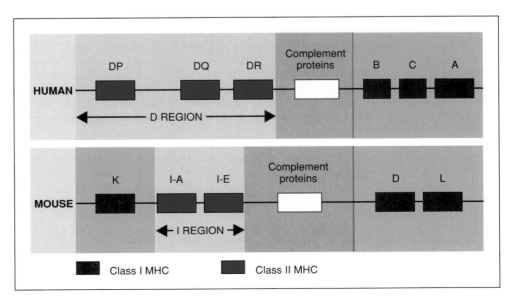

FIGURE 5-2. Schematic maps of human and mouse MHC loci. Sizes of genes and intervening distances are not shown to scale. Each class II locus, e.g., DP and DQ, consists of multiple genes. HLA-DQ is much closer to HLA-DR than to HLA-DP; in fact, HLA-DQ is in strong "linkage disequilibrium" with HLA-DR; i.e., certain DQ alleles are inherited together with particular DR alleles, well out of proportion to their frequency in the population.

short) and are said to contain **alloantibodies,** whose molecular targets are called **alloantigens.** It was presumed that these alloantigens are the products of polymorphic genes that distinguish foreign tissues from self. Panels of allosera from immunized donors, including multiparous women (who are immunized by paternal alloantigens expressed by the fetus during pregnancy) and actively immunized volunteers as well as transfusion or transplant recipients, were collected and compared for their ability to lyse panels of lymphocytes from different donors. Efforts at several international workshops, involving free exchanges of reagents among laboratories, led to the definition of at least six separate polymorphic genetic loci, clustered together in a single area of the genome, that can help to predict the strength of graft rejection. Because they are expressed on human leukocytes, the alloantigens recognized by these sera became known as **human leukocyte antigens (HLAs).** Family studies were then used to construct the map of these human genes (Fig. 5–2). The first three genes defined by purely serologic approaches were called HLA–A, HLA–B, and HLA–C. The second three to be identified mapped to an adjacent region, called HLA–D, which was originally detected by induction of proliferation of foreign T cells in the mixed leukocyte reaction (see below). The first gene product detected by alloantibodies that mapped to the HLA–D region was called "HLA–D related" or HLA–DR. The other two genes were subsequently called HLA–DQ and HLA–DP, with Q and P chosen for their proximity in the alphabet to R. *The HLA region is now known as the human MHC and is equivalent to the H-2 region of mice* (Fig. 5–2). The various HLA and H-2 loci are structurally and functionally homologous. *Specifically, human HLA–A, –B, and –C resemble mouse H-2 K, D, and L and are called class I MHC molecules, whereas human HLA–DP, –DQ and –DR resemble mouse I-A and I-E and are called class II MHC molecules.* Indeed, similar polymorphic genes and protein products have been found in every vertebrate species examined!

The studies of the mouse MHC were accomplished with a limited number of inbred and congenic strains. Although it was appreciated that mouse MHC genes were polymorphic, only 10 to 20 alleles were defined at each locus. The human serologic studies were conducted on outbred human populations. The most remarkable feature to emerge from the studies of the human MHC genes is the unprecedented and unanticipated extent of their polymorphism. More than 40 separate alleles have been identified to date for some of the HLA loci, and this is undoubtedly an underestimate resulting from the limited resolution of serology. *MHC genes are by far the most polymorphic genes present in the genome of every species analyzed.* The significance of this polymorphism will become evident when we turn to the structure and functions of MHC molecules.

The use of antibodies to study alloantigenic differences between donors and recipients in human transplantation was complemented by the mixed leukocyte reaction (MLR), a test for T cell recognition of foreign MHC molecules. The MLR is also an *in vitro* model for allograft rejection and will be discussed more fully in the context of transplantation (see Chapter 16). Analysis of the allogeneic MLR led to the conclusion that two distinct classes of T lymphocytes recognize and respond to different types of MHC gene products. CD4+ T cells, most of which are cytokine-producing helper cells, are specific for class II MHC molecules, i.e., HLA–DR, –DQ, and –DP in man and I-A and I-E in mice. CD8+ T cells, most of which are cytolytic T lymphocytes (CTLs), are specific for class I MHC molecules, namely HLA–A, –B, and –C or H-2K, D, and L. As we shall see in Chapter 6, these MHC recognition specificities of CD4+ and CD8+ T cells apply not only to recognition of allogeneic MHC molecules but also to recognition of foreign protein, e.g., microbial antigens, in every individual. Thus, *CD4+ T cells recognize foreign antigens bound to self class II MHC molecules, and CD8+ T cells recognize foreign antigens bound to class I molecules.*

The total set of MHC alleles present on each chromosome is also called an **MHC haplotype.** In humans, each HLA allele is given a numerical designation. For instance, an HLA haplotype of an individual could be HLA–A2, –B5, –DR3, and so on. All heterozygous individuals, of course, have two HLA haplotypes. Inbred mice, being homozygous, have a single haplotype. Thus, the haplotype of an H-2^k mouse is H-2K^k I-A^k I-E^k D^k L^k. In humans, certain HLA alleles at different loci are inherited together, a phenomenon called linkage disequilibrium. Such haplotypes, in which multiple HLA genes remain linked, are associated with certain autoimmune diseases (see Chapter 18).

STRUCTURE OF MHC MOLECULES

The realization that MHC molecules play an essential part in the recognition of all protein antigens by T cells has led to an enormous effort in many laboratories to elucidate the structure of these molecules. The biochemical analysis of MHC molecules has been highly successful, especially with the recent solution of the crystal structures for the extracellular portions of two human class I molecules, HLA–A2 and HLA–Aw68, by Don Wiley, Jack Strominger, and colleagues. On the basis of this new knowledge, we can now address two interrelated structural issues that are important for understanding the functions of MHC molecules:

First, how do MHC molecules bind foreign peptide antigens and how does the genetic polymorphism of MHC molecules contribute to the specificity of peptide binding?

Second, what structural features of MHC molecules underlie the specificity of CD8+ T cells for class I molecules and of CD4+ T cells for class II molecules?

We will initially consider class I and class II molecules separately but, as we shall see, many features of these molecules now point to their fundamental similarity.

Class I MHC Molecules

All class I molecules contain two separate polypeptide chains: an MHC–encoded α or heavy chain of about 44 kilodaltons (kD) in humans, or about 47 kD in mice, and a non-MHC–encoded β chain of 12 kD in both species (Fig. 5–3). The α chain is formed by a core polypeptide of about 40 kD and contains one (human) or two (mouse) N-linked oligosaccharides. Each α chain is oriented so that about three quarters of the complete polypeptide, including the amino terminus and oligosaccharide group(s), extends into the extracellular milieu, a short hydrophobic segment spans the membrane, and the carboxy terminal 30 amino acid residues are located in the cytoplasm. The β chain interacts non-covalently with the extracellular portion of the heavy chain and has no direct attachment to the cell. Based upon primary amino acid sequences of many class I molecules and upon the crystal structure of the HLA–A2 and HLA–Aw68 molecules, we can now divide class I molecules into four separate regions (Fig. 5–3): an amino terminal extracellular peptide-binding region; an extracellular immunoglobulin (Ig)-like region; a transmembrane region; and a cytoplasmic region.

THE PEPTIDE-BINDING REGION

As we noted in the introductory section of this chapter, the principal function of MHC molecules is to bind fragments of foreign proteins, thereby forming complexes that can be recognized by T lymphocytes.

The portion of class I molecules that interacts with protein antigens consists of approximately 180 amino acid residues at the amino terminus of the class I α chain. Analysis of amino acid sequences has indicated that this region is formed of two homologous segments of about 90 amino acid residues each, referred to as α1 and α2. Each human class I MHC molecule has a single N-linked oligosaccharide attached near the junction of α1 and α2. Murine class I MHC molecules contain a second oligosaccharide attached near the carboxy terminal side of α2. The α2 segment contains a disulfide bond, forming a loop of about 63 amino acid residues. Despite initial reports to the contrary, there is no evidence that the α1 or α2 segments of MHC molecules are structurally or evolutionarily related to Ig domains. Moreover, the crystal structure of class I MHC molecules has been revealed to have a unique conformation: α1 and α2 interact to form a platform of an eight-stranded, β-pleated sheet supporting two parallel strands of α-helix (Fig. 5–4 and Color Plate II, opposite page 53). Four strands of the β-pleated sheet and one of the α-helices are formed from amino acid residues of α1; the remaining four strands of the β-pleated sheet and the other α-helix are formed from amino acid residues of α2. The two α-helices form the sides of a cleft whose floor is formed by the strands of the β-pleated sheet. *The cleft is of appropriate size (25Å × 10Å × 11Å) to bind a 10 to 20 amino acid fragment of a protein folded into a single α-helix or in a flexible, extended conformation and is the presumed site where foreign peptides bind to MHC molecules for presentation to T cells.* Significantly, the cleft is too small

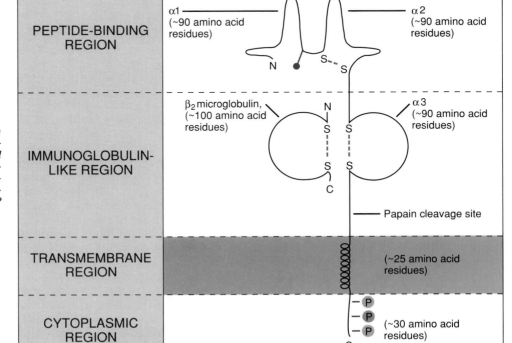

FIGURE 5–3. Schematic diagram of a class I MHC molecule. Different segments are not shown to scale. N and C refer to amino and carboxy termini of the polypeptide chains, respectively; S--S, to intrachain disulfide bonds; ↑ to carbohydrate; and P to phosphorylation sites.

PEPTIDE-BINDING REGION

α1 (~90 amino acid residues)   α2 (~90 amino acid residues)

N   S--S

IMMUNOGLOBULIN-LIKE REGION

β₂ microglobulin, (~100 amino acid residues)   N   α3 (~90 amino acid residues)

S   S

S   S

C

Papain cleavage site

TRANSMEMBRANE REGION

(~25 amino acid residues)

CYTOPLASMIC REGION

P
P
P
(~30 amino acid residues)

C

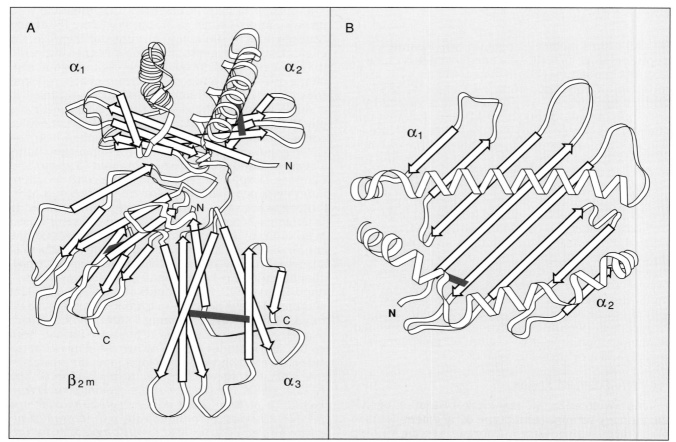

FIGURE 5–4. Polypeptide folding pattern of a human class I MHC molecule. *Panel A shows a side view and Panel B depicts a top view, revealing the peptide-binding cleft. The white arrows represent polypeptide folded as β pleated sheet, the white coils represent polypeptide folded as α helix, and the blue bars represent disulfide bonds. (Adapted with permission from Bjorkman, P. J., M. A. Saper, B. Samraoui, W. S. Bennet, J. L. Strominger, and D. C. Wiley. Structure of the human class I histocompatibility antigen HLA–A2. Nature 329:506–512, 1987. Copyright © 1987, Macmillan Magazines Ltd.)*

to bind an intact globular protein and thus differs from the more planar binding site of antibody molecules (see Chapter 3). The small size of the cleft in MHC molecules requires that native globular proteins be "processed," to produce smaller fragments that can bind to MHC molecules and be recognized by T lymphocytes (see Chapter 6). Remarkably, analysis of the HLA molecules by x-ray diffraction revealed that various extrinsic peptides were still bound in the clefts of the class I protein crystals! Presumably, this mixture of peptides had remained attached to the class I molecules through purification and crystal formation.

Comparisons of amino acid and nucleotide sequences of a large number of human and murine class I heavy chains have indicated that almost all of the polymorphic residues, i.e., those amino acids found to vary among different allelic forms, are located either in the α-helical sides of the cleft or on the β strands that form the floor of the cleft and are oriented such that the amino acid side chains point into the cleft or toward the top of the helices. Combining the information from the crystal structure and sequence analyses leads to the conclusion that *polymorphism among class I MHC alleles serves to create variation in the chemical surface of the peptide-binding cleft.* Other polymorphic residues of MHC molecules form contact with T cell antigen receptors, so that *T cells specifically interact both with MHC–associated foreign antigens and with the MHC molecules themselves* (see Chapters 6 and 7). The N-linked oligosaccharides, although located in the peptide-binding region, do not contribute to the structure of the cleft or to peptide binding.

Several inferences about the nature of peptide binding to MHC molecules can be made from these structural analyses of MHC gene products:

1. Each MHC molecule has only a single site for peptide binding, so that all peptides that bind must bind to the same site.

2. The structural polymorphism of this binding region suggests that different allelic forms of MHC molecules may differ in their ability to bind structurally distinct peptide antigens. As we discuss in Chapter 6, this is indeed the case. However, the specificity of peptide-MHC association is determined only by the MHC allele inherited in the germline. This is different from antigen binding by antibodies and T cell antigen receptors, in which specificity is determined mainly by somatic DNA recombination and, in the case of

antibodies, by mutations, but not by the inheritance of different alleles (see Chapters 4 and 8). Because MHC genes lack recombinational and mutational mechanisms for generating structural diversity in their protein products, relatively few variations in the binding sites of MHC molecules are possible. As a result, the affinity and selectivity of class I MHC molecules for foreign peptides are markedly less than those of antibodies and T cell antigen receptors.

3. It has been proposed that the extraordinary polymorphism of MHC molecules has evolved and is maintained in each species by positive natural selection, so that members of the species express different alleles capable of binding many distinct foreign peptide antigens. Otherwise, if the number of variant MHC molecules in the population were limited, a microbe could simply mutate its antigens until they attained structures incapable of binding to MHC molecules. This would prevent T cell recognition of the antigens, and the microbe would evade specific immunity. However, with so many possible MHC molecules available within the gene pool, such microbial peptides unable to bind to all MHC molecules in the population are unlikely to emerge.

THE IMMUNOGLOBULIN-LIKE REGION

The α3 segment of the heavy chain is composed of about 90 extracellular amino acid residues between the carboxy terminal end of the α2 segment and the insertion into the plasma membrane. The amino acid sequence in this region is highly conserved among all class I molecules examined and by sequence analysis is homologous to Ig constant domains. The α3 segment contains an Ig-like disulfide-linked loop.

The β chain of class I molecules, which is encoded by a gene outside the MHC, is absolutely invariant among all human class I molecules examined. (In the mouse, there are two common alleles.) This polypeptide is identical to a protein previously identified in human urine, called β_2 **microglobulin** for its electrophoretic mobility (β_2), size (micro), and solubility (globulin). The β chain of class I molecules is usually called β_2 microglobulin even when attached to the cell surface. Like the α3 segment, β_2 microglobulin is structurally homologous to an Ig constant domain and contains a disulfide-linked loop. Indeed, the HLA–A2 crystal structure has confirmed that both α3 and β_2 microglobulin are folded to form Ig-like domains and thus class I MHC molecules are considered to be part of the Ig gene superfamily (see Chapter 7, Box 7–3). These two domains interact with each other, and β_2 microglobulin also interacts with the β-pleated sheet platform of the peptide-binding region, forming extensive contacts with amino acid residues in α1 and α2. The interactions of β_2 microglobulin with the α1, α2, and α3 segments of the heavy chain appear critical for maintaining class I molecules in their native conformation. Every attempt to displace β_2 microglobulin from the class I molecule has produced loss of heavy-chain native structure.

The strong correlation of CD8 expression on T cells with specificity for class I MHC–associated peptides led to the simple proposal that CD8 might function by binding to a nonpolymorphic portion of a class I molecule. This hypothesis has now been proven by a variety of experiments (see Chapter 7). The nonpolymorphic α3 region contains the binding sites for CD8, based on mutational analysis of MHC molecules.

THE TRANSMEMBRANE REGION

The polypeptide of the α chain extends from the α3 segment into a short connecting region and then into an approximately 25 amino acid residue stretch of hydrophobic amino acids. This region is believed to form an α-helix that passes through the hydrophobic region of the plasma membrane lipid bilayer and anchors the MHC molecule in the membrane. As with all known transmembrane proteins, the hydrophobic sequence is immediately terminated at its carboxy terminal end with a cluster of basic amino acid residues that are believed to interact with the phospholipid headgroups of the inner leaflet of the membrane bilayer. Some, but not all, class I heavy chains contain a cysteine residue within the hydrophobic sequence that may be modified by esterification with myristic acid. The significance of this covalent attachment of a fatty acid is unknown.

The hydrophobic segment of the class I molecule does not affect the conformation of the extracellular portions of the molecule. For example, no alterations in structure or in the spectroscopic properties of class I molecules have been found when the enzyme papain is used to cleave the transmembrane region from the extracellular portion. Papain treatment does affect the solubility of the molecule; after removal of the transmembrane region, the extracellular portions of class I molecules are soluble in aqueous buffers without detergents. The form of HLA–A2 and HLA–Aw68 used to solve the crystal structure was actually prepared by papain treatment to remove the transmembrane region.

THE CYTOPLASMIC REGION

The extreme carboxy terminal portion of class I α chains contains approximately 30 amino acids. This region is believed to be located in the cytoplasm. The overall sequence of this region is not conserved among different class I MHC molecules, but several specific features are highly conserved. For example, all class I α chains contain amino acid residues that form consensus phosphorylation sites for cyclic adenosine monophosphate (cAMP)–dependent protein kinase (protein kinase A), and for pp60 *src* tyrosine kinase. The extreme carboxy terminal region of all known class I molecules undergoes endogenous phosphorylation at yet a third conserved site. In addition, all class I heavy chains contain in their carboxy termini a glutamine residue that is a suitable substrate for transpeptidation by the enzyme transglutaminase. The functional significance of these structural features is unknown, but they may play a role in regulating the interaction of class I MHC molecules with other membrane proteins or with cytoskeletal elements. Furthermore, deletion of portions of the carboxy terminus has been found to inhibit internalization of class I molecules, directly implicating the carboxy terminal region in intracellular trafficking.

Class II MHC Molecules

All class II MHC molecules are composed of two non-covalently associated polypeptide chains (Fig. 5–5). In general, the two class II chains are similar to each other in overall structure. The α chain (32 to 34 kD) is slightly larger than the β chain (29 to 32 kD) as a result of more extensive glycosylation. In class II molecules, both polypeptide chains contain N-linked oligosaccharide groups, both polypeptide chains have extracellular amino termini and intracellular carboxy termini, and over two thirds of each chain is located in the extracellular space. The two chains of class II molecules are encoded by different MHC genes, and, with few exceptions, both class II chains are polymorphic.

The three-dimensional structure of class II molecules has not yet been solved by x-ray crystallography. However, the nucleotide and amino acid sequences of many class II molecules are known and reveal certain structural similarities between class I and class II molecules. Recent spectroscopic studies have also indicated an overall similarity in structure. These structural data, combined with functional similarities between class I and class II molecules, have

led to the construction of a model of class II folding drawn from the known class I structure (Fig. 5–6). In parallel with the structural features of the class I molecules, it is useful to divide class II MHC molecules into a peptide-binding region, an Ig-like region, a transmembrane region, and an intracytoplasmic region.

THE PEPTIDE-BINDING REGION

The extracellular portions of both the α and β chains have been subdivided into two segments of about 90 amino acid residues each, called α1 and α2 or β1 and β2, respectively. The peptide-binding region is formed by an interaction of both chains involving the α1 and β1 segments. This is different from class I MHC molecules, in which only the α chain is involved in forming the peptide-binding cleft. According to the proposed model of class II molecules, α1 and β1 fold to form an eight-stranded, β-pleated sheet platform supporting two α-helices; four strands of the β-pleated sheet and one of the α-helices are formed by α1, whereas the other four strands and the other α-helix are formed by β1. Class II α1 (like class I α1) does not contain a disulfide-linked loop, whereas class II β1 (like class I α2) does; in this model, the class II β1 disulfide-linked loop is in the same position as the class I α2 disulfide-linked loop. As in the class I structure, the class II model uses α-helices and β strands to form the sides and floor, respectively, of the peptide-binding cleft.

One of the strongest arguments in favor of this model of class II structure is the remarkable fact that,

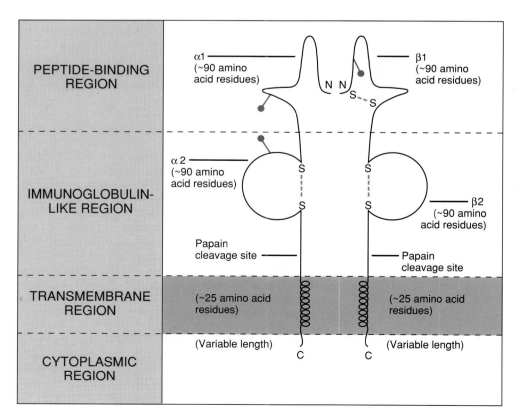

FIGURE 5–5. Schematic diagram of a class II MHC molecule. Different segments are not shown to scale. N and C, amino and carboxy termini of the polypeptide chains; S--S, intrachain disulfide bonds and ❘ to carbohydrate.

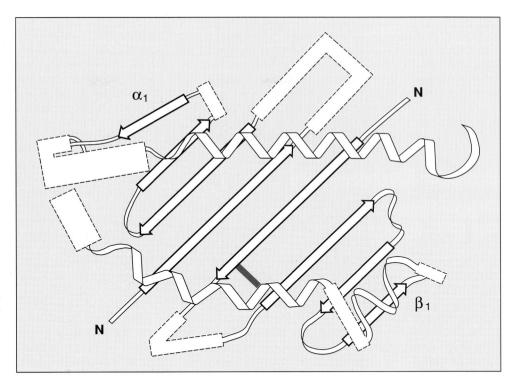

FIGURE 5–6. Polypeptide folding pattern proposed for the peptide-binding cleft of class II MHC molecule. Note the similarities to the class I peptide-binding cleft (see Fig. 5–4B). The white arrows represent polypeptide folded as β pleated sheet, the white coils represent polypeptide folded as α helix, and the blue bar represents a disulfide bond. The dotted boxes on the edge refer to uncertainties about how these regions fold. (Adapted with permission from Brown, J. H., T. Jardetzky, M. A. Saper, B. Samraoui, P. J. Bjorkman, and D. C. Wiley. A hypothetical model of the foreign antigen binding site of class II histocompatibility molecules. Nature 332:845–850, 1988. Copyright ©1988, Macmillan Magazines Ltd.)

as in the case of class I molecules, the polymorphic residues are concentrated in $\alpha 1$ and $\beta 1$ in locations such that they lie in the α-helical sides or β-pleated sheet floor of the peptide-binding cleft, with their side chains pointing into the cleft or toward the top of the helices. *Thus, as for class I molecules, genetic polymorphism of class II MHC molecules determines the chemical surface of the cleft and is the principal determinant of the specificity and affinity of peptide-binding and T cell recognition.* Again, both specificity and affinity for foreign antigens are much lower for class II molecules than for true antigen receptors such as antibody or the T cell antigen receptor. As with class I, the use of inherited polymorphisms to determine antigen binding provides an explanation for the evolutionary drive to generate and maintain such polymorphism: a high level of polymorphism is needed to prevent the emergence of microbial peptides that cannot bind to any class II MHC molecule.

THE IMMUNOGLOBULIN-LIKE REGION

Both the $\alpha 2$ and $\beta 2$ segments of class II molecules contain internal disulfide bonds and by amino acid sequence belong to the Ig gene superfamily. It is presumed that these segments, like class I $\alpha 3$ and β_2 microglobulin, are actually folded into Ig domains within the native MHC molecule. The class II $\alpha 2$ and $\beta 2$ segments are essentially nonpolymorphic among various alleles of a particular class II gene but show some differences among the different genetic loci. Thus, the $\alpha 2$ regions of all DR alleles are similar, but DR$\alpha 2$ differs from DP$\alpha 2$ or DQ$\alpha 2$. The correlation of CD4 expression on T cells with specificity for class II MHC

molecules has been proposed to arise from binding of the CD4 molecule with the Ig-like nonpolymorphic domain of the class II molecules.

The Ig-like regions of the class II molecules are probably important for non-covalent interactions between the two chains, although other portions of the polypeptide chains no doubt contribute as well. These interactions are quite strong and can be disrupted only by harsh denaturing conditions. In general, α chains of one locus (e.g., DR) pair only with β chains of the same locus and less commonly with β chains of other loci (e.g., DQ or DP).

THE TRANSMEMBRANE AND CYTOPLASMIC REGIONS

The carboxy terminal sides of the $\alpha 2$ and $\beta 2$ segments extend into short connecting regions followed by approximately 25 amino acid stretches of hydrophobic residues, likely to span the membrane. Extended cleavage with papain can separate the extracellular portions of the molecule from the transmembrane region without loss of structure. In both chains, the hydrophobic transmembrane region ends with a cluster of basic amino acid residues; these are followed by short, hydrophilic cytoplasmic tails, which form the carboxy terminal ends of the polypeptides. Less is known about the intracellular regions of class II molecules than of class I. It is likely that the transmembrane and cytoplasmic sequences of the class II chains will determine intracellular distributions and trafficking of these molecules through their interactions with other cellular proteins. It should be noted that patterns of intracellular trafficking differ between class I and class II molecules, and this may eventually be explained by the divergent structures of the intracytoplasmic regions. These differences in intracellular trafficking may underlie the fact, as will be described in Chapter 6, that class I and class II molecules preferentially bind foreign proteins found in different cellular compartments. It is also possible that class II molecules may act as signal-transducing molecules and that the intracellular regions play a role in transfer of information across the membrane.

GENOMIC ORGANIZATION

Organization of the MHC Gene Loci

In humans, the MHC is located on the short arm of chromosome 6. β_2 microglobulin is encoded by a gene on chromosome 15. The human MHC occupies a large segment of DNA, extending about 3500 kilobases (kb). (For comparison, a large human gene may extend up to 50 to 100 kb, and 3500 kb is the size of the entire *Escherichia coli* genome!) In classical genetic terms, it extends about 4 centimorgans, meaning crossovers within the MHC occur with a frequency of over 4 per cent at each meiosis. A recent molecular map of the human MHC is shown in Figure 5–7. The class II genes are located closest to the centromere in the order DP, DQ, and DR. A surprise from these gene-mapping studies is that there may be two or three functional β chain genes for some class II loci but usually only one functional α chain gene. The use of more than one β chain gene allows some class II gene products, especially HLA–DR, to be expressed in more than two "allelic" forms on a single cell. This contributes to an important difference between class I and class II loci. For class I, *a heterozygous individual expresses six different*

polymorphic alleles (three from each parent) and six class I MHC molecules per cell. For class II, although the individual also inherits only six different polymorphic loci, more than six class II MHC $\alpha\beta$ heterodimers can be expressed per cell. Some class II molecules are formed by more than one functional polymorphic β chain within the same allelic locus. Additional class II heterodimers are produced by the combination of the α chain from one allele and the β chain of the other allele. *Usually, individuals can express 10 to 20 different class II gene products per cell; the variation in number depends upon which alleles have been inherited.* This increases the potential number of foreign protein antigens that can bind to and be presented in association with class II molecules. In addition, there are several pseudo(defective) genes and additional class II–like sequences called DZ (linked closely to DP), DO, and DX (linked closely to DQ), which may be pseudogenes or may encode protein products not yet identified.

The complement or so-called "class III" region is telomeric to the class II region and encodes components of the complement system (C2 and C4, which are homologous to the S or serum proteins of the mouse MHC) as well as the enzyme steroid 21-hydroxylase. The most telomeric portion of the MHC contains the class I α chain genes in the sequence B, C, and A. The genes for the cytokines, tumor necrosis factor (TNF) and lymphotoxin (LT), map between the complement and class I regions. The large space located between the C and A genes contains additional genes that are class I–like. Many more class I–like genes have been found telomeric to HLA–A outside of the true MHC; these genes occupy another 11 centimorgans! Some of these class I–like sequences are pseudogenes, but some encode nonpolymorphic proteins that are expressed in association with β_2 microglobulin.

The function of the nonpolymorphic class I–like

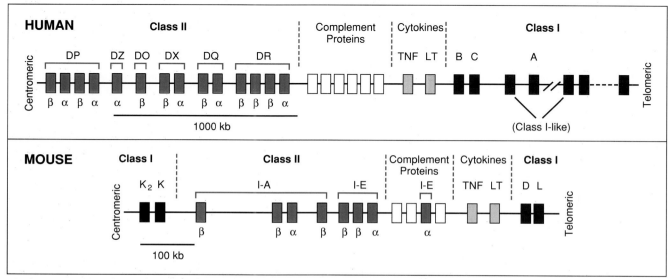

FIGURE 5–7. Genomic organization of human and mouse MHC loci. *Genes comprising each locus and intervening distances are of approximate relative size. The number of α and β genes in each human class II locus varies among alleles. The mouse cytokine genes (TNF and LT) are assigned tentatively based upon the location in humans. Note that each class Iα or class IIα or β gene consists of multiple exons that are not shown (see Fig. 5–8.). TNF, tumor necrosis factor; LT, lymphotoxin.*

genes and their products is largely unknown. In mice, one such gene, called Tla, is expressed on thymocytes and leukemic T cells. Recently, another class I–like product has been described to function as an Fc receptor, binding and transporting IgG molecules across an epithelial barrier; however, the gene for this product has not yet been mapped. Rare T cells may recognize variant class I molecules instead of the conventional polymorphic class I molecules. (This has been shown most convincingly for a subset of T cells, discussed in Chapter 7, that recognizes CD1 molecules, class I–like proteins that are encoded on a different chromosome from the HLA complex.) An alternative proposal for the function of the nonpolymorphic class I–like genes and pseudogenes is that these genes serve as a repository of alternative nucleic acid sequences to be used for generating polymorphic sequences in the true class I molecules. According to this hypothesis, the process of **gene conversion** (that is, incorporation of variant sequences into the true class I and class II genes without reciprocal crossing over) has occurred during evolution to generate the extraordinary polymorphism of the MHC alleles. Moreover, ongoing gene conversion events would provide a source of new mutations, constantly introducing new alleles into the population. Gene conversion would be far more efficient than point mutations because (1) several changes can be introduced at once, and (2) amino acids necessary for maintaining structure can remain unchanged if identical amino acids at those positions are encoded by both the genes involved in the conversion event.

The murine MHC, located on chromosome 17, occupies a somewhat smaller region than the human MHC, and the genes are organized in a slightly differ-ent order (see Fig. 5–7). Specifically, one of the class I genes (H2-K) is located centromeric to the class II region, but the other class I genes and the nonpolymorphic genes are telomeric to the class II region. A possible interpretation of this variant arrangement is that the basic form of the MHC, namely class II, complement, cytokines, and class I, arose prior to speciation between mouse and man. Subsequent to speciation, the murine MHC is presumed to have undergone a rearrangement, which resulted in dividing the class I genes. The molecular structure of the murine class II region has also revealed some surprises not fully anticipated by classical genetics. The I-A subregion, originally defined by classical genetics, codes for the α and β chains of the I-A molecule as well as the highly polymorphic β chain of the I-E molecule. The I-E subregion of classical genetics codes only for the less polymorphic α chain of the I-E molecule. As in the human, β_2 microglobulin is not coded for by the MHC, but is located on a separate chromosome (chromosome 2).

Organization of Individual Class I and Class II MHC Genes

The general patterns of intron-exon organization of the individual class I and class II genes are similar to each other. Schematic examples of class I α, class II α, and class II β genes are depicted in Figure 5–8. In all MHC genes, the first exon encodes the leader or signal sequences that target the nascent proteins to the endoplasmic reticulum. These amino acid residues are not found on mature, cell surface MHC molecules (see

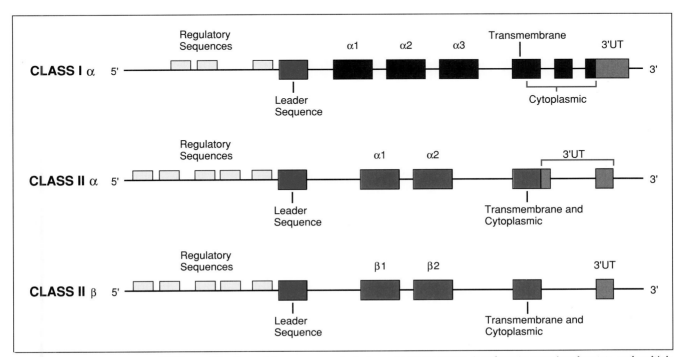

FIGURE 5 – 8. Exon-intron structures of MHC genes. *The 5′ regulatory sequences include promoter sequences, interferon-responsive elements, and multiple DNA sequences unique to class I or class II genes. 3′ UT indicates the 3′ untranslated sequence. Note that exons and introns are not shown to scale.*

the discussion of biosynthesis later in this chapter). Each of the extracellular approximately 90 amino acid residue segments (e.g., class I α1, α2, and α3) is coded for by a separate large exon. The transmembrane and cytoplasmic regions are encoded by several small exons. For class I α chains, each of the intracellular conserved phosphorylation sites is encoded by a separate small exon, emphasizing the probable importance these sites play in the intracellular trafficking of class I molecules.

Many *cis*-regulatory sequences that function to control MHC gene transcription are located in the 5′ flanking regions of the exons that code for the MHC molecules. These nucleotide sequences act as molecular targets for DNA–binding proteins that function as *trans*-acting transcriptional regulators. The general principles of transcriptional regulation of MHC genes are similar to those for other genes such as Ig (see Box 4–5, Chapter 4). Promoter and enhancer elements have been identified for class I genes. In addition, all class I loci contain nucleotide sequences that are required for responding to cytokines, particularly interferon, by increasing class I gene transcription. Class II loci contain three conserved nucleotide sequences, called W (or H), X, and Y boxes, that are necessary for expression of these genes. Class II genes with these regulatory elements can be expressed in transgenic mice. Deletions or mutations involving W, X, or Y boxes usually abolish expression completely. Nuclear factors that control class II gene expression are incompletely defined as yet.

EXPRESSION OF MHC MOLECULES

The expression of MHC molecules on different cell types determines whether or not T lymphocytes can interact with foreign antigens present on the surface of these cells. CD8+ CTLs recognize foreign antigens such as viral polypeptides when they are bound to class I MHC molecules. The ability of CTLs to lyse a virally infected cell is a direct function of the quantity of class I molecules expressed. In contrast, CD4+ helper T lymphocytes recognize antigens bound to class II MHC molecules. Class II MHC molecules are expressed by fewer cell types than class I MHC molecules and are under different regulation. As a consequence, fewer cell types can present antigens to helper T cells. Furthermore, the ability to present antigen to helper T cells is, in large part, a function of the level of class II MHC molecule expression. The concluding portion of this chapter describes the biosynthesis of class I and class II MHC molecules common to all cells and the cellular patterns of MHC molecule expression and their regulation by cytokines.

Biosynthesis of MHC Molecules

MHC molecules are translated from messenger RNA (mRNA) molecules on membrane-bound ribosomes and co-translationally inserted into the membrane of the endoplasmic reticulum. The signal or leader sequence, responsible for targeting to the endoplasmic reticulum, is removed from the nascent polypeptide during translation. N-linked high-mannose oligosaccharides are added in the endoplasmic reticulum, either during or immediately after translation. The MHC molecules then pass through to the Golgi apparatus, where the oligosaccharides are converted from high mannose to complex form. Finally, the mature glycoproteins are translocated to the plasma membrane by vesicular transport. For class I molecules, association of the α chain with β_2 microglobulin occurs intracellularly, probably within the endoplasmic reticulum. Studies of a human B cell line called Daudi have been particularly informative about the importance of β_2 microglobulin for class I MHC molecule expression. Daudi lacks the genetic information for synthesizing β_2 microglobulin, and although it transcribes class I genes and translates class I mRNA, only unstable intracellular translation products appear. Upon transfection of a functional β_2 microglobulin gene into Daudi cells or fusion with a β_2 microglobulin–expressing partner, class I products derived from the Daudi line are "rescued" and appear on the cell surface. Similarly, as discussed in Chapter 8, transgenic mice which lack β_2 microglobulin fail to express class I molecules. The surface expression of class I molecules may also be stimulated by or dependent on the binding of the newly synthesized molecules to peptides being produced within the cell. Association of such peptides with the peptide-binding cleft may promote association of the α chain with β_2 microglobulin and correct folding of the complete class I molecule.

For class II molecules, the α and β chains must also be coordinately synthesized and presumably must associate within the endoplasmic reticulum. Certain inbred mouse strains lack functional I-E α chains, and I-E β products appear only as unstable intracellular proteins because cell surface expression requires covalently linked α and β chains. Upon interstrain breeding, a functional I-E α chain synthesized from the gene of the other parent can "rescue" these I-E β products, leading to cell surface expression of I-E from both parental alleles.

Within a cell, recently synthesized class II gene products are associated with a third, nonpolymorphic chain not encoded by the MHC. This peptide has been called either γ **or invariant,** because upon migration in two-dimensional gels it is "invariant" among different individuals and inbred strains, a reflection of nonpolymorphism. The γ chain is about 30 kD in size and is a member of the Ig gene superfamily. Its orientation is reversed, in contrast to most transmembrane proteins, so that the amino terminus is intracellular and the carboxy terminus is extracellular. The γ chain separates from the mature class II $\alpha\beta$ heterodimer before it reaches the cell surface. It has been speculated that the γ chain either alters the nature of post-translational processing of α and β chains or is involved in directing intracellular trafficking of class II molecules, perhaps related to the function of class II molecules in the presentation of foreign antigens to helper T cells. The definitive function of γ is still unknown, but it does not appear to be essential for class II molecule synthesis or expression. A recent proposal is that the γ chain functions to prevent association of endogenously synthesized peptides with class II molecules so that the peptide binding site remains available for peptides derived from exogenous antigens.

Regulation of MHC Molecule Expression

The expression of class I and class II MHC molecules is regulated both by differentiation, in a cell- and tissue-specific manner, and by extrinsic immune and inflammatory stimuli. There are four important features of MHC molecule expression:

1. *The constitutive expression of class I molecules is distinct from that of class II molecules.* In general, class I molecules are present on virtually all nucleated cells, whereas class II molecules are normally expressed only on B lymphocytes, macrophages, dendritic cells, endothelial cells, and a few other cell types.

2. *The rate of transcription is the major determinant of MHC molecule expression on the cell surface.*

3. *Transcription and expression of the various class I genes and molecules are coordinately regulated; similarly, the transcription and expression of different class II genes and their products are also coordinately regulated.* In many cells, β_2 microglobulin is coordinately regulated with class I α chains, and the γ chain is coordinately regulated with class II α and β chains, despite the fact that β_2 microglobulin and the γ chain genes are not located within the MHC.

4. *Cytokines can modulate the rate of constitutive transcription of class I and class II genes in a wide variety of cell types.* This is an important amplification mechanism for T cell responses, because most of the cytokines that enhance MHC expression are secreted by T cells and MHC molecules are components of the ligands that T cells recognize and respond to. On almost all cell types examined, γ-interferon (IFN-γ) increases the level of expression of class I molecules. Other cytokines (α- and β-interferons, TNF, and lymphotoxin) can also increase class I molecule expression. (The biologic activities of cytokines are discussed in detail in Chapter 11.) These cytokine effects are mediated by increased levels of gene transcription and probably result from cytokine-activated transcription factors binding to regulatory DNA sequences in class I genes.

In contrast to class I molecules, class II molecules show marked differences in cell expression among various cell types and in their responses to cytokines (Table 5-1). Among the cells that commonly present antigen to T cells, mononuclear phagocytes express only low levels of class II molecules, until stimulated to do so by IFN-γ or certain other cytokines. Epidermal Langerhans cells, also like mononuclear phago-

TABLE 5-1. Patterns of Class II MHC Molecule Expression

Mononuclear phagocyte	Weak; increased by IFN-γ
Langerhans cell	Constitutive; increased by IFN-γ
Dendritic cell	Constitutive; no cytokine response
Endothelial cell	Negative; induced by IFN-γ
B cell	Constitutive; increased by IL-4, diminished by IFN-γ
Epithelial and stromal cells	Negative; induced by high levels of IFN-γ
Neurons	Negative; no cytokine response
T cell	Upon activation in humans and rats, not in mice; no cytokine response

Abbreviations: IFN, interferon; IL, interleukin.

cytes, increase class II expression in response to IFN-γ, whereas lymphoid dendritic cells are constitutively positive for class II expression and do not appear to respond to cytokines. Vascular endothelial cells, like monocytes and Langerhans cells, readily express class II molecules in response to IFN-γ. B lymphocytes constitutively express class II molecules and can respond to cytokines. However, resting B cells in mice increase expression of class II molecules in response to interleukin-4 and decrease expression in response to IFN-γ. Most non-immune cell types express little if any class II MHC molecules unless exposed to high levels of IFN-γ. In some cases, such as pancreatic islet cells, additional cytokines like TNF may be necessary as co-signals for induction. These cells are unlikely to present antigens to T cells except in unusual circumstances. Some cells, such as neurons, do not respond to any known cytokine treatment and remain class II-negative. Finally, human but not mouse T cells express class II molecules upon activation; however, no cytokine has been identified in this response, and its functional significance is unknown.

Non-MHC Genes Involved in the Assembly and Functions of MHC Molecules

Recently, a number of non-MHC genes have been identified within the human and murine MHC complexes that are mutated or defective in cell lines that fail to express MHC molecules or to present peptide antigens in association with MHC molecules. Several of these genes are homologous to genes encoding transmembrane pumps. Such genes were initially identified as being responsible for multiple drug resistance in a variety of cells. It is thought that the products of these genes act as peptide transporters to carry peptides (derived from self or viral antigens) from the cytoplasm of cells into the endoplasmic reticulum, where the peptides complex with the α chains of class I MHC molecules and β_2 microglobulin. This tri-molecular complex of class I molecules is conformationally stable and is expressed on the cell surface. Thus, the binding of peptides not only is the function of class I MHC molecules but also is required for efficient assembly and cell surface expression of class I MHC. Although this is an intriguing hypothesis, the protein products of these putative peptide transport genes have not been identified yet, so that their function is not established. It may be that similar gene products are involved in the assembly of and antigen presentation by class II MHC molecules.

Another set of genes within the MHC codes for proteins that function as multicatalytic proteinases. These enzymes may play a role in degrading proteins to generate peptides of a size that can fit in the peptide-binding clefts of MHC molecules. Again, however, the function of these putative proteinases is not yet established. Nevertheless, the identification of additional genes within the MHC suggests that this genetic locus may encode the full machinery needed to process protein antigens, transport peptides to appropriate intracellular sites, and present MHC–associated peptides to T cells.

SUMMARY

The MHC is a large genetic region coding for the class I and class II MHC molecules as well as other proteins. MHC molecules are extremely polymorphic, with more than 40 common alleles for each individual gene. Both class I and class II molecules were originally recognized for their role in triggering T cell responses that caused the rejection of transplanted tissue. It is now appreciated that MHC–encoded class I and class II molecules bind foreign protein antigens and form complexes that are recognized by antigen-specific T lymphocytes. Antigens associated with class I molecules are recognized by CD8[+] CTLs, whereas class II–associated antigens are recognized by CD4[+] helper T cells. The class I products are composed of a 44 kD transmembrane glycoprotein in a non-covalent complex with a nonpolymorphic 12 kD polypeptide (β_2 microglobulin). The class II products contain two MHC–encoded polymorphic chains (about 31 to 34 kD and 29 to 32 kD). It has been proposed that the three-dimensional structures of both classes of MHC molecules are similar and may be divided into an amino terminal extracellular peptide-binding region, an extracellular nonpolymorphic immunoglobulin-like region, a transmembrane region, and a cytoplasmic region. The peptide-binding region of class I molecules is formed by the α1 and α2 segments of the heavy chain. It consists of a cleft measuring approximately 25Å × 10Å × 11Å with α-helical sides and an eight-strand β pleated sheet floor. The cleft can accommodate a peptide of about 10 to 20 amino acid residues. The analogous cleft of class II molecules is formed by the α1 and the β1 domains of the two chains. In both class I and class II molecules, the polymorphic amino acid residues are located in the peptide-binding region and determine the specificity of peptide binding and T cell antigen recognition.

The human MHC is very large (about 3500 kb) and is organized as follows: (1) class II genes (HLA–DP, HLA–DQ, HLA–DR), (2) complement genes, (3) cytokine (TNF and LT) genes, and (4) class I genes (HLA–B, HLA–C and HLA–A). The mouse MHC is smaller, and the sequence of genes is (1) class I (H-2K), (2) class II (I-A, I-E), (3) complement genes, (4) cytokine genes, and (5) class I (H-2D, H-2L). All MHC genes have similar exon-intron structure, and most regulatory sequences have been located in the 5′ flanking region. The expression of the MHC gene products is highly regulated at the level of transcription both by cell type–specific factors and by inflammatory and immune stimuli, including cytokines like IFN–γ. In general, class I genes are expressed more widely, i.e., on more diverse cell types, than are class II genes. Different cell types have distinct patterns of expression of class II MHC molecules. Some cells, such as mononuclear phagocytes, can be induced to express class II molecules by cytokines, especially IFN–γ. Other cells, such as dendritic cells and B lymphocytes, constitutively express class II molecules.

SELECTED READINGS

Auffray, C., and J. L. Strominger. Molecular genetics of the human major histocompatibility complex. Advances in Human Genetics 15:197–247, 1987.

Benoist, C., and D. Mathis. Regulation of major histocompatibility complex class II genes: X, Y and other letters of the alphabet. Annual Review of Immunology 8:681–715, 1990.

Bjorkman, P. J., and P. Parham. Structure, function and diversity of class I major histocompatibility complex molecules. Annual Review of Biochemistry 59:253–288, 1990.

Bjorkman, P. J., M. A. Saper, B. Samraoui, W. S. Bennett, J. L. Strominger, and D. C. Wiley. Structure of the human class I histocompatibility antigen, HLA-A2. Nature 329:506–512, 1987.

Brown, J. H., T. Jardetzky, M. A. Saper, B. Samraoui, P. J. Bjorkman, and D. C. Wiley. A hypothetical model of the foreign antigen binding site of class II histocompatibility molecules. Nature 332:845–850, 1988.

Hood, L., M. Steinmetz, and B. Malissen. Genes of the major histocompatibility complex of the mouse. Annual Review of Immunology 1:529–568, 1983.

Strominger, J. L., V. H. Engelhard, A. Fuks, B. C. Guild, F. Hyafil, J. F. Kaufman, A. J. Korman, T. G. Kostyk, M. S. Krangel, D. Lancet, J. A. Lopez de Castro, D. L. Mann, H. T. Orr, P. R. Parham, K. C. Parker, H. L. Pleogh, J. S. Pober, R. J. Robb, and D. A. Shackelford. Biochemical analysis of products of the MHC. *In* M. E. Dorf (ed.). The Role of the Major Histocompatibility Complex in Immunobiology. Garland STPM Press, New York, 1981, pp. 115–172.

CHAPTER SIX

ANTIGEN PRESENTATION AND T CELL ANTIGEN RECOGNITION

The induction of humoral and cell-mediated immune responses to protein antigens requires the recognition of the antigens by helper T cells. The reason for this is that helper T cells are necessary for stimulating B lymphocyte growth and differentiation and for activating the effector cells of cell-mediated immunity, namely macrophages and cytolytic T lymphocytes (CTLs). Before we discuss the activation of T cells by protein antigens and the functions of various T cell subsets in subsequent chapters, we need to understand the structures of antigens that are recognized by T cells. The concept that major histocompatibility complex (MHC)–encoded molecules play an important role in antigen recognition by helper cells and CTLs was introduced in Chapter 5. This chapter describes the formation of complexes of foreign antigens and MHC molecules, which are the ligands for which T cell antigen receptors are specific, and the physiologic significance of this unusual specificity.

CHARACTERISTICS OF ANTIGEN RECOGNITION BY T LYMPHOCYTES

It is now known that CD4+ T lymphocytes, most of which are helper cells, recognize peptides that are bound to class II MHC molecules on the surfaces of other, non-T cells. Class II–associated peptides are usually derived from extracellular microbes and soluble protein antigens. Furthermore, CD8+ T cells, most of which are CTLs, recognize peptide fragments bound to class I MHC molecules on cells that are targets of the lytic action of CTLs. These class I–associated peptides are generally derived from endogenously synthesized proteins, such as viral antigens. The elucidation of these principles was one of the most impressive achievements in immunology in the 1980s. Our current understanding of T cell antigen recognition is the culmination of a vast amount of work beginning with studies on the physicochemical forms of antigens that stimulated cell-mediated immunity. These studies led to the discovery that cells other than T lymphocytes play an obligatory role in T cell activation by foreign antigens and later to the

elucidation of the function of MHC molecules in T cell antigen recognition.

Physicochemical Forms of Antigens Recognized by T Lymphocytes

The realization that humoral and cell-mediated immunity are mediated by different classes of lymphocytes, i.e., B and T cells, respectively, led many investigators to examine the properties of the antigens that stimulated these two types of immune responses. Such studies established a fundamental concept, namely that *T lymphocytes recognize different forms of antigens from B lymphocytes and secreted immunoglobulin* (Ig).

1. T lymphocytes recognize only protein antigens, whereas B cells can specifically recognize proteins, nucleic acids, polysaccharides, lipids, and small chemicals. Some T cells are specific for chemically reactive forms of haptens such as dinitrophenol. In these situations, it is likely that the haptens bind to cell surface proteins, including MHC molecules, and these hapten-protein conjugates are recognized by T cells. As we shall see later, the reason why T cells respond only to protein antigens is that only fragments of proteins can form stable complexes with MHC molecules.

2. B cells specific for protein antigens may recognize conformational determinants that exist when proteins are in their native tertiary (folded) configuration or determinants that are exposed by denaturation or proteolysis. In contrast, T cells recognize only linear determinants defined predominantly by primary amino acid sequences. Thus, when an animal is immunized with a native protein, the antibodies it produces will react only with the native protein. In contrast, the antigen-specific T cells which are stimulated by immunization with the native protein will respond to denatured or even proteolytically digested forms of that protein (Table 6–1). Consistent with this difference in the nature of antigenic determinants for T and

TABLE 6–1. Qualitative Differences in Antigen Recognition by T and B Lymphocytes

		Secondary Immune Response	
Immunizing Antigen	Secondary Antigen Exposure	B Cell–Mediated (Antibody Production)	T Cell–Mediated (Delayed Type) Hypersensitivity
Native protein	Native protein	+	+
Denatured protein	Native protein	−	+
Native protein	Denatured protein	−	+
Denatured protein	Denatured protein	+	+

Antigen recognition by T and B lymphocytes is qualitatively different. In an immunized animal, B cells are specific for conformational determinants of the immunogen and, therefore, distinguish between native and denatured protein antigens. T cells, however, do not distinguish between native and denatured protein antigens because T cells recognize non-conformational linear epitopes.

B cell recognition is the finding that T cell responses to a soluble antigen cannot be inhibited using antibodies specific for conformational determinants of that antigen, whereas antigen recognition by B cells can be competitively inhibited by such antibodies.

Role of Accessory Cells in T Cell Responses to Antigens

The second important characteristic of antigen recognition by T lymphocytes is that *T cells recognize and respond to foreign protein antigens only when the antigen is attached to the surfaces of other cells,* whereas B cells and secreted antibodies bind soluble antigens in the circulation or in the aqueous phase. Thus, CTLs recognize antigens bound to the surface of target cells and kill these targets. The activation of helper T cells by foreign antigens requires the participation of cells other than T lymphocytes; these are called **accessory cells.** These accessory cells serve two principal functions in helper T cell stimulation:

1. Accessory cells display fragments of foreign protein antigens on their surfaces in a form that can be specifically recognized by T cell antigen receptors. This phenomenon is called **antigen presentation,** and the cell populations capable of performing this function are **antigen-presenting cells** (APCs). (The term APCs is used for accessory cells that present antigens to helper T lymphocytes. Since CTLs also recognize foreign antigens bound to the surfaces of their target cells, all such target cells may be conceptually included among APCs. Conventionally, however, cells that are recognized and lysed by CTLs are called **target cells,** not APCs.)

2. Accessory cells provide stimuli to the T cell, beyond those initiated by ligand binding to the T cell antigen receptor, which are required for physiologic activation. These stimuli, referred to as **costimulator activities,** are incompletely characterized. They may be provided by membrane-bound or secreted products of accessory cells.

The antigen-presenting functions of accessory cells are described in more detail later in this chapter, and their costimulator functions are discussed in Chapter 7.

The importance of APCs in initiating T cell–dependent immune responses was first suggested in the 1950s by the demonstration that radioactively or fluorescently labeled antigens injected into animals were found in mononuclear phagocytes or follicular dendritic cells and not in lymphocytes. Later studies showed that an antigen that was bound to macrophages *in vitro* and then injected into mice was up to 1000 times more immunogenic on a molar basis than the same antigen administered by itself, in a cell-free form. The explanation for this finding is that T cells respond only to antigen associated with macrophages or other APCs, and only a small fraction of an injected soluble antigen ends up in this immunogenic cell-associated form.

The obligatory role of accessory cells in lymphocyte activation was formally established when techniques for stimulating immune responses *in vitro* were developed. For example, T cells isolated from the blood, spleen, or lymph nodes of individuals immunized with a protein antigen can be restimulated in tissue culture by that antigen. Stimulation may be measured by assaying the production of cytokines by the T cells or by the proliferation of the T cells. When contaminating macrophages and dendritic cells are removed from the cultures, the purified T lymphocytes no longer respond to antigen, and responsiveness can be restored by adding back the macrophages or dendritic cells. Such experimental approaches provide the basis for defining the accessory functions of various cell types in T lymphocyte activation. The importance of accessory cells in immune responses *in vivo* is suggested by the observation that **adjuvants** often need to be administered in addition to antigen in order to elicit an immune response to the antigen. These adjuvants are usually insoluble or undegradable substances that promote nonspecific inflammation, with recruitment of mononuclear phagocytes at the site of immunization.

The Phenomenon of MHC–Restricted Antigen Recognition by T Lymphocytes

The critical advance in our understanding of antigen recognition by helper T cells and CTLs was the discovery of the phenomenon of **self MHC restriction** in the 1970s. *MHC restriction is the requirement that an APC must express MHC molecules that the T cell recognizes as self in order for the T cell to recognize and respond to a foreign protein antigen presented by that APC.* The MHC molecules that T cells recognize as self are those that the T cells encountered during their maturation from precursors in the thymus. (The process of T cell maturation is discussed in much more detail in Chapter 8.) "Self MHC" refers not to MHC molecules expressed by the T cells themselves but to MHC molecules on the APCs or target cells. Normally, because T cells and APCs develop in the same individual, they are syngeneic and all the MHC molecules on the APCs are seen as self MHC by all the T cells in that individual. In experimental systems, T cells respond to antigens presented by a particular APC if the two cell types are at least partly syngeneic, i.e., if they are derived from individuals or inbred strains that share one or more MHC alleles. In this situation the APCs express MHC molecules that the T cells encountered and learned to see as self during their maturation.

This phenomenon of self MHC restriction was discovered when T cells from one inbred strain of animal were mixed with APCs from different inbred strains and T cell responses were assayed. Three sets of experiments established MHC restriction of antigen recognition by helper T cells and CTLs:

1. T cells from an antigen-primed guinea pig of one inbred strain proliferate in response to antigen *in vitro* only if macrophages from the same strain are present. These proliferating T cells are mostly helper cells. Subsequent analyses using inbred and congenic strains of mice revealed that in order to present antigens to helper T cells, the APCs have to express class II MHC molecules that are seen as self by the T cells (Fig. 6–1). Such experiments, and others using purified and monoclonal T cell populations from mice and humans, have established that *antigen recognition by helper T cells is class II MHC–restricted.*

2. *In vivo* experiments with inbred mice utilizing

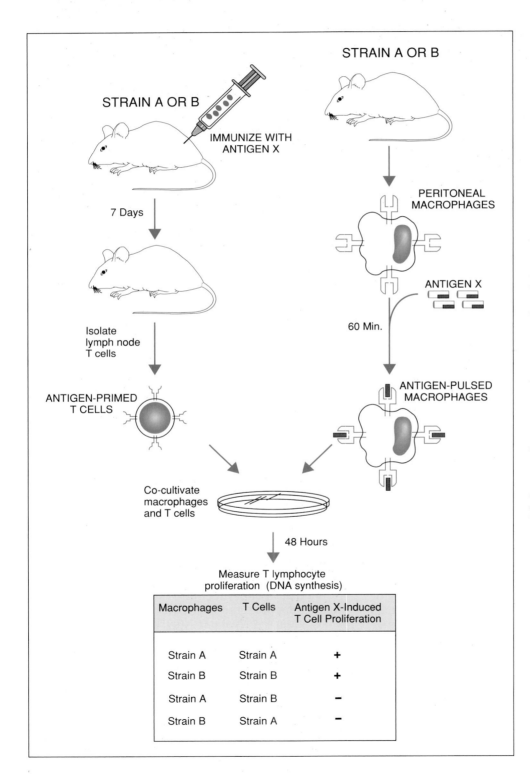

FIGURE 6–1. MHC restriction of proliferating (helper) T lymphocytes. T cells from a strain A or strain B mouse primed with an antigen X proliferate in response to that antigen only in the presence of strain A or B macrophages (or other antigen-presenting cells [APCs]), respectively. In the experiment depicted, the T cell populations are devoid of alloreactivity; i.e., strain A T cells do not respond to the foreign MHC molecules of strain B, and vice versa. The T cells also do not proliferate in the absence of antigen. Using congenic and recombinant strains of mice, it can be shown that the macrophages and T cells must come from animals that share class II MHC alleles in order for the antigen-induced T cell proliferation to occur.

adoptive transfer techniques and *in vitro* studies of antibody production showed that helper T lymphocytes and B cells cooperate to produce an antibody response to a protein antigen only if the B cells express class II MHC molecules that are seen as self by the T cells. This phenomenon is discussed in more detail in Chapter 9. It further supports the conclusion that helper T cells are class II MHC–restricted.

3. Perhaps the clearest demonstration of MHC

restriction came from assays of virus-specific CTL–mediated lysis of virally infected target cells in mice and humans. In most of these systems, the virus-infected target cells are lysed only if they express class I MHC molecules that are recognized as self MHC by the T cells (Fig. 6–2). This established that *CTL recognition of viral antigens is class I MHC–restricted.*

These experiments suggest that the MHC gene products involved in T cell antigen recognition must

FIGURE 6 – 2. MHC restriction of cytolytic T lymphocytes (CTLs). Virus-specific CTLs from a strain A or strain B mouse lyse only syngeneic target cells infected with the specific virus. The CTLs do not lyse uninfected targets and are not alloreactive. Further analysis has shown that the CTLs and target cells must come from animals that share class I MHC alleles in order for the target cell to present viral antigens to the CTLs. LCMV, lymphocytic choriomeningitis virus.

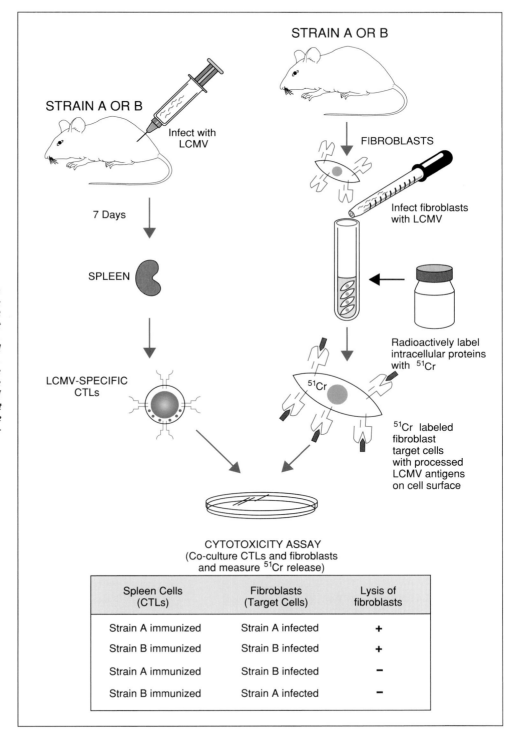

STRAIN A OR B

STRAIN A OR B

Infect with LCMV

FIBROBLASTS

Infect fibroblasts with LCMV

7 Days

SPLEEN

Radioactively label intracellular proteins with ⁵¹Cr

LCMV-SPECIFIC CTLs

⁵¹Cr

⁵¹Cr labeled fibroblast target cells with processed LCMV antigens on cell surface

CYTOTOXICITY ASSAY
(Co-culture CTLs and fibroblasts and measure ⁵¹Cr release)

Spleen Cells (CTLs)	Fibroblasts (Target Cells)	Lysis of fibroblasts
Strain A immunized	Strain A infected	+
Strain B immunized	Strain B infected	+
Strain A immunized	Strain B infected	−
Strain B immunized	Strain A infected	−

**TABLE 6–2. Major Histocompatibility Complex (MHC)
Restriction of T Cell Responses to Antigen Depends on
MHC Molecules on Antigen-Presenting Cells (APCs)**

Monoclonal T Cell Population from (A × B)F1 Mouse, Specific for Antigen X	T Cell Response to Antigen X plus APC from Strain			
	A	B	(A × B)F1	C
Clone No. 1 (MHC^B – restricted)	–	+	+	–
Clone No. 2 (MHC^A – restricted)	+	–	+	–

MHC restriction of T cell responses to antigen depends on MHC molecules on the APC. Individual T cells can be isolated from an antigen X – immunized (A × B)F1 mouse, which has both strain A and strain B MHC genes. These T cells are then propagated *in vitro*, giving rise to multiple identical progeny (monoclonal T cell populations). Recognition of antigen X by progeny of T cell clone number 1 depends on the presence of APCs from strain B, whereas T cell clone number 2 requires APCs from strain A. Both T cell clones number 1 and number 2 respond to antigen X in the presence of APCs from an (A × B)F1 mouse. Neither T cell clone will respond to antigen X alone or in the presence of APCs from a third unrelated strain (C), which has no shared MHC genes with A or B. This pattern of responses indicates that the MHC restricting element, i.e., the MHC protein which the T cell recognizes as self, must be expressed by the APC.

be expressed on the APC or on the target for CTL–mediated lysis. Several experiments have proved that this is indeed the case and that the necessary MHC molecules need not be present on the T cells themselves.

1. A monoclonal antigen-specific T cell restricted by MHC of type A responds to that antigen in the presence of APCs that express the type A MHC allele (Table 6–2). Among antigen-specific T cells derived from an (A × B)F1 individual, some of the cells are MHC^A – restricted, others are MHC^B – restricted, and a smaller subset may be restricted by hybrid MHC molecules expressed only in (A × B)F1 mice. The key point is that even though the MHC^A – restricted T cells are from an (A × B) F1 mouse, they only respond to APCs which express MHC^A (either alone or with MHC^B).

2. The response of an MHC^A – restricted T cell to an antigen is blocked by antibodies specific for type A MHC molecules. The lytic activity of CD8$^+$ T cells is inhibited by antibodies against class I MHC molecules, and the activation of CD4$^+$ T cells is inhibited by anti – class II antibodies. Such inhibition is seen only if the antibodies bind to the APC, not if they bind to the T cells (Table 6–3).

3. APCs that do not express restricting MHC molecules fail to stimulate antigen-specific T cells. For instance, in the example mentioned above, MHC^A – restricted T cells do not respond to APCs that are MHC^A – negative. If the genes coding for MHC^A are transfected into the APCs and the cells become MHC^A – positive, they also acquire the ability to stimulate the T cells (Table 6–4).

These experiments led to the fundamental concept that *helper and cytolytic T lymphocytes specific for foreign protein antigens simultaneously recognize two structures, the foreign antigen and a self MHC molecule, both of which are present on the surface of the APC or target cell* (Fig. 6–3). The experiments described above suggested that helper T cells and CTLs are ex-

TABLE 6–3. Inhibition of MHC – Restricted Antigen Presentation by Anti – MHC Antibodies

	T Cells from Immunized Mice	Macrophages	Antibody in Culture	T Cell Proliferation
A	I-A restricted helper T cell	Normal	None	–
	I-A restricted helper T cell	Ag-pulsed	None	+
	I-A restricted helper T cell	Ag-pulsed	anti – I-A	–
	I-A restricted helper T cell	Ag-pulsed	anti – I-E	+
	I-A restricted helper T cell	Ag-pulsed	anti – K/D	+
B	I-A restricted helper T cell + anti – I-A (prebound)	Ag-pulsed	None	+
	I-A restricted helper T cell	Ag-pulsed + anti – I-A (prebound)	None	–

A helper T cell population specific for I-A – associated antigen proliferates in response to the antigen presented by I-A expressing APCs. The response is blocked by anti – I-A antibody (in part *A* of table), but only if the antibody is allowed to bind to the APCs before adding the T cells (part *B*). Therefore, T cells recognize self MHC – associated antigens presented by APC.

Abbreviations: MHC, major histocompatibility complex; Ag, antigen; APC, antigen-presenting cell.

TABLE 6-4. Requirement for Class II MHC Expression in Antigen Presentation to CD4+, Antigen-Specific T Cells

APCs	Genes Transfected Into APCs	Surface Class II MHC	Surface Class I MHC	Antigen	Response of Cytochrome c–Specific, I-E^k–Restricted T Cell Line (Cytokine Secretion)
3T3 (murine fibroblast)	None	None	K^k, D^k	Cytochrome c	−
3T3 (murine fibroblast)	Murine class II Eα^k and Eβ^k	I-E^k	K^k, D^k	None	−
3T3 (murine fibroblast)	Murine class II Eα^k and Eβ^k	I-E^k	K^k, D^k	Cytochrome c	+

Class II MHC expression is required for antigen presentation to CD4+, antigen-specific T cells. In this experiment, a murine fibroblast cell line, 3T3, derived from an H-2^k mouse, which expresses class I, but not class II, MHC molecules, does not present cytochrome c to a cytochrome c–specific, I-E^k–restricted, T cell hybridoma line. When functional genes encoding the α and β chains of the I-E^k molecule are transfected into 3T3 cells, they become competent at presenting antigen to the T cell line.

Abbreviations: MHC, major histocompatibility complex; APC, antigen-presenting cell.

clusively restricted by class II and class I MHC molecules, respectively. In fact, the class I or class II restriction of T cells correlates more strongly with their expression of CD8 or CD4 than with the functional capabilities of the cells. Thus, *all CD4+ T cells are restricted by class II MHC molecules,* and in fact CD4 itself binds to class II molecules. Most CD4+ cells are helper cells, although CD4+ CTLs (again class II–restricted) have been identified in humans and mice. *Similarly, all CD8+ T cells are class I–restricted,* and the CD8 molecule binds to class I MHC molecules. Most of these cells are CTLs, although some may function as cytokine-producing helper cells. (Some CD8+ T cells suppress immune responses; the specificity of suppressor cells is a controversial issue and is discussed in Chapter 10.) The structures of CD4 and CD8 molecules and their roles in T cell antigen recognition are discussed in Chapter 7.

The molecular basis of MHC–restricted antigen recognition by T cells was elucidated by parallel studies of the structure of the T cell receptor for antigen and of antigen presentation. As we shall see in Chapter 7, T cells express a single antigen receptor that simultaneously interacts with an epitope of a protein antigen that is bound to MHC molecules and with polymorphic residues of MHC molecules. The analysis of antigen presentation being done concurrently has revealed that *foreign protein antigens are presented to T cells as peptides that are non-covalently attached to the peptide-binding clefts of MHC molecules.* As we discuss below, these studies have demonstrated how large protein antigens can physically associate with MHC molecules. Furthermore, we now understand how the vast number of protein antigens that different T cells can recognize are presented by the few (less than 20) allelic MHC molecules expressed in each individual.

MECHANISMS OF ANTIGEN PRESENTATION

The fundamental feature of antigen presentation to MHC–restricted T cells is that foreign antigens

form physical complexes with MHC molecules. The ability to generate such complexes is the essential property of all APCs or targets for CTLs. Thus, APCs are capable of converting even large globular proteins to a sufficiently small size and appropriate conformation that can non-covalently attach to the peptide-binding clefts of MHC molecules synthesized by the APCs. The conversion of native proteins to MHC–associated peptide fragments is called **antigen processing.** Foreign antigens that are synthesized outside the APCs, such as bacterial proteins and soluble protein antigens that are administered to individuals, first bind to APCs and are then endocytosed. At this stage, the proteins may be in their native tertiary forms. They are then partly degraded, and fragments derived from the antigens usually bind to the peptide-binding clefts of class II MHC molecules. Complexes of processed antigens and class II MHC molecules are displayed on the surfaces of APCs, where they are recognized by class II MHC–restricted T lymphocytes. Foreign proteins that are synthesized within a cell, such as viral proteins and tumor antigens, are also processed, but they enter a different intracellular compartment from endocytosed antigens. Peptides derived from endogenously synthesized proteins generally associate with class I MHC molecules, although some endogenously synthesized, e.g., viral, proteins may be processed and may become bound to class II molecules. Complexes of peptides and class I MHC molecules are displayed on the cell surface, where they are recognized by class I–restricted T cells.

This portion of the chapter describes the cell types that can function as APCs, the mechanisms of antigen processing, and the characteristics of peptide-MHC association.

Types of Antigen-Presenting Cells

The two requisite properties that allow a cell to function as an APC for class II MHC–restricted helper T lymphocytes are the ability to process endocytosed antigens and the expression of class II MHC gene products. Most mammalian cells appear to be capable of endocytos-

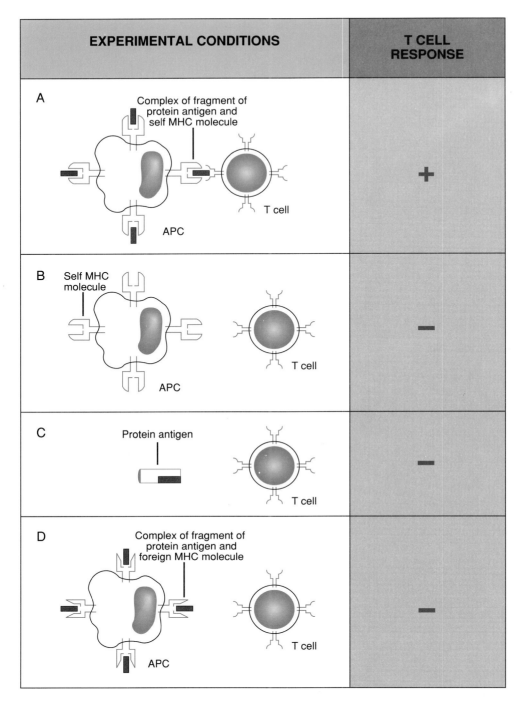

EXPERIMENTAL CONDITIONS	T CELL RESPONSE
A Complex of fragment of protein antigen and self MHC molecule · APC · T cell	+
B Self MHC molecule · APC · T cell	−
C Protein antigen · T cell	−
D Complex of fragment of protein antigen and foreign MHC molecule · APC · T cell	−

FIGURE 6–3. Specificity of MHC–restricted T cells. *Helper T cells and cytolytic T lymphocytes (CTLs) recognize complexes of self MHC molecules and peptide fragments of foreign antigens (A). MHC–restricted T cells do not recognize self MHC molecules alone or self MHC with self peptide (B), foreign antigens without MHC molecules (C), or complexes of foreign MHC molecules and peptide fragment of antigen (D). APC, antigen-presenting cell; MHC, major histocompatibility complex.*

ing and processing protein antigens, so that the critical property that enables a particular cell to function as an APC is the expression of class II MHC molecules.

The best-defined APCs for helper T lymphocytes include: (1) mononuclear phagocytes, (2) B lymphocytes, (3) dendritic cells, (4) Langerhans cells of the skin, and (5) in humans, endothelial cells.

Macrophages and other cells of the **mononuclear phagocyte system** actively phagocytose large parti-

cles. Therefore, they probably play an important role in presenting antigens derived from infectious organisms such as bacteria and parasites.

B lymphocytes specific for a protein antigen are very efficient at presenting that antigen to helper T lymphocytes *in vitro* and may serve as APCs *in vivo*, particularly when the concentration of available antigen is low. The reason why antigen-specific B cells are uniquely efficient APCs is that their membrane Ig molecules can bind the antigen with high affinity and, therefore, at low concentrations. The antigen-presenting function of B cells may be particularly important in helper T cell–dependent antibody production (see Chapter 9).

Dendritic cells of the spleen and lymph nodes are irregularly shaped, nonphagocytic cells making up a small fraction (<1 per cent) of the total cell population of these organs. They are derived from the bone marrow and may be related to the mononuclear phagocytic lineage. Dendritic cells are competent at presenting protein antigens to helper T cells. It is also believed that dendritic cells are important for inducing T cell responses to foreign (allogeneic) MHC molecules in tissue allografts. Consistent with this hypothesis is the observation that dendritic cells are potent stimulators of mixed lymphocyte reactions (see Chapter 16).

Langerhans cells are specialized epidermal cells with a dendritic morphology. They are derived from bone marrow progenitors, express the CD1 marker, and contain an unusual cytoplasmic organelle called the Birbeck granule. Langerhans cells may be related in lineage to the dendritic cells of spleen and lymph nodes. They are the only resident epidermal cells known to be capable of antigen presentation and, therefore, may be important in presenting the anti-

gens responsible for cutaneous contact sensitivity reactions.

In humans, *venular endothelial cells* express class II MHC molecules and may also interact with T cells. This may be particularly important in cell-mediated immune reactions, such as delayed type hypersensitivity reactions in peripheral tissues (see Chapter 12).

In addition to cells that express class II MHC molecules constitutively, many cell types can be induced to express their class II MHC genes by the T lymphocyte–derived cytokine γ interferon (IFN–γ) (Fig. 6–4). Epithelial, glial, mesenchymal, and vascular endothelial cells may acquire antigen-presenting capabilities *in vitro* when they are induced to express class II MHC molecules. The physiologic role of these cell types in immune responses to protein antigens *in vivo* is not well defined. It is likely that immune responses are initiated by APCs that express class II molecules constitutively. This may result in the activation of T cells at the site of antigen exposure, local production of IFN–γ, and increased class II MHC expression on resident APCs as well as on endothelial or mesenchymal cells that normally cannot present antigens. As a result, more cell populations begin to function as APCs, and this may lead to enhanced antigen presen-

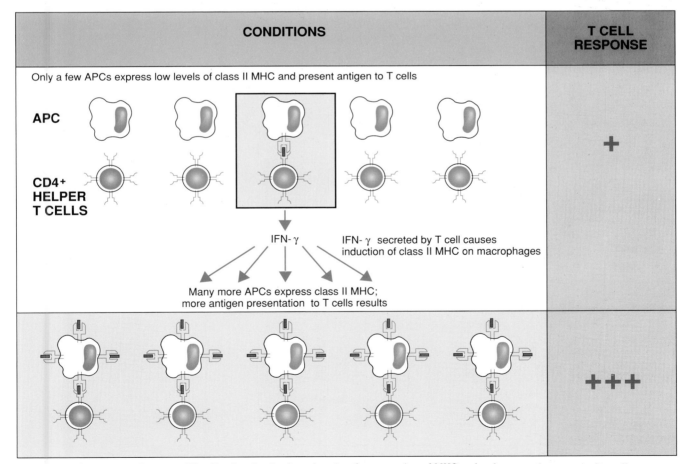

FIGURE 6–4. *Gamma interferon amplifies T cell activation by enhancing the expression of MHC molecules on antigen-presenting cells.*

tation and T cell activation. Thus, the ability of IFN – γ to stimulate the expression of class II MHC molecules may be an important amplification mechanism for T cell – mediated immune responses.

Since virtually all nucleated cells express class I MHC molecules, all such cells can present endogenously produced foreign protein antigens to class I MHC – restricted CTLs and, therefore, can serve as targets for CD8+ CTLs. This is an important defense mechanism against viruses, which can infect many types of nucleated cells. Various T cell – derived cytokines, particularly IFN – γ and tumor necrosis factor (TNF), augment the expression of class I MHC molecules. Both these cytokines are produced by CTLs, suggesting that cytokine regulation of class I expression may serve to amplify CTL – target interactions.

The mechanisms of antigen processing and presentation have been most thoroughly analyzed for extracellular antigens that are recognized by CD4+ class II MHC – restricted helper T cells. Less is known about antigen presentation to CD8+ class I – restricted CTLs. Therefore, much of the subsequent discussion will focus on the class II – associated presentation of extracellular antigens by APCs. Antigen presentation to CTLs is described separately on p. 131.

Uptake and Processing of Extracellular Protein Antigens by Antigen-Presenting Cells

The initial step in the presentation of a foreign protein antigen is the binding of the native antigen to an APC. Different APCs can bind protein antigens in several ways and with varying efficacies and specificities. Macrophages and dendritic cells bind many different antigens with little or no specificity to surface molecules that are undefined. There are, however, special cases in which the surface molecule on the APC that mediates binding and subsequent internalization of the antigen is identified. For example, specific receptors for the Fc portions of immunoglobulins and receptors for the complement protein C3b, which are present on the surface of macrophages, can efficiently bind opsonized antigens and enhance their internalization. This may partially explain why secondary immune responses require lower doses of antigen than primary responses, since at the time of secondary immunization pre-existing specific antibody may augment binding of the antigen to APCs.

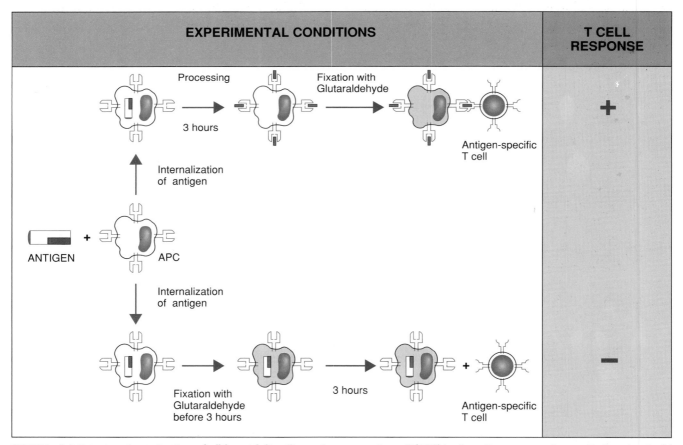

FIGURE 6 – 5. Antigen processing requires time and cellular metabolism. If an antigen-presenting cell (APC) is allowed to process antigen and is then chemically fixed (rendered metabolically inert) 3 hours or more after antigen internalization, it is capable of presenting antigen to T cells. Antigen is not processed or presented if APCs are fixed less than 1 to 3 hours after antigen uptake. Effective antigen presentation is assayed by measuring a T cell response, such as cytokine secretion.

Another example of specific receptors on APCs is the surface Ig on B cells, which can bind antigens at low concentrations in a highly specific and efficient manner and internalize these antigens for processing.

Within minutes after antigens bind to APCs, they enter the cells, usually by phagocytosis or by receptor-mediated endocytosis in clathrin-coated vesicles. Soluble protein antigens may also be internalized into APCs by fluid phase pinocytosis, without actually binding to the cell surface. Such internalized antigens become localized in intracellular membrane–bound vesicles called **endosomes**. The next step in antigen presentation is the processing of the antigen that was internalized in its native form. Several characteristics of the processing of protein antigens are known:

1. *Antigen processing is a time- and metabolism-dependent phenomenon that takes place subsequent to internalization of antigen by APCs.* If macrophages (or other APCs) are incubated briefly ("pulsed") with a protein antigen such as ovalbumin (OVA), rendered metabolically inert by chemical fixation at various times thereafter, and tested for their ability to stimulate OVA–specific T cells, functional antigen presentation occurs only if 1 to 3 hours elapse between the antigen pulse and fixation (Fig. 6–5). This time is required for the APCs to process the antigen and present it in association with class II MHC molecules on the cell surface. Processing of antigen is inhibited by maintaining the APCs below physiologic temperatures, by adding metabolic inhibitors such as azide, or by fixation before or less than 1 hour after the antigen pulse.

2. *Antigen processing takes place in acidic intracellular compartments.* Chemical agents that increase the pH of intracellular acid vesicles, such as chloroquine and ammonium chloride, are potent inhibitors of antigen processing.

3. *Cellular proteases are required for the processing of many protein antigens.* Protease inhibitors, such as leupeptin, block the presentation of protein antigens by APCs. The function of proteases is to cleave native protein antigens into small peptides. Many cellular proteases function optimally at acid pH, and this is the likely reason why antigen processing occurs best in acidic endosomes.

4. *The processed forms of most protein antigens that T cells recognize are proteolytically cleaved fragments presented on the surface of APCs.* Macrophages that are fixed or that are treated with chloroquine before exposure to antigen can effectively present pre-digested peptide fragments of that antigen, but not the intact protein, to specific T cells (Fig. 6–6). This phenomenon has proved to be extremely useful in analyzing the minimal features of a peptide required for binding to MHC molecules and recognition by T cells. Peptides generated by the *in vitro* proteolysis of a complex globular protein or produced synthetically are capable of stimulating antigen-specific T cells in the presence of fixed APCs, and such peptides can be analyzed for amino acid sequence and secondary structure. Immunogenic peptides derived from many complex globular proteins, such as cytochrome

c, ovalbumin, myoglobin, and lysozyme, have been characterized in detail in this way. Immunogenic fragments of **hen egg lysozyme** (HEL), generated by proteolytic cleavage, have been analyzed extensively by Emil Unanue and his associates. We will refer to HEL–derived peptides later in this chapter as prototypical examples for our discussion of the biology of antigen processing and presentation.

In summary, the intracellular proteolysis of endocytosed protein at acid pH generates peptide fragments that can bind to MHC molecules and can be presented to T cells. This type of processing is required for MHC–associated presentation of most protein antigens, because the peptide-binding cleft of MHC molecules is of a size that accommodates peptides that are only 10 to 20 amino acids long (see Chapter 5). Proteolysis may not be necessary for proteins that can bind to MHC molecules in an unfolded configuration even if their size is such that the ends hang out of the binding clefts of MHC molecules. One example of such a protein is fibrinogen, a 30 kD molecule that can be presented by fixed APCs, i.e., without processing. The carboxy terminal end of this protein contains a hydrophilic portion that has no identifiable secondary structure and may be capable of binding to MHC molecules in its native form.

The requirement for antigen processing prior to T cell stimulation explains why T cells recognize linear but not conformational determinants of protein and why T cells cannot distinguish between native and denatured forms of a protein antigen (see Table 6–1). Moreover, in mammalian cells, polysaccharides and lipids cannot be processed to a form that can associate with MHC molecules. This is the reason why polysaccharides and lipids are not recognized by MHC–restricted T lymphocytes and fail to stimulate cell-mediated immunity. It is also likely that most types of APCs, including macrophages, B cells, and dendritic cells, are qualitatively similar in their ability to process endocytosed antigens; however, there may be quantitative differences. For instance, macrophages contain many more proteases than do B cells and are more actively phagocytic, so that macrophages may be more efficient than B cells at internalizing and processing large particulate antigens and presenting peptide fragments of these antigens. It is also possible that different APCs generate distinct sets of peptides from the same native protein because of differences in their endosomal proteases. Although there are no clearly documented examples, this raises the possibility that the APCs involved in presenting a particular protein antigen can influence which T cells are activated by that antigen.

Association of Processed Peptides with Class II MHC Molecules

After protein antigens are processed, they remain sequestered in membrane-bound vesicles and bind to class II MHC molecules within the APCs. The exact site

EXPERIMENTAL CONDITIONS	T CELL RESPONSE

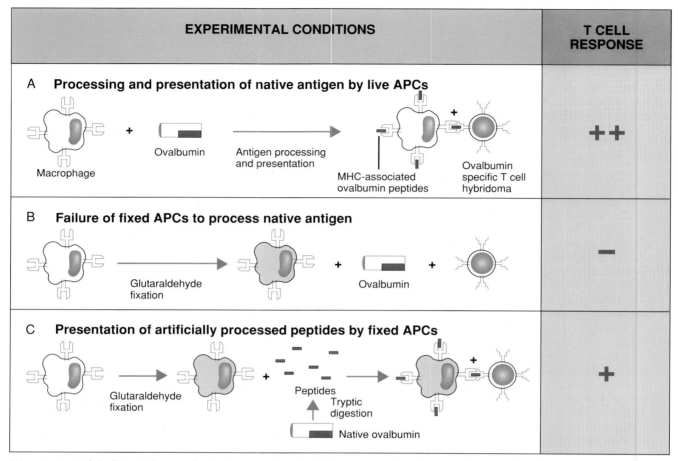

A   Processing and presentation of native antigen by live APCs

Macrophage + Ovalbumin → Antigen processing and presentation → MHC-associated ovalbumin peptides + Ovalbumin specific T cell hybridoma

++

B   Failure of fixed APCs to process native antigen

→ Glutaraldehyde fixation → + Ovalbumin +

−

C   Presentation of artificially processed peptides by fixed APCs

→ Glutaraldehyde fixation → + Peptides ← Tryptic digestion ← Native ovalbumin → +

+

FIGURE 6 – 6. *Metabolically inert (chemically fixed) antigen-presenting cells (APCs) present proteolytic fragments of antigens. A native antigen is processed and presented by viable APCs (A) but not by fixed APCs (B). Fixed APCs bind and present proteolytic fragments of antigens to specific T cells (C). The artificial proteolysis, therefore, mimics physiologic antigen processing by APCs. (Note that T cell hybridomas respond to processed antigens on fixed APCs, but growth factor–dependent T cells may require costimulators that are destroyed by certain types of fixation. This is discussed fully in Chapter 10.)*

of this association is not known. It has been suggested that class II MHC molecules are synthesized and transported to the cell surface in post-Golgi vesicles. According to this model, the vesicles containing MHC molecules physically intersect endosomes containing processed antigens during their intracellular traffic, and the MHC molecules and processed peptides form non-covalent bonds (Fig. 6-7). The complexes of peptides and class II molecules are then transported to and expressed on the surface of the APCs. It is not known how a protein antigen endocytosed by an APC escapes complete proteolytic degradation during processing and is prevented from entering the lysosomal compartment of the cell. One possibility is that binding of a peptide to an MHC molecule prevents further enzymatic hydrolysis of the peptide. Purified peptides bound to MHC molecules are resistant to destruction by proteases *in vitro*, whereas the same peptides in the absence of MHC molecules are readily hydrolyzed into amino acids by proteolytic enzymes.

The formal experimental demonstration that *an-tigenic peptides bind to purified MHC molecules even in cell-free solutions* has provided important new approaches for defining the structural basis of MHC–associated antigen recognition. Peptide-MHC binding was first demonstrated by the technique of equilibrium dialysis (see Chapter 3). Purified class II MHC molecules were enclosed within a semipermeable membrane through which they could not diffuse and were incubated with an excess of a freely diffusible fluorescently labeled peptide fragment of HEL. The accumulation of fluorescent label in the compartment containing peptide and MHC molecules was compared with the amount of label in the compartment with peptide alone. Such analyses showed that peptide-MHC binding is saturable, and the dissociation constant (K_d) of the interaction was calculated to be about 10^{-6} M (Fig. 6-8). Other techniques have been developed to measure the physical association of peptides and MHC molecules. These include the use of radioactively labeled peptides and gel filtration to separate unbound peptide from the larger peptide-

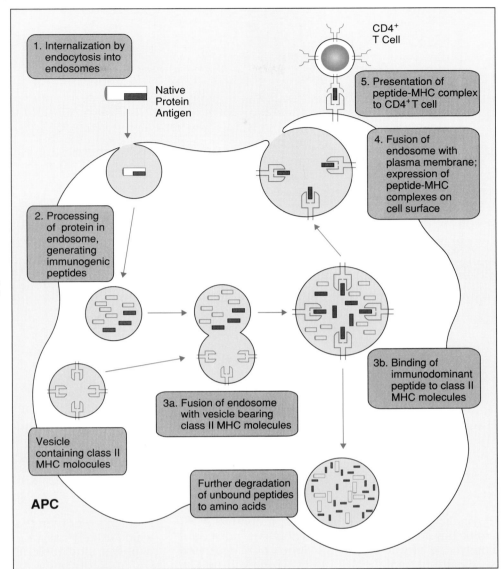

FIGURE 6-7. Pathway of class II MHC-restricted presentation of an extracellular protein antigen.

1. Internalization by endocytosis into endosomes

Native Protein Antigen

2. Processing of protein in endosome, generating immunogenic peptides

CD4+ T Cell

5. Presentation of peptide-MHC complex to CD4+ T cell

4. Fusion of endosome with plasma membrane; expression of peptide-MHC complexes on cell surface

3b. Binding of immunodominant peptide to class II MHC molecules

3a. Fusion of endosome with vesicle bearing class II MHC molecules

Vesicle containing class II MHC molecules

Further degradation of unbound peptides to amino acids

APC

MHC complexes and the measurement of fluorescence resonance energy transfer between the two sets of interacting proteins labeled with different fluorochromes. Based on such studies, several important characteristics of the binding of antigenic peptides to class II MHC molecules are known. Following are the main features of this association; its physiologic and functional significance are discussed later in the chapter.

1. *Multiple peptide antigens can bind to the same MHC molecule.* This was first suggested by functional assays of antigen competition, before purified MHC molecules were available for direct analyses. For instance, structurally similar amino acid polymers compete with one another for presentation to a T cell specific for either one. Such competition occurs if the competing antigen is added before or together with the antigen that is recognized by the T cell (Table 6-5). These experiments suggested that an MHC molecule can bind more than one antigen but that a T cell is specific for only one of these. Competition between antigens for binding to a particular MHC molecule has been definitively established by direct physical measurements. Thus, many peptides compete with one another for binding to the same MHC molecule. Somewhat surprisingly, these antigenic peptides often show little sequence homology (Table 6-6). Formal proof of a single peptide-binding cleft in each MHC molecule came with the solution of the crystal structure of the HLA-A2 molecule (see Chapter 5). These observations, together with the limited number of MHC alleles expressed in each individual, support the hypothesis that *MHC molecules show a broad specificity for peptide binding, and the fine specificity of antigen recognition resides largely in the antigen receptors of*

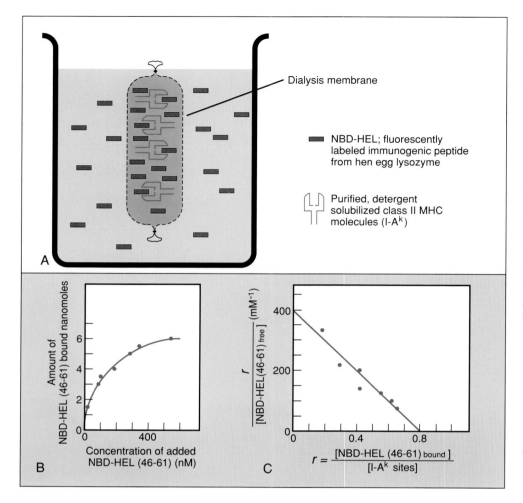

FIGURE 6–8. Demonstration of peptide binding to MHC molecules by equilibrium dialysis. *Purified I-A^k class II MHC molecules bind a peptide fragment of hen egg lysozyme (HEL), HEL (46–61), that is labeled with a fluorescent marker (NBD), which allows the concentration of the peptide to be determined (A). Analysis of the amount of HEL bound (i.e., the concentration within the dialysis membrane minus the concentration outside) at varying concentrations of peptide shows that the binding is saturable (B). Scatchard analysis shows that each I-A^k molecule has approximately one binding site (X-axis intercept), and the dissociation constant (K$_d$) is approximately 1×10^{-6} M (calculated from the slope of the line). In this plot, r represents the number of peptide molecules bound to each MHC molecule when there is an excess of peptide (C). Note that HEL (46–61) is known to be presented in association with I-A^k molecules. (Modified with permission from Babbitt, B. P., P. M. Allen, G. Matsueda, E. Haber, and E. R. Unanue. Binding of immunogenic peptides to Ia histocompatibility molecules. Nature 317:359–361, 1985. Copyright © 1985, Macmillan Magazines Limited.)*

T lymphocytes. On the other hand, individual MHC molecules do not bind all foreign peptides indiscriminately; the physiologic implications of this limited specificity of peptide-MHC associations will be discussed later.

2. *The association of antigenic peptides and MHC molecules is a low-affinity interaction (K$_d$ ≅ 10^{-6} M) with a slow "on rate" and a very slow "off rate."* This affinity is much lower than that of antigen-antibody binding, which usually has a K$_d$ of 10^{-7} to 10^{-11} M. In solution, peptides bind to MHC molecules, reach saturation within 15 to 30 minutes, and remain bound for as long as 6 hours at neutral pH. Dissociation occurs more rapidly at acidic pH. The slow on rate suggests that conformational changes, probably in the peptide, are needed to permit binding. The very slow off rate may

TABLE 6–5. Competition of Antigens for Presentation by Antigen-Presenting Cells (APCs)*

	APC	Antigen (Amino Acid Polymer)	Time of Addition of Excess Competing Antigen, GT	Stimulation of GAT–Specific, I-A^d Restricted T Cells
A	I-A^d expressing macrophage	GAT	None added	+/No competition
B	I-A^d expressing macrophage	GAT	GT same time as GAT	−/Competition
C	I-A^d expressing macrophage	GAT	GT 3 hours after GAT	+/No competition

The random amino acid polymer GAT is effectively presented by I-A^d expressing macrophages to GAT–specific, I-A^d restricted T cells, stimulating them to secrete cytokines (A). When an excess of a structurally similar amino acid polymer, GT, is added to the APCs at the same time as the GAT, there is competition so that GAT is not presented and there is no T cell response (B). If, however, GAT is added to the APC first and time is allowed for processing, latter addition of GT does not block presentation of GAT (C). In these experiments, processed forms of both GAT and GT bind to the I-A^d molecule, but only GAT–I-A^d complexes stimulate the T cells.

Abbreviations: GAT, glutamic acid–alanine–tyrosine; GT, glutamic acid–tyrosine.

TABLE 6-6. Binding of Unrelated Peptides to an MHC Molecule: Correlation with Inhibition of Antigen Presentation

Competing Peptide	Ability of Peptide to Compete with OVA(323-339) for Binding to I-A^d	Ability of Peptide to Inhibit Presentation of OVA(323-339) by I-A^d Expressing APC to OVA-Specific, I-A^d Restricted T Cells
Ovalbumin OVA(323-339)	++++	NA
Influenza virus hemagglutinin Ha(130-142)	++++	++++
Hen egg lysozyme HEL(74-86)	++	+++
λ-repressor protein λ-(12-26)	++	++
Sperm whale myoglobin Myo(132-153)	±	±
Herpes simplex virus glycoprotein HSV(8-23)	±	±

Peptide binding to purified MHC molecules correlates with MHC-restricted presentation of peptide to T cells. Binding of ^{125}I-labeled ovalbumin-derived peptide, OVA(323-339), to purified, detergent solubilized murine I-A^d was measured by gel filtration in the presence of varying concentrations of unlabeled peptides. Presentation of OVA(323-339) by paraformaldehyde fixed, I-A^d expressing APC to an OVA(323-339)-specific, I-A^d-restricted T cell line, in the presence of varying concentrations of competing peptides, was assayed by measuring antigen-induced T cell cytokine secretion. The results indicate that the ability of a competing peptide to block OVA(323-339) binding to purified I-A^d correlates well with the ability of the same competing peptide to block I-A^d-restricted presentation of OVA(323-339) to T cells. Numbers following abbreviations of proteins refer to the amino acid residues of the native protein.

Adapted from Buus, S., A. Sette, S. M. Colon, C. Miles, and H. M. Grey: The relationship between major histocompatibility (MHC) restriction and the capacity of Ia to bind immunogenic peptides. Science 235:1353-1358, 1987. Copyright 1987 by the AAAS.
Abbreviations: MHC, major histocompatibility complex; NA, not applicable.

be responsible for peptide-MHC complexes persisting long enough to interact with T cells, despite the low affinity of peptide-MHC association.

3. *The association of peptides with MHC proteins is determined by the primary and secondary structures of both molecules.* The crystal structure of class I MHC molecules and the model of class II molecules based on the known class I structure were described in Chapter 5 (see Figs. 5-4 and 5-6). The single predicted peptide-binding cleft of a class II molecule has a β-pleated sheet floor and α-helical sides made up of the N-terminal domains of the two chains of the heterodimeric class II protein. Polymorphic amino acid residues are concentrated in this peptide-binding region. Processed antigenic peptides are thought to lie within the cleft in molecular contact with the floor and the α-helical sides. Some peptides may assume α-helical configurations. All immunogenic peptides contain some amino acids that form contacts with the MHC molecule and other amino acids that point away from the cleft and are presumably recognized by T cells. Mutational analysis of antigenic peptides is a useful method for defining which residues bind to MHC molecules and compete with other antigens for presentation and which residues are recognized by T cells (Table 6-7). Such studies indicate that in order to stimulate T cells, peptides must be capable of forming non-covalent bonds with MHC molecules. This binding, however, is not sufficient for immunogenicity because each peptide must contain residues that are recognized by specific T cells as well.

4. *The association of antigenic peptides with MHC molecules is stabilized by the interaction of antigen-specific, MHC-restricted T cells with the peptide-MHC complexes.* This has been directly demonstrated by measuring the strength of interactions between antigenic peptides and MHC molecules in the presence and absence of specific T cells. For instance, a peptide fragment of ovalbumin (OVA) binds to the mouse class II molecule, I-A^d, incorporated in synthetic lipid membranes. The proximity of the two can be estimated by attaching fluorescent labels to each and measuring resonance energy transfer. The resonance energy transfer is markedly increased if an OVA-specific, I-A^d-restricted T cell population is added. Based on these findings it has been postulated that *in vivo* protein antigens are continuously endocytosed by APCs, processed, associated with class II MHC molecules, and expressed on the cell surface. If these surface complexes are not recognized by a T cell, they recycle back into endosomes, where the acidic pH dissociates the peptide from the MHC molecules. The peptide may be degraded in lysosomes, and the MHC molecules may become available for binding another processed antigen. If, on the other hand, the peptide-MHC molecule complex is recognized on the surface of the APCs by an antigen-specific, MHC-restricted T cell, the complex is prevented from recycling because of the stabilizing influence of the T cell antigen receptor. This leads to activation of the T cell.

5. *The bimolecular complex of processed antigen and MHC molecules is the specific ligand for T cell anti-*

TABLE 6–7. Identification of MHC–Binding and T Cell Receptor–Binding Residues in Peptide Antigens

	HEL Peptide										Stimulation of HEL–Specific T Cells	Binding to Purified I-Aᵏ	Competition with Native HEL for T Cell Stimulation
	Amino Acid Residue Position No.												
	52	53	54	55	56	57	58	59	60	61			
1	Asp	Tyr	Gly	Ile	Leu	Gln	Ile	Asn	Ser	Arg	+	+	NA
2	Asp	Tyr	Gly	Ile	Ala	Gln	Ile	Asn	Ser	Arg	–	+	+
3	Asp	Ala	Gly	Ile	Leu	Gln	Ile	Asn	Ser	Arg	–	+	+
4	Asp	Tyr	Gly	Ala	Leu	Gln	Ile	Asn	Ser	Arg	–	–	–
5	Asp	Tyr	Ala	Ile	Leu	Gln	Ile	Asn	Ser	Arg	+	+	NA

Synthetic peptides were produced that differed from the native hen egg lysozyme peptide HEL(52–61) (peptide 1) by substitutions for single residues, and the functional consequences of these engineered mutations were analyzed. Substitutions at positions 56 and 53 (peptides 2 and 3) result in loss of T cell stimulation, but retain I-Aᵏ binding. The amino acids at these positions in the native peptide are part of the epitope recognized by the T cell receptor. Substitution of residue 55 (peptide 4) results in loss of T cell stimulation and I-Aᵏ binding. This residue is in part of the peptide that binds to the class II MHC molecule. A substitution at position 54 (peptide 5) has no effect, and therefore this residue is not essential for binding of the peptide to either the MHC or T cell receptor molecules.

Adapted from Unanue, E. R., and P. M. Allen: The basis for the immunoregulatory role of macrophages and other accessory cells. Science 236:551–557, 1987. Copyright 1987 by the AAAS.
Abbreviations: MHC, major histocompatibility complex; HEL, hen egg lysozyme; NA, not applicable.

gen receptors. Complexes of OVA peptide + I-Aᵈ incorporated in synthetic lipid membranes induce the activation of OVA–specific, I-Aᵈ–restricted monoclonal T cell hybridomas. Similar results have been obtained with many other antigen-MHC combinations.

6. *Peptide-MHC complexes are produced in intact cells as they are in cell-free experimental systems.* If an APC is incubated with a radioactively labeled protein antigen, radioactive complexes composed of antigen fragments and class II MHC molecules can be isolated from the plasma membranes of the APC.

7. *Autologous peptides bind to self MHC molecules.* Equilibrium dialysis experiments (Fig. 6–8) first showed that the binding of an HEL peptide to the mouse class II molecule, I-Aᵏ, could be competitively inhibited by a homologous mouse lysozyme peptide. Complexes of autologous peptides with self MHC molecules are also formed *in vivo.* This was formally demonstrated using two MHC identical strains of mice that express different allelic versions of the hemoglobin β chain, called *Hbbᵈ* and *Hbbˢ.* Cloned T cell lines specific for *Hbbᵈ* were generated from *Hbbˢ* mice after immunizing them with hemoglobin from the *Hbbᵈ* strain. Freshly isolated macrophages from unimmunized mice of the *Hbbᵈ* strain could activate these T cells specific for *Hbbᵈ* without the addition of hemoglobin (Fig. 6–9). Since no exogenous hemoglobin was added, processed class II MHC–associated self hemoglobin must have been present on the surface of the macrophages of the *Hbbᵈ* strain.

These findings, that self peptides can be bound by MHC molecules, raise two important questions. First, if individuals process their own proteins and present them in association with their own MHC molecules, why do we normally not develop immune responses against self proteins? It is likely that self-

tolerance is mainly due to the absence of lymphocytes capable of recognizing and responding to self antigens, and this is why self peptide-MHC complexes do not induce autoimmunity (see Chapter 8). Second, if MHC molecules are bathed in processed autologous proteins, how can they ever bind and present foreign antigenic peptides? It has been postulated that the constant recycling of MHC molecules from the cell surface to acidic endosomes and back again ensures that self MHC molecules will be stripped of bound self peptides long enough to allow binding of foreign peptides. Engagement of the T cell receptor may stabilize peptide-MHC interactions, as discussed above, and this can happen only with foreign peptide–self MHC complexes, since T cells normally recognize only foreign antigens.

In summary, the principal steps in class II MHC–associated antigen presentation (see Fig. 6–7) are the following:

1. Internalization of native protein antigens from the extracellular environment into APCs.
2. Processing of the antigen in acidic endosomes, leading to the generation of peptide fragments.
3. Low-affinity binding of peptides to class II MHC molecules within the APCs.
4. Expression of peptide-MHC complexes on the cell surface.
5. Recognition of the complexes by T cells that are specific for the foreign peptide and the self MHC molecule.

The broad specificity of MHC molecules for peptides accounts for the ability of an APC with a limited number of allelic forms of MHC proteins to present many different antigens.

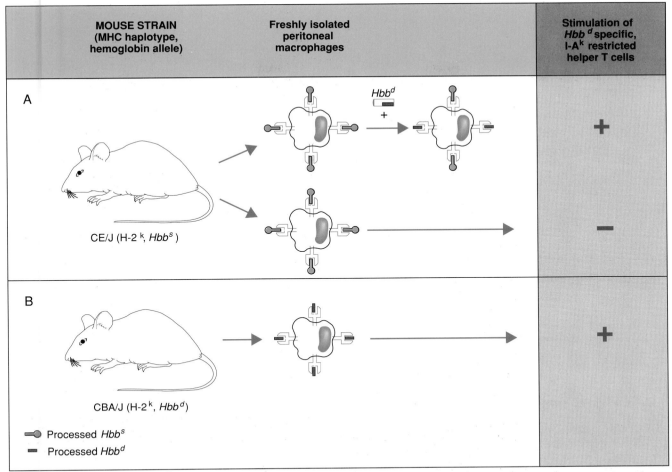

FIGURE 6–9. *Macrophages present self hemoglobin in association with self MHC molecules in vivo. Macrophages from Hbbˢ-expressing mice will stimulate Hbbᵈ-specific I-Aᵏ–restricted T cells only if the antigen, Hbbᵈ, is added (A). However, freshly isolated macrophages from Hbbᵈ-expressing mice stimulate the same T cells without any requirement for exogenous antigen (B). Therefore, the freshly isolated macrophages from Hbbᵈ-expressing mice must bear processed Hbbᵈ on their surface.*

Class I MHC – Associated Antigen Presentation

As we have mentioned previously, CD8⁺ T cells, most of which are CTLs, recognize class I MHC–associated foreign protein antigens. Furthermore, CD8⁺ T cells usually recognize protein antigens that are synthesized within APCs and subsequently expressed on the surface in association with class I MHC molecules. Examples of endogenously synthesized foreign proteins are viral proteins and tumor antigens. CTLs are the principal immunologic defense mechanisms against viruses and may be important in the immune destruction of tumors.

In vitro analyses of the binding of foreign peptides to class I MHC molecules indicate that it is essentially similar to peptide–class II binding. Each class I MHC molecule has a single binding cleft that accommodates peptides that are 10 to 20 amino acids long. The affinity of class I–peptide association is in the order of 10^{-6} M. Different peptides can bind to the same site in

a class I MHC molecule and compete with one another for presentation. Any one peptide can also bind to class I and class II MHC molecules, and there are no structural motifs that confer specificity for class I or class II MHC association on an antigenic peptide. Whether a particular antigen will be presented by an APC in association with class I or class II MHC molecules is apparently determined by the intracellular compartmentalization of the protein. Antigens that are synthesized endogenously within the APCs generally traverse different compartments from those antigens that are endocytosed from the extracellular environment. This is supported by several studies:

1. If a viral protein, such as influenza nucleoprotein, or a protein like ovalbumin is added in soluble form to a cell that expresses class I and class II MHC molecules, the antigen is internalized, processed, and presented only in association with class II MHC molecules. Such exogenously added antigens will be recognized by class II–restricted, antigen-specific CD4⁺ T cells but will not sensitize the APC to lysis by CD8⁺ cells. On the other hand, if the gene encoding the viral

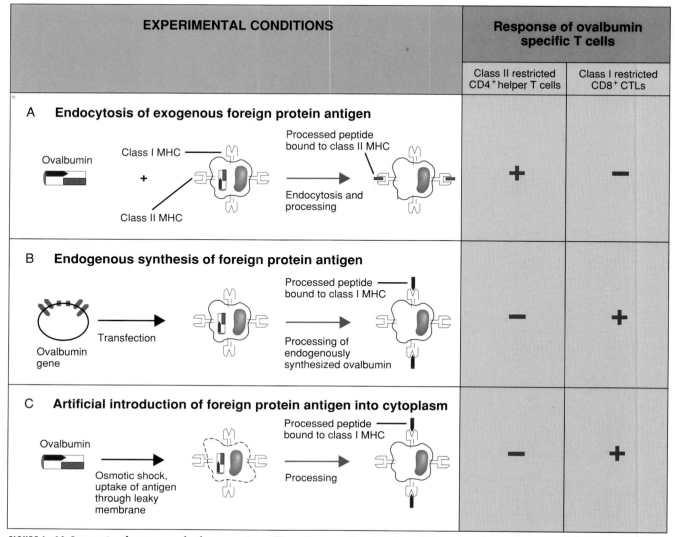

EXPERIMENTAL CONDITIONS	Response of ovalbumin specific T cells	
	Class II restricted CD4$^+$ helper T cells	Class I restricted CD8$^+$ CTLs
A Endocytosis of exogenous foreign protein antigen	+	−
B Endogenous synthesis of foreign protein antigen	−	+
C Artificial introduction of foreign protein antigen into cytoplasm	−	+

FIGURE 6–10. Presentation of exogenous and endogenous antigens. *The antigen, ovalbumin, when added to an antigen-presenting cell (APC) that expresses class I and class II MHC molecules, is presented only in association with class II (A). The same ovalbumin synthesized intracellularly as a result of transfection of its gene (B) or introduced into the cytoplasm by osmotic shock (C) is presented in association with class I MHC molecules. The measured response of class II restricted helper T cells is cytokine secretion and the measured response of class I–restricted cytolytic T lymphocytes (CTLs) is killing of the APCs.*

protein or ovalbumin is transfected into the APCs so that the antigen is synthesized endogenously, the cell becomes sensitive to lysis by specific class I–restricted CD8$^+$ cells (Fig. 6–10). APCs that express these transfected gene products do not stimulate CD4$^+$ T cells. Intracellular localization rather than endogenous synthesis may be the critical factor determining the class I association of antigenic peptides. For instance, if an antigen is introduced into the cytoplasm of a cell by making the plasma membrane transiently permeable to macromolecules, the antigen is subsequently processed and peptides associate only with class I MHC molecules (Fig. 6–10). This further supports the concept that the traffic patterns of intracellular and endocytosed proteins are different.

2. Presentation of some endogenously synthesized viral antigens to CD8$^+$ CTLs cannot be inhibited by chloroquine, whereas presentation of exogenously added viral proteins to CD4$^+$ T cells is chloroquine-sensitive. This suggests that processing of endogenously produced antigens may not occur in acidic endosomes.

3. *Class I–restricted presentation of endogenously synthesized viral antigens requires association of antigen with newly synthesized class I MHC molecules in the endoplasmic reticulum (ER).* This has been demonstrated in two ways. First, a pharmacologic inhibitor of protein transport out of the ER, called Brefeldin A, can block the post-translational processing and transport of all newly synthesized proteins including self class I and class II MHC and foreign viral proteins. This drug treatment inhibits the class I–restricted presentation of endogenously synthesized viral protein, more than the class II–restricted presentation of

exogenously encountered proteins. Second, the adenovirus E19 protein specifically binds to and prevents transport of class I MHC molecules out of the ER. The ability of E19 to block nascent class I transport correlates with its ability to block class I–restricted antigen presentation.

Thus, the association of antigens with class I versus class II MHC molecules is due to the trafficking of the antigens through different intracellular compartments (Fig. 6–11). In most cases, the commitment to one or another traffic pattern is determined by where the antigen comes from; endogenously synthesized antigens end up associated with class I MHC and exogenously synthesized and endocytosed antigens end up associated with class II MHC. There are exceptions, however, when endogenously synthesized proteins do end up being presented in association with class II MHC molecules.

Many unanswered questions remain about the cell biology of class I–restricted antigen presentation. The site at which antigens are processed into peptides before association with class I MHC molecules is not known, nor is it understood how the processed peptides get into the rough ER, where nascent class I MHC molecules are being synthesized. There is some evidence that the ER itself may contain proteolytic enzymes that could generate immunogenic peptides. Since both class I and class II MHC molecules are produced in the rough ER and both have a natural affinity for peptides, there must also be some mechanism that prevents peptides from binding to class II molecules in the ER. This may be accomplished by the class II–associated invariant or γ chains that may interfere with the peptide-binding clefts. Class I MHC molecules do not have invariant chains when they are synthesized and are therefore free to bind peptides produced within the cell. This may be one reason why

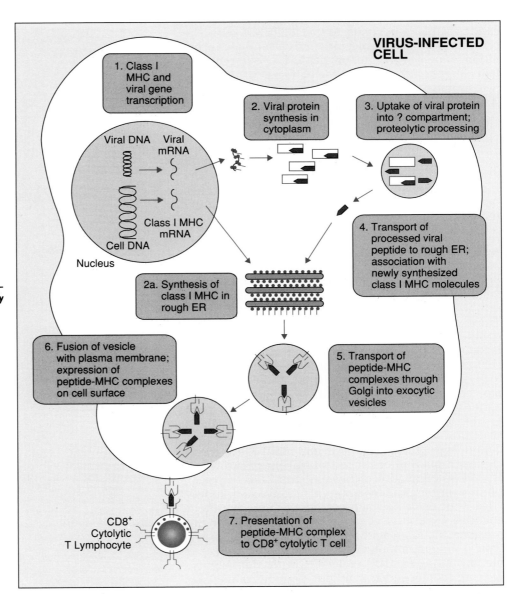

FIGURE 6–11. *Pathway of class I MHC–restricted presentation of an endogenously synthesized (e.g., viral) antigen.*

endogenously synthesized antigens become class I–associated. As the class II MHC molecules are being transported in vesicles to the cell surface, they shed the invariant chain. At this stage, the vesicles containing MHC molecules may intersect with endosomes containing internalized, processed antigens. Since the binding clefts of the class I molecules are already occupied by peptides, the endocytosed and processed antigens bind to the only available MHC molecules, which are now the class II molecules.

PHYSIOLOGIC SIGNIFICANCE OF MHC–ASSOCIATED ANTIGEN PRESENTATION

So far we have discussed the specificity of CD4+ and CD8+ T lymphocytes for MHC–associated foreign protein antigens and the mechanisms by which complexes of peptides and MHC molecules are produced. It is important to also consider the physiologic implications of this rather unusual specificity of T cells. The central role of MHC molecules in T cell antigen recognition influences the immunogenicity of different protein antigens and the response patterns of the T cells.

Immunogenicity of Protein Antigens

Our present understanding of the role of MHC genes in determining the ability of protein antigens to induce specific immunity is limited largely to exogenous antigens. MHC molecules may determine the immunogenicity of protein antigens in two related ways:

1. *The immunodominant epitopes of complex proteins are often the peptides that bind most avidly to MHC molecules.* If an individual is immunized with a multideterminant protein antigen, in many instances the majority of the responding T cells are specific for one or a few linear amino acid sequences of the antigen. These are called the "immunodominant" determinants or epitopes. For instance, in H-2k mice immunized with HEL, more than half the HEL–specific T cells are specific for the epitope formed by residues 46 to 61 of HEL in association with the I-Ak but not the I-Ek molecule. This is because HEL(46–61) binds to I-Ak better than do other HEL peptides and does not bind to I-Ek. However, it is not yet known exactly which structural features of a peptide determine immunodominance. The question is an important one because an understanding of these features may permit the efficient manipulation of the immune system with synthetic peptides. An obvious application of such knowledge is the design of vaccines. For example, a protein encoded by a viral gene could be analyzed for the presence of amino acid sequences that would form a typical immunodominant secondary structure capable of binding to MHC molecules with high affinity. Vaccines composed of synthetic peptides mimicking

this region of the protein theoretically would be effective in eliciting T cell responses against the viral peptide expressed on an infected cell, thereby establishing protective immunity against the virus.

2. *The expression of particular class II MHC alleles in an individual determines the ability of that individual to respond to particular antigens.* The phenomenon of immune response (Ir) gene–controlled immune responsiveness was mentioned in Chapter 5. We now know that Ir genes that control antibody responses are class II MHC genes. They influence immune responsiveness in part because various allelic class II MHC molecules differ in their ability to bind different antigenic peptides and, therefore, to stimulate specific helper T cells. For instance, H-2k mice are re-

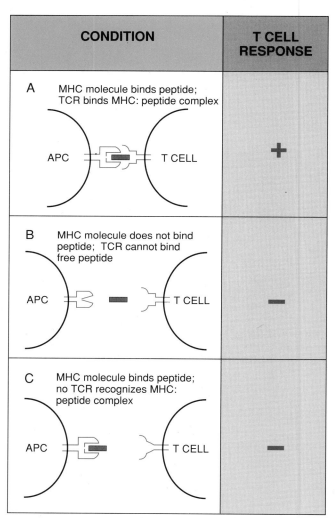

FIGURE 6–12. Mechanisms of MHC–linked immune response (Ir) gene function. *Antigen presentation and T cell activation occur when an individual expresses MHC molecules that can bind peptides derived from the processed antigen and T cells are present that specifically recognize complexes of these MHC molecules with the peptides (A). If an individual does not inherit genes encoding MHC molecules that can bind the peptides, no T cell response occurs (B). Alternatively, if no T cells are present which recognize the MHC molecules as self, no T cell response occurs (C). The development of self-restricted T cells is discussed in Chapter 8.*

sponders to HEL(46–61) but H-2^d mice are non-responders to this epitope. Equilibrium dialysis experiments have shown that HEL(46–61) binds to I-A^k but not to I-A^d molecules (see Fig. 6–8). A possible molecular basis for this difference in MHC association is suggested from the model of the class II molecule and the known amino acid sequences of I-A^k and I-A^d proteins. If the HEL(46–61) peptide in the form of an α-helix is hypothetically placed in the predicted binding cleft of the I-A^k molecule, charged residues of the HEL peptide become aligned with oppositely charged residues of the MHC molecule. This would presumably stabilize the bimolecular interaction. In contrast, the I-A^d molecule has different amino acids in the binding cleft that would result in the aligning of similarly charged residues with the HEL peptide. Therefore, HEL(46–61) would not bind to or be presented in association with I-A^d and the H-2^d mouse would be a non-responder. Similar results have been obtained with numerous other peptides. MHC–linked immune responsiveness may also be important in humans. For instance, Caucasians who are homozygous for an extended HLA haplotype containing HLA-B8,DR3,DQw2a are low responders to hepatitis B virus surface antigen. Individuals who are heterozygous at this locus are high responders, presumably because the other alleles contain one or more HLA genes that confer responsiveness to this antigen. Thus, HLA typing may prove to be valuable for predicting the success of vaccination. These findings support the **determinant selection model** of MHC–linked immune responses. This model, which was proposed many years before the demonstration of peptide-MHC binding, states that the products of MHC genes in each individual select which determinants of protein antigens will be immunogenic in that individual. We now understand the structural basis of determinant selection and Ir gene function in antigen presentation. Most Ir gene phenomena have been studied by measuring helper T cell function, but the same principles apply to CTLs. Individuals with certain MHC alleles may be incapable of generating CTLs against some viruses. In this situation, of course, the Ir genes may map to one of the class I MHC loci.

Although these concepts are based largely on studies with simple peptide antigens and inbred strains of mice, they are also relevant to the understanding of immune responses to complex multideterminant protein antigens in outbred species. It is likely that all individuals will express at least one MHC molecule capable of binding at least one determinant of a complex protein, so that all individuals will be responders to such antigens. As stated in Chapter 5, this may be the evolutionary pressure for maintaining MHC polymorphisms.

This discussion of the influence of MHC gene products on the immunogenicity of protein antigens has focused on antigen presentation and has not considered the role of the T cells. We have mentioned earlier that the exquisite specificity and diversity of antigen recognition are attributable to antigen receptors on T cells. MHC–linked immune responsiveness is also dependent, in part, on the presence and absence of specific T cells. In fact, some peptides bind to MHC molecules in a particular inbred mouse strain but do not activate T cells in that strain (Table 6–7). It is likely that these mice lack T cells capable of recognizing the particular peptide-MHC complexes. *Thus, Ir genes may function by determining antigen presentation or by shaping the repertoire of antigen-responsive T cells* (Fig. 6–12). The development of the T cell repertoire and the role of the MHC in T cell maturation are discussed in Chapter 8.

Nature of T Cell Responses

Based on this knowledge of antigen presentation to T cells, we can now explain other physiologic consequences of MHC–restricted antigen recognition that were introduced in Chapter 5.

1. Because T cells recognize only MHC–associated protein antigens, they can respond only to antigens associated with other cells (the APCs) and are unresponsive to soluble or circulating proteins. *This unique specificity for cell-bound antigens may be essential for the functions of T lymphocytes, which are largely mediated by cell-cell interactions and by cytokines that act at short distances.* For instance, helper T cells help B lymphocytes and activate macrophages. Not surprisingly, B lymphocytes and macrophages are two of the principal cell types that express class II MHC genes, function as APCs for CD4$^+$ helper T cells, and focus helper T cell effects to their immediate vicinity. Similarly, CTLs can lyse any nucleated cell producing a foreign antigen and all nucleated cells express class I MHC molecules, which are the restricting elements for antigen recognition by CD8$^+$ CTLs.

2. The patterns of MHC association of different forms of antigens determine which subset of T cells is preferentially or selectively activated (Fig. 6–13). Extracellular antigens activate class II–restricted CD4$^+$ T cells, which function as helpers to stimulate effector mechanisms such as antibodies and phagocytes that serve to eliminate extracellular antigens. Conversely, endogenous antigens activate class I–restricted CD8$^+$ CTLs, which lyse cells producing these intracellular antigens. *Thus, different forms of antigens selectively stimulate the T cell population that is most effective at eliminating that type of antigen.* This is particularly significant because neither the antigen receptors of helper T cells and CTLs nor class I and class II MHC molecules themselves have the ability to distinguish between extracellular (e.g., bacterial) and intracellular (e.g., viral) protein determinants.

SUMMARY

T cells recognize antigens only on the surface of accessory cells in association with the product of a self MHC gene. CD4$^+$ helper T lymphocytes recognize

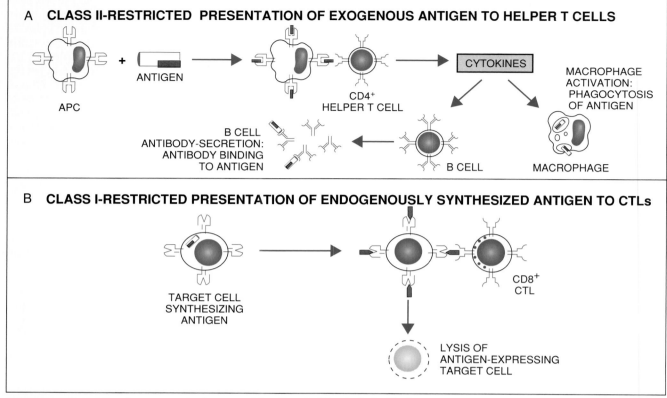

FIGURE 6–13. *Presentation of exogenous and endogenous protein antigens to different subsets of T cells.*
A. *Exogenous antigens are presented to class II–restricted CD4+ helper cells, which stimulate B cells and macrophages to mediate elimination of extracellular antigens.*
B. *Endogenously synthesized antigens (e.g., derived from intracellular microbes) are presented to class I–restricted CD8+ cytolytic T lymphocytes (CTLs), which kill cells harboring intracellular microbes.*

antigens in association with class II MHC gene products (class II MHC–restricted recognition), and CD8+ CTLs recognize antigens in association with class I gene products (class I MHC–restricted recognition). Exogenous foreign proteins are internalized in APCs, where they undergo processing in an acid vesicular compartment. Processing ensures that portions of a protein (the immunodominant peptides) will bind to class II MHC molecules and form immunogenic complexes. These complexes are expressed on the surface of APCs, where they are recognized by CD4+ T cells. Class II MHC genes function as Ir genes; their products selectively bind and present some antigens but not others. The target antigens for CD8+ CTLs are endogenously synthesized proteins, such as viral antigens, which are processed and associate with class I MHC molecules. Many cell types have the capacity to present antigens to CD4+ helper T cells; a minimal requirement is the expression of class II MHC genes. The regulation of class II MHC gene expression is an important control point for immune responses.

SELECTED READINGS

Allen, P. M. Antigen processing at the molecular level. Immunology Today 8:270–273, 1987.

Babbitt, B. P., P. M. Allen, G. Matsueda, E. Haber, and E. R. Unanue. Binding of immunogenic peptides to Ia histocompatibility molecules. Nature 317:359–361, 1985.

Benacerraf, B. A hypothesis to relate the specificity of T lymphocytes and the activity of I-region–specific Ir genes in macrophages and B lymphocytes. Journal of Immunology 120:1809–1812, 1978.

Buus, S., A. Sette, S. M. Colon, C. Miles, and H. M. Grey. The relationship between major histocompatibility complex (MHC) restriction and the capacity of Ia to bind immunogenic peptides. Science 235:1353–1358, 1987.

Germain R. N., and B. Malissen. Analysis of the expression and function of class II major histocompatibility complex–encoded molecules by DNA mediated gene transfer. Annual Review of Immunology 4:281–316, 1986.

Harding, C. V., and E. R. Unanue. Cellular mechanisms of antigen processing and the function of class I and class II major histocompatibility complex molecules. Cell Regulation 1:499–509, 1990.

Moore, M. W., F. R. Carbone, and M. J. Bevan. Introduction of soluble protein into the class I pathway of antigen processing and presentation. Cell 54:777–785, 1988.

Rock, K. L., and B. Benacerraf. Inhibition of antigen-specific T lymphocyte activation by structurally related Ir gene controlled polymers. Journal of Experimental Medicine 157:1618–1634, 1983.

Rosenthal, A. S., and E. M. Shevach. Function of macrophages in antigen recognition by guinea pig T lymphocytes. Journal of Experimental Medicine 138:1194–1212, 1973.

Schwartz, R. H. Immune response (Ir) genes of the murine major histocompatibility complex. Advances in Immunology 38:31–201, 1986.

Townsend, A., J. Rothbard, F. Gotch, B. Bahadur, D. Wraith, and

A. McMichael. The epitopes of influenza nucleoprotein recognized by cytotoxic T lymphocytes can be defined with short synthetic peptides. Cell 44:959–968, 1986.

Unanue, E. R., and P. M. Allen. The basis for the immunoregulatory role of macrophages and other accessory cells. Science 236:551–557, 1987.

Watts, T. H., H. E. Gaub, and H. M. McConnell. T-cell-mediated association of peptide antigen and major histocompatibility complex protein detected by energy transfer in an evanescent wave-field. Nature 320:179–181, 1986.

Zinkernagel, R. M., and P. C. Doherty. Activity of sensitized thymus-derived lymphocytes in lymphocytic choriomeningitis reflects immunological surveillance against altered self components. Nature 251:547–548, 1974.

CHAPTER SEVEN

MOLECULAR BASIS OF T CELL ANTIGEN RECOGNITION AND ACTIVATION

In Chapter 6 we introduced the concept that helper and cytolytic T lymphocytes (CTLs), unlike B cells, recognize fragments of foreign protein antigens that are physically associated with self major histocompatibility complex (MHC) molecules on the surfaces of antigen presenting cells (APCs) or target cells. Antigen recognition by T cells is the initiating stimulus for T cell activation. In different T cells, activation leads to the secretion of cytokines, proliferation, and the performance of regulatory or cytolytic effector functions. The elucidation of the structure and function of the molecules involved in T cell antigen recognition is one of the most important advances in immunology in the last decade. This relatively new knowledge has provided a molecular basis for the study of normal and pathologic immune responses in which the T cell plays a central role.

The receptors on T cells which are responsible for the highly specific recognition of and response to antigen plus MHC are composed of a complex of several integral plasma membrane proteins. Some of the proteins in this complex mediate specific binding to antigen-MHC complexes on the surface of APCs or target cells, and therefore the binding portions of these proteins differ among T cells with different antigen-MHC specificities. Other proteins in the complex are invariant among all T cells, and they probably function in signal transduction into the interior of the T cell. In addition to the receptor for antigen plus MHC, T cells express a number of other cell surface proteins, which are collectively called **accessory molecules.** These molecules are important in the cognitive, activation, and effector phases of T cell responses. Several of these accessory molecules function to strengthen the adhesion of the T cells to other cells, thereby promoting maximally effective interactions between helper T cells and APCs or between CTLs and their targets. Several of these same accessory molecules may transduce signals in addition to signals transduced by the antigen receptor that are important for activation of the T cells.

In this chapter, we describe the structure of the T cell antigen receptor proteins as well as the structure and function of the accessory molecules on T cells and how they may act coordinately with the antigen receptor to ensure a functional T cell response to antigen. In addition, we describe the intracellular events that occur in response to antigen binding to the T cell surface. The early biochemical changes inside the T cell are considered to be the "second messengers" that link the binding of antigen to the functional responses of the T cell. Later biochemical events, such as cytokine synthesis, mark the beginning of the effector phase of the T cell response to antigen.

THE $\alpha\beta$ T CELL RECEPTOR FOR ANTIGEN AND MHC MOLECULES

Identification of the T Cell Antigen Receptor

The molecular nature of the T cell receptor (TCR) responsible for MHC–restricted antigen recognition

---

B O X   7 – 1.   MONOCLONAL T CELL POPULATIONS

The development of techniques for propagating monoclonal T cell populations *in vitro* has been crucial to many of the recent advances in our understanding of T cell recognition of antigen and T cell activation. By definition, all the T cells in a monoclonal population are genetically identical to one another (except for rare spontaneous mutants) and therefore express identical TCR. This provides a homogeneous population of cells for functional, biochemical, and molecular analyses. Three types of monoclonal T cell populations have been frequently utilized in experimental immunology.

1. *Antigen-specific T cell clones* are derived by *in vivo* immunization of an individual with a particular antigen, isolation of T cells from either blood or lymphoid tissue, repetitive *in vitro* stimulation with the immunizing antigen plus MHC–matched APCs (which drive proliferation of T cells only with the appropriate specificities), and cloning single antigen–MHC–responsive cells in semisolid media or in liquid media by **limiting dilution.** Permanent lines can be expanded and maintained by periodic *in vitro* restimulation with antigen and MHC–matched APCs. Antigen-specific responses can be easily measured in these populations, since all the cells in a cloned line have the same receptors and have been selected for growth in response to a known antigen-MHC complex. The full range of activation events, including early signal transduction, proliferation, and differentiation to effector function, can be observed in T cell clones. Both helper and CTL clones have been established from mice and humans.

2. *Antigen specific T-T hybridomas* are created in a way similar to that for B cell hybridomas (see Box 3–1, Chapter 3). Mice are immunized with the antigen of interest, lymph nodes draining the site of immunization are removed, and T cells are purified. These cells are fused with an autonomously growing T cell tumor line, and metabolic selection is applied so that only the fused cells grow. From the resultant hybridomas, cells responding to the desired antigen:APC combination are selected and cloned. TCR–mediated activation events ranging from early signal transduction to cytokine secretion can be measured in T-T hybridomas. Since hybridomas are already autonomously growing, stimulation of proliferative responses cannot be observed. Murine T-T hybridomas can be easily made, including those derived from both mature T cells and thymocytes. Human T-T hybridomas have also been made recently.

3. *Tumor lines derived from T cells* have been established *in vitro* after removal of malignant T cells from animals or humans with T cell leukemias or lymphomas. Some tumor-derived lines express functional cell surface TCR molecules. Even though the antigen specificities of these lines are not known, they can be activated via their TCRs in other ways, e.g., with anti-TCR antibodies or lectins, leading to early signal events, gene transcription, and cytokine secretion.

was elucidated in the 1980s, several years after immunoglobulin (Ig) molecules and their genes were described. After the phenomenon of MHC restriction of antigen-specific T cells was discovered, two alternative theories about the structure of the T cell antigen receptor were proposed. One hypothesis was that T cell antigen recognition required the simultaneous binding of two independent receptors, one to foreign antigen and the other to self MHC. The alternative postulate, which we now know to be correct, was that *a single T cell receptor specifically recognizes MHC associated antigen.* The evidence that processed antigen and MHC molecules are expressed as complexes on the APC surface, prior to involvement of the T cell (see Chapter 6), is most consistent with a single receptor model. A more complete understanding of T cell recognition required analysis of the structure and specificity of the relevant molecules on the T cell surface.

An important advance in the study of T cell receptors was the development of technologies for propagating monoclonal T cell populations *in vitro,* including T-T hybridomas and antigen specific T cell clones (Box 7–1, p. 139). All the cells in a clonal T cell population are derived from a single cell, are genetically identical, and therefore express identical TCRs that are different from the receptors produced by all other clones. Therefore, TCRs produced by any one clone express unique determinants, or idiotypes, in their antigen-binding regions that are not present on the antigen receptors of any other clone. Idiotypic determinants on T cells are analogous to idiotypic determinants of antibodies, described in Chapter 3 (Box 3–2). Monoclonal antibodies against these clone-specific T cell idiotypic determinants (anti-idiotypic or anti-clonotypic antibodies) were generated by immunizing animals with cloned T cells and creating B cell hybridomas from the spleen cells of these animals. (See Box 3–1, Chapter 3, for a description of monoclonal antibody production.) The hybridomas were then screened for the production of antibodies that bound only to the immunizing T cell clone and not to any other T cells. Anti-idiotypic antibodies generated in this way have served as powerful tools for analyzing the structure and function of TCR molecules. Such antibodies are used to specifically immunoprecipitate and purify TCR molecules from membranes of T cells, and the isolated TCR molecules can be characterized biochemically, including partial amino acid sequencing. These antibodies can also produce functional effects when they bind to the antigen receptors on T cells, either mimicking or blocking the activation of T cells by antigen-MHC complexes on APCs.

A seminal accomplishment of modern molecular immunology was the isolation and characterization of TCR genes at a time when the biochemical analysis of the proteins was largely incomplete. In fact, most of the fine details of the structure of TCR molecules discussed below are predicted from the nucleotide sequences of the cloned genes. The strategy behind the first successful identification of TCR genes was based on the following three assumptions:

1. The TCR genes would be uniquely expressed in T cells.
2. Like immunoglobulin genes (see Chapter 4), the functional TCR genes would undergo somatic

---

BOX 7–2. THE ISOLATION OF T CELL RECEPTOR GENES

The first reported isolations of TCR genes were accomplished by creating complementary DNA copies (cDNAs) of mRNA expressed in T cells and not B cells. Clones of these cDNAs were then analyzed for the properties expected of an antigen receptor. A powerful modification of this approach was the use of **subtractive hybridization** (see figure). This strategy, developed by Mark Davis, was based on the assumption that T cell receptor genes should only be transcribed into mRNA in T cells and that most of the other transcripts in T cells would also be found in B cells. In fact, it is now known that T and B cells differ in less than 1 per cent of their mRNAs. With the expectation that the nascent polypeptide of an integral plasma membrane antigen receptor molecule should be found on rough endoplasmic reticulum, ^{32}P-labeled cDNA copies of membrane-bound polysomal RNA from an antigen-specific T cell hybridoma were synthesized. Sequences that were not T cell–specific were discarded by hybridization with B cell mRNA and physical separation of these DNA–RNA duplexes. This left a small group of cDNA sequences that could be used as specific probes for the very small fraction of the total genes transcribed in T cells that are not transcribed in B cells. These probes were used to screen, by hybridization, a library of cDNAs from the same T cell hybridoma. In this way, an individual gene was found that was somatically rearranged in this and several other T cell lines (but not in B cell lines) compared to the "germ line" configuration found in non-lymphoid, e.g., liver, DNA. In addition, different rearrangements of this gene were found in T cells with different antigen specificities as detected by restriction fragment length polymorphism. These findings immediately suggested that T cell receptor genes, like Ig genes, utilize somatic rearrangement as a mechanism of generating diversity. A thymocyte genomic DNA library was subsequently screened with the original hybridoma-derived probe, and nucleotide sequences of cross-reacting (hybridizing) clones were compared. This analysis revealed variable (V), constant (C), and joining (J) segments remarkably similar in size and organization to those found in Ig genes. N-terminal amino acid sequencing of proteins precipitated from T cells by anti-TCR antibodies revealed that the cDNA clones described above encoded the β chain of the TCR heterodimer. The same approach was used to isolate a TCR α chain gene, except that subtractive hybridization of cDNAs from one clonal T cell population was performed with RNA from two other T cell clonal populations (rather than a B cell population). This variation in the approach was based on the assumption that in each clonal T cell population, the unique mRNA sequences would encode the variable parts of the TCR molecule that differ among TCRs of different specificities. Therefore, the "T cell clone" minus "T cell clone" subtraction would enrich for TCR cDNAs and eliminate cDNAs encoding other invariant T cell specific molecules.

Continued

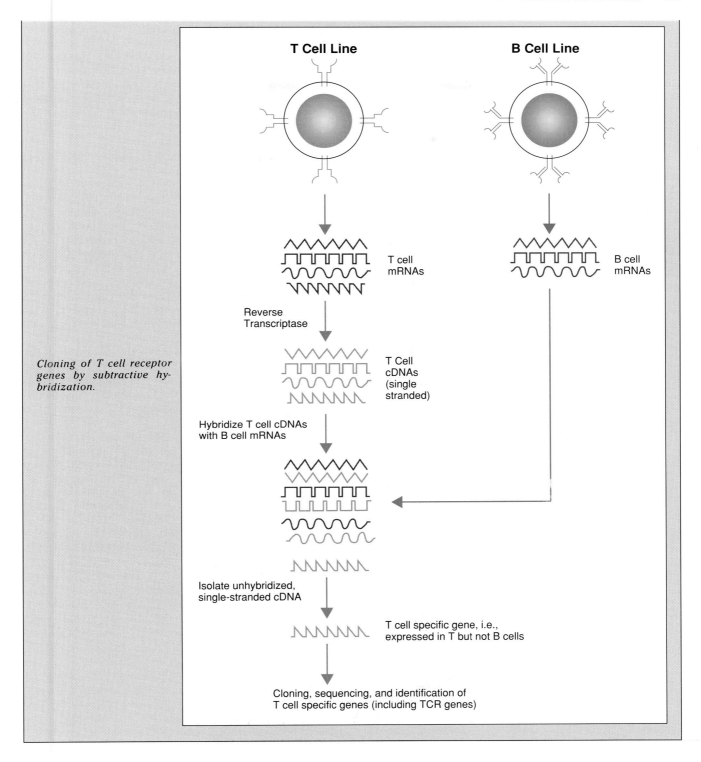

Cloning of T cell receptor genes by subtractive hybridization.

rearrangement during T cell development and would therefore appear different, by Southern analysis, in mature T cells compared to the germline configuration seen in non-T cells.

3. The TCR genes would have some homology to Ig genes.

T cell receptor genes were first identified by preparing complementary DNA (cDNA) clones of messenger RNA (mRNA) from clonal T cell populations and testing these cDNAs for the properties listed above (Box 7–2, p. 140). The predicted amino acid sequences from the cloned TCR genes matched the limited amino acid sequence data that had been obtained from purified TCR proteins. The characteristics of TCR proteins are discussed in the following sections. The genomic organization of these TCR genes and the mechanisms of their rearrangements leading to TCR diversity are discussed in detail in Chapter 8, in the context of development of T cells from bone marrow–derived precursors.

Biochemical Characteristics of the $\alpha\beta$ T Cell Receptor

The antigen-MHC receptor on the majority of T cells, including MHC–restricted helper T cells and CTLs, is a heterodimer consisting of two polypeptide chains, designated α and β, covalently linked to each other by disulfide bonds (Fig. 7–1). (Another less common type of TCR, found on a small subset of T cells, is composed of γ and δ chains and is discussed later.) The α **chain** is a 40 to 50 kilodalton (kD) acidic glycoprotein and the β **chain** is a 40 to 45 kD uncharged or basic glycoprotein. The α chain contains only complex N-linked oligosaccharides; the β chain contains both complex N-linked sugars and simple

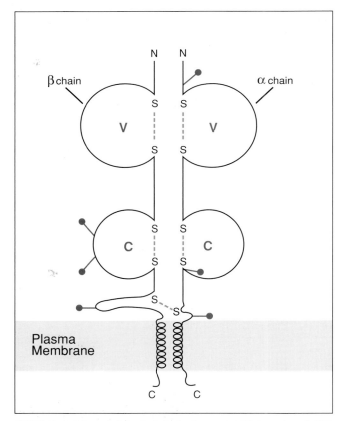

FIGURE 7–1. Schematic diagram of the T cell receptor (TCR) for antigen + MHC molecules. V and C refer to Ig-like variable and constant domains, respectively, of the α and β chains; N and C refer to the amino and carboxy termini of the polypeptides, respectively. S--S indicates a disulfide bond, and ——• indicates approximate location of carbohydrate groups.

high-mannose glycan side chains. There are striking structural similarities between the α and β chains and Ig. Both α and β chains have variable (V) and constant (C) regions. The C-terminal end of the V region, i.e., the junction between V and C regions, is encoded by a joining (J) segment gene, and, in the case of the β chain only, a diversity (D) segment gene (Fig. 7–2). The presence of V, D, J, and C regions is also characteristic of Ig (see Chapter 4).

The V regions of α and β chains are 102 to 119 amino acids long and contain two cysteine residues spaced appropriately to allow the formation of an intrachain disulfide bonded loop. Furthermore, there are many amino acid residues that are conserved between the V regions of TCR and Ig molecules. These residues in the TCR V region may contribute to the formation of a tertiary structure like the Ig V domain. The similarities in amino acid sequences and conformation between TCR and Ig V regions probably reflect the fact that both molecules have the similar function of binding extremely diverse foreign antigens. In Chapters 3 and 4 we introduced the concept that membrane proteins which contain domains that are structurally homologous to Ig V and C domains are members of a family of molecules that constitute the **Ig gene superfamily** (Box 7–3). Proteins belonging to this family are thought to have evolved from one ancestral gene. Many of these proteins play important roles in cell-cell interactions.

The C regions of the α and β chains range in length from 138 to 179 amino acids, and each consists of four functional domains that are usually encoded by separate exons. The most amino-terminal domain contains two cysteine residues spaced appropriately for the formation of an intrachain disulfide bonded loop, which also probably folds into a tertiary structure similar to an Ig constant region domain. A short hinge region or connecting peptide comprises the second part of the C region and contains a cysteine residue most likely involved in the disulfide linkage of the two chains. The third part of the C region of both α and β chains is the transmembrane domain, composed of 20 to 24 predominantly hydrophobic amino acid residues. An unusual feature of these transmembrane portions is the presence of a lysine residue (β chain) or a lysine and an arginine residue (α chain), the positively charged side chains of which may be crucial for interactions with negatively charged residues found in the transmembrane portions of the CD3 polypeptides (see below). The carboxy terminal part of the C region of both α and β chains forms a 5 to 12 amino acid long cytoplasmic tail. These cytoplasmic regions are thought to be too small to have intrinsic signal transducing properties, and other molecules physically associated with the TCR, such as the CD3 complex, most likely provide signal-transducing functions. Unlike Ig, the TCR α and β chains do not undergo changes in C region expression, i.e., "isotype switching," during T cell differentiation. Also, the C regions of TCR molecules are not known to participate in effector functions as do the C regions of antibodies.

Since the TCR has not yet been crystallized, the

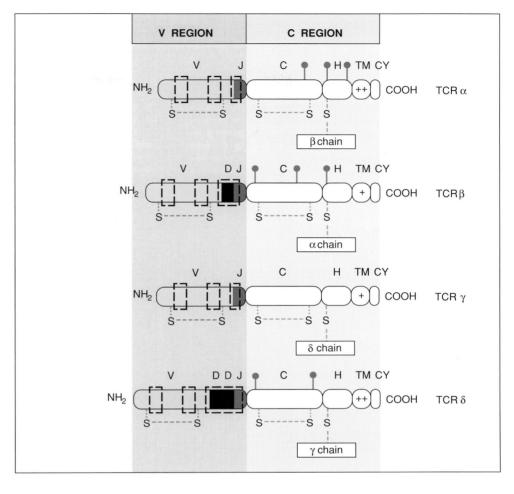

FIGURE 7–2. Relation of T cell receptor (TCR) gene segments to domains of polypeptide chains. The V region is encoded by variable (V), diversity (D), and joining (J) gene segments. Locations of disulfide bonds (S--S) and carbohydrates (——•) are approximate. Areas in dashed boxes are hypervariable (complementarity-determining) regions, "+" refers to positively charged amino acids in the transmembrane region. H, hinge region; TM, transmembrane domain; CY, cytoplasmic domain. (Modified with permission from Davis, M., and P. J. Bjorkman. T cell antigen receptor genes and T cell recognition. Nature 334:395–402, 1988. Copyright © 1988, Macmillan Magazines Limited.)

three-dimensional structure of the site for peptide-MHC complexes can only be inferred from sequence homologies with antibody molecules and the known three-dimensional structure of Ig and MHC molecules. Although amino acid variability from one receptor to another appears to be more spread out over the TCR molecule compared with Ig, there are at least three highly diverse regions in both the α and β chains of the TCR that correspond to the antigen-binding complementarity-determining regions (CDRs) of Ig. These hypervariable regions are presumed to form the contact points for the binding of complexes of foreign antigen and self MHC molecules. Two of these TCR hypervariable regions are encoded by V gene segments, and one is composed of sequences encoded by V and J gene segments (in the α chain) or V, D, and J segments (in the β chain) (Fig. 7–2).

Role of the $\alpha\beta$ Receptor in Recognition of MHC–Associated Antigen

The $\alpha\beta$ heterodimer recognizes complexes of processed peptides, generated from foreign protein anti-gens, bound to self MHC molecules. This has been demonstrated by several experimental approaches:

1. Anti-idiotypic antibodies generated against clones of antigen-specific, MHC–restricted T cells recognize only the $\alpha\beta$ heterodimer.

2. When an anti-idiotypic antibody raised against one clonal T cell population with a defined antigen-MHC specificity was used to screen hundreds of other randomly generated clonal T cell populations, the only one that bound the antibody had the same antigen and MHC specificities as the original clone.

3. The key features of T cell specificity, namely self MHC restriction and foreign antigen recognition, are always linked and do not segregate independently. For example, when two T cells with different antigen specificities and MHC restrictions are fused, the hybrid cell line recognizes each of the antigens recognized by the two parent T cell fusion partners, but only with the same independent MHC restrictions as the parent T cells (Fig. 7–3). Therefore, a single receptor confers specificity for both antigen and MHC.

4. Definitive proof that the $\alpha\beta$ heterodimer is responsible for both the antigen (peptide) specificity and the self MHC restriction of a T cell came from experiments with isolated TCR genes. In these experi-

BOX 7 – 3. THE Ig GENE SUPERFAMILY

Many of the cell surface and soluble molecules that mediate recognition, adhesion, or binding functions in the vertebrate immune system are evolutionarily derived from a common precursor. In addition, several molecules found outside the immune system, but often with similar functions, are also apparently derived from the same precursor. The genes encoding all these molecules comprise the **Ig gene superfamily,** and the protein molecules encoded by these genes are referred to as members of the Ig superfamily. Members of a gene superfamily are evolutionarily related and are therefore structurally homologous, but they do not necessarily share similar functions or proximity in the genome. *The criterion for inclusion of a protein in the Ig superfamily is the presence of one or more **Ig domains (homology units),** which are regions 70 to 110 amino acid residues long homologous to either Ig V or C domains.* The Ig domain contains conserved residues that permit the polypeptide to assume a globu-

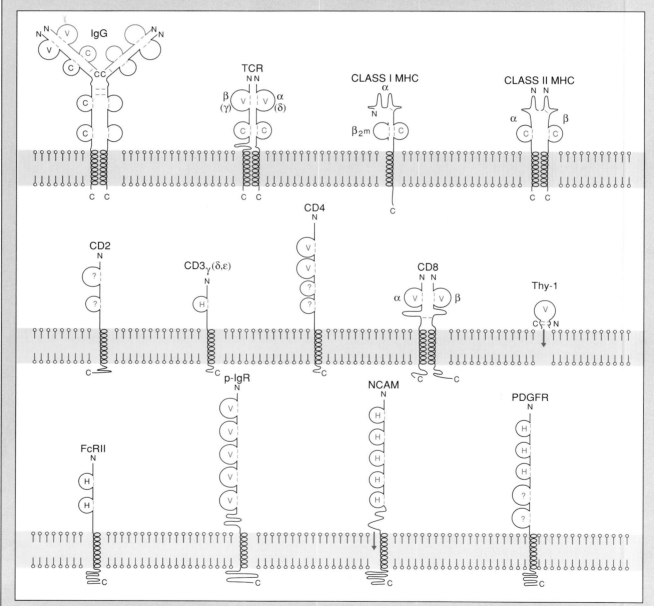

Examples of proteins in the Ig gene superfamily.

V, Ig variable-like domain; C, Ig constant-like domain; H, primordial Ig-like domain; ?, disulfide bonded loop of uncertain relationship to Ig domains; FcRII, Fc receptor II; p-IgR, poly-Ig receptor (transports antibodies across epithelial cells); NCAM, neural cell adhesion molecule; PDGFR, platelet-derived growth factor receptor. Modified from Hunkapiller, T., and L. Hood. Diversity of the immunoglobulin gene superfamily. Advances in Immunology 44:1 – 63, 1989. Courtesy of Academic Press, Orlando.

Continued

lar tertiary structure called an **antibody fold** (see Chapter 3), composed of a sandwich arrangement of two β-sheets, each made up of three to four antiparallel β-strands of five to ten amino acid residues. The sandwich-like structure is stabilized by hydrophobic amino acid residues on the β-strands pointing inward, which alternate with hydrophilic residues pointing out. In addition, conserved cysteine residues contribute to the formation of an intrachain disulfide-bonded loop of 55 to 75 amino acids (approximately 90 kD). Ig domains are classified as V-like or C-like on the basis of closest homology to either Ig V or C domains. V domains are formed from a longer polypeptide than C domains and contain an extra pair of β-strands within the β-sheet sandwich. A third type of Ig domain, called either C2 or H, is shorter and more compact than the C domain and may be derived from an evolutionary precursor of both V and C domains.

Using several criteria of evolutionary relatedness, such as primary sequence, intron-exon structure, and ability to undergo DNA rearrangements, molecular biologists have postulated a scheme, or family tree, depicting the evolution of members of the Ig gene superfamily. In this scheme, a very early event was the duplication of a gene for a primordial surface receptor followed by divergence of V and C exons. Modern members of the superfamily contain different numbers of V and/or C domains. The early divergence is reflected by the lack of significant sequence homology in Ig and TCR V and C units, although they share similar tertiary structures. A second early event in the evolution of this family was the acquisition of the ability to undergo DNA rearrangements, which has remained a unique feature of the antigen receptor gene members of the family.

Members of the Ig gene superfamily (shown in the accompanying figure) are for the most part unlinked, being present on many different chromosomes. This is true even for different members which form functional complexes with one another, such as the CD3 γ, δ, and ϵ protein genes (on human chromosome 11) and the TCR α and β chain genes (on human chromosomes 14 and 7, respectively). There are, however, important exceptions in which groups of genes encoding Ig homology units are closely linked. These include the linkage of the rearranging V, D, and J gene segments of all the antigen receptors to C domain genes on the same chromosome, the linkage of the members of the MHC, the linkage of the two CD8 chain genes and the V_κ locus, and the linkage of the CD3, NCAM, and Thy-1 genes. A consistent feature of the gene structure of Ig superfamily members is that most of the sequence for each homology unit is encoded by a single exon.

Most identified members of the Ig superfamily are integral plasma membrane proteins with Ig domains in the extracellular portions, transmembrane domains composed of hydrophobic amino acids, and widely divergent cytoplasmic tails with no homology to one another or to previously identified signal-transducing structures. There are exceptions to these generalizations. For example, the platelet-derived growth factor receptor has a cytoplasmic tail with tyrosine kinase activity and the Thy-1 molecule has no cytoplasmic tail but, rather, is anchored to the membrane by a phosphatidyl inositol linkage.

One recurrent characteristic of the Ig superfamily members is that interactions between Ig domains on different polypeptide chains are essential for the function of the molecules. These interactions can be homophilic, occurring between identical domains on opposing polypeptide chains of a multimeric protein, as in the case of C_H:C_H pairing to form functional Fc regions of Ig molecules. Alternatively, they can be heterophilic, as occurs in the case of V_H:V_L or V_β:V_α pairing to form the antigen binding sites of Ig or TCR molecules, respectively. Heterophilic interactions can also occur between homology units on entirely distinct molecules expressed on the surfaces of different cells. Such interactions provide adhesive forces that stabilize immunologically significant cell:cell interactions. For example, the presentation of an antigen to a helper T cell by an APC probably involves heterophilic intercellular Ig domain interactions between at least three pairs of Ig superfamily molecules, including TCR:Class II MHC, CD4:Class II MHC, and CD2:LFA – 3. The importance of all these interactions is demonstrated by the observation that antibodies that block the binding of these molecules to one another also block antigen plus APC – induced T cell activation. Several Ig superfamily members have been identified on cells of the developing and mature nervous system, consistent with the functional importance of highly regulated cell-cell interactions in these sites.

---

ments, functional TCR genes from a T cell clone of defined specificity were transfected into another T cell. For example, when the α and β genes isolated from a cytochrome c-specific, I-E^k restricted murine T cell clone were transfected into a T cell with an unknown specificity, the transfectants began to respond to cytochrome c plus I-E^k. Neither the TCR α gene nor the TCR β gene alone confers antigenic specificity or MHC restriction upon a cell.

Based on the predicted tertiary structure of the TCR and the sequencing of TCR genes from a large number of monoclonal T cells, the following important features of TCR specificity have been established:

1. In most cases both α and β chains are involved in binding both foreign peptide and self MHC molecules; i.e., neither chain is independently specific for antigen or MHC (Fig. 7 – 4).

2. Different portions of the hypervariable regions of α and β chains, i.e., V, D, or J segments, may interact with the helical sides of the peptide-binding cleft of MHC molecules or with the foreign peptide resting in the floor of this cleft. These fine structural details can be definitively resolved only by crystallographic analyses of isolated TCR molecules bound to peptide-MHC complexes. Such analyses have not been done yet.

3. Whether a particular T cell is class I or class II MHC – restricted is not determined by the V, D, J, or C genes used by the α or β chain of the antigen receptor of that cell. In other words, the same sets of TCR genes can be expressed in class I – and class II – restricted T cells and no TCR genes are exclusive for one subpopulation. As we discussed in Chapter 6, the ability of a particular T cell to respond to either class I – or class II – associated antigen is determined mainly by the expression of CD8 or CD4, respectively.

THE CD3 COMPLEX

The TCR $\alpha\beta$ heterodimer provides T cells the ability to recognize antigen-MHC complexes, but both the cell-surface expression of TCR molecules and their function in activating T cells are dependent on a group

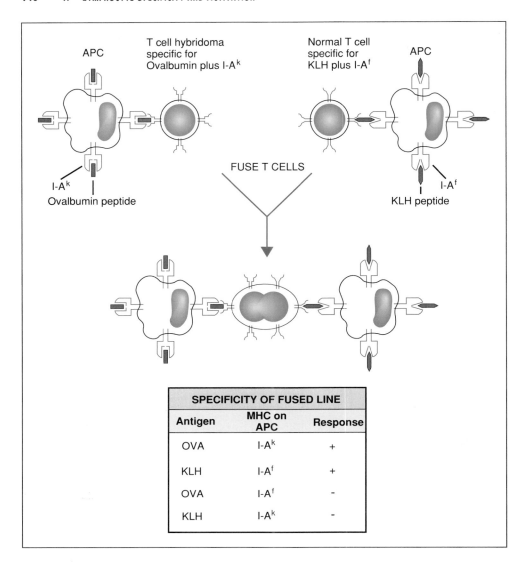

FIGURE 7–3. Antigen specificity and MHC restriction are linked properties of one TCR molecule. If an ovalbumin (OVA) + I-A^k–specific T cell is fused with a keyhole limpet hemocyanin (KLH) + I-A^f–specific T cell, the resultant hybrid recognizes both OVA + I-A^k and KLH + I-A^f but not either antigen in association with the other MHC molecule. Thus, antigen specificity and MHC restriction of the receptors on the two parent T cells are linked and do not segregate independently in the hybrid.

SPECIFICITY OF FUSED LINE		
Antigen	MHC on APC	Response
OVA	I-A^k	+
KLH	I-A^f	+
OVA	I-A^f	–
KLH	I-A^k	–

of associated proteins that form the CD3 complex. The CD3 complex consists of at least five distinct integral membrane proteins non-covalently associated with one another and with the TCR $\alpha\beta$ heterodimer (Fig. 7–5). These proteins were first identified, before the $\alpha\beta$ heterodimer, by the use of monoclonal antibodies raised against T cells. Anti-CD3 antibodies react with 100 per cent of peripheral T cells isolated from the blood or lymphoid tissues.

The $\alpha\beta$ heterodimer and the CD3 complex are physically associated with one another, and this association is required for surface expression of both $\alpha\beta$ and CD3 proteins. This has been demonstrated in several ways.

1. Antibodies against the TCR $\alpha\beta$ heterodimer or the CD3 complex co-precipitate both the heterodimer and the CD3 complex from solubilized cell membrane preparations.

2. When intact T cells are treated with either anti-CD3 or anti-TCR heterodimer antibodies, both structures are endocytosed and disappear from the cell surface; i.e., they are co-modulated.

3. T cell tumor lines that have lost cell surface expression of the TCR heterodimer because of mutations in α or β chain genes also do not express CD3 molecules on their surface. When functional TCR genes are transfected into these cells to replace the mutated genes, expression of both the TCR heterodimer and CD3 is restored (Fig. 7–6).

Five distinct members of the CD3 complex have been defined in humans and mice (Table 7–1). These include a 25 to 28 kD glycosylated γ **chain,** a 20 kD glycosylated δ **chain,** a 20 kD nonglycosylated ϵ **chain,** a 16 kD nonglycosylated ζ **chain,** and a 21 kD nonglycosylated η **chain.**

The CD3 γ, δ, and ϵ chains exist as monomers in the TCR:CD3 complex. In contrast, the ζ chain is expressed as a homodimer in 90 per cent of TCRs, and as a $\zeta\eta$ heterodimer in the remaining 10 per cent of TCRs. Thus, the minimal stoichiometry of the most common TCRs is $\alpha\beta:\gamma\delta\epsilon\zeta_2$.

The structures of all these chains have been predicted from the sequences of cDNA clones.

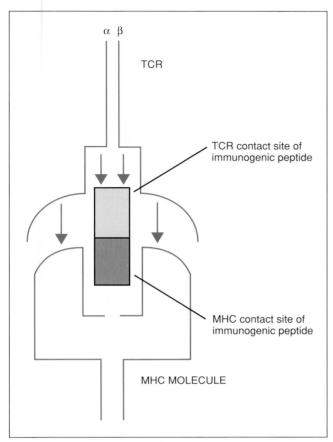

α β

TCR

TCR contact site of
immunogenic peptide

MHC contact site of
immunogenic peptide

MHC MOLECULE

FIGURE 7–4. Contacts between the T cell receptor (TCR) and MHC–associated peptide. *Every immunogenic peptide contains sites that bind to MHC molecules and other sites that are recognized by the T cell. The TCR molecule has regions that contact the foreign peptide and other regions that recognize polymorphic determinants of the MHC molecules (both shown by bold arrows).*

The γ, δ, and ϵ chain genes are highly homologous to each other, are located on chromosome 11 in humans (chromosome 9 in mice), and probably all arose from a common ancestral gene by gene duplication. The γ, δ, and ϵ chain proteins each include an N-terminal extracellular region, a short connecting peptide, a transmembrane segment, and a cytoplasmic tail. The extracellular region of γ, δ, and ϵ chains each contains a single Ig–like domain, and therefore these three proteins are members of the Ig gene superfamily. There is no variability or polymorphism identified in the extracellular domains of the CD3 proteins or their genes, and therefore it is not likely that these proteins contribute to the specificity of antigen recognition. The transmembrane segments of all three chains contain a negatively charged aspartic acid residue. This unusual feature may be important for the physical association or functional interactions of the CD3 proteins with the TCR α and β chains, since the latter polypeptides each contain a positively charged lysine residue in their transmembrane domains. The cytoplasmic domains of the CD3 γ, δ, and ϵ proteins range from 44 to 81 amino residues long and, there-

fore, are of sufficient size to transduce signals to the cell interior. There are, however, no homologies shared between these cytoplasmic domain sequences and the cytoplasmic domains of identified growth factor receptors or other well-characterized signal-transducing membrane proteins.

The structures of the ζ and η chains are similar to one another, and unrelated to the γ, δ, and ϵ proteins. Both ζ and η chains have identical amino acids in their extracellular and transmembrane domains, but differ in their cytoplasmic tails. The extracellular domains are short (nine amino acids), the transmembrane domains contain a negatively charged aspartic acid residue (similar to the CD3 γ, δ, and ϵ chains), and the cytoplasmic domains are long (113 and 155 amino acids for ζ and η chains, respectively). Both chains have multiple possible sites for tyrosine phosphorylation in their cytoplasmic tails. As we will discuss in Chapter 12, the ζ chain may be associated with other receptors such as the Fcγ receptor in natural killer (NK) cells.

When antigen binds to the TCR, the associated CD3 complex most likely transduces the activating signals to the cytoplasm of the T cell. Antibodies against CD3 proteins can often stimulate T cell functional responses that are identical to antigen-induced responses. However, unlike antigens, which stimulate only specific T cells, anti-CD3 antibodies stimulate all T cells in a mixed population, regardless of antigen specificity. This hypothetical role of the CD3 complex in mediating T cell responses to antigens is further supported by the observation that several of the CD3 proteins become phosphorylated when T cells are stimulated by TCR–binding ligands or by pharmacologic agents that activate T cell responses. Phosphorylation of cytoplasmic amino acid residues of transmembrane proteins is a phenomenon common to many growth factor receptors and is thought to play a role in the signal-transducing functions of these molecules. Phosphorylated serine residues appear on γ and δ chains, and phosphorylated tyrosines are identifiable on the ζ chain upon T cell stimulation. There is some evidence that TCR:CD3 complexes that contain $\zeta\zeta$ homodimers serve a different signaling function than the 10 per cent of complexes that contain $\zeta\eta$ heterodimers.

In the subsequent discussion we will refer to T cell antigen recognition or activation being mediated by the "TCR:CD3" complex. It should be noted, however, that recognition of antigen is due to the TCR only, and the signals that initiate activation are most likely transduced by the associated CD3 complex. It should also be noted that although the signals transduced by the TCR:CD3 complex are necessary for initiating the activation of normal T cells, they are usually not sufficient. Additional "costimulators," which interact with T cell surface molecules other than the TCR:CD3 complex, are also required, as we will discuss later.

It is clear that the TCR $\alpha\beta$ heterodimer and the CD3 proteins are mutually dependent upon one another for surface expression and function. The synthesis of the components of the TCR:CD3 complex, their assembly,

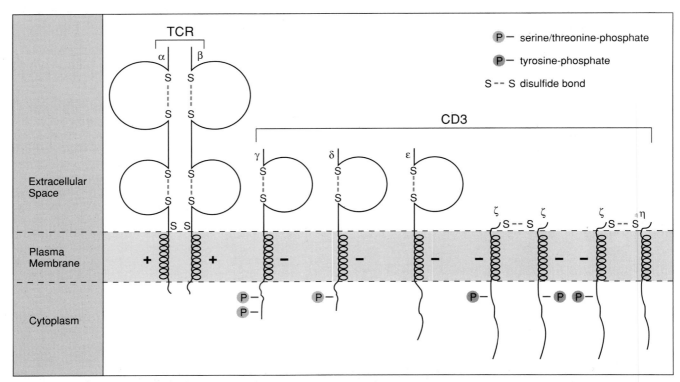

FIGURE 7 – 5. Components of the TCR:CD3 complex. *The γ, δ, and ε chains are present as monomers, non-covalently associated with the T cell receptor αβ heterodimer and with one another. ζ and η chains are present as ζζ homodimers or as ζη heterodimers, and these chains may also physically associate with the TCR or with other CD3 chains. Disulfide-bonded loops of Ig-like domains are indicated in the extracellular regions of the TCR α and β chains and the CD3 γ, δ, and ε chains. The + and − symbols refer to charged residues in the transmembrane regions that probably mediate association of chains. Approximate sites where the proteins may be phosphorylated are indicated.*

TABLE 7 – 1. Proteins in T Cell Antigen Receptor Complexes

Name	Function	Size (kD) Human	Size (kD) Mouse	Multimeric Form	Comments
TCR α	One chain of receptor for recognition of antigen-MHC complexes	45 – 60	44 – 55	αβ	Ig superfamily member; rearranging genes; on CD4+ or CD8+ T cells
TCR β	One chain of receptor for recognition of antigen-MHC complexes	40 – 50	40 – 55	αβ	Ig superfamily member; rearranging genes; on CD4+ or CD8+ T cells
TCR γ	One chain of receptor for unknown forms of antigen	45 – 60	45 – 60	γδ or γγ	Ig superfamily member; rearranging genes, predominantly on CD4−CD8− T cells
TCR δ	One chain of receptor for unknown forms of antigen	40 – 60	40 – 60	γδ	Ig superfamily member; rearranging genes, predominantly on CD4−CD8− T cells
CD3 γ	Signal transduction for αβ and γδ TCR	25 – 28	21		Ig superfamily member; phosphorylated on serine residues
CD3 δ	Signal transduction for αβ and γδ TCR	20	28		Ig superfamily member; phosphorylated on serine residues
CD3 ε	Signal transduction for αβ and γδ TCR	20	25		Ig superfamily member; phosphorylated on serine residues
CD3 ζ	Signal transduction for αβ and γδ TCR	16	16	ζζ or ζη	Phosphorylated on tyrosine residues
CD3 η(p21)	Signal transduction for αβ and γδ TCR	?	21	ζη	
CD3 ω or TRAP	Assembly of CD3 proteins in ER	28	28		Not expressed on cell surface TCR:CD3 complex

Abbreviations: TRAP, T cell receptor–associated protein; TCR, T cell receptor; ER, endoplasmic reticulum.

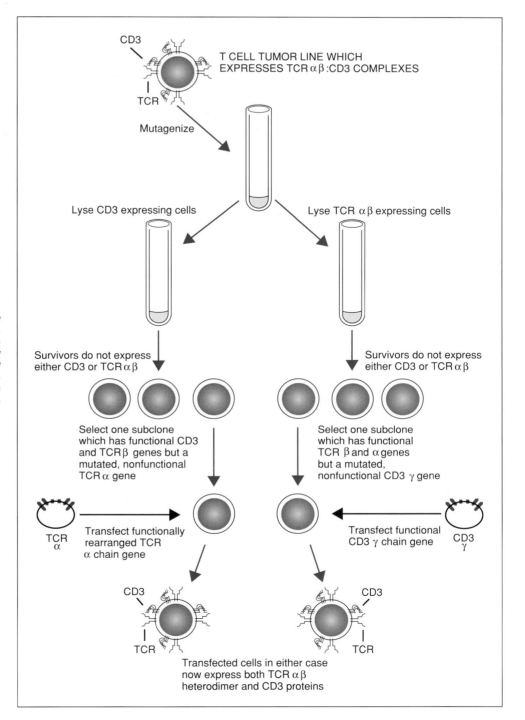

FIGURE 7–6. Co-expression of T cell receptor (TCR) and CD3 molecules. *If T cell mutants are selected for loss of either TCR or CD3, the surviving cells do not express either. In individual mutants lacking one functional TCR or CD3 chain gene, transfection of a normal gene encoding this chain restores expression of the entire TCR:CD3 complex.*

and their surface expression are tightly regulated and coordinated phenomena that occur during the maturation of T cells in the thymus (see Chapter 8). The CD3γ, δ, and ε genes are expressed by very immature thymocytes, before TCR α or β chain genes are expressed. Furthermore, the protein products of the CD3 genes are post-translationally modified and form γδε core structures in the absence of TCR α or β chains. The association of the TCR αβ heterodimer with the CD3γδε complex takes place in the endoplasmic retic-

ulum, after which the complex is transported to the Golgi, where further modification of N-linked oligosaccharides takes place. Incomplete complexes do not make their way to the plasma membrane, probably because some mechanism inhibits transport of these proteins out of the Golgi to the plasma membrane until they are all physically associated with one another. TCR–α, TCR–β, CD3–γ, CD3–δ, and CD3–ε chains are all synthesized in great excess over the quantity that is expressed on the cell surface, whereas CD3–ζ, in contrast, is synthesized in limiting amounts. There is evidence that $\zeta\zeta$ homodimers must associate with a TCR$\alpha\beta$–CD3$\gamma\delta\epsilon$ complex in order for the entire assembly of proteins to be routed to the plasma membrane. Recently, a 28 kD cytoplasmic protein has been identified that associates with incompletely assembled components of the TCR:CD3 complex but is not present as part of the mature complex on the surface of T cells. This protein, called ω or T cell receptor-associated protein (TRAP), is hypothesized to control assembly and transport of the TCR:CD3 complex, but its mechanism of action is not yet defined.

THE $\gamma\delta$ T CELL RECEPTOR

The $\gamma\delta$ TCR is a second type of highly diverse, CD3–associated disulfide linked heterodimer expressed on a small subset of $\alpha\beta$-negative peripheral T cells and immature thymocytes. (It is completely distinct from the γ and δ components of the CD3 complex.) Its existence was first suggested when the γ chain gene was cloned and characterized as an Ig-like gene that is somatically rearranged and expressed only in T cells, but with no sequences compatible with the N-linked glycosylation sites known to exist on TCR α and β chains. Subsequent cloning of the Ig-like δ chain gene, and concurrent immunochemical identification of a CD3–associated heterodimeric protein on cells not expressing α or β chains, confirmed the existence of the $\gamma\delta$ receptor. As is the case with the $\alpha\beta$ receptor, much of the information available about the protein structure of the $\gamma\delta$ receptor is predicted from the sequences of the cloned genes. Although the function of this receptor is not known, there are several interesting properties of the genes encoding it and the cells on which it is expressed that are areas of active investigation. The protein structure, specificity, and function of $\gamma\delta$ receptors are discussed below. The genomic organization, rearrangement, and generation of diversity of $\gamma\delta$ receptor genes are described in Chapter 8.

Biochemical Characteristics of the $\gamma\delta$ T Cell Receptor

The γ and δ proteins are present on T cells which express the CD3 proteins but do not produce $\alpha\beta$ receptors. γ and δ chains are transmembrane glycoproteins with structures similar to the the α and β chains. Both γ and δ chains include extracellular Ig-like V and C regions, short connecting or hinge regions, hydrophobic transmembrane segments, and short cytoplasmic tails (Fig. 7–2). The hinge regions usually contain cysteines involved in interchain disulfide linkages. Like the α and β chains, the transmembrane regions of both γ and δ chains each contain a positively charged lysine residue that may be important in interacting with the negatively charged aspartic acid residues found in the transmembrane regions of the

CD3 polypeptides. In addition, the transmembrane region of the δ chain (like the α chain) contains a second positively charged arginine residue. The amino acid sequence of γ chains is most like that of TCR β chains, and δ chains are most like α chains. In humans, the $\gamma\delta$ heterodimers are found in both disulfide-linked and noncovalently linked forms. The human γ chain is a glycoprotein with a size varying from 36 to 55 kD glycoprotein, depending on differences in both polypeptide backbone length and extent of glycosylation. The human δ chain is a 40 to 60 kD glycoprotein. In the mouse, only disulfide-linked $\gamma\delta$ heterodimers have been identified.

Specificity and Function of $\gamma\delta$ Receptors

Our current understanding of the structure of the $\gamma\delta$ receptor is a tribute to modern molecular biology, in that the information about the genes encoding the molecule is available well before any understanding of the molecule's function. Two interrelated approaches to analyzing the function of the $\gamma\delta$ receptor have been (1) characterization of the location and function of cells that express the receptor, and (2) determination of what $\gamma\delta$ receptors recognize.

Initial studies of TCR gene expression in the thymus established that γ and δ gene rearrangements occurred earlier than α and β gene rearrangements. However, $\gamma\delta$-expressing T cells are a distinct lineage from $\alpha\beta$-expressing cells. Mature $\alpha\beta$-expressing T cells contain either unrearranged γ and δ genes or genes that are aberrantly rearranged and incapable of giving rise to functional TCR γ and δ proteins (see Chapter 8). Furthermore, most $\gamma\delta$ T cells do not express CD4 or CD8 and are not restricted by polymorphic self MHC molecules as are $\alpha\beta$-producing helper cells and CTLs. One intriguing finding is the predominance of $\gamma\delta$ receptor-bearing cells among certain populations of lymphocytes found within epithelia. For example, lymphocytes within the small bowel mucosa in mice and chickens, called **intraepithelial lymphocytes,** are almost all $\gamma\delta$-expressing T cells. In addition, the population of T cells within the mouse epidermis, called **dendritic epidermal cells,** expresses predominantly $\gamma\delta$ receptors. Equivalent cell populations are not as abundant in human epithelial tissues. Although the functions of these cell populations are not known, their location suggests that the $\gamma\delta$ receptor may be involved in the recognition of a class of antigens that contact the epithelial boundaries between an individual and the external environment.

Functional studies of $\gamma\delta$-expressing T cells derived from various sources have demonstrated that many of them display nonspecific cytolytic activities against tumor cells. The role of the $\gamma\delta$ receptor in this type of cytolysis is not known. However, $\gamma\delta$-expressing T cell lines that display antigen-specific CTL–like activity which does depend on the $\gamma\delta$ receptor have also been described. The fact that $\gamma\delta$ receptors are associated with the CD3 molecule suggests that the signaling events and subsequent functional activation of $\gamma\delta$-bearing cells are similar to $\alpha\beta$-expressing cells.

The question of what the $\gamma\delta$ receptor recognizes remains unresolved. There is some evidence that these cells may recognize or are restricted by nonpolymorphic class I MHC–related molecules such as the Tla molecules (in mice) or CD1 molecules in humans (see Chapter 5). The cellular infiltrates seen in some infections and immunologic diseases contain a high frequency of $\gamma\delta$-expressing cells that recognize certain antigens such as *Mycobacterium tuberculosis* heat shock proteins, in a manner apparently unrestricted by polymorphic MHC molecules. A working hypothe-

sis for the function and specificity of $\gamma\delta$ receptor–expressing T cells is that they initiate immune responses to a small number of commonly encountered microbial antigens, perhaps at epithelial boundaries.

ACCESSORY MOLECULES ON T CELLS

The TCR heterodimer and the associated CD3 complex are the key molecules involved in specific antigen recognition by and antigen-induced activation of MHC–restricted helper T lymphocytes and CTLs. In addition, several other integral membrane proteins that play significant roles in both antigen

TABLE 7–2. T Cell Accessory Molecules

Name	Synonyms	Biochemical Characteristics	Gene Family	Cellular Distribution	Ligand	Function in T Cells Adhesion	Function in T Cells Signal Transduction
CD4	T4 (human), L3T4 (mouse)	55 kD monomer	Ig	TCR $\alpha\beta$ positive Class II MHC–restricted T cells; macrophages	Class II MHC molecules	+	+
CD8	T8 (human), Lyt-2 (mouse)	$\alpha\alpha$ homodimer with 78 kD α chain or $\alpha\beta$ heterodimer	Ig	TCR $\alpha\beta$ positive class I MHC–restricted T cells	Class I MHC molecules	+	+
CD2	T11, LFA–2, Leu-5 SRBC receptor	55 kD monomer	Ig	>90% mature human T cells, >70% human thymocytes	CD58 (LFA–3)	+	+
CD11aCD18	LFA–1	$\alpha\beta$ heterodimer (180 kD, 95 kD)	Integrin	All bone marrow–derived cells	CD54 (ICAM–1), ICAM–2	+	?
CDW49CD29	VLA-4,5,6	$\alpha\beta$ heterodimer	Integrin	Leukocytes, other cells	Matrix molecules, VCAM–1	+	+
CD28	Tp44	80–90 kD homodimer	Ig	All CD4+ cells; 50% CD8+ T cells	?	?	+
CD44	PgP-1, Hermes, Ly-24	80–200 kD monomer; variably glycosylated, chondroitin sulfated	Cartilage link proteins	Thymocytes, T cells, granulocytes, macrophages, erythrocytes, fibroblasts	? Collagen, fibronectin, HEV addressin, hyaluronate	+	?
CD45R	T200, leukocyte common antigen; B220 (on B cells)	180–220 kD monomers; cytoplasmic tyrosine phosphatase domain	Protein-tyrosine phosphatase	All immature and mature leukocytes	?	?	+
CD5	T1, Leu-1 (humans), Lyt-1 (mice)	67 kD monomer	Unknown	All T cells and thymocytes; subset of B cells	?	?	+
Thy-1		25–30 kD monomer; glycophospholipid membrane anchor	Ig	Murine thymocytes and mature T cells (not human); various other tissues, including neurons (mouse and man)	?	?	+
Ly-6	TAP	10–18 kD monomers; glycophospholipid membrane anchor	Unknown	Immature and mature T and B cells; various other tissues	?	?	+

Abbreviations: HEV, high endothelial venule; kD, kilodalton; MHC, major histocompatibility complex; TCR, T cell receptor; ICAM, intracellular adhesion molecule; LFA, lymphocyte function–associated antigen; VCAM, vascular cell adhesion molecule; VLA, very late activation.

recognition and functional responses are expressed on the surface of T cells (Table 7–2). These proteins, often collectively called **accessory molecules,** were initially discovered and characterized by the use of monoclonal antibodies raised against T cells. The antibodies were first used to identify T cell surface molecules by immunofluorescence and immunoprecipitation techniques. These antibodies were also used to block or initiate functional responses of T cells and thus served as probes for studying the physiologic roles of accessory molecules. There are several common properties shared by these accessory molecules:

1. *Accessory molecules on T cells specifically bind other molecules (ligands) present on the surface of other cells, such as APCs or target cells.*

2. *Accessory molecules are nonpolymorphic and invariant.* Thus, unlike the TCR or MHC molecules, accessory molecules are essentially identical on all T cells in all individuals of a species. This implies that these molecules have no capacity to specifically recognize many different, variable ligands, such as antigens.

3. As a consequence of binding their specific ligands on the surfaces of other cells, *accessory molecules increase the strength of adhesion between a T cell and an APC or target cell.* This property helps to ensure that the concurrent interaction between the TCR and peptide-MHC complexes is stable enough to result in activation of the T cell.

4. *Many accessory molecules may transduce biochemical signals* to the interior of the T cell that are important in regulating functional responses. Signal transduction presumably occurs as a consequence of ligand binding and may act in concert with other signals generated by the TCR:CD3 complex.

5. *Many T cell accessory molecules are members of the Ig gene superfamily or the integrin gene family.*

6. *T cell accessory molecules are useful cell surface "markers" that facilitate immunocytochemical identification of T cells in pathologic lesions, such as T cell lymphomas and leukemias.* In addition, antibodies against these markers can be used to physically isolate T cells for experimental or diagnostic procedures.

Accessory molecules on T cell surfaces may contribute to the regulation of immune responses in various ways. The intercellular adhesion roles of many of these molecules serve to localize the T cell interaction with foreign antigen to cell surfaces, where the ligands of the accessory molecules are also expressed (Fig. 7–7). Thus, cells that express ligands for accessory molecules may function more efficiently as APCs or CTL target cells. In addition, the expression and affin-

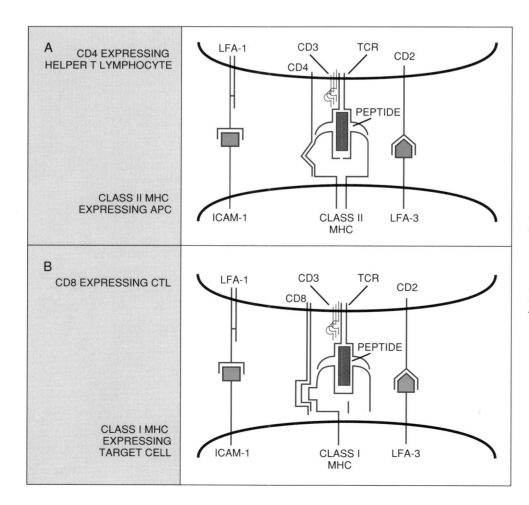

FIGURE 7–7. T lymphocyte surface molecules and their ligands involved in antigen recognition and T cell responses. Interactions between a CD4+ T cell and an antigen-presenting cell (APC) (A) or a CD8+ cytolytic T lymphocyte (CTL) and a target cell (B) involve multiple T cell surface proteins that recognize different ligands on the APC or target cell.

ity for ligand of some of these accessory molecules and their ligands are enhanced by different cytokines and by TCR–mediated stimulation, in contrast to TCR:CD3 expression, which is relatively constant. Cytokines are produced by T cells, and their ability to increase the expression of accessory molecules or their ligands may be a positive amplification mechanism in immune responses. Thus, changes in accessory molecules can serve to regulate the efficiency of antigen recognition.

The importance of accessory molecules in T cell activation is suggested by many experiments showing that antibodies against one or more of these molecules can block T cell responses to antigens. The current view is that the TCR:CD3 complex and accessory molecules function cooperatively in the interactions of T cells with antigens. According to one postulated model, the initial binding of T cells to APCs or target cells is mediated by accessory molecules and is antigen-independent. Thus, helper T cells may transiently bind to APCs or CTLs to target cells by their accessory molecules, without involvement of the TCRs or antigen. If the particular APC or target cell also expresses the MHC–associated antigen that the T cell recognizes, the binding is stabilized and the T cell responds. The alternative hypothesis is that the first interaction between a T cell and an APC or target cell is a specific but weak interaction mediated by the TCR, and in order for functional responses to occur, it needs to be stabilized by the accessory molecules. In fact, it has recently been shown that when a TCR binds an activating ligand, such as anti-CD3 antibody, a signal(s) is generated that leads to a marked increase in the avidity with which the T cell accessory molecules bind to their ligands on APCs. Clearly, the two models are not mutually exclusive.

Accessory molecules may also bind to extracellular matrix components or to molecules expressed on vascular endothelium. This may be important for the homing to, and retention of, lymphocytes at peripheral sites of antigen exposure and inflammation.

CD4 and CD8: Accessory Molecules Involved in MHC–Restricted T Cell Activation

CD4 and CD8 are T cell surface glycoproteins that are expressed on mutually exclusive subsets of mature T cells with distinct patterns of MHC restriction. CD4 and CD8 serve as accessory molecules by facilitating interactions of T cells with APCs or CTL target cells. Both molecules are members of the Ig gene superfamily, but they are no more related to one another than to other members of the family. Nonetheless they have very similar functions. Approximately 65 per cent of peripheral $\alpha\beta$-positive T cells express CD4 and 35 per cent express CD8. (Altered ratios of CD4+:CD8+ peripheral T cells are often used as a clini-

cal parameter for immune dysfunction, although the informational value of this parameter is very limited.)

STRUCTURE OF CD4

CD4 is a transmembrane glycoprotein, approximately 55 kD in size, which is expressed as a monomer on the surface of both peripheral T cells and thymocytes. In humans, it is also present on macrophages. The molecule was first defined by monoclonal antibodies and is commonly referred to as Leu-3 or T4 in humans, and L3T4 in mice. The predicted structure from the sequences of cDNA clones indicates that CD4 has an extracellular region with four Ig V-like domains. In addition there is a hydrophobic transmembrane region, and a highly basic cytoplasmic tail 38 amino acids long. The CD4 gene is on the same chromosome as, but it is not closely linked to, the CD8 and Igκ genes, in both humans (chromosome 2) and mice (chromosome 6).

FUNCTIONS OF CD4

The CD4 molecule is thought to have two important functions in immune responses.

First, *CD4 serves as a cell-cell adhesion molecule*, by virtue of its specific affinity for class II MHC molecules (Fig. 7–7). Several experiments have shown that the binding of CD4 to class II MHC molecules stabilizes the interaction of a class II MHC–restricted T cell with an APC–bearing class II MHC–associated antigen.

1. Class II MHC–expressing cell lines bind to monolayers of fibroblasts that express transfected CD4 genes, but no such binding occurs with untransfected fibroblasts or with mutant cell lines not expressing class II MHC (Fig. 7–8).
2. The ability of T cells to functionally respond to class II MHC–expressing APCs requires the presence of CD4 on the T cell surface (Fig. 7–9).

Because the CD4 molecule is invariant, it is assumed that it binds to a nonpolymorphic part of the class II MHC molecule, probably in the immunoglobulin-like $\alpha2$ or $\beta2$ domains. It is clear that there is a wide spectrum of affinities of TCR for their specific antigen-MHC molecule ligands. The adhesive role of CD4 may be most critical when the TCR affinity is low.

Second, *the CD4 molecule may transduce signals* or facilitate TCR:CD3 mediated signal transduction upon binding class II MHC molecules, thereby promoting the subsequent functional responses of class II–restricted T cells. The signal transducing role of CD4 has been suggested by a variety of experimental observations.

1. Monoclonal antibodies against CD4 have stimulatory or inhibitory effects on MHC–independent T cell activation induced by binding of anti-TCR or anti-CD3 antibodies. Such activation is independent of recognition of MHC molecules.
2. Phosphorylation of serine residues in the cy-

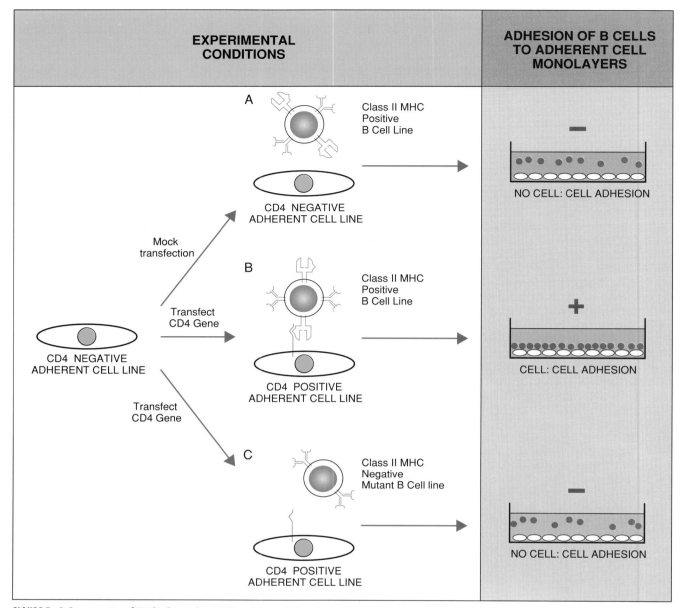

EXPERIMENTAL CONDITIONS	ADHESION OF B CELLS TO ADHERENT CELL MONOLAYERS

A
Class II MHC
Positive
B Cell Line

CD4 NEGATIVE
ADHERENT CELL LINE

−

NO CELL: CELL ADHESION

Mock
transfection

CD4 NEGATIVE
ADHERENT CELL LINE

Transfect
CD4 Gene

B
Class II MHC
Positive
B Cell Line

CD4 POSITIVE
ADHERENT CELL LINE

+

CELL: CELL ADHESION

Transfect
CD4 Gene

C
Class II MHC
Negative
Mutant B Cell line

CD4 POSITIVE
ADHERENT CELL LINE

−

NO CELL: CELL ADHESION

FIGURE 7 – 8. Demonstration of CD4 binding to class II MHC molecules. *A class II MHC – positive B cell tumor line binds to CD4+ fibroblasts (B) but not to CD4− fibroblasts (A). A mutant B cell line that does not express class II molecules also fails to bind to CD4+ fibroblasts (C).*

toplasmic tail of the CD4 molecule occurs rapidly upon stimulation of T cells by antigen plus MHC or by anti-TCR antibodies. Furthermore, a lymphocyte-specific protein tyrosine kinase, called p55 ^{lck}, is physically associated with the CD4 molecule. The possible role of such protein kinases in T cell activation is discussed later in this chapter.

3. On the basis of antibody-induced co-modulation of both CD4 and TCR, some investigators believe that CD4 molecules are physically associated with the TCR:CD3 complex. Bifunctional antibodies which bind simultaneously to both CD4 and CD3 proteins are more potent activators of T cell responses than are antibodies reactive with CD3 alone.

In addition to its physiologic roles, CD4 is the receptor for the human immunodeficiency virus (see Chapter 19).

STRUCTURE OF CD8

The structure of the CD8 molecule varies among species and in T cells at different stages of maturity. On peripheral human T cells, the CD8 molecule consists of either a homodimer of a 34 kD polypeptide chain called CD8α or as complexes (heterodimers or multimers) composed of CD8α and a second, less well characterized chain called CD8β. Most of the commonly used monoclonal antibodies against human

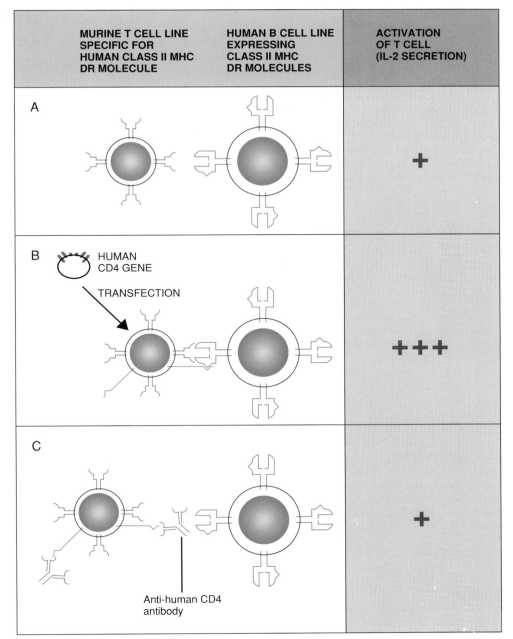

	MURINE T CELL LINE SPECIFIC FOR HUMAN CLASS II MHC DR MOLECULE	HUMAN B CELL LINE EXPRESSING CLASS II MHC DR MOLECULES	ACTIVATION OF T CELL (IL-2 SECRETION)
A			+
B	HUMAN CD4 GENE TRANSFECTION		+++
C		Anti-human CD4 antibody	+

FIGURE 7 – 9. Role of CD4 molecules in T cell activation. *A monoclonal mouse T cell specific for human class II MHC (DR) molecules responds weakly to a human DR+ B cell line (A). (Note that the mouse T cell may express mouse CD4 that does not bind to human MHC molecules.) If the mouse T cell line is made to express human CD4 by gene transfection, it responds well to the human DR+ cell line (B). This response is blocked by an antibody against human CD4 (C).*

CD8 recognize epitopes on CD8α, and the entire CD8 molecule is often referred to by the names of these antibodies, e.g., Leu-2 or T8. On human thymocytes, CD8α is expressed both as a homodimer and as a higher-molecular-weight multimer containing a disulfide-linked polypeptide chain called CD1, which is closely related in structure to class I MHC molecules. In the mouse, CD8 is expressed as a disulfide linked heterodimer of α and β chains (homologous to their human counterparts) on peripheral T cells and thymocytes.

The genes encoding CD8α and CD8β are closely linked to one another and to the Igκ gene on human chromosome 2 and on mouse chromosome 6. Both CD8α and CD8β are members of the Ig superfamily with N-terminal extracellular Ig V-like domains, connecting peptides, hydrophobic transmembrane regions, and highly basic cytoplasmic tails that are 25 to 27 amino acid residues long.

FUNCTIONS OF CD8

The CD8 molecule is thought have the same two important functions as CD4, namely in cell-cell adhesion and in signal transduction.

First, *CD8 serves as a cell-cell adhesion molecule,* by binding to nonpolymorphic immunoglobulin-like α3 domains of class I MHC molecules, thereby stabilizing the interaction of a class I MHC–restricted T cell (usually a CTL) with a target cell bearing class I–MHC associated antigen (Fig. 7–7). This has been established by experiments similar to the ones described above for CD4.

1. Anti-CD8 antibodies can block the formation of conjugates between class I MHC–restricted CTLs and class I MHC–expressing target cells, thereby inhibiting cytolytic activity.

2. Fibroblast monolayers expressing transfected CD8α genes tightly bind class I MHC–expressing cells, whereas untransfected fibroblast monolayers do not.

3. If the TCR α and β genes are isolated from a CD8+ CTL clone and transfected into another T cell line that does not express CD8, the transfected line will not kill target cells bearing the relevant MHC–associated antigen. Cytolytic activity against such targets is restored, however, if the CD8α gene is co-transfected along with the TCR genes.

Experiments utilizing α3 domain mutant class I MHC molecules demonstrate that in order for a CTL to recognize its specific target, the TCR and CD8 molecules must bind to the same class I MHC molecule. As with CD4, the adhesive role of CD8 is probably most important when T cells express antigen receptors with low affinity for specific antigen-MHC complexes or when the concentration of these complexes expressed on the surface of target cells is low.

Second, *the CD8 molecule may transduce signals* or may facilitate TCR:CD3–mediated signal transduction upon binding class I MHC molecules, thereby promoting subsequent functional responses of class I–restricted T cells. The signal-transducing role of CD8 has been suggested by a variety of experimental observations.

1. Binding of monoclonal antibodies to CD8, or cross-linking of CD8 and the TCR:CD3 complex, either enhances or inhibits the ability of the T cell to be activated.

2. Antibodies specific for CD8 block CTL killing of target cells, and this occurs even when the antibodies are added after the CTLs bind to their targets. This is consistent with a role of the CD8 molecule in CTL activation beyond target cell adhesion.

3. The cytoplasmic domain of the CD8 molecule becomes rapidly phosphorylated upon ligand binding to the TCR. Furthermore, as with the CD4 molecule, the tyrosine kinase called p55^{lck} is physically associated with the CD8 molecule.

Although experimental observations demonstrate that CD4 and CD8 can be signal-transducing molecules under some conditions, it is not yet clear whether CD4–mediated and CD8–mediated signals are normally activating and/or inhibitory or whether such signals play an obligatory role in the physiologic responses of T cells to recognition of antigen plus MHC.

Other Accessory Molecules Involved in T Cell Activation and Cell-Cell Interactions

In addition to CD4 and CD8, several other T cell integral membrane proteins can influence T cell activation and/or the functional interactions of T cells with other cells. The precise roles of these accessory molecules in antigen-driven activation of T cells are not completely understood, and in several cases the ligands to which they bind are not known. Nonetheless, monoclonal antibodies specific for these proteins have profound effects on T cells, raising the possibility that these T cell surface molecules may serve significant physiologic functions. The major characteristics of these molecules are described below. We will begin by describing three types of molecules—CD2, LFA–1 **(lymphocyte function–associated antigen–1)**, and VLA (very late activation) molecules—for which naturally occurring ligands have been clearly identified. Next, we will describe two molecules—CD28 and CD44—with less well characterized ligands. Finally, we will describe four molecules—CD45, CD5, Thy-1, and Ly-6—with unknown natural ligands.

CD2

The CD2 protein, also called T11, LFA–2, Leu-5, Tp50, sheep red blood cell (SRBC) receptor, is a 45 to 50 kD glycoprotein that is present on >90 per cent of mature T cells and on 50 to 70 per cent of thymocytes. CD2 is also present on natural killer (NK) cells. CD2 may be a member of the Ig gene superfamily on the basis of sequence homologies. The molecule contains two extracellular globular domains that are distantly related to Ig homology units, followed by a hydrophobic transmembrane region and a long (116 amino acid residue) cytoplasmic tail.

CD2 functions as an intercellular adhesion molecule. An identified ligand for CD2 is the structurally similar molecule called **leukocyte function–associated antigen-3** (LFA–3, CD58). LFA–3 is a 55 to 70 kD surface glycoprotein expressed on a wide variety of hematopoietic and nonhematopoietic cells. It has a similar extracellular domain structure to CD2, but in contrast to CD2 it can be expressed either as a typical transmembrane protein or as a phosphatidyl inositol-anchored surface molecule. CD2 binding to LFA–3 promotes cell-cell adhesion. This may be critical for the functional binding of helper T cells to APCs, CTLs to their target cells, and maturing thymocytes to thymic epithelial cells (see Fig. 7–7). Consistent with this hypothesis is the finding that anti-CD2 antibodies can block conjugate formation between T cells and other LFA–3 expressing cells, and, perhaps as a consequence of diminishing cell-cell adhesion, these antibodies can block both CTL activity and antigen-stimulated helper T cell responses.

Mature human T lymphocytes form rosettes with SRBCs, and SRBC rosetting is used as a technique to purify T cells from other leukocytes in the blood. *It is now known that CD2 is the SRBC receptor* and binds to an LFA-3 homolog on the surface of SRBC.

In addition to its adhesive function, CD2 is also a signal-transducing molecule. Certain combinations of anti-CD2 antibodies can activate T cells to secrete cytokines and to proliferate. This has led to the hypothesis that a *CD2-dependent alternative pathway of T cell activation may co-exist with the TCR:CD3 pathway in normal T cells.* The relationship of these two pathways remains unclear. CD2 is expressed on developing T cells in the thymus earlier than the TCR:CD3 complex, and therefore it has been suggested that CD2 is important for mitotic stimulation of immature T cells. It is possible that CD2 transduces negative or inhibitory signals as well as activating signals, since some anti-CD2 antibodies can block T cell activation induced by anti-TCR or anti-CD3 antibodies. Thus, the consequence of CD2 binding to LFA-3 may depend on the nature of other concurrent stimuli to the T cell.

LFA-1 (CD11aCD18)

LFA-1 is a member of the integrin family of heterodimeric leukocyte surface proteins, which function primarily as adhesion molecules (Box 7-4). LFA-1 is expressed on virtually all bone marrow-derived cells, including more than 90 per cent of thymocytes and mature T cells, B cells, polymorphonuclear leukocytes, and monocytes.

Anti-LFA-1 antibodies inhibit a wide variety of adhesion-dependent lymphocyte functions, including antigen and APC-induced helper T cell stimulation, CTL-mediated killing of target cells, and lymphocyte adhesion to high endothelial venules (see Chapter 2). This effect is presumably due to the ability of these antibodies to block conjugate formation between the T lymphocytes and other cells.

One specific ligand for LFA-1 is **intercellular adhesion molecule-1** (ICAM-1), an 80 to 114 kD integral membrane glycoprotein that contains five extracellular Ig-like domains and is thus a member of the Ig gene superfamily. ICAM-1 is expressed on a variety of hematopoietic and nonhematopoietic cells, including B and T cells, fibroblasts, keratinocytes, and endothelial cells, and the level of expression on these cells can be upregulated by various cytokines. Recently, ICAM-1 has been shown to be a specific receptor both for rhinoviruses—the etiologic agents of many cases of the common cold—and for malarial parasites.

Some LFA-1-dependent cell adhesion phenomena cannot be blocked by anti-ICAM-1 antibody or by soluble ICAM-1; in fact, another LFA-1-binding molecule called ICAM-2 has been identified. ICAM-2 is also an Ig superfamily member, with two extracellular Ig-like domains; it has a similar tissue distribution to ICAM-1, but is apparently expressed constitutively and is not upregulated by cytokines.

VLA MOLECULES

The VLA molecules, or $\beta1$ integrins, all share the same β chain (CD29), as described in Box 7-4. Three members of this family, VLA-4, VLA-5, and VLA-6, are expressed on resting T cells. Like LFA-1, these molecules are increased in number, and their affinity for specific ligands also increases, upon T cell activation. Interactions of these molecules with their extracellular matrix ligands (fibronectin for VLA-4 and VLA-5, laminin for VLA-6) provide costimulator signals to T cells. VLA-4 also mediates binding of lymphocytes to high endothelial venules of Peyer's patch (see Chapter 2, Box 2-2) and to endothelium at inflammatory sites. In this case, the ligand may be an endothelial cell surface protein called vascular cell adhesion molecule-1 (VCAM-1).

OTHER T CELL ACCESSORY MOLECULES (CD28, CD44, CD45, CD5, Thy-1, Ly-6)

Immunologists have identified several additional T cell surface proteins that may transduce activating signals, but their natural ligands and their relationship to the physiology of antigen-induced T cell activation are less well defined. Like the accessory molecules already discussed, these molecules were also initially discovered by raising antibodies against T cells. Subsequent studies showed that antibodies reactive with some surface molecules would induce functional responses in T cells. The principal characteristics of some of these molecules are summarized below.

CD28. CD28 (Tp44) is an 80 to 90 kD, disulfide-linked homodimer expressed on all CD4+ and 50 per cent of CD8+ human T cells. CD28 is a member of the Ig gene superfamily since the predicted amino acid sequence from the cloned gene indicates the presence of an extracellular Ig-like domain. A murine homolog has recently been identified. An anti-CD28 monoclonal antibody can synergize with other stimuli, such as anti-TCR antibodies, in inducing CD28 expressing T cells to secrete cytokines and proliferate. A ligand on B cells for CD28, called B7 or BB1, has recently been identified.

CD44. CD44 (Pgp-1, Ly-24, extracellular matrix receptor III, Hermes) is an acidic sulfated integral membrane glycoprotein ranging in molecular weight from 80 kD up to 200 kD, depending on the degree of glycosylation and addition of chondroitin sulfate. CD44 is expressed on a wide variety of cell types, including T cells, thymocytes, B cells, granulocytes, macrophages, erythrocytes, neural cells, epithelial cells, and fibroblasts. A soluble form of CD44 also circulates in the plasma. The amino terminal portion of CD44 is homologous to cartilage link proteins, which promote proteoglycan- and collagen-dependent extracellular matrix adhesion. Furthermore, CD44 has been shown to be associated with the cytoskeleton in some cells and can bind extracellular matrix components such as hyaluronate, collagen, and fibronectin.

BOX 7-4.   THE INTEGRIN GENE FAMILY OF ADHESION PROTEINS

The specific (nonrandom) adhesion of cells to other cells or to extracellular matrices is a basic component of cell migration and recognition and underlies many biologic processes, including embryogenesis, tissue repair, and immune responses. It is, therefore, not surprising that many different proteins have evolved with specific adhesive functions. Many of the genes encoding these proteins display homologies indicative of a common ancestral gene. *The integrin gene family consists of homologous genes encoding molecules that promote cell-cell or cell-matrix interactions.* The Ig gene superfamily (see Box 7-3) is another set of homologous genes encoding proteins with adhesive and recognition functions.

All integrins are heterodimeric cell surface proteins composed of two noncovalently linked polypeptide chains, α and β. The two chains consist of extracellular and transmembrane segments and cytoplasmic tails 30 to 46 amino acids long. The extracellular domains of the two chains bind to various ligands, including extracellular matrix glycoproteins, complement components, and proteins on the surface of other cells. Many of the integrins bind to **Arg-Gly-Asp (R-G-D) sequences** in the ligands, but this is not always the case. The relative contributions of the α and β chains to binding of ligand is not known. The cytoplasmic domains of the integrins interact with cytoskeletal components (including vinculin, talin, actin, α-actinin, and tropomyosin), and it is hypothesized that the integrins coordinate (i.e., "integrate") the binding

of cells to extracellular proteins with cytoskeleton-dependent motility, shape change, and phagocytic responses.

Three integrin subfamilies were originally defined on the basis of which of three β subunits were used to form the heterodimers. In general, each β chain pairs with a distinct set of α chains but some β chains have been found to associate with more than one kind of α chain. Furthermore, additional β chains have now been identified. The major members of the family are listed in the table.

The β1-containing integrins are also called "very late activation" (VLA) molecules because VLA-1 was first shown to be expressed on T cells 2 to 4 weeks after stimulation *in vitro*. They are also expressed on other leukocytes and non-blood cells. The VLA proteins mediate attachment of leukocytes to extracellular matrices and vascular endothelium.

The β2 integrins, also known as the LFA-1 family, were identified by monoclonal antibodies that blocked adhesion-dependent lymphocyte function, such as killing of target cells by CTLs. LFA-1 plays an important role in the adhesion of lymphocytes with other cells, such as accessory cells and vascular endothelium. This family is also called CD11 CD18, with CD11 referring to different α chains and CD18 to the common β subunit. LFA-1 itself is termed CD11aCD18. Other members of the family include CD11bCD18 (Mac 1, CR3) and CD11cCD18 (p150,95, CR4), both of which have the same β subunit as LFA-1. CD11bCD18 and

Integrins

Name	Cell Distribution	Subunit Composition	Defined Ligands	Functions
VLA-1 (CD$_w$49aCD29)	Leukocytes, other cells	$\alpha1\beta1$ ($\beta1$ = CD29)	Laminin collagen	Cell-matrix adhesion
VLA-2 (CD$_w$49bCD29)	Leukocytes, other cells	$\alpha2\beta1$ ($\beta1$ = CD29)	Laminin collagen	Cell-matrix adhesion
VLA-3 (CD$_w$49cCD29)	Leukocytes, other cells	$\alpha3\beta1$ ($\beta1$ = CD29)	Fibronectin, laminin, collagen	Cell-matrix adhesion
VLA-4 (CD$_w$49dCD29)	Leukocytes, other cells	$\alpha4\beta1$ ($\beta1$ = CD29)	Fibronectin, VCAM-1	Cell-matrix adhesion; T cell homing
VLA-5 (CD$_w$49eCD29)	Leukocytes, other cells	$\alpha5\beta1$ ($\beta1$ = CD29)	Fibronectin	Cell-matrix adhesion
VLA-6 (CD$_w$49fCD29)	Leukocytes, other cells	$\alpha6\beta1$ ($\beta1$ = CD29)	Laminin	Cell-matrix adhesion
LFA-1 (CD11aCD18)	Leukocytes	$\alpha L\beta2$ ($\beta2$ = CD18)	ICAM-1 ICAM-2	Leukocyte adhesion
Mac-1 (CD11bCD18)	Macrophages, granulocytes	$\alpha M\beta2$ ($\beta2$ = CD18)	iC3b	iC3b receptor; leukocyte adhesion
p150,95 (CD11cCD18)	Macrophages, granulocytes	$\alpha X\beta2$ ($\beta2$ = CD18)	iC3b	Leukocyte adhesion
Vitronectin receptor (CD51CD61)	Endothelium	$\alpha V\beta3$ ($\beta3$ = CD61)	Vitronectin, fibrinogen, von Willebrand factor, thrombospondin	?
Glycoprotein IIb/IIIa	Platelets	$\alpha IIb\beta3$ ($\beta3$ = CD61)	Fibronectin, laminin, vitronectin, von Willebrand factor, ?thrombospondin, collagen	Platelet adhesion, aggregation

Abbreviations: VLA, "very late activation"; LFA, leukocyte function-associated antigen.

Continued

CD11cCD18 both mediate leukocyte attachment to endothelial cells and subsequent extravasation. CD11bCD18 and CD11cCD18 also function as complement receptors on phagocytic cells, binding solid particles opsonized with a by-product of complement activation called the inactivated C3b fragment. An autosomal recessive inherited deficiency in LFA–1, Mac–1 and p150,95 proteins, called leukocyte adhesion deficiency, has been identified in a few families and is characterized by recurrent bacterial and fungal infections, lack of polymorphonuclear leukocyte accumulations, and defects in adherence-dependent immune functions (see Chapter 19). The disease is a result of a mutation in the CD18 gene, which encodes the β chain of LFA–1 subfamily molecules, and it demonstrates the physiologic importance of the LFA–1 related proteins, the functions of which have otherwise been identified only *in vitro.*

Other integrins expressed on non-lymphoid cells contain $\beta3$ chains (see table), and yet other β chains may be present in additional less well defined molecules that are involved in the adhesion of cells to one another or to extracellular matrices.

These properties suggest that CD44 may functionally link the cytoskeleton with cellular adhesion to extracellular matrix (similar to the structurally distinct integrins). Many other functional roles of CD44 have been inferred from the effects of anti-CD44 antibodies *in vitro.* CD44 on T and B cells apparently serves as one of several homing receptors that bind to molecules on high endothelial venules, prerequisite to organ specific extravasation of lymphocytes from blood into peripheral lymphoid tissues (see Box 2–2, Chapter 2). CD44 is also involved in the activation of T cells mediated by other surface molecules. For example, antibodies against CD44 augment the responses of T cells to anti-CD2 and anti-CD3 antibodies. Some anti-CD44 antibodies also increase CD2–LFA–3 dependent adhesion of T cells and monocytes. In mice, CD44 is present on bone marrow derived precursors of T cells, before they enter the thymus. CD44 expression declines during murine T cell maturation, and only a small subset of mature peripheral T cells, believed to be memory T cells, express high levels of the molecule. In man, memory T cells express higher levels of CD44 than naive T cells.

CD45. CD45 (T-200, leukocyte common antigen) consists of a group of integral membrane glycoproteins, ranging in molecular weight from 180 to 220 kD, which are expressed only on immature and mature leukocytes, including T and B cells, thymocytes, mononuclear phagocytes, and polymorphonuclear leukocytes. The CD45 family consists of multiple members that are all products of a single complex gene on chromosome 1 of mice and humans. This gene contains 34 exons, three of which are alternatively spliced at the primary RNA transcript level to generate up to eight different mRNAs and eight different protein products. The predicted amino acid sequences of the protein products include external domains varying in length from 391 to 552 amino acids, a transmembrane region, and a 705 amino acid, highly conserved cytoplasmic domain, which is the largest yet identified among all membrane proteins. Different glycosylation patterns of the same peptide backbone also contribute to heterogeneity of the members of this protein family. Several different monoclonal antibodies that recognize individual members have been useful in the study of the distribution and functions of CD45 proteins. Isoforms of CD45 proteins that are expressed on a restricted group of cell types are designated CD45R.

CD45R expression on T cells is of interest for several reasons. First, the expression of different forms of CD45R is developmentally regulated during the process of maturation of T cells. Distinct subsets of CD4 expressing T cells at different stages of maturation or with different functional capabilities *in vitro* have been discerned on the basis of expression of different forms of CD45R. As discussed in Chapter 2, naive T cells express a form of CD45R called CD45RA, and memory T cells induced by prior exposure to antigen express a different isoform called CD45Ro. Second, the large *cytoplasmic domain of CD45 contains an intrinsic tyrosine phosphatase activity,* which may be important in the regulation of various activation pathways that involve tyrosine kinase activity (discussed later in this chapter). *In vitro,* purified CD45 can remove phosphates from tyrosine residues on the p55^{lck} protein. This may be why anti-CD45 antibodies can either inhibit or enhance various functional responses of T lymphocytes.

CD5. CD5 (also called T1, Tp67, or Leu-1 in humans and Ly-1 in mice) is a 67 kD protein expressed on all T cells and thymocytes and a small subset of B cells. cDNA cloning indicates a large extracellular domain, a transmembrane region, and a long cytoplasmic domain. Monoclonal antibody binding to CD5 on T cells can enhance the response to TCR–binding or CD3–binding ligands.

Thy-1. Thy-1 was one of the first differentiation antigens to be discovered on thymocytes and T cells. It was originally identified in the mouse and anti–Thy-1 antibodies were the first reagents used to separate T lymphocytes from other cells. The Thy-1 molecule is a 25 to 30 kD glycoprotein with two intrachain disulfide bonds and an extracellular Ig V-like domain. The protein has no cytoplasmic tail, but is attached to the plasma membrane by a C-terminal covalent glycophosphatidylinositol linkage. In mice, Thy-1 is expressed on thymocytes, mature T cells, pluripotent stem cells, fibroblasts, epithelial cells, and brain neurons. The brain expression is conserved in other species, including humans, but T cell expression is variable. In rats, thymocytes express the antigen, but mature T cells do not. In man, Thy-1 is expressed on very few thymocytes or mature T cells. In mice, some monoclonal anti–Thy-1 antibodies can act as potent stimulators of T cells, causing cytokine secretion and proliferation. The physiologic significance of this activation pathway is unknown.

Ly-6. Ly-6 proteins are a group of at least five

distinct cell surface molecules, ranging from 10 to 18 kD, found on mouse T and B lymphocytes at various developmental stages as well as on polymorphonuclear leukocytes. The mouse Ly-6 proteins are encoded by genes in a single complex locus located on chromosome 2. A homologous gene has been identified in humans, but little information is available yet on patterns of expression. The Ly-6 proteins are attached to the plasma membrane by a glycophosphatidylinositol linkage (as are Thy-1 and some forms of LFA-3). Some antibodies specific for Ly-6 proteins can activate T cells to secrete cytokines, and this activation pathway may be dependent on the coexpression of TCR:CD3 complexes.

Requirement for Costimulators in TCR:CD3-Mediated T Cell Activation

The functional activation of helper T cell populations, particularly normal resting T cells, requires more than binding of a ligand (anti-TCR antibody or MHC-associated antigen) to the TCR:CD3 complex. For example, highly purified normal T cells do not respond to lectins that cross-link CD3 or to anti-TCR:CD3 antibodies alone. Additional signals are required, and they can be provided in several ways. Accessory cells, such as monocytes, macrophages, dendritic cells, and B lymphocytes, can provide such signals in addition to serving as APCs. This has been shown *in vitro* by thoroughly depleting contaminating accessory cells from T cell populations. These purified populations show markedly reduced proliferative responses to lectins or anti-TCR:CD3 antibodies, and normal responses can be restored by adding back macrophages or B cells. Since lectins or anti-TCR antibodies provide MHC-independent stimuli, it is clear that the role of accessory cells goes beyond antigen presentation. The ability of accessory cells to complement TCR:CD3-mediated signals for the induction of T cell activation is attributed to largely uncharacterized **costimulator molecules,** produced by the accessory cell, which act on the T cell. The requirement for adjuvants in eliciting a primary immune response to a protein antigen may be a reflection of the requirement for costimulators as well as antigen presenting function, since adjuvants promote the migration of macrophages to the site of antigen administration and macrophages provide excellent costimulators for T cell activation.

Some cytokines, including **interleukin-1** (IL-1), **tumor necrosis factor** (TNF), and **interleukin-6** (IL-6), have demonstrable costimulator activities on certain T cell populations *in vitro*. They may function either by enhancing the production of the T cell autocrine growth factor interleukin-2 (IL-2), or by acting more directly as growth factors themselves (see Chapter 11). There is very little information on the intracellular signals generated by these cytokines when they bind to their specific receptors. It is also clear that co-stimulators distinct from these known cytokines are necessary for the activation of some T cells.

Many of these costimulators may be membrane-bound and not secreted molecules. *It is possible that some costimulator activity may be provided by signals transduced by T cell accessory molecules when these molecules interact with their ligands on the surface of APCs.*

The physiologic role of costimulators is not known, but they could have at least two regulatory functions.

1. *Costimulators may be important in determining whether the interaction of T cells with MHC-associated antigens leads to activation or tolerance.* For example, the absence of costimulators at the time of TCR binding of antigen can lead to unresponsiveness of a T cell to either growth factors or to subsequent antigen presentation (see Chapter 10). This has been demonstrated *in vitro* by exposing T cells to antigen plus MHC on artificial membranes or by the use of anti-TCR antibodies in the absence of costimulators. This may be an important mechanism of self-tolerance, because T cells that see a self antigen presented by APCs that lack costimulators may be rendered unresponsive to that antigen.

2. Costimulators may play a role in determining the nature of the cytokines secreted by antigen stimulated T cells, and this, in turn, can determine the characteristics of the immune response (e.g., humoral versus cell-mediated). For instance, an individual helper T cell may secrete different panels of cytokines, depending on what costimulators are present during antigen presentation. Alternatively, functionally distinct subsets of helper T cells may require different costimulators in order to be activated. Because APCs may be the major source of costimulators, the type of APC that presents the antigen to the T cell may be an important determinant of the type of immune response that ensues.

T Cell Activation

So far in this chapter, we have discussed the cell surface proteins that are involved in T lymphocyte antigen recognition. The consequence of T cell antigen recognition is the generation of biologic responses of the T cell, including the following (Fig. 7-10).

1. *Effector functions of T cells* initiated by antigen recognition are the biologic activities that enable T cells to mount a useful immune response to foreign antigen. *The major effector function of CD4-expressing helper T cells is the secretion of cytokines,* which act on the same T cells and on other cells, including B cells, macrophages, other T cells, inflammatory leukocytes, and vascular endothelium. These cytokines exert various effects that promote and regulate humoral and cell-mediated immune responses and inflammation. *The major effector function of CTL is to lyse antigen bearing target cells;* in addition, CTLs secrete some cytokines. The details of these various effector func-

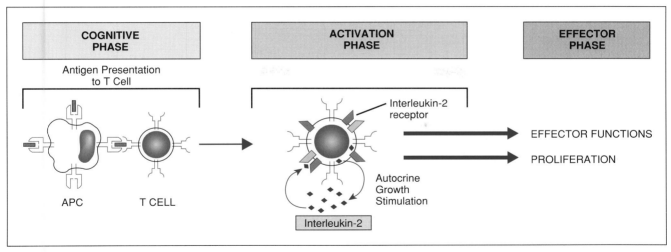

FIGURE 7–10. Functional responses of T cells. *Antigen recognition by a T cell (in this example a CD4+ cell) leads to cytokine (e.g., interleukin-2) production, proliferation as a result of autocrine stimulation, and effector functions (e.g., macrophage activation and B cell stimulation). CD8+ cytolytic T lymphocytes (CTLs) show less autocrine growth, and their principal effector function is cytolysis mediated by discharge of granule contents. APC, antigen-presenting cell.*

tions of helper and cytolytic T cells are discussed in Chapters 9 and 12.

2. *Proliferation of T cells,* in response to antigen recognition, is mediated primarily by an **autocrine growth** pathway, in which the responding T cell secretes its own growth-promoting cytokines and also expresses cell surface receptors for these cytokines. The principal autocrine growth factor for T cells is IL–2. Some T cells may exclusively use a different autocrine growth factor, interleukin-4 (IL–4); this subset has been clearly identified among mouse CD4+ T cell clones, but its existence in other species is not as well established. The result of the proliferative response is **clonal expansion** of antigen-specific T cells, which are necessary in large numbers to handle foreign antigen. Some of the progeny of antigen-responsive cells develop into **antigen-specific memory T cells,** which initiate larger secondary immune responses upon subsequent exposures to the antigen.

The response of T cells to antigen plus MHC consists of a series of cellular events collectively called **T cell activation.** The binding of antigen-MHC complexes to the TCR:CD3 complex generates intracellular signals that transiently increase the transcription of several genes that are quiescent in unstimulated T cells. This, in turn, leads to the transient production of proteins that are essential for T cell mitosis and function. (In contrast, some cell types, including CTLs and mast cells, show transient responses to external stimuli by releasing pre-formed molecules; this is a fundamentally different type of response pattern from cytokine secretion by T cells.) Thus, T cell activation includes the following interrelated steps:

1. Early signal transduction events.
2. Transcriptional activation of a variety of genes.
3. Expression of new cell surface molecules.

4. Secretion of cytokines.
5. Induction of mitotic activity.

Functional and mitotic responses of T cells to antigenic stimulation last only for brief periods, and the responses quickly wane as the antigen is eliminated.

The early events of T cell activation have largely been defined by *in vitro* models, often using monoclonal T cell populations, in which the molecular consequences of ligand binding to TCR:CD3 complexes are analyzed (Box 7–5). A great deal of recent research has been directed at understanding how stimulation of the TCR leads to transcriptional activation of genes. Although the early events after receptor stimulation may vary in different T cells, *a key step in all these cells may be phosphorylation of proteins that regulate transcription.* It is becoming clear that transcription of many genes is regulated by *trans*-acting DNA–binding proteins (nuclear factors), which bind to DNA sequences in the enhancer or promoter regions of the genes (see Box 4–5, Chapter 4). Nuclear factors may be rendered active, or freed of inhibition, by phosphorylation catalyzed by enzymes called **protein kinases.** There are different kinds of protein kinases in lymphocytes as well as in other cells, and each type may be responsible for phosphorylating different transcriptional regulatory proteins. Thus, a probable sequence of early events in T cell activation may be: generation of intracellular second messengers — activation of protein kinases — synthesis of, or phosphorylation of nuclear factors — functional activation of nuclear factors — stimulation of gene transcription. In the remainder of this chapter, we discuss some of the intracellular events in T cell activation, concentrating mainly on cytokine-secreting CD4+ helper T cells. The activation of CTLs, leading to granule discharge and cytolytic activity, may be basically similar but is not as well understood (see Chapter 12).

Early Membrane/Intracellular Signal Events in T Cell Activation

When antigen is presented to a T cell or when the TCR is bound by an activating antibody or a lectin (Box 7–5), a series of membrane and cytoplasmic events rapidly occur. These events are hypothesized to be causally related to the more distal events of T cell activation, such as cytokine production and mitosis. These early "signal" events are similar to those that cell biologists have described in the stimulus-response physiology of a variety of non-lymphoid cells, such as mast cells, platelets, endocrine secretory epithelium, and muscle (Fig. 7–11). Increased intracellular concentrations of several ions and biochemicals are critical to the signaling events; these ions and biochemicals are often called "second messengers." The three major categories of early activation events are (1) plasma membrane inositol phospholipid hydrolysis, (2) increases in cytoplasmic ionized calcium concentrations, and (3) phosphorylation of membrane and cytoplasmic proteins.

Inositol Phospholipid Hydrolysis and Increased Calcium

Within seconds of binding of ligands to the TCR, there is an increased rate of phospholipase C catalyzed hydrolysis of a plasma membrane phospholipid called phosphatidylinositol 4,5-bisphosphate (PIP_2). This results in increased cytoplasmic levels of two PIP_2 breakdown products: **diacylglycerol** (DAG) and **inositol 1,4,5-trisphosphate** (IP_3) (Fig. 7–11). PIP_2 breakdown is followed by a rapid rise in the cytoplasmic ionized calcium concentration, thought to be a result of the IP_3-stimulated release of membrane sequestered intracellular calcium stores. A sustained increase in cytoplasmic calcium is often maintained for over an hour, and this is dependent on influx of extracellular calcium. **Protein kinase C** (PKC) is activated, presumably as a result of the increases in DAG and calcium, which have been shown to activate purified PKC. Elevated calcium concentrations also favor the formation of complexes of this ion with the ubiquitous calcium-dependent regulatory protein called calmodulin. This leads to the activation of calcium-calmodulin–dependent protein kinases, which have distinct substrates from PKC. The relevance of these biochemical changes to the functional activation of T cells is supported by the fact that PKC activators (such as phorbol myristate acetate [PMA]) and calcium ionophores (such as ionomycin, which raise cytoplasmic calcium concentrations) act synergistically to promote the later differentiative and mitotic events normally seen in T cells in response to TCR–binding ligands. There is evidence that a **GTP–binding protein** (G protein) transduces signals from the TCR:CD3 complex to phospholipase C. For example, cholera toxin, which acts by chemically modifying certain G proteins, inhibits TCR:CD3–mediated increases in IP_3 and cytoplasmic free calcium and the G protein activating agent aluminum fluoride has been shown to increase inositol phosphate turnover, cytoplasmic free calcium, and CD3 phosphorylation.

The fact that neither PKC activators nor calcium ionophores are sufficient alone for T cell activation (but their combination is) has been interpreted as

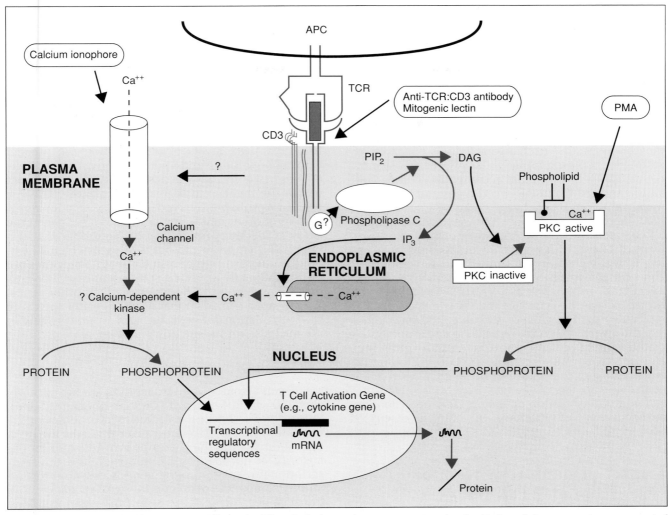

FIGURE 7 – 11. Intracellular second messengers in T cell activation. *The principal second messenger systems involved in the cellular response to engagement of the TCR:CD3 complex are shown. Various components of this response are mimicked by calcium ionophores and phorbol esters (e.g., PMA).*

evidence for a **two-signal model of T cell activation.** In this model, T cells require at least two different signals, generated by two different cell surface-binding events, in order to generate a full response. One signal may be provided by binding of MHC – associated antigen to the TCR and is transduced by the CD3 complex. The second signal may be triggered by accessory molecules on T cells binding to ligands on APC, or by co-stimulators produced by the APCs binding to specific receptors on T cells. Many questions, however, remain unanswered. It is not clear why two such sets of signals are necessary, which T cell surface proteins generate which signals, and what is the relationship between the signals generated by physiologic T cell activation and those triggered by pharmacologic agents that induce similar responses in T cells.

PHOSPHORYLATION OF PROTEINS

The phosphorylation of several different T cell membrane and cytoplasmic proteins occurs within sec-

onds following ligand binding to the TCR. The enzymes that may catalyze serine and threonine phosphorylations in T cells include PKC and calcium:calmodulin – dependent kinases. Other, less well defined biochemical signals may lead to the phosphorylation of tyrosine residues. As mentioned earlier, there is also a lymphocyte-specific, CD4 – and CD8 – associated tyrosine kinase, p55 ^{lck}. Furthermore, the presence of a tyrosine phosphatase domain in the cytoplasmic tail of the CD45 proteins may be important in the regulation of some T cell activation events by dephosphorylating, thereby deactivating, proteins that were previously activated by tyrosine kinases. Examples of protein kinase activity following TCR perturbation are the phosphorylation of serine residues on the cytoplasmic tail of the CD3 γ and δ chains and of tyrosine residues in the ζ chain. Other examples of T cell surface molecules that become phosphorylated during T cell activation are CD4, CD8, and CD45. Furthermore, as discussed above, direct phosphorylation of DNA – binding proteins, or the phosphorylation-induced release of inhibitory subunits from DNA – binding proteins, may be a mechanism for the transcriptional regulation of genes that are essential to T cell activation.

OTHER EARLY EVENTS IN T CELL ACTIVATION

Several other changes in membrane function occur within minutes of stimulation of the T cell antigen receptor, but their causal relation to functional activation of T cells is not clear. Increased plasma membrane Na^+/H^+ exchange activity is observed, resulting in increased intracellular pH. Increased intracellular pH is an event that accompanies cellular activation and growth in many cell types and the plasma membrane Na^+/H^+ exchanger may be a substrate for PKC. Increased numbers of open voltage–dependent K^+ channels are observed within 1 minute after treatment of T cells with mitogenic lectins. Increased cation fluxes including Na^+ influx and K^+ efflux with concomitant increase in oubain sensitive Na^+/K^+ adenosine triphosphatase (ATPase) activity also occur. Increased plasma membrane transport of small molecules such as glucose, amino acids, and nucleosides has been observed. Changes in cyclic nucleotide metabolism have been reported to occur within minutes of exposure of T cells to TCR:CD3–binding ligands, although the nature of these changes remains controversial. These changes may be involved in T cell gene transcription or may merely be secondary consequences of $PtdInsP_2$ breakdown discussed above.

Transcriptional Activation and Expression of T Cell Genes

Within minutes of the binding of ligands to the TCR:CD3 complex, T cells begin transcribing a variety of genes whose protein products are assumed or known to be essential for functional activation to proceed. These genes, which number more than 70, have been categorized as immediate, early, and late on the basis of the time course of their activation (Table 7–3). Transcription of immediate genes does not require protein synthesis, whereas early and late gene transcription does. Immediate and early genes are transcribed prior to mitosis, and late genes are transcribed after mitosis. The genes transcribed in activated T cells can also be categorized on the basis of the functions of their protein products. Three main functional categories of genes that are expressed early during T cell activation are (1) cellular proto-oncogenes, (2) cytokine genes, and (3) cytokine receptor genes.

CELLULAR PROTO-ONCOGENES

Cellular proto-oncogenes are normal cellular genes whose products are involved at various cellular sites in the regulation of cell growth and differentiation. They are so named because overexpression of these genes, or expression of mutated forms of these genes or their viral homologs, leads to malignant transformation of cells. Several cellular proto-oncogene transcripts are significantly elevated in T cells after TCR:CD3–mediated stimuli, as they are in many non-lymphoid cell types that are stimulated by external ligands. Two of the most frequently studied genes are c-fos and c-myc. Both are in the immediate gene category; transcripts are first detectable within 15 minutes and 1 hour, respectively, after T cell stimulation, and peak levels of transcription are present within 1 hour for fos and 6 hours for myc. The products of these two cellular oncogenes are believed to act within the nucleus to regulate cell growth. The Fos protein is probably involved in the transcriptional regulation of other genes, including the IL–2 gene (see below). The Myc protein may be required for the initiation of DNA synthesis, but the way in which it functions is unknown. Other cellular proto-oncogenes are transcriptionally activated at later stages of T cell activation and require prior expression of other genes. For example, c-myb is transcribed only after autocrine IL–2 stimulation of T cells; the Myb protein is found in the nucleus, but its function is not known.

CYTOKINE GENES

T cell cytokine gene transcripts are significantly elevated within 4 hours of TCR:CD3–mediated stimulation. The IL–2 gene has served as a paradigm for the regulation of cytokine gene transcription during T cell activation. IL–2 is the autocrine growth factor for the majority of normal T cells, and therefore the transcriptional regulation of its gene is essential for the mitotic component of functional T cell activation. The transcription of the IL–2 gene (and other cytokine genes such as γ-interferon) begins within 1 hour following TCR–mediated stimulation of normal human lymphocytes. The elevation in RNA transcripts of cytokine genes is largely due to increased transcription as opposed to decreased RNA degradation.

The IL–2 gene contains an enhancer located 5′ of the transcriptional initiation site, which operates in a tissue-specific manner to direct IL–2 gene transcription only in T cells. Several DNA–binding proteins that bind to the IL–2 gene enhancer region are believed to be important links between antigen plus MHC binding to the TCR and transcriptional regulation of the IL–2 gene. Some sequences in this enhancer region specifically bind a transcription-activating protein complex called AP–1. AP–1 has been found in many different cell types, and AP–1 binding sites have been identified in the regulatory regions of many different genes. AP–1 is largely composed of the protein products of the c-jun oncogene, but its DNA binding affinity is greatly increased when it forms a complex with the protein product of the c-fos oncogene. The Fos and Jun proteins apparently bind to one another by hydrophobic interactions of multiple interdigitating leucine residues, a structure referred to as a "leucine zipper." Certain T cell tumor lines have proven useful in analyzing the role of AP–1 in tran-

TABLE 7–3. Representative Molecules Expressed by Activated T Lymphocytes

Name	Functional Category	Time of Earliest Detection of mRNA After T Cell Stimulation	Location	Fold Increase After Activation
		Immediate		
c-fos	Nuclear-binding protein	15 min	Nucleus	<100
c-myc	Cellular oncogene	30 min	Nucleus	20
NF–AT	Nuclear-binding protein	20 min	Nucleus	50
NF–κB	Nuclear-binding protein	30 min	Nucleus	>10
		Early		
IFN–γ	Cytokine	30 min	Secreted	>100
IL–2	Cytokine	45 min	Secreted	>1000
TGF-β	Cytokine	≤2 hr	Secreted	>10
IL–2 receptor (p55)	Cytokine receptor	2 hr	Plasma membrane	>50
IL–3	Cytokine	1–2 hr	Secreted	>100
Lymphotoxin	Cytokine	1–3 hr	Secreted	>100
IL–4	Cytokine	<6 h	Secreted	>100
IL–5	Cytokine	<6 hr	Secreted	>100
IL–6	Cytokine	<6 hr	Secreted	>100
c-myb	Cellular oncogene	16 hr	Nucleus	100
Transferrin receptor	Receptor	14 hr	Plasma membrane	5
GM–CSF	Cytokine	<20 hr	Secreted	?
		Late		
HLA–DR	Class II MHC molecule	3–5 days	Plasma membrane	10
VLA–1	Adhesion molecule	7–14 days	Plasma membrane	?

Modified from Crabtree, G. R. Contingent genetic regulatory events in T lymphocyte activation. Science 243:355–361, 1989. Copyright 1989 by the AAS.

Abbreviations: IL, interleukin; VLA, "very late activation"; mRNA, messenger RNA; IFN–γ, interferon γ; TGF, transforming growth factor; NF–AT, nuclear factor of activated cell; GM–CSF, granulocyte-monocyte–colony-stimulating factor; HLA, human leukocyte antigen.

scriptional regulation of the IL–2 gene. These cell lines transcribe the IL–2 gene only in response to the combined action of a TCR–mediated signal (e.g., generated by binding of the lectin phytohemagglutinin [PHA] to the cell surface) and IL–1 serving as a costimulator. In these cells, PHA stimulates *c-fos* transcription and IL–1 stimulates *c-jun* transcription so that the combination of PHA and IL–1 induces the appearance of the AP–1 nuclear factor (Fig. 7–12). Thus, in this experimental model, ligand binding to the TCR and IL–1 binding to its receptor cooperate to stimulate the formation of a nuclear factor required for IL–2 gene transcription. The situation in normal T cells may be more complex, requiring other nuclear factors. This is suggested by the presence of other, non-AP–1 binding sequences in the IL–2 enhancer region that are required for TCR–mediated activation of IL–2 gene transcription in other T cell lines. Nonetheless, it is likely that antigen-MHC binding to the TCR and costimulators induce (or activate) two or more distinct sets of DNA–binding proteins, which function in concert to turn on the transcription of the IL–2 gene. Thus, the two-signal requirement for T cell activation mentioned above may be based on the requirement for different types of DNA–binding proteins which are induced by two different stimuli at the cell surface. The mechanisms of transcriptional regulation of other cytokine genes, e.g., IL–4 and γ-interferon, are not well characterized but may be fundamentally similar.

A characteristic feature of cytokine gene transcription in T cells is its sensitivity to inhibition by the immunosuppressive drug **cyclosporin A.** This drug is the most useful available treatment for allograft rejec-

tion (e.g., heart and kidney transplant rejection, see Chapter 16), and it works principally by inhibiting T cell cytokine production, thus preventing T cell growth and the development of effector functions. The IL–2 gene enhancer region is the site of action of cyclosporin A inhibition of IL–2 gene transcription, and the drug presumably interferes with the action of one or more of the transcription-activating DNA-binding proteins.

CYTOKINE (AUTOCRINE GROWTH FACTOR) RECEPTOR GENES

The transcription of **IL–2 receptor** genes is another component of the T cell activation process, which is necessary for the autocrine growth of the T cell in response to the IL–2 that it secretes. IL–2 induced growth of T cells requires the formation of a trimolecular complex composed of the cytokine and two integral membrane receptor proteins, which are 55 and 70 to 75 kD in size. TCR–mediated stimulation of T cells leads to increased expression of the p55 subunit of the IL–2 receptor. This response is due, in part, to increased gene transcription and is not dependent on new protein synthesis. The gene encoding the IL–2 receptor p55 polypeptide has a 5′ enhancer region that can bind PMA–inducible nuclear factors. The gene encoding the larger chain of the IL–2 receptor has been recently cloned, but analysis of transcriptional regulation is not yet available. Production and association of the two chains lead to the formation of a high-affinity IL–2 receptor that binds IL–2 and stimulates mitosis. The interaction of IL–2 with

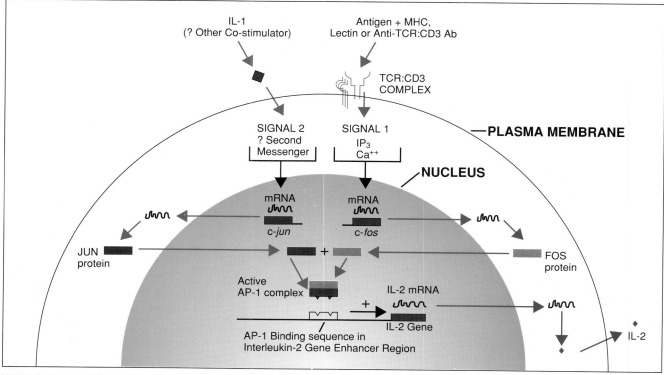

FIGURE 7–12. *A model for the transcriptional regulation of the IL–2 gene. In this model, based on studies with a T cell tumor cell line, TCR:CD3–mediated stimulation (signal 1) and costimulators such as IL–1 (signal 2) each increase synthesis of a different intracellular protein; the two proteins combine to form a transcription-activating complex. The complex binds to 5' regulatory sequences in the IL–2 gene to initiate and/or enhance IL–2 gene transcription. The model illustrates how two signals initiated at the cell surface may act together to generate a functional T cell response (e.g., cytokine synthesis). Stimulation of IL–2 gene transcription in normal T cells may be more complex, involving other nuclear binding proteins and 5' regulatory sequences.*

its receptor is discussed in more detail in Chapters 11 and 12. Genes encoding receptors for other cytokines, e.g., IL–4, are also transcriptionally activated upon T cell stimulation and may be regulated in a similar manner to the IL–2 receptor gene.

Proliferation of T Cells

Mitotic division of activated T cells results in the expansion of clones of cells with the same antigen specificity and thereby augments the immune response to a particular antigen. Along with cytokine assays, the measurement of mitotic activity by ^{3}H-thymidine incorporation into newly synthesized DNA is one of the most frequently used assays for T cell activation. When T cells are stimulated through the TCR:CD3 complex, mitotic activity can be measured within 48 to 72 hours *in vitro*. Depending on the T cell population, this induction of mitosis reflects cell cycle transition from either G_0 or G_1 to the S phase of the cell cycle. The binding of T cell growth factors, particularly IL–2 or IL–4, to their receptors initiates a series of poorly understood events that culminate in mitotic activity. No rapid change in cytoplasmic ionized calcium has been observed after IL–2 or IL–4 binding, and there are no clear indications that membrane phospholipid hydrolysis or PKC activation occurs in

response to IL–2 or IL–4 binding to cells. By analogy with studies of fibroblast growth physiology, ligands that bind the TCR:CD3 complex have been referred to as competence factors, meaning they allow cells to enter the cell cycle but not to progress through G_1 to S phase. In contrast, IL–2 has been called a progression factor, because it does allow cells to reach S phase.

Sᴜᴍᴍᴀʀʏ

MHC–restricted T cells express clonally distributed, disulfide-linked heterodimeric protein receptors ($\alpha\beta$ TCR) that are homologous to Ig molecules. These receptors specifically bind processed antigen complexed to MHC molecules as well as polymorphic determinants of self MHC molecules on the surface of APCs. The $\alpha\beta$ heterodimer is noncovalently associated with a complex of up to five distinct, invariant membrane proteins, collectively called the CD3 complex, which may function as the signal-transducing component for the TCR. The $\gamma\delta$ receptor is another clonally distributed, CD3–associated heterodimer that is expressed on a small subset of $\alpha\beta$-negative T cells. The nature of the ligand of the $\gamma\delta$ receptor and the functions of $\gamma\delta$-expressing cells are unknown. In addition to the TCR:CD3 complex, several accessory molecules are important in antigen-induced T cell activation. Some of these molecules bind ligands on APCs or target cells and thereby provide stabilizing adhesive forces. In addition, accessory molecules may transduce activating or regulatory signals. CD4 and CD8 are accessory molecules expressed on mutually exclusive subsets of mature T cells and bind nonpolymorphic determinants of class II and class I MHC molecules, respectively. CD4 is expressed on class II–restricted T cells, and CD8 is expressed on class I–restricted CTLs. Other T cell accessory molecules with known adhesion properties include CD2, which binds LFA–3, and LFA–1, which binds ICAM-1 and ICAM-2. The result of antigen-MHC binding to T cells is a series of intracellular events, collectively called T cell activation, beginning with second messenger generation and ending with the development of effector functions and T cell proliferation. The earliest events in this cascade include membrane phospholipid breakdown, elevated protein kinase C activity, and rises in cytoplasmic calcium. Several proteins are subsequently phosphorylated. These second messengers stimulate the transcription of genes required for the proliferative and effector responses of the T cell.

SELECTED READINGS

Ashwell, J. D., and R. D. Klausner. Genetic and mutational analysis of the T-cell antigen receptor. Annual Review of Immunology 8:139–167, 1990.

Bierer, B. E., B. P. Sleckman, S. E. Ratnofsky, and S. J. Burakoff. The biologic roles of CD2, CD4 and CD8 in T-cell activation. Annual Review of Immunology 7:579–600, 1989.

Clevers, H., B. Alarcon, T. Wileman, and C. Terhorst. The T cell receptor/CD3 complex: a dynamic protein ensemble. Annual Review of Immunology 6:629–662, 1988.

Crabtree, G. R. Contingent genetic regulatory events in T lymphocyte activation. Science 243:355–361, 1989.

Doyle, C., and J. L. Strominger. Interaction between CD4 and class II MHC molecules mediates cell adhesion. Nature 330:256–259, 1987.

Hedrick, S. M., D. I. Cohen, E. A. Nielsen, and M. M. Davis. Isolation of cDNA clones encoding T cell-specific membrane-associated proteins. Nature 308:149–153, 1984.

Hemler, M. E. VLA proteins in the integrin family: structure, functions, and their role on leukocytes. Annual Review of Immunology 8:365–400, 1990.

Hunkapillar, T., and L. Hood. Diversity of the immunoglobulin gene superfamily. Advances in Immunology 44:1–63, 1989.

Kappler, J. W., B. Skidmore, J. White, and P. Marrack. Antigen-inducible, H-2 restricted, interleukin-2–producing T cell hybridomas: lack of independent antigen and H-2 recognition. Journal of Experimental Medicine 153:1198–1214, 1981.

Kishimoto, T. K., R. S. Larson, A. L. Corbi, M. L. Dustin, D. E. Staunton, and T. A. Springer. The leukocyte integrins. Advances in Immunology 46:149–182, 1989.

Marrack, P., and J. W. Kappler. The antigen-specific, major histocompatibility complex–restricted receptor on T cells. Advances in Immunology 38:1–30, 1986.

Parnes, J. R. Molecular biology and function of CD4 and CD8. Advances in Immunology 44:265–312, 1989.

Raulet, D. H. The structure, function, and molecular genetics of the γ/δ T cell receptor. Annual Review of Immunology 7:175–208, 1989.

Saito, T., A. Weiss, J. Miller, M. A. Norcross, and R. N. Germain. Specific antigen-Ia activation of transfected human T cells expressing murine Ti $\alpha\beta$-human T3 receptor complexes. Nature 325:125–130, 1987.

Weiss, A., and J. B. Imboden. Cell surface molecules and early events in human T lymphocyte activation. Advances in Immunology 41:1–38, 1987.

Yanagi, Y., Y. Yoshikai, K. Leggett, S. P. Clark, I. Aleksander, and T. W. Mak. A human T cell–specific clone encodes a protein having extensive homology to immunoglobulin chains. Nature 308:145–148, 1984.

CHAPTER EIGHT

T CELL

MATURATION

IN THE

THYMUS

The total number of T lymphocyte specificities for different antigens in an individual is called the T cell repertoire. Any individual's repertoire of mature helper and cytolytic T lymphocytes (CTLs) has two fundamental properties. First, as discussed in Chapter 6, *antigen recognition by T cells is self MHC restricted;* i.e., T cells in each individual can recognize and respond to foreign antigens only in association with self major histocompatibility complex (MHC) molecules. Second, *the mature T cell repertoire is self-tolerant;* i.e., T cells in each individual do not recognize self MHC molecules alone or self antigens in association with self MHC molecules. Failure to maintain self-tolerance leads to immune responses against one's own tissue antigens and autoimmune diseases. Therefore, understanding how the mature T cell repertoire develops is important for understanding the specificity of T cells and may help us unravel the pathogenesis of autoimmune diseases.

The thymus is the major site of selection and maturation of both helper T cells and CTLs. This was first suspected because of immunologic deficiencies associated with the lack of a thymus. An adult mouse whose thymus is removed shortly after birth has very few T lymphocytes within the peripheral lymphoid tissues and is unable to mount immune responses to a variety of foreign protein antigens. The congenital absence of the thymus, as occurs in the di George syndrome in humans or in the "nude" mouse strain, is characterized by low numbers of mature T cells in the circulation and peripheral lymphoid tissues and severe functional deficiencies in T cell – mediated immunity. The fact that some functional T cells with a mature phenotype do exist in athymic individuals suggests that extrathymic sites of T cell maturation may exist, but the location of these sites is unknown and their contribution to the development of T cell immunity is apparently minor. Furthermore, although the thymus is clearly the principal site of T cell maturation, the organ involutes with age and is virtually undetectable in postpubertal humans. Nevertheless, at least some maturation of T cells continues throughout adult life. It may be that the remnant of the involuted thymus is adequate for some T cell maturation or that other tissues can assume the role of the thymus. Since memory T cells have a long life span (perhaps longer than 20 years in humans), the need for generating new T cells decreases with age.

This chapter describes the development of the mature T cell repertoire. T cell maturation consists of three closely related processes:

1. Migration and proliferation: *Pre-T cell populations arising in the bone marrow migrate through the thymus, where some cells are stimulated to grow and others die.* The surviving progeny eventually return to the blood and peripheral tissues as functional T cells. Immature T cells that have recently arisen from precursors in the bone marrow are committed to the T lymphocyte lineage but do not express TCR or accessory molecules, and they have no capacity to recognize antigens or perform effector functions. These precursors leave the bone marrow and enter the thy-

mus. They migrate from the thymic cortex to the medulla and are finally released as mature T cells into the periphery. During this intrathymic migration, some cells proliferate rapidly after entering the thymic cortex and many cells die in the cortex. The cell death ensures that only MHC – restricted and self-tolerant mature T cells exit the thymus.

2. Differentiation: *The mature phenotype of T cells develops in the thymus.* TCR:CD3 complexes are expressed early during intrathymic T cell maturation, after the formation of functional TCR genes by somatic rearrangement of different gene segments. In addition to the TCR:CD3 complex, surface expression of a variety of accessory molecules occurs during thymic maturation, some of which — including CD4 and CD8 — play important roles in antigen recognition and T cell activation. Functional maturation, which is the ability to perform helper or cytolytic functions, occurs simultaneously with, and in large part depends on, the expression of these T cell surface molecules.

3. Selection: *The mature repertoire of foreign antigen – specific, self MHC – restricted T cells is selected in the thymus.* All individuals contain essentially the same full sets of T cell receptor (TCR) genes in their genomes. These TCR genes can code for receptors that can recognize many different antigens in association with many MHC molecules. Therefore, in every individual, as T cells arise from bone marrow precursors, they have the potential of expressing receptors that can recognize any antigen (self or foreign) in association with any MHC molecule (also self or foreign). After different receptors are expressed on the surface of different clones of developing T cells, the repertoire is modified or shaped by two related selection processes (Fig. 8 – 1). The **positive selection** process by which the T cell repertoire becomes self-MHC restricted is also called **thymic education.** A second **negative selection** process eliminates or inactivates potentially autoreactive clones, ensuring that mature T cells are self-tolerant. These selection processes occur at the level of the entire population of developing T cells, and are due to selective growth or death of individual cells.

MIGRATION AND PROLIFERATION OF MATURING T CELLS IN THE THYMUS

T lymphocytes, like B lymphocytes, originate from precursors in the bone marrow. At present, little is known about the marrow stem cells that give rise to T or B lymphocytes or when and why they become committed to mature along a particular lineage. We also do not know why T cell precursors selectively migrate to the thymus. In mice, immature lymphocytes are first detected in the thymus on the 11th day of a normal 21-day gestation. This corresponds to about week 7 or 8 of gestation in humans. The cells

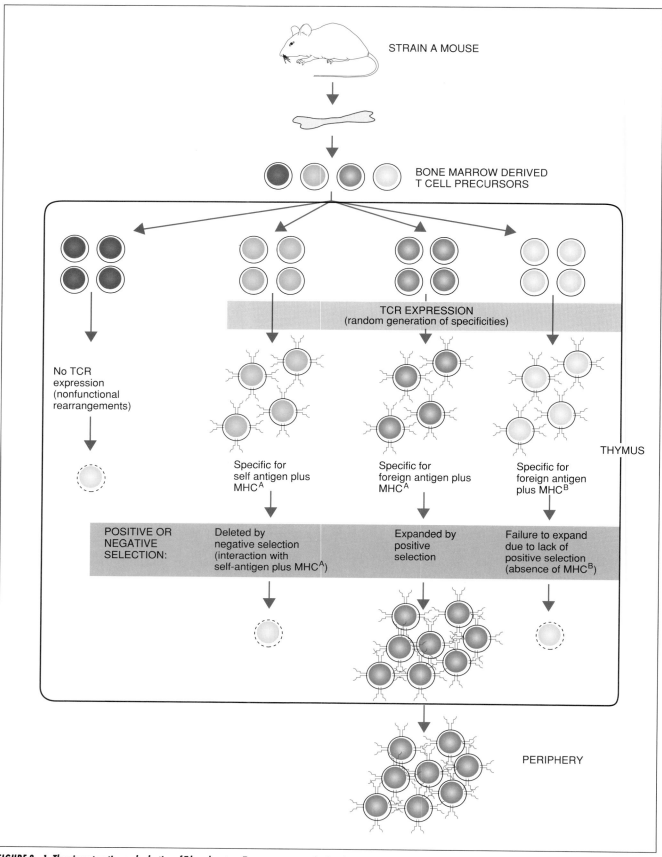

FIGURE 8 – 1. Thymic maturation and selection of T lymphocytes. *Bone marrow – derived precursors have unrearranged T cell receptor (TCR) genes and do not express TCRs. During intrathymic maturation, TCR gene rearrangements occur and maturing thymocytes express TCRs with random specificities. Only those clones specific for foreign antigen peptides bound to self MHC molecules are selected to mature and leave the thymus to populate peripheral lymphoid tissues.*

that first appear in the fetal thymus do not express TCR molecules, CD3, CD4, or CD8 and are incapable of recognizing or responding to antigen or performing effector functions. T cells in the thymus are also called **thymocytes.** The most immature thymocytes are found in the cortex, and the most mature thymocytes are detected in the medulla, from where they leave the thymus on their way to the peripheral lymphoid tissues. Immature cortical thymocytes are killed by high doses of corticosteroids, and this is one reason why chronic steroid therapy for a variety of diseases can cause a state of immunodeficiency. There is a high rate of mitosis in the cortex, with each bone marrow–derived precursor giving rise to multiple progeny. *Nonetheless, more than 95 per cent of the cortical thymocytes die before reaching the medulla.* This is probably due to the selection processes that preserve the minority of developing T cells that express self MHC–restricted, foreign antigen–specific TCRs, and eliminate the cells that express receptors of all other specificities. Consistent with this view that thymic selection processes occur in the cortex is the fact that TCR expression, as well as CD4 and CD8 expression, is first detected on cortical thymocytes. These selection processes are considered in more detail later in the chapter.

As they are maturing, thymocytes come into close physical contact with a variety of non-lymphoid cells in the thymus. These include thymic epithelial cells along with bone marrow–derived macrophages and dendritic cells (see Fig. 2–9, Chapter 2). The superficial cortical thymic epithelial cells include **nurse cells,** which surround thymocytes within membrane invaginations. Deeper within the cortex, epithelial cells form a meshwork of long cytoplasmic processes, around which thymocytes must pass in order to reach the medulla. Epithelial cells are also present in the medulla. Bone marrow–derived dendritic cells are present at the corticomedullary junction and within the medulla, whereas macrophages are present primarily within the medulla. The migration through this anatomic arrangement allows sequential interactions between thymocytes and these other cells, and such interactions are necessary for the maturation of T lymphocytes.

Two types of molecules produced by the non-lymphoid thymic cells may be important for T cell maturation. The first are **MHC molecules,** which are expressed by many of the non-lymphoid cells in the thymus. Cortical macrophages, epithelial cells, and dendritic cells express high levels of class II MHC molecules; medullary epithelial and dendritic cells express both class I and class II MHC molecules; and medullary macrophages express high levels of class I MHC molecules. The interaction of maturing thymocytes with these MHC molecules within the thymus may be important for the selection of the mature T cell repertoire, as will be discussed in detail later. Second, thymic epithelial cells produce **thymic hormones,** which are postulated to promote T cell maturation. These hormones include a variety of proteins that have been well characterized biochemically but whose physiologic roles are largely unknown. They have been given various names, including thymosin, thymopoietin, thymulin, and thymic humoral factor. Thymic hormones have been shown to induce the appearance of some T lymphocyte lineage specific surface molecules on bone marrow cells or immature thymocytes *in vitro* and to enhance T cell functional responses, such as proliferative responses to polyclonal activators. Some of these hormones have also been used in clinical trials for the treatment of immunodeficiency states in humans. Thymic stromal cells may also secrete interleukin-7 (IL–7), a cytokine that may stimulate the proliferation and maturation of developing T cells in the thymus. However, no thymic hormone or cytokine has been shown to support the extrathymic development of immunocompetent, TCR–expressing, MHC–restricted and self-tolerant T cells from bone marrow precursors or from immature cortical thymocytes *in vitro.*

T Cell Receptor Genes: Organization, Rearrangements, and Generation of Diversity

The selection processes that shape the mature T cell repertoire begin only after developing T cells first express randomly generated TCR molecules with diverse specificities. The expression of TCRs is necessary for both positive and negative selection because both processes are dependent on specific recognition of self MHC and/or self antigens on the surfaces of thymic epithelial cells, dendritic cells, and macrophages. This portion of the chapter describes the organization of TCR genes and the mechanisms for generating the diverse repertoire of TCR specificities prior to selection.

Genomic Organization of T Cell Receptor α and β Genes

Functional TCR α and β chain genes, which are capable of being expressed as polypeptides, are normally present only in cells of the T lymphocyte lineage. *These functional TCR genes are formed by somatic rearrangement of germline gene segments,* by a process that is very similar to Ig gene rearrangements (see Chapter 4). The genomic organization of TCR α and β genes is fundamentally the same in all species studied (Figs. 8–2 and 8–3) and is similar to the organization of Ig genes. Each TCR locus consists of variable (V), joining (J), and constant (C) region genes, and the β chain locus also contains diversity (D) gene segments. Complete mapping of the unrearranged β chain locus has been achieved in mice; other TCR loci in mouse and man are still incompletely described. The β chain locus is on chromosome 7 in humans and on

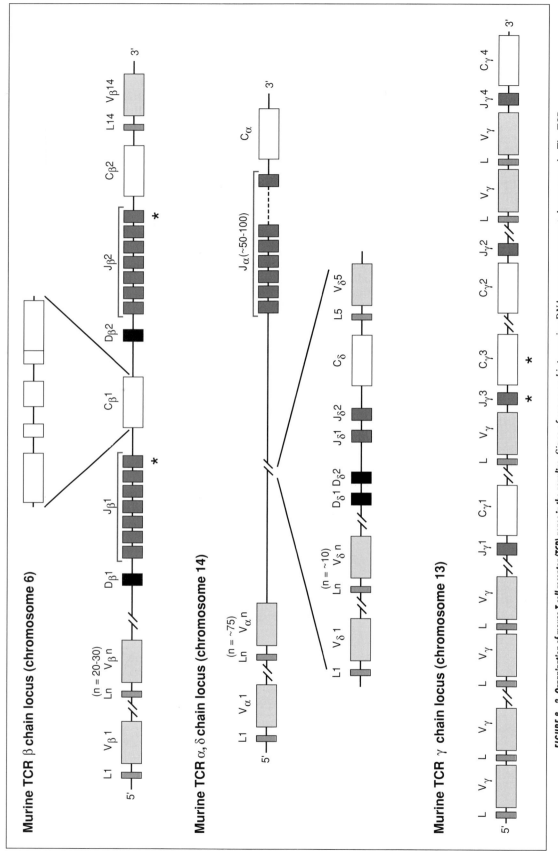

Murine TCR β chain locus (chromosome 6)

Murine TCR α, δ chain locus (chromosome 14)

Murine TCR γ chain locus (chromosome 13)

FIGURE 8 – 2. Organization of mouse T cell receptor (TCR) genes in the germline. Sizes of exons and intervening DNA sequences are not shown to scale. The TCR β locus has been completely sequenced; other loci are incompletely defined. Note that the δ locus is located within the α chain locus. All of the C genes are actually composed of multiple exons, as shown for the $C_\beta 1$ gene. * indicates nonfunctional pseudogenes. The numbering of V_γ genes is not yet uniformly defined.

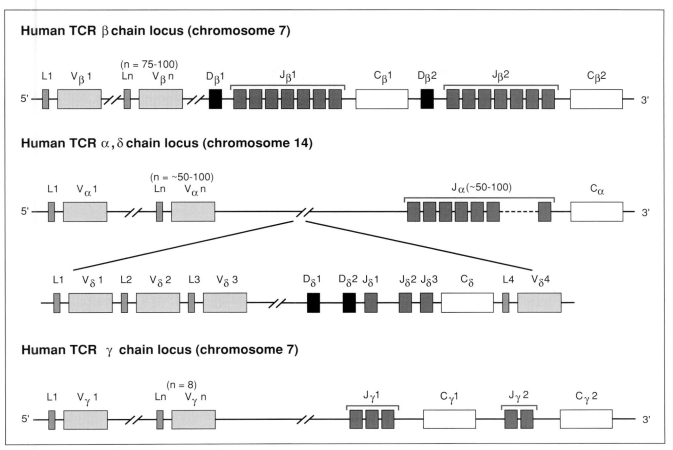

FIGURE 8 – 3. Organization of human T cell receptor (TCR) genes in the germline. *The genomic organization of human TCR loci is similar to that of the mouse (see Fig. 8–2); the human loci have not been completely sequenced.*

chromosome 6 in mice. There are two nearly identical C_β genes, each containing four exons. Each C_β gene is associated with a 5' cluster of six or seven J segments and one D segment. In mice there are 20 to 30 V_β segments that can be grouped into 20 families, members of which are more than 75 per cent homologous in DNA sequence. Most V_β segments are located 5' of the two clusters of C and J segments, although at least one V_β gene, which is used in mature T cells, is 3' to and in the opposite transcriptional orientation to the C_β genes. Interestingly, some strains of mice have deletions of up to half of the V_β segments or half of the D_β and J_β segments, and yet they are immunologically normal. Genomic sequences encoding the α chain are present on chromosome 14 in both humans and mice. There is a single C_α gene of four exons associated with a large 5' cluster of up to 60 different J segments. D segments have not been identified in the α locus. There are about 75 V_α gene segments, grouped into at least 12 families, all located 5' of the J and C regions. The α locus also contains all the coding sequences for the TCR δ chain (see below).

Rearrangement and Expression of T Cell Receptor α and β Chain Genes

The TCR genes in the earliest T cell precursors are in the nonfunctional germline configuration, which is characterized by the spatial separation of V, D, J, and C gene segments on the chromosome. During maturation of T cells in the thymus, the TCR gene segments are rearranged in a defined order, resulting in the formation of functional TCR α and β genes in which V, D, J, and C segments are in close proximity to one another (Fig. 8–4). This process of somatic rearrangement is a prerequisite to TCR gene expression and is important for the generation of TCR diversity, as we will discuss below. The basic sequence of TCR gene rearrangements and expression is quite similar to that of Ig.

Somatic rearrangements of TCR V, D, and J genes are mediated by recombinases, which are thought to

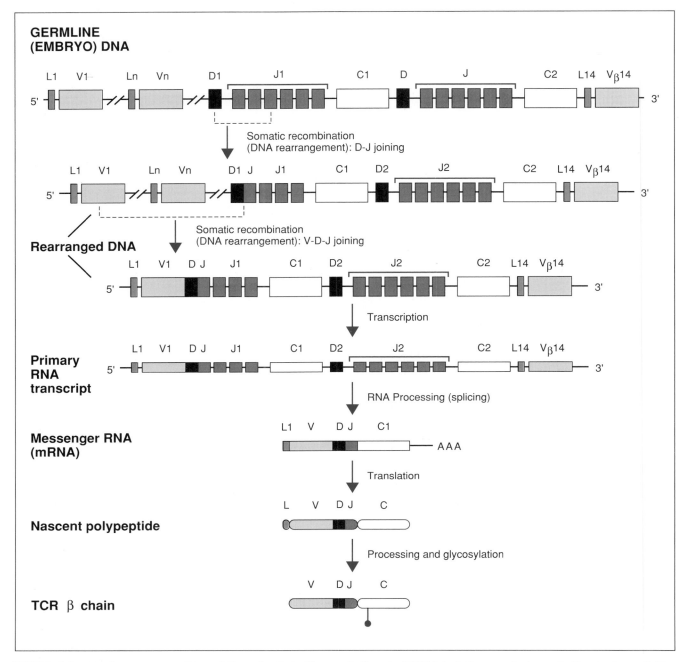

FIGURE 8 – 4. Sequence of gene rearrangement, transcription, and synthesis of the mouse T cell receptor (TCR) β chain. In the example shown, the V region is encoded by exons V1, D1, and the third exon in the J1 cluster; the C region is encoded by C1. Each C gene consists of multiple exons that are not shown. Unused V and J segments located between rearranged V and J genes are deleted. Note that in this example the DNA rearrangement involves DJ, followed by V joining to DJ, but direct VJ joining may also occur in the β chain locus.

recognize specific sequences of nucleotides in the genome adjacent to each rearranging segment (see Chapter 4). Since these recognition sequences are essentially the same in Ig and TCR gene segments, it is likely that the same recombination mechanism mediates both types of receptor gene rearrangements. In fact, germline TCR genes transfected into immature B cell lines are efficiently rearranged. The recognition sequences include a conserved heptamer and nonamer separated by either a 12-base pair (bp) or 23-bp

nonconserved spacer sequence. The location of heptamer, nonamer, and spacer sequences flanking the V, D, and J gene segments in the β chain locus are such that either VDJ joining or (unlike Ig) direct VJ joining can occur. As a result, T cell receptor β transcripts do not always contain D sequences. The mechanisms that have been proposed for Ig DNA rearrangements, including excision and inversions, may all be operational in T cell receptor DNA rearrangements.

The β chain locus rearranges prior to the α locus,

and the process begins with the joining of one D_β segment with one J_β segment. This is followed by a second rearrangement in which the newly formed DJ segment is joined to a V_β segment, resulting in a VDJ gene. The genomic sequences between the rearranging elements, including D, J, and possibly $C_\beta 1$ genes (if $C_\beta 2$ is used), are deleted during this rearrangement process.

The primary nuclear transcripts of the TCR β genes contain noncoding sequences (introns) between the recombined VDJ and C genes. These are spliced out to form a mature messenger RNA (mRNA) in which the VDJ complex is juxtaposed to either one of the two C_β genes. The two C_β genes may be thought of as structurally analogous to the Ig heavy chain isotype genes; however, unlike Ig heavy chain genes, the use of $C_\beta 1$ versus $C_\beta 2$ appears to be random and there is no evidence that an individual T cell ever switches from one C_β gene to another. Furthermore, there is no known association of the use of either C_β gene segment with a particular function or specificity of the TCR. It is clear that β chain transcription is activated by rearrangement of the β chain gene segments, and this may be due to the presence of an enhancer element in the region of the β chain constant genes, analogous to the location of Ig gene enhancers in heavy and light chain Ig genes. A putative β chain enhancer has been identified 3' of the $C_\beta 2$ gene in the mouse. DNA sequences that serve as β chain promoters have not yet been clearly defined, and β chain gene-specific nuclear-binding proteins have not been well characterized.

Functional rearrangement, and probably expression, at the β chain locus stimulates the rearrangement of the α chain locus. The rearrangement of the α chain gene segments is basically similar to the β chain gene rearrangements. Since there are no D segments in the α locus, rearrangement consists solely of the joining of V and J segments. Once VJ joining has occurred, transcription of the α chain gene ensues. A promoter has been identified 5' of a V_α transcriptional initiation site in the mouse, and an enhancer has been identified 3' to the C_α gene, which stimulates expression from the V_α promoter in T cells. This enhancer is unusual in its ability to act over large distances. For example, the distance between the α chain promoter and this enhancer can be up to 70 kb in rearranged TCR α genes. In addition, near the α chain enhancer, there are "silencer sequences" that can inhibit α chain transcription in non-T cells as well as in cells of the $\gamma\delta$ lineage. There is only one C_α gene, so that once the primary transcript is formed, RNA processing gives rise to only one possible complete α chain mRNA.

Only one of the two inherited α chain loci and one of the two inherited β chain loci are functionally rearranged and expressed in any one T cell. This is the phenomenon of **allelic exclusion,** and, as in Ig genes, it occurs because the productive rearrangement of a TCR locus on one chromosome inhibits the rearrangement of the corresponding allelic locus on the other chromosome. Allelic exclusion of TCR genes has been demonstrated by transfection and transgene experiments, in which the introduction of an exogenous, functionally rearranged TCR α or β chain gene into immature T cells inhibits the rearrangement and expression of the endogenous genes. In normal development, nonproductive rearrangements of one or both alleles of the α and β chain locus are quite common. When the β chain gene locus on one chromosome is nonfunctionally rearranged, such that it cannot be transcribed or its transcript cannot be translated, rearrangement of the other β chain locus proceeds. Successful rearrangement of the second locus does not shut off transcription of non-functional products at the first locus to have attempted rearrangement. Therefore, mature T cells often contain truncated, nonfunctional β chain transcripts as well as a functional, full-length mRNA. If both alleles of the β chain locus are nonproductively rearranged, the developing T cell will die. The rearrangement and expression of α chain loci proceed in a similar manner in those cells that have produced functional β chains.

Estimates of the potential size of the unselected immature T cell repertoire range from 10^{10} to 10^{15} specificities. As discussed in Chapter 7, homologies of the TCR to Ig molecules suggest that the peptide-MHC binding site of a TCR $\alpha\beta$ heterodimer is formed by the V, D, and J regions of both chains. The structural diversity of the TCR heterodimers is generated by molecular mechanisms that are essentially similar to the mechanisms that generate antibody diversity (Table 8–1). These include the following:

1. *Multiple germline V, D, and J segments* can be used to create TCRs of different specificities. Although there are fewer V genes in TCR α and β loci than in Ig, the much greater number of J gene segments more than compensates for this. For instance, in mice there are at least 12 J_β and up to 50 J_α segments compared with only 4 in the IgH and κ chain loci.

2. During TCR gene rearrangements, *combinatorial associations of different V, D, and J gene segments generate TCR diversity.*

3. *Junctional diversity,* involving coding sequences at VJ, VD, and DJ junctions, contributes significantly more to TCR diversity than to Ig diversity. Several different mechanisms are involved in TCR junctional diversity. First, the random addition of nucleotides that are not part of the genomic sequence, at VD, DJ, and VJ junctions, called **N-region diversification,** occurs in both α and β genes but only in Ig heavy chain and not light chain genes. N-region diversification may be catalyzed by the enzyme terminal deoxyribonucleotidyl transferase (TdT). Second, the joining of TCR gene segments can be imprecise and still result in functionally rearranged genes, a phenomenon called "flexibility." For example, more than one 3' position of V_α genes can join to J_α segments, and more than one 5' position of J_β segments can join with D_β segments. Third, many D_β segments can be translated in all three possible reading frames, an uncommon

TABLE 8-1. Contribution of Different Mechanisms to Generation of Diversity of T Cell Receptor (TCR) and Immunoglobulin (Ig) Genes

Mechanism	Immunoglobulin		TCR $\alpha\beta$		TCR $\gamma\delta$	
	Heavy Chain	κ	α	β	γ	δ
Variable segments	250-1000	250	75	25	7	10
Diversity (D) segments	12	0	0	2	0	2
D segments read in all three reading frames	Rare	—	—	Often	—	Often
N region diversification	V-D, D-J	None	V-J	V-D, D-J	V-J	V-D$_1$, D$_1$-D$_2$, D$_1$-J
Joining segments	4	4	50	12	2	2
Variable segment combinations	62,500-250,000		1875		70	
Total potential repertoire with junctional diversity	~10^{11}		~10^{16}		~10^{18}	

The mechanisms are described in the text. TCR loci have fewer V gene segments than Ig loci, but there is potentially much greater junctional diversity in TCR genes. The contribution of somatic mutation, which occurs in the Ig but not the TCR genes, is not included in the table, since these mutations tend to increase affinities of Ig molecules for antigen but may or may not change specificity.

Adapted from Davis, M. M., and P. J. Bjorkman. T-cell receptor antigen genes and T-cell recognition. Nature 334:395-402, 1988. Copyright © 1988, Macmillan Magazines Ltd.

feature for Ig heavy chain genes. Because of this, imprecise VD joining more often results in functional rearrangements.

4. The *pairing of α and β chains* serves to multiply the diversity generated for each chain. For example, there are up to 75 V$_\alpha$ and 25 V$_\beta$ genes in the human genome, contributing up to 10,000 potential V$_\alpha$V$_\beta$ region combinations.

In summary, TCR genes fundamentally resemble Ig genes in their mechanisms of diversity generation and expression, but they also differ from Ig genes in several respects. Although there are far fewer TCR V genes than Ig V genes, the potential diversity of TCR molecules has been estimated to be greater than that for Ig, largely because of the greater junctional diversity in TCR genes (Table 8-1). Once a TCR gene is functionally rearranged, however, there are no further genetic alterations leading to changes in function or affinity of the protein receptor. Thus, unlike Ig genes, there is no isotype switching in TCR. Furthermore, *there is no evidence of somatic mutation of TCR genes;* consequently, affinity maturation of the TCR is not observed in secondary T cell immune responses as is observed in secondary antibody responses.

T Cell Receptor γ and δ Genes

The γ chain locus is located on the short arm of chromosome 7 in humans and on chromosome 13 in mice, distinct from either TCR α or β loci. The human γ locus is organized similarly to the TCR β chain locus (Figs. 8-2 and 8-3) with two JC clusters containing five J segments and two C segments in total, located 3′ of multiple V$_\gamma$ gene segments (up to 14 in total, including six nonfunctional "pseudogenes"). In mice, the arrangement is more complex, with up to seven V$_\gamma$ gene segments interspersed with four JC clusters. (One of the murine V$_\gamma$ gene segments and one of the

JC$_\gamma$ clusters are nonfunctional.) No D$_\gamma$ segments have been identified. One striking difference in the γ chain locus compared with the TCR α and β chain loci is the variation among the multiple C$_\gamma$ gene segments, including differences in sequence, length, and number of the exons encoding the hinge region (connecting peptide) of the protein. This variation results in different molecular weights and different N-linked glycosylation patterns of the expressed γ chain proteins on different cells as well as the presence of both disulfide and non-covalent linkages of the γ chain with the δ chain.

The δ chain locus is unusual in that it is located entirely within the α chain locus between the V$_\alpha$ gene segments and the JC$_\alpha$ clusters (see Figs. 8-2 and 8-3). In humans, the δ locus consists of up to four V gene segments and one C gene segment associated with three J and two D segments. The arrangement in mice is fundamentally similar, but up to eight murine V$_\delta$ families (and more than ten individual V$_\delta$ gene segments) have been identified.

Rearrangements of γ and δ genes occur by the same mechanism as Ig and TCR α and β genes, utilizing the same recombinases and recognition signals as the other antigen receptor loci. Since the δ locus lies between the V$_\alpha$ and C$_\alpha$ genes, functional rearrangements of the α locus will delete the δ locus. It is apparent, however, that several murine V$_\delta$ genes are identical or very similar to V$_\alpha$ genes, and thus some of these V gene segments can be joined to either J$_\alpha$ or J$_\delta$ segments to produce either functionally rearranged α or δ genes. On the other hand, four of the murine V$_\delta$ subfamilies are significantly different from V$_\alpha$ gene segments and are used preferentially in δ chains. The molecular basis for the exclusive use of these V$_\delta$ genes in δ and not α chains is not understood. It appears that in the mouse there is a strong preference for the use of V$_\gamma$ and V$_\delta$ segments most proximal to C genes early in fetal life and for more distal V segments later. This is reflected in a highly limited usage of only certain V$_\delta$

and V_γ genes in adult $\gamma\delta$ receptor–expressing T cell populations.

The small number of γ and δ V gene segments suggests a limited amount of combinatorial diversity among $\gamma\delta$ receptors. The limitations are even greater because of the selective use of certain V_γ segments during different stages of life. There is, however, an enormous potential diversity of $\gamma\delta$ receptors as a result of variations in junctional sequences, especially in the δ chain. This potential junctional diversity is largely due to the unique feature that either one or both D_δ segments in tandem can be used within a single rearranged δ gene. Because imprecise joining of V, D, and J segments and N-region diversification also occur in rearranging δ and γ genes, there are theoretically more possible $\gamma\delta$ molecules than $\alpha\beta$ or Ig molecules (Table 8–1).

ONTOGENY OF T CELL RECEPTOR AND ACCESSORY MOLECULE EXPRESSION

The rearrangement and expression of TCR genes during intrathymic maturation are the necessary first steps in the development of the T cell repertoire. TCR gene expression occurs coordinately with the expression of other proteins, including CD3, CD4, and CD8, which are important for the selection of MHC–restricted helper T cells and CTLs. Our current understanding of T lymphocyte maturation is based largely on the analysis of the expression of TCR, CD4, and CD8 molecules on thymocytes. As part of this analysis, immunologists have defined subpopulations of thymocytes that differ in their cell surface phenotypes. The anatomic locations, sizes, and functional properties of these subpopulations—and changes induced in them by experimental manipulations—provide important insights into the mechanisms of thymic selection. We next discuss the ontogeny of T cell surface molecule expression and the characteristics of the best-defined thymocyte subsets.

Ontogeny of T Cell Receptor Expression

Most studies of T cell ontogeny have relied on fetal murine thymuses, in which distinct populations of developing T cells can be identified on the basis of surface molecule expression at various times of gestation. The events that occur in these fetal organs are similar to what has been found in adult murine, fetal human, and adult human thymuses. As described above, T cell precursors are first detected in the fetal thymus on the 11th day of gestation in mice and these cells do not express TCR:CD3 complexes. Organ culture of embryonic thymuses, in which there is no ongoing influx of bone marrow precursors, has demon-

TABLE 8–2. Some Surface Molecules Used for Defining Thymocyte Subsets

Surface Molecule	Comments
CD1	Expressed before TCR:CD3, class I–like molecule, paired with CD8 polypeptide on immature thymocytes
CD2	Expressed before TCR:CD3, binds LFA-3 on thymic epithelium, may deliver activating signal
CD5	Expressed before TCR:CD3
Thy-1	Expressed before TCR:CD3 on murine, may deliver activating signal
Peanut agglutinin (PNA) receptor	Lectin, present on CD4+CD8+ (double-positive) cells, but not single-positive cells
CD44 (Pgp-1)	Present on earliest bone marrow immigrants (as well as memory T cells), may serve as homing/adhesion molecule

strated that these CD3⁻ cells are the precursors to all more mature forms. Surface molecules that are expressed on this immature population of thymocytes prior to or shortly after their entry into the thymus include CD44 (Pgp-1), Thy-1 (in mice), and the class I MHC–like molecule CD1 (Table 8–2). The functions of these molecules are not known; CD44 may play a role in the migration of T cell precursors to the thymus.

In mouse thymocytes, TCR genes are in the germline configuration until day 13 or 14 of fetal life (corresponding to about 8 to 9 weeks' gestation in humans). The first TCR gene rearrangements are detected at this time and involve the γ and δ genes (Figs. 8–5 and 8–6). Full-length mRNA transcripts of the γ and δ genes are detectable by day 14, and surface expression of a CD3–associated $\gamma\delta$ heterodimeric protein occurs by day 14 or 15. The genes encoding the CD3 polypeptides are first transcribed concomitantly with the $\gamma\delta$ genes and are expressed on the surface of thymocytes in association with $\gamma\delta$ heterodimers. *Thus, the $\gamma\delta$ receptor is the first TCR to be expressed during T cell development.*

Although nonfunctional DJ rearrangements at the β chain locus begin simultaneously with γ and δ chain rearrangements on day 13 or 14, functional β chain VDJ rearrangements and full-length 1.3 kb transcripts are first detectable on day 16. The α chain genes are the last to rearrange and to generate functional mRNA, on day 17 of fetal life. Surface expression of CD3–associated $\alpha\beta$ heterodimers is first detected on day 17, about 2 days after $\gamma\delta$ expression. Expression of $\alpha\beta$ receptors rapidly overtakes expression of $\gamma\delta$ receptors, so that by birth most TCR:CD3–expressing thymocytes have $\alpha\beta$ receptors. This is consistent with the fact that more than 90 per cent of mature peripheral T cells express only the $\alpha\beta$ form of antigen receptors.

There is strong evidence that $\gamma\delta$ and $\alpha\beta$ expressing thymocytes are separate lineages with a common precursor. Southern blot analysis of mature $\alpha\beta$-express-

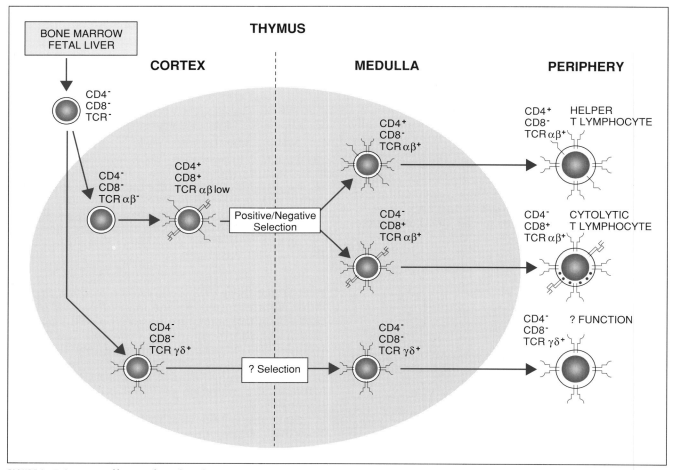

FIGURE 8 – 5. Ontogeny and lineage relationships of maturing T cells. *TCRγδ – and TCRαβ – expressing cells are separate lineages that develop from a common precursor. In the αβ lineage, the majority of thymocytes express both CD4 and CD8. TCR expression commences in this double-positive stage, beginning with low numbers of receptors on each cell and increasing as maturation proceeds. Single-positive, i.e., CD4⁺ or CD8⁺ TCRαβ – expressing mature cells are selected from this population. Some γδ cells express CD4 or CD8.*

ing T cells often show out-of-frame rearrangements of γ genes that are incapable of being transcribed, indicating that these cells could never have expressed γδ receptors. The δ chain gene segments are located between the V_α and J_α gene segments (see Figs. 8 – 3 and 8 – 4), and they are deleted in a circle of DNA when the α chain gene rearranges. Analysis of these deleted DNA circles from murine thymuses shows that the δ chain gene is in the germline configuration in cells which have rearranged their α chain genes. This finding also indicates that αβ-expressing T cells have never expressed γδ receptors and that the two types of antigen receptors are produced by two distinct lineages of T cells. A hypothetical scheme of these lineage relationships is shown in Figure 8 – 5.

This temporal pattern of early γδ gene expression followed by αβ expression is seen in chickens, mice, and humans. In human fetal thymuses, γδ receptor expression begins at about 9 weeks of gestation, followed by TCR αβ expression at 10 weeks. This evolutionary conservation of the sequence of receptor expression suggests that the presence of thymocytes expressing γδ receptors prior to αβ-expressing cells

may play an important role in the normal development of T cells. We can only speculate on that role, since the functions of mature γδ-bearing T cells and the nature of the ligand that the γδ receptor binds are as yet largely known.

The TCR gene rearrangements described above take place in a rapidly dividing population of cells. A single primitive T cell precursor that enters the thymus can generate multiple cells, each with a unique TCR conferring a distinct antigen-binding specificity. This has been demonstrated by an experiment in which a single precursor cell with unrearranged TCR genes was introduced into a thymus previously depleted of thymocytes. The progeny of this cell showed multiple, different β chain rearrangements after 12 days. As discussed in the previous section, N-region diversification significantly contributes to the diversity of TCR and is most likely catalyzed by the enzyme TdT. It is interesting to note that in murine fetal thymuses TdT is not expressed until after the earliest rearranged δ chain genes have already been transcribed; as a result, the first δ chains expressed show far less diversity than later ones. TdT activity was

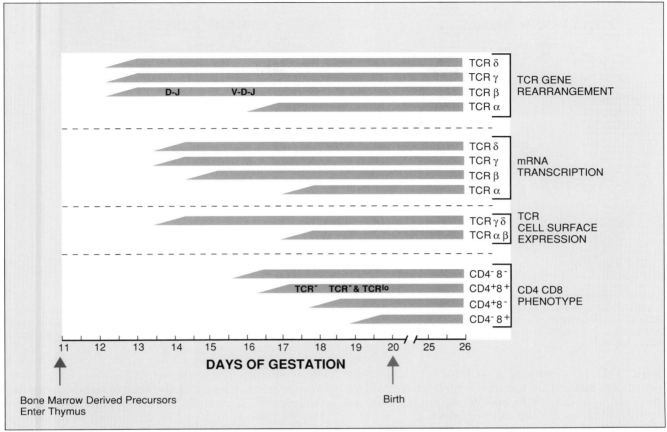

FIGURE 8 – 6. *Chronology of expression of TCR, CD4, CD8, and effector functions in the fetal mouse thymus. Note that TCRαβ heterodimers and TCRγδ heterodimers are expressed on different cells. (Modified with permission from Fowlkes, B. J., and D. M. Pardoll. Molecular events in T cell development. Advances in Immunology 44:207–264, 1989. Courtesy of Academic Press, Orlando.)*

used as a marker of lymphocyte lineage in phenotypically immature cells, such as certain leukemias, long before the significance of this enzyme in the generation of receptor diversity was understood.

Ontogeny of CD4 and CD8 Expression and Thymocyte Subsets

CD4 and CD8 molecules are commonly used as markers to categorize subsets of thymocytes and to define the sequence of thymocyte maturation. Furthermore, recent experiments indicate that the expression of these molecules may be important in the selection processes that shape the T cell repertoire. Thymocytes can be divided into four groups on the basis of CD4 and CD8 expression (Fig. 8–7). These groups include (1) CD4−CD8− "double-negative" cells; (2) CD4+CD8+ "double-positive" cells; and (3) CD4+CD8− or CD4−CD8+ "single-positive" cells.

In addition, several other surface molecules are used to further subdivide populations of thymocytes (Table 8–2). The significance of these smaller subsets

is not completely known and they will not be discussed further.

The most immature cells in the thymic cortex, which are also the precursors of all T cells, do not express CD4 or CD8 (see Fig. 8–5). These double-negative cells are a heterogeneous group making up about 5 per cent of the total thymocytes in an adult (Fig. 8–7). Most (80 per cent) of these cells are rapidly dividing cortical thymocytes that are actively rearranging TCR genes but are not yet expressing TCR:CD3 complexes. The remaining double-negative cells are more mature and consist mainly of γδ-positive thymocytes (most of which will never express CD4 or CD8). Little is known about the stimuli that drive the proliferation and maturation of immature double-negative thymocytes. Many of these cells have been shown to express transcripts for IL–2 and IL–4. In addition, double-negative cells express receptors for IL–2 and proliferate *in vitro* in response to IL–7, a cytokine first identified as a B cell–specific lymphopoietic factor. Therefore, cytokines produced by the T cells themselves or by non-lymphoid cells in the thymus may function as growth and differentiation factors for these immature thymocytes. The CD2 molecule is also present on most CD4−CD8− human thymo-

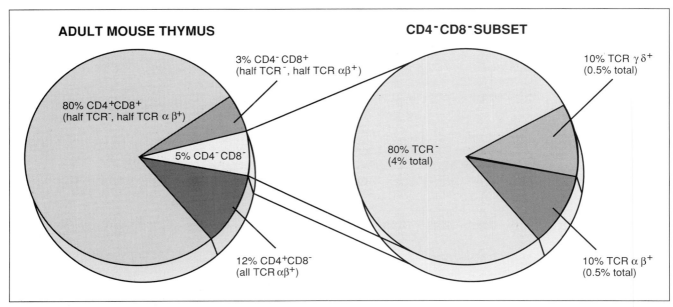

FIGURE 8 – 7. Subpopulations of thymocytes in the adult mouse thymus. *T cell maturation continues throughout life, so that even in adults the thymus contains different populations of thymocytes, which represent different stages in T cell development identified in the fetal thymus. (Modified with permission from Fowlkes, B. J., and D. M. Pardoll. Molecular events in T cell development. Advances in Immunology 44:207–264, 1989. Courtesy of Academic Press, Orlando.)*

cytes. This may provide a TCR:CD3 – independent growth and maturation stimulus, which is triggered by the binding of CD2 to its specific ligand, LFA – 3, on thymic epithelial cells or macrophages.

Double-negative thymocytes mature along different pathways. The majority of the double-negative cells begin to express both CD4 and CD8 and will later give rise to CD4+ or CD8+, TCR αβ-expressing, MHC – restricted mature T cells (see Fig. 8 – 5). Double-positive cells are detected by day 16 or 17 of gestation in the fetal mouse thymus and make up about 80 per cent of the cells in the adult thymus (see Fig. 8 – 7). Some immature double-negative cells may transiently express only CD8 at day 15 or 16 of gestation in the mouse and then become CD4+CD8+. Small numbers of double-negative cells remain CD4−CD8− and this population includes cells with rearranged γδ TCR.

The rearrangement of αβ TCR genes occurs in the double-positive population as these cells migrate from the cortex to the medulla (see Fig. 8 – 5). By day 17 or 18 of gestation, the mouse thymus contains CD4+CD8+ cells, which also express TCR αβ:CD3 complexes. In the adult thymus, about half the double-positive cells are TCR αβ:CD3 – positive and half are TCR αβ:CD3 – negative (see Fig. 8 – 7). The great majority of double-positive cells die *in vivo*, because selection processes act at this stage of maturation. Furthermore, unproductive TCR gene rearrangements, leading to a failure to express TCR molecules, result in the death of cells because there is no mechanism for continued growth stimulation and maturation.

The CD4+CD8+ cells give rise to mature CD4+ and CD8+ (single-positive) peripheral T cells (Fig. 8 – 5). This has been established by a variety of experiments. For instance, if neonatal mice are injected with anti-CD4 antibody, the numbers of both CD4+ and CD8+

cells in the periphery are reduced. This is interpreted to indicate that the antibody bound to and induced the complement-dependent lysis of double-positive thymocytes and inhibited the maturation of all single-positive cells. CD4+CD8−TCR αβ-expressing thymocytes are first detected at day 18 of gestation in mice and make up about 12 per cent of adult thymocytes (see Fig. 8 – 7). These cells display functional helper activity in *in vitro* assays and migrate to the circulation and peripheral lymphoid tissues to constitute the mature, class II MHC – restricted helper T cell subset. CD4−CD8+TCR αβ-expressing cells appear by day 19 of gestation and make up about 3 per cent of thymocytes in the adult. They display cytolytic activity *in vitro* and migrate out of the thymus to become mature, class I MHC – restricted CTLs in the periphery. Single-positive thymocytes express higher levels of TCR αβ heterodimers per cell than αβ-expressing, double-positive cells. We do not know the stimuli that induce a particular CD4+CD8+ cell to selectively express either CD4 or CD8 and to simultaneously acquire the functional capabilities of a helper or cytolytic cell, respectively.

This sequence of T cell maturation—from CD4−CD8−TCR− to CD4+CD8+TCR−, to CD4+CD8+-TCR+, and finally to CD4+CD8−TCR+ or CD4−CD8+-TCR+ cells—has been most clearly established in mice. It is difficult to examine the maturation pathway of T cells during fetal life in humans because of many obvious limitations. The information that is available suggests that the same sequence of maturation events occurs in humans as in mice. It is clear that in both mouse and man, TCR αβ receptors are first expressed on double-positive cortical thymocytes. This is when the selection processes that determine the specificities of the mature T cell repertoire begin to occur.

Thymic Selection Processes Leading to T Cell MHC Restriction and Self-Tolerance

The next important event in intrathymic T cell maturation is the selection of cells that will make up the repertoire of mature T cells in the periphery. Selection processes act on thymocytes after they express TCR molecules and are responsible for the survival of T cells which express only "useful" TCRs, i.e., TCRs that recognize foreign antigens in association with self MHC molecules. Although the cellular and biochemical mechanisms of selection are not well understood, the current model of this process has the following general features.

1. Before selection can begin, TCRs must be expressed on the developing thymocytes. This is because thymocytes are selected to survive or to be eliminated on the basis of their specificities, determined by the binding of the TCRs to MHC molecules and antigens expressed in the thymus.

2. Because of the random nature of the molecular events in TCR gene expression, all possible antigen and MHC specificities are represented in the TCR-expressing, preselected, immature thymocyte population.

3. Positive selection of self MHC-restricted T cells and negative selection of self antigen specific T cells represent two sequential processes (see Fig. 8-1). It is likely that positive selection precedes negative selection.

4. **Positive selection** is the process in which thymocytes whose TCRs bind self MHC molecules are permitted to survive and all those that have no affinity for self MHC die. This step eliminates all non-self MHC-restricted T cells, which would be incapable of recognizing antigen in the periphery because the APCs obviously only express self MHC. Positive selection leaves both useful foreign antigen specific self MHC-restricted T cells and potentially harmful self antigen-specific, self MHC-restricted T cells.

5. During **negative selection,** clones of thymocytes whose TCRs bind with high affinity to self antigens in association with self MHC molecules are eliminated **(clonal deletion)** or inactivated **(clonal anergy).** After this step, the only thymocytes that are left are those whose TCRs bind foreign antigens in association with self MHC molecules, so that mature T cells are self MHC-restricted and self-tolerant.

Positive Selection Processes in the Thymus: Development of the Self MHC-Restricted T Cell Repertoire

Once a thymocyte expresses a T cell receptor, it cannot change its specificity. Therefore, *MHC restric-* *tion must develop at a population level during thymic T cell ontogeny,* not at the level of individual cells, and reflects selective survival and expansion of thymocytes with self MHC-restricted specificities characteristic of mature peripheral T cells. This positive selection may be a result of the activation of thymocytes after the binding of their TCRs with self MHC molecules. It is hypothesized that such stimulation may be necessary to rescue the thymocyte from biologically programmed death. Thus, thymocytes whose TCR have no affinity for self MHC molecules will die.

In theory, T cells could be self MHC-restricted either because during development they themselves express self MHC molecules or because they encounter these molecules on other cells during maturation. Bone marrow chimeras were used to first demonstrate that *the MHC genes of the host animal in which T cells develop determine the MHC restriction pattern of the mature T cells.* In these experiments, chimeras were created by transferring the bone marrow–derived hematopoietic stem cells from a mouse with one MHC haplotype into a lethally irradiated mouse of a partially different MHC haplotype (Table 8-3). By immunizing these mice and defining the MHC restrictions of the CTLs and helper T cells, it was found that the T cells that matured in these chimeras recognized antigen only in association with MHC molecules of the host strain.

Further analysis showed that *the thymus is the critical host element for the development of MHC-restriction patterns of T cells.* This was accomplished by creating bone marrow plus thymic chimeras. These host animals were prepared by removing the thymuses, lethally irradiating adult mice of one MHC haplotype, and transplanting into them different combinations of bone marrow and thymuses from mice with other MHC haplotypes (Table 8-4). The transplanted thymuses were also either irradiated or treated with cytotoxic drugs (such as deoxyguanosine) to kill all bone marrow–derived resident macrophages, dendritic cells, and lymphoid cells, leaving only the ra-

TABLE 8-3. Development of MHC Restriction in Bone Marrow Chimeric Mice

Marrow Donor Strain	Host	Specific Killing of Virus Infected Targets From	
		Strain A	*Strain B*
(A × B)F1	(A × B)F1	+	+
(A × B)F1	A	+	−

Bone marrow chimeras are created as described in Figure 2-2. Strain A and B mice have different class I MHC alleles. The MHC restriction specificity of mature T cells in these mice is tested by assaying the ability of CTLs generated in response to viral infection to kill virus-infected target cells from different mouse strains *in vitro*. These experiments demonstrate that the host MHC type, and not the bone marrow donor type, determines the restriction specificity of the mature T cells.

Abbreviation: MHC, major histocompatibility complex; CTL, cytolytic T lymphocyte.

TABLE 8-4. Development of MHC Restriction Patterns in Bone Marrow Plus Thymic Chimeras

Chimera			Stimulation of Mature T Cells		
Host	Bone Marrow Donor	Thymus Donor	Antigen	Strain of APC	Response
A	(A × B)F1	A	+	A	+
A	(A × B)F1	A	+	B	−
A	(A × B)F1	A	−	A	−
A	(A × B)F1	B	+	B	+
A	(A × B)F1	B	+	A	−
A	(A × B)F1	B	−	B	−

In the chimeric mice, the mature T cells that develop respond to foreign antigen in association with the MHC allele expressed on the thymic epithelial cells.

Abbreviations: APC, antigen-presenting cell; MHC, major histocompatibility complex.

dioresistant **thymic epithelial cells.** Again, mature T cells developed in these mice and their MHC restriction was examined after immunization and *in vitro* restimulation of T cells with antigen plus APCs. Antigen recognition by these T cells was always restricted by MHC gene products expressed on the transplanted thymic epithelial cells and not necessarily by MHC gene products expressed on extrathymic cells (Table 8-4).

Positive selection of self MHC-binding thymocytes has also been demonstrated by creating transgenic mice (see Box 4-2, Chapter 4) that express an αβ TCR of known specificity, derived from a single T cell clone (Table 8-5). Since virtually all developing T cells in these transgenic mice express this transgenic TCR and endogenous TCR gene rearrangements are blocked (by allelic exclusion), it is relatively simple to study the selection and maturation of the T cells in these mice. When the transgenic α and β TCR genes encode a TCR that recognizes a foreign peptide in association with a particular allelic MHC molecule, the transgenic T cells will mature and will populate peripheral lymphoid tissue only in mice expressing that MHC allele. If the mouse has another MHC haplotype and does not express the MHC molecule that the transgenic TCR recognizes, no transgenic TCR-expressing T cells mature. This result shows that de-

veloping T cells must express TCRs that can bind self MHC molecules in order to survive. As we shall see later, the same experimental system has been used to study negative selection.

The studies using chimeras demonstrate the central role of thymic epithelium in positive selection of T cells but do not indicate where, how, or when, during T cell maturation such selection occurs. As stated previously, positive selection must occur after the expression of TCR αβ proteins, in or after the CD4+CD8+ stage of T cell maturation. It is hypothesized that if the antigen receptor of a developing thymocyte binds MHC molecules on thymic epithelial cells, even with low affinity, that thymocyte survives and continues to mature. Thus, positive selection ensures survival of T cells restricted to the MHC encountered during development, which, of course, is self MHC in the normal situation. These same T cells, which were selected because of a low-affinity interaction with self MHC molecules in the thymus, may be capable of high-affinity interactions with complexes of foreign peptides and self MHC molecules in the periphery. According to such a postulate, foreign antigens need not be present in the thymus in order for positive selection to occur.

In Chapter 6 we discussed the phenomenon of MHC-linked immune responsiveness (Ir genes), and

TABLE 8-5. The Use of T Cell Receptor (TCR) Transgenic Mice to Study Thymic Selection Processes

Transgenic Mouse			Selection		Presence of Mature Peripheral T Cells Expressing Transgenic TCR
Specificity of Transgenic TCR	MHC D Allele	Sex/H-Y Antigen Expression	Positive	Negative	
H-Y antigen/MHC D^b	D^b	Male/H-Y-positive	Yes	Yes	No
H-Y antigen/MHC D^b	D^b	Female/H-Y-negative	Yes	No	Yes (CD8+, H-Y-specific)
H-Y antigen/MHC D^b	D^k	Female/H-Y-negative	No	No	No

The transgenic mice express a TCR specific for a D^b-associated H-Y (male-specific) antigen, which is, in effect, a foreign antigen for a female mouse. T cells expressing the transgene mature in female mice expressing the D^b allele, but not in H-Y+ male mice (because of negative selection as a result of self-antigen recognition), nor in female mice not expressing D^b (because of lack of positive selection of the D^b-restricted TCR-expressing cells).

Abbreviations: MHC, major histocompatibility complex.

how MHC genes can function as immune response genes because MHC molecules can bind some epitopes of protein antigens and not others. Another way by which MHC molecules can control immune responsiveness is by determining which T cells are positively selected in the thymus. Thus, in some individuals the T cells that are selected by self MHC molecules may not contain cells capable of recognizing particular foreign antigens. Individuals expressing such MHC alleles will show an MHC–linked unresponsiveness to these antigens because they will lack mature T cells with specific receptors.

Another important feature of positive selection is that CD4+ cells become exclusively class II MHC–restricted and CD8+ cells become class I MHC–restricted. It has been proposed that these restrictions arise as a consequence of the ability of CD4 and CD8 to bind to class II and class I molecules, respectively, and thereby promote effective interactions of thymocytes with epithelial cells expressing these MHC molecules. Thus, if a developing T cell expresses a TCR with low affinity for class II MHC molecules, it may continue to be positively selected beyond the CD4+CD8+ stage only if it also continues to express CD4. The converse would, of course, be true for CD8. In fact, in transgenic mice expressing a class I MHC–restricted transgenic TCR, most of the T cells that develop express the transgene and are CD8+ (Table 8–5). This is presumably because both the TCR and CD8 are required for binding to class I MHC molecules on thymic epithelium and, therefore, for positive selection to proceed. Similarly, experimentally created lines of mice that lack class I MHC expression fail to develop CD8+ mature T cells.

Negative Selection Processes in the Thymus: Development of Self-Tolerance

The importance of self-tolerance to the health of all individuals has been mentioned previously, and the development of autoimmunity as a result of the breakdown of self-tolerance will be described in Chapter 18. Individuals may be tolerant to self antigens because they lack B and/or T lymphocytes specific for these antigens or because such lymphocytes are present but cannot respond to self antigens. *It is now clear that tolerance to self proteins is largely due to T cell tolerance, and a principal mechanism for inducing T cell tolerance is the deletion or inactivation of self-reactive clones of T cells during their maturation in the thymus.* This process, which we have referred to as negative selection, is discussed here because it is closely related to positive selection of T cells. Other mechanisms of tolerance induction are described in Chapter 10.

The possibility that self-reactive clones of T cells are deleted in the thymus was suggested many years ago, when the role of the thymus in the development of mature T cells was first appreciated. Formal proof for clonal deletion of T cells in the thymus has come from two recently developed experimental approaches, both of which allow investigators to observe the effects of self antigen recognition by a large number of developing T cells in the thymus. One approach is based on the observation that TCRs utilizing certain V_β genes specifically bind particular MHC–antigen complexes, irrespective of which D_β and J_β gene segments are used or which α chains are present. (Antigens that bind to all TCRs utilizing a particular V_β gene segment, regardless of the other components of the heterodimeric antigen receptor, have been called "superantigens" and are discussed in Chapter 15.) For example, in mice the use of the $V_\beta17a$ gene imparts a TCR with specificity for an uncharacterized "self" antigen associated exclusively with I-E class II MHC molecules. In strains of mice that express I-E class II MHC molecules, there are virtually no $V_\beta17a$-expressing T cells in the peripheral lymphoid organs or in the thymic medulla but there are $V_\beta17a$-expressing thymocytes in the cortex. In contrast, strains of mice that do not express I-E molecules, because of a defect in the class II I-E$_\alpha$ gene, have readily detectable $V_\beta17a$-expressing T cells in the thymic medulla and periphery (Table 8–6). This suggests that as T cells mature in the thymus of an I-E+

TABLE 8–6. Clonal Deletion of $V_\beta17a$–Positive T Cells in I-E Expressing Mice

Mouse Strain	I-E Expression	Peripheral T Cells Expressing TCRs Utilizing $V_\beta17a$ (Per Cent)
A. SWR	None	14.2
SJL	None	9.4
SJA	None	8.5
B. C57BR	Yes	0.1
BALB/c	Yes	0
AKR	Yes	0
B10.TL	Yes	0

Mature T cells with $V_\beta17a$-containing TCRs are present in I-E– (A) but not in I-E+(B) inbred mouse strains, because these TCRs recognize an I-E-associated self antigen and are deleted in I-E+ mice.

Adapted from Kappler, J., N. Roehm, and P. Marrack. T cell tolerance by clonal elimination in the thymus. Cell 49:273, 1987. Copyright by Cell Press.
Abbreviations: TCR, T cell receptor; MHC, major histocompatibility complex.

mouse, all $V_\beta 17a$-expressing thymocytes encounter a self antigen complexed with I-E molecules and are deleted. If they do not encounter this self antigen-I-E complex, as would be the case in the I-E–deficient mice, they may mature normally. It is not clear how $V_\beta 17a$-expressing thymocytes are positively selected in I-E⁻ mice, but it is possible that they may also bind less strongly to other self MHC molecules such as I-A molecules.

A second approach that also suggests that T cell tolerance results from intrathymic deletion of self-reactive clones employs TCR transgenic mice mentioned earlier in the discussion of positive selection. In one such study, transgenic mice were made that expressed a class I MHC–restricted transgenic TCR specific for the sex associated H-Y molecule. H-Y is a self antigen abundantly expressed on many cell types in male mice but not in female mice (see Table 8–5). Female mice with this transgenic TCR had normal numbers of CD8⁺ T cells expressing the transgene in the periphery and normal numbers of thymocytes in the thymic medulla. In contrast, male transgenic mice had very few mature peripheral T cells and very few TCR–expressing, single-positive thymocytes in the medulla. There was an apparent block of T cell maturation after the cortical double-positive stage, presumably because all the maturing T cells expressed a transgenic TCR that recognized the self H-Y antigen on thymic cells and thus were deleted before they could mature into single-positive cells.

The clonal deletion of self-reactive T cells presumably occurs when the TCR on a CD4⁺CD8⁺ thymocyte binds to a self antigen presented by another thymic cell. There is strong evidence that bone marrow–derived cells within the thymus, such as dendritic cells and macrophages, can present self antigens to and cause the deletion of self antigen–reactive T cell clones. As with positive selection, the CD4 and CD8 molecules likely play a role in negative selection because they promote effective interactions between the developing thymocyte and the "tolerizing" thymic antigen-presenting cell (APC). For example, in vivo administration of anti-CD4 antibody to I-E expressing mice blocks the elimination of $V_\beta 17a$-expressing CD4⁺CD8⁻ thymocytes. Thus, the interaction of both CD4 and $V_\beta 17a^+$ TCR with the I-E class II MHC molecule is necessary for deletion of the $V_\beta 17a$-expressing T cell.

Recent experiments suggest that some self antigens may not induce deletion of specific T cell clones. Instead, the self-reactive T cells may be rendered permanently unresponsive, or anergic, by encounter with self antigens on non-lymphoid thymic cells. The net result of clonal deletion and clonal anergy is the same, because both make the individual incapable of responding to self antigens.

This model of T cell tolerance induced by deletion or anergy of self-reactive clones raises at least two unanswered questions. First, the mechanism by which self-reactive thymocytes are deleted or inactivated upon binding self antigens is entirely unknown. It may be that of the positively selected self MHC–

recognizing thymocytes, those that recognize complexes of self antigens and self MHC in the thymus with high affinity are deleted. Such a postulate suggests that the affinity with which the TCR of a developing thymocyte binds to its ligand may be a critical determinant of the fate of the cell expressing that TCR. Recent experiments have shown that immature CD3⁺ T cells exposed to anti-CD3 antibody, an analog of antigen, undergo DNA fragmentation followed by nuclear fragmentation **(apoptosis)** and cell death. Thus, it may be that high-affinity engagement of the TCR:CD3 complex in immature T cells generates biochemical alterations that lead to cell death, whereas the same external stimulus in mature T cells initiates the program of activation.

The second obvious problem in this postulated model of negative selection is that in order to delete or inactivate self-reactive T cells, self antigens must be present in the thymus and they must be processed and associated with MHC molecules. It is not known how (or indeed whether) the large numbers of self antigens to which an individual is normally tolerant gain access to developing T cells in the thymus. Experiments with hemoglobin allele-specific T cells (described in Chapter 6) indicate that thymic epithelial cells, dendritic cells, and macrophages do process and present self hemoglobin in vivo, and the same may be true of many other self antigens. On the other hand, some T cells reactive with self antigens not present in the thymus may mature and exit the thymus but may be rendered anergic by exposure to self antigens in the periphery (see Chapter 10).

From the discussion above, it is clear that the MHC plays a critical role in the development of the T cell repertoire, since thymocyte recognition of self MHC molecules is part of both positive and negative selection processes. Furthermore, as we have emphasized in Chapters 6 and 7, MHC molecules are critical to immune responses of mature peripheral T cells to foreign protein antigens. An understanding of these roles of the MHC in T cell antigen recognition has many potentially important medical implications. For example, the development of autoimmune diseases is often associated with a particular pattern of MHC gene inheritance (see Chapter 18). This may reflect the fact that T cells with specificities for some self antigens in association with certain MHC molecules are not clonally deleted during T cell maturation.

Summary

Stem cells committed to developing into T cells first arise in the bone marrow and migrate to the thymus during both fetal and adult life. The earliest T lineage immigrants to the thymus have unrearranged TCR genes and do not express CD4 or CD8 molecules. The developing T cells within the thymus, called thymocytes, initially populate the outer cortex, where they undergo population growth, rearrangement of TCR genes, and surface expression of CD3, TCR, CD4, and CD8 molecules. The TCR α and β polypeptides are encoded by functional genes that are created only in T cells by the somatic rearrangement of variable, diversity (β only) and joining gene segments, bringing them in the vicinity of C gene segments. Multiple combinatorial possibilities for the joining of the different gene segments, as well as several mechanisms that generate junctional diversity, result in the generation of a large repertoire of T cell specificities. Unlike Ig genes, there is no somatic mutation or affinity maturation in TCR genes. The functional genes encoding the TCR γ and δ polypeptides are also formed by somatic rearrangement of germline genes. The mechanisms of generation of TCR $\gamma\delta$ diversity are similar to those described for the $\alpha\beta$ receptor, except that there are fewer V genes in the γ and δ loci and significantly more potential junctional diversity. TCR $\gamma\delta$ receptors are the first receptors to be expressed on a small subset of cortical thymocytes, followed by the more abundant expression of TCR $\alpha\beta$ receptors on a distinct lineage of developing T cells. The TCR $\alpha\beta^+$,CD4$^+$CD8$^+$ cortical thymocytes interact with MHC–expressing cortical epithelial cells and bone marrow–derived, nonlymphoid cells and undergo selection processes that shape the T cell repertoire toward self MHC restriction and self-tolerance. T cell tolerance is at least in part due to clonal deletion of self-reactive T cells during the TCR $\alpha\beta^+$,CD4$^+$CD8$^+$ stage of development. Most of the cortical thymocytes do not survive these selection processes. As the surviving TCR $\alpha\beta^+$ thymocytes mature, they move into the medulla and become either CD4$^+$CD8$^-$ or CD4$^-$CD8$^+$. Medullary thymocytes acquire helper or cytolytic functional capabilities and finally emigrate to peripheral lymphoid tissues, where they reside as self MHC–restricted, foreign antigen–responsive helper T cells and CTLs.

SELECTED READINGS

Adkins, B., C. Mueller, C. Y. Okada, R. Reichert, I. L. Weissman, and G. J. Spangrude. Early events in T-cell maturation. Annual Review of Immunology 5:325–365, 1987.

Blackman, M., J. Kappler, and P. Marrack. The role of the T cell receptor in positive and negative selection of developing T cells. Science 248:1335–1341, 1990.

Davis, M. M., and P. J. Bjorkman. T-cell antigen receptor genes and T-cell recognition. Nature 334:395–402, 1988.

Fink, P. J., and M. J. Bevan. H-2 antigens of the thymus determine lymphocyte specificity. Journal of Experimental Medicine 148:766–775, 1978.

Fowlkes, B. J., and D. M. Pardoll. Molecular and cellular events of T cell development. Advances in Immunology 44:207–264, 1989.

Kappler, J. W., N. Roehm, and P. Marrack. T cell tolerance by clonal elimination in the thymus. Cell 49:273–280, 1987.

Ransdell, F., and B. J. Fowlkes. Clonal deletion versus clonal anergy: The role of the thymus in inducing self tolerance. Science 248:1342–1348, 1990.

Sprent, J., E.-K. Gao, and S. R. Webb. T cell reactivity to MHC molecules: Immunity versus tolerance. Science 248:1357–1363, 1990.

Strominger, J. L. Developmental biology of T cell receptors. Science 244:943–950, 1989.

von Boehmer, H. Developmental biology of T cells in T cell-receptor transgenic mice. Annual Review of Immunology 8:531–556, 1990.

von Boehmer, H., and P. Kisielow. Self-nonself discrimination by T cells. Science 248:1369–1373, 1990.

Zinkernagel, R. M., A. Althage, E. Waterfield, B. Kindred, R. M. Welsh, G. Callahan, and P. Pincetl. Restriction specificites, alloreactivity, and allotolerance expressed by T cells from nude mice reconstituted with H-2–compatible or –incompatible thymus grafts. Journal of Experimental Medicine 151:376–399, 1980.

CHAPTER NINE

B CELL ACTIVATION

AND

ANTIBODY

PRODUCTION

Humoral immunity is mediated by antibodies, which are produced by cells of the B lymphocyte lineage. The physiologic function of antibodies is to neutralize and eliminate the antigen that induced their formation. The elimination of different antigens requires several effector mechanisms, which are dependent on distinct classes, or isotypes, of antibodies (see Chapter 3). The humoral immune response is also different at various anatomic sites. For instance, mucosal lymphoid tissues are uniquely adapted to produce high levels of IgA in response to the same antigens that stimulate other antibody isotypes in non-mucosal lymphoid tissues.

A fundamental feature of humoral immunity is that production of all these varied classes of antibodies is initiated by the interaction of antigens with a small number of mature IgM and IgD-expressing B lymphocytes specific for each antigen. Mature antigen-responsive B lymphocytes develop in the bone marrow prior to overt antigenic stimulation. Such cells enter peripheral lymphoid tissues, which are the sites of interaction with foreign antigens. An antigen binds to the membrane IgM and IgD on specific B cells and initiates a series of responses which lead to two principal changes in that clone of B cells: **proliferation,** resulting in expansion of the clone, and **differen-** tiation, resulting in the progeny of the membrane Ig-expressing, antigen-responsive B cells actively secreting antibodies of different heavy chain isotypes (Fig. 9–1). Therefore, the analysis of humoral immune responses is, in essence, an analysis of the growth and differentiation of B lymphocytes that occur following specific antigenic stimulation. The molecular mechanisms that regulate the expression of immunoglobulin genes have been described in Chapter 4. This chapter describes the cellular basis of the humoral immune response, in particular the stimuli that induce B cell growth and differentiation and the patterns of responses of B lymphocytes.

FEATURES OF HUMORAL IMMUNE RESPONSES

The earliest studies of specific immunity were devoted to analyses of antibody responses. As a result, until the 1960s, much of our knowledge of the immune system was based on our understanding of humoral immunity. The basic features of humoral immune responses were established before it was known that B lymphocytes and their progeny were the only

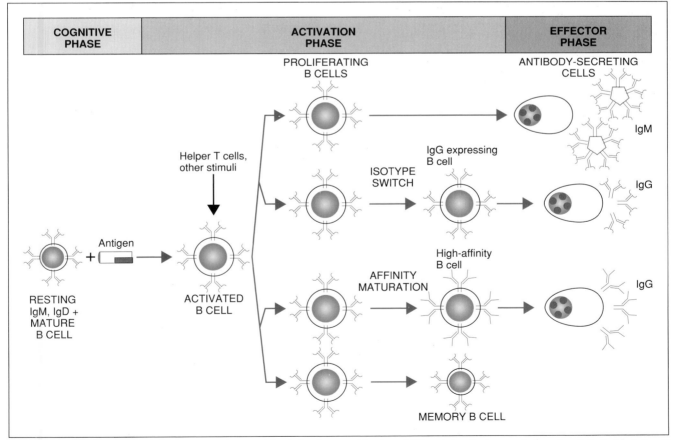

FIGURE 9–1. The humoral immune response: sequence of antigen-induced B lymphocyte proliferation and differentiation. *Antigen and other stimuli, including helper T cells, stimulate the proliferation and differentiation of a specific B cell clone. Progeny of the clone may produce IgM or other Ig isotypes (e.g., IgG), may undergo affinity maturation, or may persist as memory cells.*

cells capable of producing antibodies. The most important general properties of antibody responses are the following:

1. Protein antigens do not induce antibody responses in the absence of T lymphocytes, for instance, in T cell–deficient individuals. For this reason proteins are classified as "thymus-dependent" or "T-dependent" antigens. This observation led to the hypothesis that antibody production in response to protein antigens requires Ig-producing B cells as well as T cells, which are called **helper T cells.** As we shall see later in this chapter, a great deal is now known about the specificity and functions of helper T cells. The demonstration of their role in antibody responses is the basis of the concept that *resting B cells, which have not been previously exposed to antigen, require two distinct types of signals or stimuli for their proliferation and differentiation.* One type of signal is provided by the antigen, which interacts with membrane Ig molecules on specific B cells. The second type of signal is provided by helper T lymphocytes and their secreted products. The "two-signal" theory of lymphocyte activation may apply to most or all lymphocytes, because antigen-specific helper and cytolytic T lymphocytes (CTLs) also need other stimuli, in addition to antigens, for their full growth and differentiation (see Chapters 7 and 12).

2. Non-protein antigens like polysaccharides and lipids induce antibody responses without a requirement for antigen-specific helper T lymphocytes, e.g., in T cell–deficient individuals. Therefore, polysaccharide and lipid antigens are called "thymus-independent."

3. *Primary and secondary antibody responses differ qualitatively and quantitatively in several respects* (Table 9–1). First, the secondary response develops more rapidly than the primary response and larger

amounts of antibodies are produced in the secondary response. This is a clear example of immunologic **memory.** Primary antibody responses result from the activation of previously unstimulated B cells, whereas secondary responses are due to stimulation of expanded clones of memory cells. Second, the dominant class of secreted antibody in the primary response is usually IgM because resting B cells express only IgM (and IgD, which is rarely secreted). In contrast, other Ig isotypes, such as IgG, IgA, and IgE, are relatively increased in secondary responses. This change results from **heavy chain class** or **isotype switching.** Third, the average affinity of specific antibodies produced in a secondary response is higher than in the primary response. This is called **affinity maturation,** and results from somatic mutations in Ig genes and selective activation by antigen of those B cells whose membrane Ig molecules have increased affinity for that antigen. Affinity maturation is seen in both the membrane Ig on specific memory B cells and in the secreted antibodies. Affinity maturation of membrane Ig explains why the optimal antigen doses required for stimulating secondary antibody responses are lower than those for primary responses.

4. Memory cell generation, heavy chain class switching and affinity maturation are typical of humoral immune responses to proteins, but generally do not occur following immunization with thymus-independent antigens. This finding suggests that the characteristics of secondary antibody responses are due to helper T cells and/or their secreted products.

Much of our understanding of the activation of B lymphocytes and the induction and regulation of antibody responses has evolved from attempts to explain these features of humoral immunity. Among the most useful analytical approaches are *in vitro* experiments, in which different stimuli are used to activate B cells and their proliferation and differentiation can be measured accurately (Box 9–1). The current view of the mechanisms of B cell activation is based largely on these *in vitro* studies, and defining the cell interactions in humoral immune responses *in vivo* remains a challenge for immunologists.

EFFECTS OF ANTIGENS ON B LYMPHOCYTES

Foreign antigens that are introduced into an individual interact with specific B lymphocytes mostly in peripheral lymphoid tissues, such as the spleen, lymph nodes, and mucosal immune system, and at the sites of antigen entry. *The binding of an antigen to membrane Ig on B cells is the initiating event in B lymphocyte activation* and, therefore, in humoral immunity. Thymus-dependent protein antigens are thought to initiate two distinct types of responses in B cells. First, these antigens stimulate intracellular second messengers that stimulate the entry of resting B cells into the cell cycle. Interaction with antigen may also

TABLE 9–1. Features of Primary and Secondary Antibody Responses

	Primary Response	Secondary Response
Lag after immunization	Usually 5–10 days	Usually 1–3 days
Peak response	Smaller	Larger
Antibody isotype	Usually IgM > IgG	Relative increase in IgG and, under certain situations, in IgA or IgE
Antibody affinity	Lower average affinity, more variable	Higher average affinity ("affinity maturation")
Induced by	All immunogens	Only protein antigens
Required immunization	Relatively high doses of antigens, optimally with adjuvants	Low doses of antigens, adjuvants usually not necessary

Abbreviation: Ig, immunoglobulin.

BOX 9–1.   ASSAYS FOR B LYMPHOCYTE ACTIVATION

The responses of B lymphocytes to antigens and other stimuli that are described in this chapter consist of the following:

1. Early intracellular alterations, including the generation of "second messengers."
2. Proliferation, leading to expansion of the stimulated clone(s) of B cells.
3. Differentiation from membrane Ig-expressing cells to cells that actively secrete Ig of different heavy chain classes.

The most frequently used assays for B cell responses measure cellular proliferation and antibody secretion.

ASSAYS FOR PROLIFERATION. The proliferation of B lymphocytes, like that of other cells, is measured *in vitro* by determining the amount of ^{3}H-labeled thymidine incorporated into the replicating DNA of cultured cells. Thymidine incorporation provides a quantitative measure of the rate of DNA synthesis, which is usually directly proportional to the rate of cell division. Cellular proliferation *in vivo* can be measured by injecting ^{3}H-thymidine into animals and determining the number of cells with radioactively labeled nuclei (called the "labeling index").

ASSAYS FOR ANTIBODY PRODUCTION. Antibody production is measured in two different ways: assays for **cumulative Ig secretion**, which measure the amount of Ig that accumulates in the supernatant of cultured lymphocytes or in the serum of an immunized individual, and **single-cell assays**, which determine the number of cells in an immune population that secrete Ig of a particular specificity and/or isotype.

The most accurate, quantitative and widely used techniques for measuring the total amount of Ig in a culture supernatant or serum sample are radioimmunoassay (RIA) and enzyme-linked immunosorbent assay (ELISA), described in Chapter 3. By using antigens bound to solid supports, it is possible to use RIA or ELISA to quantitate the amount of a specific antibody in a sample. In addition, the availability of anti-Ig antibodies that detect immunoglobulins of different heavy or light chain classes allows one to measure the quantities of different isotypes in a sample. Other techniques for measuring antibody levels include hemagglutination for anti-erythrocyte antibodies, and complement-dependent lysis for antibodies specific for known cell types. Both assays are based on the demonstration that if the amount of antigen (i.e., cells) is constant, the concentration of antibody determines the amount of antibody bound to cells, and this is reflected in the degree of cell agglutination or subsequent binding of complement and cell lysis. Results from these assays are usually expressed as antibody titers, which are the dilutions of the sample giving half-maximal effects or the dilution at which the end-point of the assay is reached.

The most widely used single-cell assay for antibody secretion is the **hemolytic plaque assay**, in which the antigen is either an erythrocyte surface protein(s) or a molecule covalently coupled to an erythrocyte surface. Such erythrocytes serve as "indicator cells." They are mixed with lymphocytes, among which are the specific antibody-producing cells, and incubated in a semisolid supporting medium to allow secreted antibody to bind to the erythrocyte surface. If the antibody binds complement avidly, the subsequent addition of complement leads to lysis of the indicator cells that are coated with specific antibody. As a result, clear zones of lysis, called **plaques**, are formed around individual B lymphocytes or plasma cells that secrete the specific antibody. These antibody-secreting cells are also called **plaque-forming cells** (PFCs). This assay can also be used to detect antibodies that do not fix complement by incorporating into the medium a complement-binding anti-Ig antibody that will coat indicator cells to which the specific Ig is bound first. In another refinement, the same basic method can be used to detect PFCs that secrete Ig of a particular isotype irrespective of antigenic specificity. Hemolytic plaque assays provide a measure of the numbers of Ig-secreting cells, but they cannot accurately quantitate the amount of Ig secreted by each cell or by the total population. These assays can be applied to B cells stimulated *in vitro* or isolated from animals immunized with particular antigens.

---

prepare the B cells for subsequent responses to helper T lymphocytes. Second, protein antigens are internalized and processed by the B cells and presented to antigen-specific helper T cells, which are thus activated at the sites of specific antigen-B cell interactions. The subsequent growth and differentiation of B cells in response to protein antigens are actually stimulated by helper T lymphocytes and their secreted products. Thymus-independent antigens stimulate B cell responses without specific T cell help. Their mechanisms of action are less well understood and are discussed later in the chapter.

It is technically difficult to study the effects of antigens on normal B cells because, as the clonal selection hypothesis predicts, very few lymphocytes in an individual are specific for any one antigen. It is estimated that less than 1 in 10^5 B cells in an unimmunized individual binds any one antigenic determinant. In order to examine the effects of antigen binding to B cells, investigators have attempted to isolate antigen-specific B cells from complex populations of normal lymphocytes or to produce cloned B cell lines with defined antigenic specificities. The latter effort has met with limited success, so far. Another approach to circumventing this problem is to use anti-Ig antibodies as analogs of antigens, with the assumption that anti-Ig will bind to constant regions of membrane Ig molecules on all B cells and have the same biologic effects as an antigen that binds to the hypervariable regions of membrane Ig molecules only on the antigen-specific B cells. To the extent that precise comparisons are feasible, this assumption appears generally correct, indicating that anti-Ig antibody is a valid model for antigens. Thus, anti-Ig antibody is frequently used as a polyclonal activator of B lymphocytes. The same concept underlies the use of antibodies against framework determinants of T cell receptors or against receptor-associated CD3 molecules as polyclonal activators of T lymphocytes (see Chapter 7). Much of our knowledge of the effects of antigens on B lymphocytes is actually deduced from experiments using anti-Ig antibodies.

Functional Effects of Antigens on B Cells

A bivalent anti-Ig antibody or an antigen that contains two or more identical determinants is capable of cross-linking, i.e., bringing together, membrane Ig molecules on a B cell. When such a cross-linking ligand interacts with a B cell, it triggers a series of biochemical and cellular responses (Fig. 9–2).

1. Within minutes there is phospholipase C-catalyzed hydrolysis of membrane inositol phospholipids, an increase in the cytoplasmic ionized Ca^{++} concentration, and activation of protein kinases, similar to the changes detected in T cells stimulated via their receptors (see Chapter 7).

2. Within 30 minutes to 1 hour, levels of messenger RNA (mRNA) for *c-fos* and *c-myc* are increased. Transcription of these cellular proto-oncogenes often correlates with subsequent mitotic division in many cell types, including T lymphocytes.

3. Beginning at about 12 hours, B cells enlarge in size, show an increase in cellular RNA content, and are thought to move from the resting or G_0 stage to the G_1 stage of the cell cycle. Thus, they are poised to proliferate once they receive additional signals.

4. Within 12 to 24 hours after anti-Ig stimulation, B cells express increased levels of membrane receptors for helper T cell–derived cytokines compared to resting or unstimulated B cells. In addition, Ig-mediated stimulation may lead to an increase in the expression of class II MHC molecules. *Such changes make antigen-stimulated B cells better able to interact with and respond to helper T lymphocytes and their secreted mediators.*

The molecular mechanisms and physiologic significance of these effects of antigen or anti-Ig binding to B cells are not yet completely understood. Membrane IgM and IgD, which are the antigen receptors on resting B cells, have short cytoplasmic domains composed of only three amino acids, lysine-valine-lysine. It is unlikely that these Ig molecules themselves transduce signals generated by binding of an antigen or an anti-Ig antibody. Membrane Ig molecules may be coupled to other proteins that actually function as the signal transducers. These other proteins may include G proteins and proteins homologous to one or more components of the CD3 complex that is present in T cells (see Chapter 7). Furthermore, most of the available evidence indicates that the consequences of anti-Ig binding to membrane IgM and IgD are similar. Because IgD appears later in B cell maturation and correlates with functional responsiveness (see Chapter 4), it has been postulated that antigen interaction with membrane IgM may inhibit B cell activation but interaction with IgD may be stimulatory. There is, however, no clear evidence to support this hypothesis. Perhaps most important, it is not clear if the biochemical changes detected after antigen binding to B cells are always necessary for the subsequent prolifer-

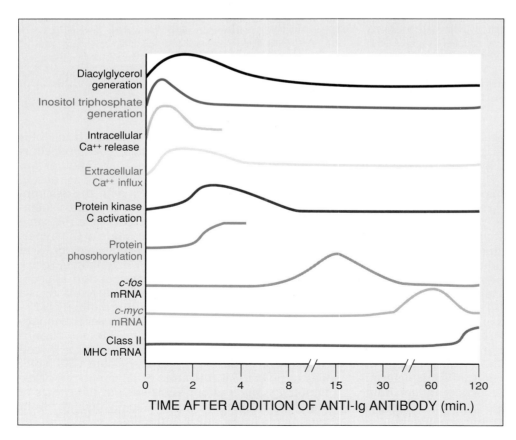

FIGURE 9–2. *Intracellular second messengers and biochemical changes induced in B lymphocytes by anti-Ig antibody. Some of the changes detected in mature mouse B lymphocytes exposed to cross-linking $F(ab')_2$ anti-Ig antibodies are shown. The same changes are presumed to occur as a result of the binding of multivalent antigens. (Courtesy of Dr. John Cambier, National Center for Immunology and Respiratory Medicine, Denver, Colo.)*

Diacylglycerol generation
Inositol triphosphate generation
Intracellular Ca^{++} release
Extracellular Ca^{++} influx
Protein kinase C activation
Protein phosphorylation
c-fos mRNA
c-myc mRNA
Class II MHC mRNA

0   2   4   8   15   30   60   120

TIME AFTER ADDITION OF ANTI-Ig ANTIBODY (min.)

ation and differentiation of the cells. Some recent data suggest that helper T cells and their cytokines may be able to activate B cells without actual cross-linking of membrane Ig by antigen. In this situation, the helper T cells may be providing signals that duplicate or circumvent the second messengers activated by antigen-Ig interactions. On the other hand, responses to thymus-independent antigens, which do not stimulate specific T cell help, may require Ig-mediated signal transduction in order to initiate B cell growth and differentiation. Thus, the importance of second messengers induced by antigen binding to B cell Ig may vary, depending on the nature of the antigen and the presence or absence of helper T cells.

Presentation of Antigens by B Cells to Helper T Lymphocytes

Following the binding of a multideterminant antigen or a bivalent anti-Ig antibody to a B cell, the mem-

brane Ig molecules are cross-linked and the complexes first aggregate and then migrate to one pole of the cell, forming a polar "cap" (Fig. 9–3). The complex of bound ligand and Ig molecules is internalized by receptor-mediated endocytosis. If the ligand is a protein, it is subsequently processed as in other antigen-presenting cells (see Chapter 6). This results in the generation of peptide fragments of the antigen that are re-expressed on the cell surface non-covalently attached to class II MHC molecules. These peptide-MCH molecule complexes can subsequently be recognized by antigen-specific, MHC–restricted helper T lymphocytes. As we shall discuss in detail later, antigen-specific B cells are extremely efficient at presenting the antigen they recognize, because membrane Ig molecules function as high-affinity receptors that enable the cells to bind, internalize and present very low concentrations of antigens. Antigen processing and presentation occur within 1 to 6 hours of binding of a protein antigen to B cells *in vitro.* Over the next 8 to 24 hours, new membrane Ig molecules are synthesized and re-expressed, so that the B cell is able to bind

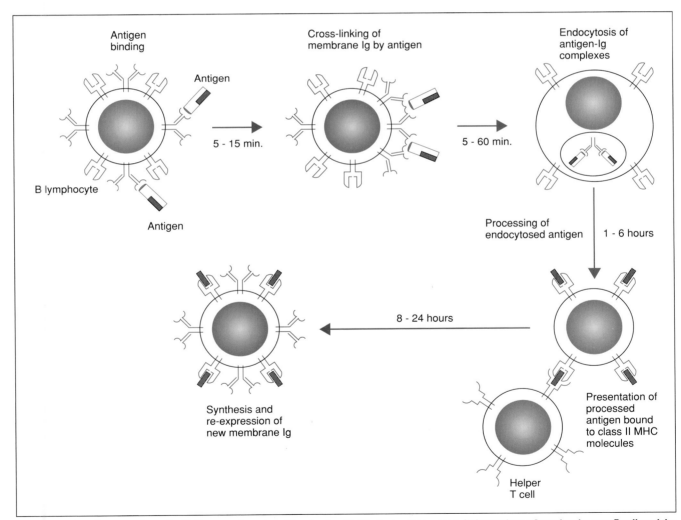

FIGURE 9 – 3. Fate of protein antigens after binding to membrane Ig on B lymphocytes. *Multivalent antigens cross-link membrane Ig molecules on a B cell, and the complexes are endocytosed. The antigen is processed inside the cell, and peptide fragments bound to class II MHC molecules are presented to helper T cells. Some of the membrane Ig may recycle back to the surface, but most of it is replaced by newly synthesized Ig molecules.*

more antigen molecules. Thymus-independent antigens such as polysaccharides and glycolipids may also be endocytosed following binding to Ig on specific B cells, but these antigens cannot be processed and associated with MHC molecules and, therefore, are not recognized by specific class II MHC–restricted helper T cells.

It is also of interest that monovalent anti-Ig antibodies and, presumably, monovalent protein antigens are internalized (without cap formation), processed, and presented by B cells and generate helper T cell–dependent antibody responses *in vitro*. However, such monovalent ligands cannot cross-link membrane Ig and, therefore, do not directly stimulate the biochemical changes in B cells that have been described above. This is one piece of experimental evidence suggesting that receptor-mediated second messenger activation may not be obligatory for B cell growth and differentiation and can be replaced or bypassed by helper T lymphocytes.

ROLE OF HELPER T LYMPHOCYTES IN ANTIBODY RESPONSES

The second signals for B lymphocyte activation that have been most thoroughly investigated are provided by contact with helper T cells and by cytokines secreted by these cells. A role for T lymphocytes in antibody responses was formally demonstrated by experiments done in the late 1960s, even before the classification of lymphocytes into T and B cell subsets was established. These experiments showed that if mouse bone marrow lymphocytes, which we now know contain mature B cells but few or no T cells, were adoptively transferred into irradiated syngeneic recipients, they would not produce specific antibody upon immunization with sheep red blood cells (SRBCs), a model protein antigen. If, however, thymic or thoracic duct lymphocytes (which contain T lymphocytes but few or no antibody-producing B cells) were transferred at the same time, antibody responses did develop following immunization (Table 9–2). This result, and later *in vitro* experiments in which purified T and B cells were mixed and stimulated with antigens, showed that B cells would proliferate and differentiate in response to soluble and particulate protein antigens only if helper T lymphocytes were also present. Subsequent studies have established that *most helper T cells are CD4+, CD8−, and class II MHC–restricted* in their recognition of foreign protein antigens (see Chapters 6 and 7). There are two important questions about the functions of helper T cells in antibody responses:

1. How are these helper T cells stimulated by antigens?
2. What are the mechanisms by which helper T cells induce the growth and differentiation of B lymphocytes?

Mechanisms of Helper T Cell–B Cell Interactions

The sequence of events leading to helper T cell–dependent antibody responses to protein antigens is best understood by considering the immune response to hapten-protein conjugates. Haptens, such as dini-

TABLE 9–2. Identification of Helper T Cells in Antibody Responses to Protein Antigens

A.   Adoptive Transfer

Cells Transferred into Irradiated Recipient			
SOURCE OF B CELLS	*SOURCE OF T CELLS*	*Antigen*	*Anti-SRBC Antibody-Producing Cells in Spleen*
Bone marrow cells	None	SRBC	—
None	Thoracic duct cells	SRBC	—
Bone marrow cells	Thoracic duct cells	SRBC	+
Bone marrow cells	Thoracic duct cells	—	—

B.   Cell Culture

Cells Cultured	*Antigen*	*Anti-SRBC Antibody-Producing Cells in Culture*
Unfractionated spleen cells	SRBC	+
Splenic B cells	SRBC	—
Splenic T cells	SRBC	—
Splenic B cells and T cells	SRBC	+
Splenic B cells and T cells	—	—

Mouse B lymphocytes by themselves do not produce antibody against a T cell–dependent antigen, SRBCs, *in vivo* (A) or *in vitro* (B). The addition of T cells allows the B cells to respond to SRBC. A response does not occur in the absence of antigen.

Abbreviation: SRBC, sheep red blood cells.

trophenol, are small chemicals that can be bound by B cell membrane Ig and by secreted antibodies but are not immunogenic by themselves. If, however, the haptens are coupled to proteins, which serve as carriers, the conjugates are able to induce antibody responses against the haptens.

There are three important characteristics of anti-hapten antibody responses stimulated by hapten-protein conjugates. First, such responses require cooperation between hapten-specific B cells and protein (carrier)-specific helper T cells. Second, in order to stimulate a response, the hapten and carrier portions have to be physically linked and cannot be administered separately. Third, the interaction is class II MHC–restricted; i.e., the helper T cells cooperate only with B lymphocytes that express class II MHC molecules recognized as self by the T cells. Such T-B interactions are also called "cognate" because the two participating cell types specifically recognize distinct antigenic determinants that are physically linked. Furthermore, the same characteristics apply not only to hapten-protein conjugates but to all protein antigens, in which one intrinsic determinant is recognized by B cells (and is, therefore, analogous to the hapten), and the same or another determinant is recognized by the helper T cells (and is analogous to the carrier).

The mechanism of T cell–B cell cooperation in the generation of antibody responses to protein antigens and hapten-protein conjugates became clear when it was appreciated that B lymphocytes are extremely efficient antigen-presenting cells. When an individual is exposed to an antigen, *membrane Ig molecules on specific B cells bind the native antigen (e.g., via the hapten determinant), process it, and present peptide fragments (carrier determinants) of the antigen associated with class II MHC molecules to specific helper T cells* (Fig. 9–4). Thus, in the generation of an antibody response, B and T cell epitopes of the same protein antigen are recognized at different times and in different forms. According to this model, the preferential recipients of T cell help are the same antigen-specific B cells that present the antigen, because these B cells are of necessity in close proximity to the helper T cells. The antigen-presenting B cells may receive additional signals from direct contact with the T cells. This would result in activation of the B cells that bound the native antigen and an antibody response that is specific for this antigen.

The significance of the antigen-presenting function of B lymphocytes in antibody responses to thymus-dependent antigens has been recognized relatively recently. Early studies examining the requirements for antibody production showed that primary antibody responses to antigens such as sheep red blood cells *in vitro* could be abolished by the depletion of adherent accessory cells such as macrophages and dendritic cells. This led to the hypothesis that antibody responses were initiated by helper T cell recognition of antigens presented by accessory cells other than B lymphocytes. However, *many of the*

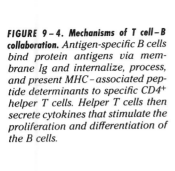

FIGURE 9–4. Mechanisms of T cell–B collaboration. *Antigen-specific B cells bind protein antigens via membrane Ig and internalize, process, and present MHC–associated peptide determinants to specific CD4+ helper T cells. Helper T cells then secrete cytokines that stimulate the proliferation and differentiation of the B cells.*

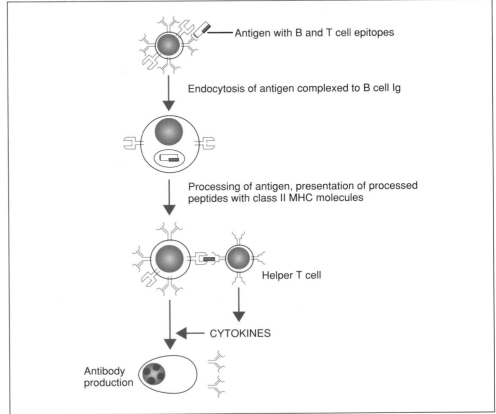

features of antibody responses to thymus-dependent proteins, especially of secondary responses, may reflect the central role of B cells as antigen-presenting cells (APCs).

1. The antigenic specificity and MHC restriction of cognate T cell–B cell interactions are best explained by postulating that antigen-specific B cells bind and present the antigen to specific, MHC–restricted helper T cells. This would also account for the observation that in order to stimulate secondary antibody responses to hapten-carrier conjugates, the hapten and carrier determinants must be physically linked. In this situation, a function of the hapten would be to focus the antigen on to hapten-specific B cells. Thus, only the hapten-specific B lymphocytes would present carrier epitopes to helper T cells, leading ultimately to stimulation of hapten-specific antibody production.

2. The optimal antigen concentrations required to stimulate secondary antibody responses *in vitro* are in the range of 1 to 100 ng/ml. At such low concentrations, antigen-binding B cells are the most efficient APCs for stimulating CD4$^+$ T cells because of the high affinity of membrane Ig molecules for antigens. In contrast, other APCs, such as macrophages and dendritic cells, which pinocytose protein antigens nonspecifically, generally require 10^4 to 10^6-fold higher concentrations of antigen to activate specific CD4$^+$ T cells. Therefore, in antibody responses to antigen at low concentrations, it is likely that the B cells that express membrane Ig capable of specifically binding that antigen will be the principal APCs.

3. Affinity maturation in secondary antibody responses may occur because the B cells producing Ig that binds antigen with the highest affinity will be the most efficient APCs and, therefore, will be maximally stimulated by the helper T cells. Thus, affinity maturation may result from two sets of events. First, somatic mutations in Ig V genes (see Chapter 4) generate B cells whose membrane Ig molecules have a wide range of affinities for the antigen. At the same time, antibody formed in the primary response neutralizes or eliminates a portion of the antigen, leading to a progressive decline in the concentration of available antigen. B cells whose receptors are of high affinity bind low concentrations of antigen and present it to helper T cells. As a result, high-affinity B cells are more likely to interact with and to be stimulated by specific helper T cells. This would also explain why affinity maturation is a T cell–dependent phenomenon that is seen with protein antigens but does not occur with T cell–independent antigens, responses to which do not require antigen presentation to specific helper T cells.

There are, however, situations in which APCs other than B lymphocytes are necessary for the induction of antibody responses. For instance, in unimmunized individuals there may be so few B cells specific for a particular antigen that they cannot effectively initiate a T cell response. B lymphocytes may also be less efficient than macrophages at processing particulate antigens (such as microbes) because B cells have fewer lysosomes and degradative enzymes.

Therefore, the induction of primary antibody responses, especially against particulate protein antigens, may require antigen presentation by other APCs such as macrophages. Once lymphocyte clones are expanded by immunization, the specific B cells may be the major APCs, i.e., in secondary antibody responses. Consistent with this hypothesis is the observation that secondary antibody responses *in vitro* require only B cells, helper T cells, and antigen. Depletion of macrophages does not abrogate antibody production by previously immunized lymphocytes, whereas macrophage depletion does reduce or abolish primary antibody responses. Finally, accessory cells such as macrophages may serve functions other than antigen presentation in humoral immunity; these functions are described later in this chapter.

Cytokines (Helper Factors) in Antibody Responses

The recognition of processed antigen by CD4$^+$ helper T cells leads to the activation of these cells at sites of immunization or in peripheral lymphoid organs, where B cells have first encountered the antigen. Helper T cells, in turn, induce the proliferation and differentiation of B cells, and these responses are mediated by cell-cell contact and by the protein hormones or cytokines that the helper cells secrete.

Cytokines secreted by T lymphocytes and by other cell types, in response to activating stimuli, mediate many of the effector functions of the cells that produce them. Cytokines are also the principal mechanisms by which various immune and inflammatory cell populations communicate with one another. Their general properties, structural features, and functional effects are described in Chapter 11. The role of these secreted proteins in humoral immunity was first demonstrated by experiments showing that lymphocyte populations depleted of T cells could not be stimulated to secrete antibodies *in vitro* when cultured with a T cell–dependent antigen like sheep red blood cells. If, however, supernatants taken from cultures of activated T cells were added, an antibody response did develop (Table 9–3). T cell supernatants also stimulated the proliferation of purified B cells cultured with polyclonal activators, such as anti-Ig antibody, or a protein called pokeweed mitogen (for human peripheral blood B lymphocytes). These results again demonstrated that two signals were required for B cell activation—antigen (or polyclonal activator) and soluble T cell–derived factor(s). They also established that *cytokines that are present in the T cell supernatants can replace intact T lymphocytes in providing some helper functions for B cells.*

These cytokines were originally classified as "B cell growth factor" (BCGF), "B cell differentiation factor" (BCDF), or "T cell (thymus) replacing factor" (TRF), based largely on the functional activities that were detected in partially purified T cell culture supernatants. It is now possible to study the activities of

TABLE 9–3. Identification of Helper Factors in Antibody Responses

Cultured Cells		Supernatant of Activated T Cells	Antigen or Polyclonal Activator	B Cell Response
A.	B cells	−	SRBC	−
	B cells + T cells	−	SRBC	+*
	B cells	+	SRBC	+*
	B cells	+	−	−
B.	B cells	−	Anti-Ig antibody	−
	B cells	+	Anti-Ig antibody	+†

Mouse B lymphocytes cultured by themselves do not respond to a T cell–dependent antigen, SRBCs (A) or to an antigen analog, anti-Ig antibody (B). The addition of cytokine-containing culture supernatants of activated T cells stimulates B cell responses to antigen and to anti-Ig antibody.

* Anti-SRBC antibody production.
† Proliferation.
Abbreviation: SRBC, sheep red blood cell; Ig, immunoglobulin.

pure, recombinant DNA–derived cytokines, so that operational designations such as BCGF, BCDF, and TRF are being replaced by names that identify distinct structurally defined molecules. Moreover, in some cases the same cytokine can induce both B cell growth and differentiation, indicating that the original classifications may not be valid. The functions of cytokines in antibody responses have been analyzed by several different experimental approaches. For example, recombinant DNA–derived cytokines stimulate the growth and/or differentiation of T cell–depleted B lymphocytes or B cell tumor lines cultured with antigens or polyclonal activators. Furthermore, antibodies that specifically recognize and neutralize cytokines or block their binding to cellular receptors can inhibit humoral immune responses *in vitro* and *in vivo*, demonstrating the obligatory role of cytokines in such responses. Transgenic mice in which cytokine genes are overexpressed also show changes in B cell growth and differentiation that are similar to the effects of cytokines on B cells *in vitro*.

The cytokines that function as helper factors in antibody responses have the following general properties:

1. *Cytokines are neither antigen-specific nor MHC-restricted,* in contrast to the helper T cells that produce them. As we discussed above and in Chapter 6, helper T cells are activated by the recognition of a specific antigenic determinant associated with class II MHC molecules on B cells or other APCs. But once they are stimulated, these helper cells secrete cytokines that can act on B cells of any antigenic specificity and MHC haplotype.

2. *Different cytokines may function in different phases of the response of B cells,* depending on whether their major effects on B cells are on proliferation, secretion of various Ig isotypes, or both (see below). Particular combinations of cytokines may be synergistic or antagonistic in their effects on B cells.

3. The effects of different cytokines may vary in different species.

4. The production of cytokines contributes to the activation of "bystander" B cells that are not specific for the antigen initiating the response but are present in the vicinity of antigen-stimulated cells. Bystander B cell activation is readily observed *in vitro* and is presumably also responsible for the production of nonspecific antibody following exposure to potent immunogens. For instance, infection with helminthic parasites stimulates 100-fold or greater increases in serum IgE, and only a small fraction of this IgE (probably less than 5 per cent) is specific for the particular helminth.

5. Some of the cytokines that stimulate B cell growth and differentiation are produced by macrophages and other non–T cells.

6. The mechanisms by which various cytokines stimulate B cell growth and differentiation are largely unknown. None of the T cell–derived helper factors has been shown to induce changes in known intracellular second messengers, such as inositol phospholipid metabolites, cytoplasmic Ca^{++}, cyclic nucleotides, or protein kinases, in B cells. Receptors for many of these cytokines have been identified, but the mechanisms by which binding of a cytokine to its receptor leads to B cell activation are not yet defined.

The activation of B cells by cytokines is an evolving story, since new factors and new effects of previously described mediators continue to be discovered. Nevertheless, it is possible to construct a basic scheme of the stages of B cell activation and to identify cytokines that act at each of these stages (Fig. 9–5).

1. *Entry of resting B cells into the cell cycle.* As stated above, high concentrations of anti-Ig antibody (and, presumably, specific antigens) initiate the transition of B cells from the G_0 to G_1 stage of the cell cycle. This is detected by an increase in cell size and cytoplasmic RNA and precedes commitment to DNA synthesis. At low concentrations, however, anti-Ig and protein antigens do not have this effect, and different cytokines may be required to initiate the entry of resting B cells into the cell cycle. In the mouse, interleukin-4 (IL–4), which is produced by CD4+ helper T cells, has been shown to have this effect. Such results suggest that even the early events of B cell activation may be mediated by helper T cell–derived factors.

2. *Proliferation.* Proliferation of B cells cultured with low concentrations of protein antigens or anti-Ig antibodies is absolutely dependent on cytokines, and many factors appear to be capable of stimulating the entry of B cells into the S phase of the cell cycle. IL–4 was identified in mice by its ability to stimulate B cell proliferation *in vitro* when added with anti-Ig antibody. Interleukin-5 (IL–5), also a helper T cell–derived cytokine, stimulates the proliferation of certain mouse B cell–derived tumor lines and normal B cells incubated with some polyclonal activators but has less of an effect on human B cells. Interleukin-2 (IL–2), which was identified first as a T cell growth

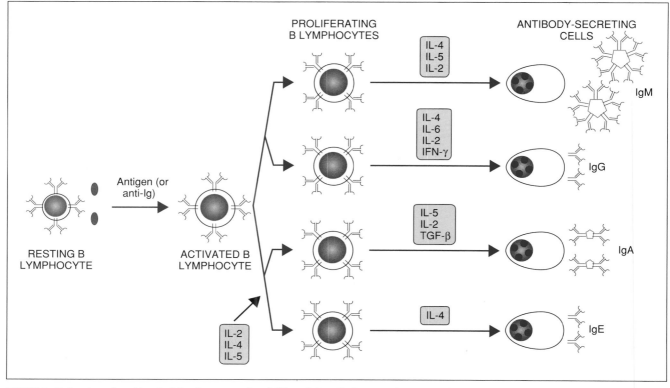

FIGURE 9-5. Functions of cytokines in B lymphocyte growth and differentiation. *Various cytokines stimulate different stages of B cell proliferation and differentiation in humans and mice. The same cytokines may have less striking effects at other stages that are not shown, and there may be differences among species.*

factor, at high concentrations induces B cell growth and differentiation, its effects being most marked on human B cells. *In vitro* experiments using anti-cytokine antibodies indicate that IL–2, IL–4 and IL–5 can all contribute to the proliferation of mouse B cells stimulated with thymus-dependent antigens in the presence of specific helper T cells. This is one example of the synergistic effects of three different cytokines. Recent experiments suggest that IL–4 and IL–5 separately increase the expression of the two polypeptide chains that make up the high-affinity receptor for IL–2 (see Chapter 11), and this may be the molecular basis of the observed synergy. Macrophage-derived cytokines, including interleukin-1 (IL–1), tumor necrosis factor (TNF), and interleukin-6 (IL–6), may also be growth and differentiation factors for B cells, particularly in primary antibody responses when the numbers of stimulated helper T cells are generally small.

3. *Ig secretion.* Antibody synthesis and secretion in response to protein antigens, like B cell proliferation, are also dependent on cytokines. In the mouse, IL–4 and IL–5 are the most potent inducers of antibody secretion by B cells. Human B cells cultured with polyclonal activators secrete high levels of antibody if IL–2 or IL–6 is added. It is not clear whether these differences in the cytokine responses of human and mouse B cells are due to true species variations, or reflect differences in experimental conditions that

lead to the preferential or selective stimulation of distinct subpopulations of B cells.

4. *Isotype switching.* We have mentioned previously that heavy chain isotype switching is typically seen with protein antigens and requires helper T cells. It is now known that different T cell–derived cytokines can selectively induce switching to particular Ig isotypes. For instance, *IL–4 is the only identified switch factor for IgE in all species examined.* IgE production appears to depend on IL–4, since IgE responses to antigen-specific or polyclonal stimulation *in vitro,* and to infection by helminthic parasites *in vivo,* are abrogated by antibodies that neutralize IL–4. These findings have many practical implications. IgE antibodies are not only important for host defense against parasitic infestations, but immediate hypersensitivity (allergic) reactions are due to IgE production (see Chapter 14). Therefore, therapeutic control of IL–4 secretion or function is potentially a powerful approach for the treatment of allergy. IL–4 also enhances the secretion of IgG1 antibodies by murine B cells. Similarly, the production of IgG2a in mice is enhanced by γ-interferon (IFN–γ) which is also secreted by T cells. Therefore, addition of IL–4 or IFN–γ induces specific isotype switching in cultures of mature IgM and IgD expressing B cells stimulated with antigens or polyclonal activators (Table 9–4). The mechanisms by which these cytokines alter Ig gene expression are being actively investigated. As men-

TABLE 9-4. Heavy Chain Isotype Switching Induced by Cytokines

B Cells Cultured with		Ig Isotype Secreted (Per Cent of Total Ig)				
Polyclonal Activator	*Cytokine*	*IgM*	*IgG1*	*IgG$_{2a}$*	*IgE*	*IgA*
LPS	None	85	2	<1	<1	<1
LPS	IL-4	70	20	<1	5	<1
LPS	IFN-γ	80	2	10	<1	<1
LPS	TGF-β and IL-2	75	2	<1	<1	15

Purified IgM$^+$ IgD$^+$ mouse B cells cultured with the polyclonal activator LPS, and various cytokines show selective switching to different heavy chain isotypes. (The values of the isotypes shown are approximations, and do not add up to 100 per cent because not all were measured.)

Courtesy of Dr. Robert Coffman, DNAX Research Institute, Palo Alto, California.

Abbreviations: Ig, immunoglobulin; LPS, lipopolysaccharide; IL, interleukin; TGF, transforming growth factor; IFN, interferon.

tioned in Chapter 4, IL-4 may function by making the C$_\epsilon$ gene accessible to transcriptional activators and by promoting switch recombination with the rearranged VDJ complex. This recombination is necessary for transcription of the complete ϵ heavy chain gene, synthesis of the ϵ heavy chain, and subsequent production of the complete IgE molecule. Interestingly, IFN-γ inhibits IL-4 induced B cell proliferation and switching to IgE and IgG1 secretion, and, conversely, IL-4 reduces IgG2a production. These are among the clearest examples of the antagonistic effects of different cytokines. IL-5 enhances the production of IgA and, therefore, may be particularly important in secretory mucosal immunity. Recent studies suggest that other cytokines, such as transforming growth factor-β (TGF-β), produced by T cells and by non-lymphoid stromal cells, may play a role in stimulating IgA production in mucosal lymphoid tissues.

5. *Affinity maturation and the generation of memory B cells.* Affinity maturation in secondary antibody responses and the generation of memory B cells are both helper T cell–dependent phenomena that occur only after immunization with protein antigens. However, the cytokines involved in these aspects of humoral immune responses have not been identified. We also do not know why, after stimulation by antigen and helper T cells, some B lymphocytes actively secrete antibodies whereas others develop into memory cells. Heavy chain isotype switching and somatic mutations of Ig V genes are readily detected in the memory cell population, but little else is understood about the physiology of these cells.

The important general principle that emerges from these findings is that *the nature and magnitude of a humoral immune response may be influenced by the relative amounts of different cytokines produced at sites of T and B cell stimulation.* However, many of our current concepts of cytokine effects are based on *in vitro* studies. Much remains to be learned about the cytokines that play obligatory roles in antibody re-

sponses to immunization with defined microbial or protein antigens *in vivo.*

Different antigens and immunization conditions induce different types of antibody responses, in part by stimulating the secretion of different cytokines. One possible explanation for this is that any T cell population can secrete distinct cytokines, depending on the nature of the antigenic stimulus. Alternatively, different antigens or conditions of immunization may selectively stimulate distinct subsets of helper T cells that produce different cytokines. In fact, the analysis of mouse CD4$^+$ T cell clones has revealed the existence of subpopulations that vary in profiles of cytokine production. One subset, called "Th1," secretes IL-2, IFN-γ, and TNF (lymphotoxin); the other, called "Th2," produces IL-4, IL-5, IL-6 and low levels of TNF. Th2 cells are the most efficient helpers for resting B lymphocytes *in vitro,* and Th1 clones are potent inducers of delayed type hypersensitivity reactions, one form of cell-mediated immunity (see Chapter 12). These results suggest that IL-4, IL-5, and IL-6, produced by Th2 clones, are most important for humoral immunity, whereas IL-2, IFN-γ, and TNF are the major cytokines involved in cell-mediated immune responses. IgE responses to parasites and some allergens may involve preferential activation of helper cells of the Th2 subset, and microbes that induce granulomatous inflammation (see Chapter 12) may stimulate mostly Th1 cells. However, at present it is not known to what extent such results with cloned cell lines can be extrapolated to uncloned, heterogeneous populations of helper T lymphocytes. It is also not clear whether these subsets represent distinct lineages or different stages of T cell maturation. Moreover, many T cell clones, particularly in humans, produce multiple cytokines, such as IL-2, IL-4, and IFN-γ, and cannot be unambiguously classified into non-overlapping groups.

The Role of T Cell–B Cell Contact

In addition to cytokine-mediated effects, *the physical or cognate interaction of antigen-specific helper T cells with antigen-presenting B lymphocytes* also appears to deliver a necessary stimulus that is not mediated by a known secreted factor. This is suggested by the finding that supernatants of helper T cells are rarely, if ever, as effective in inducing antibody production by B cells as the helper T lymphocytes themselves, especially in cultures of B cells stimulated with low concentrations of soluble protein antigens. The importance of physical contact between B and helper T lymphocytes has been most clearly demonstrated by experiments in which cells can be cultured while separated from one another by semipermeable membranes that allow passage of soluble materials but not intact cells. B cells, antigen, and helper T cells are placed on one side of the membrane and only B cells on the other side. Although all the B cells have equal access to antigen and cytokines, only the B cells cultured with the T lymphocytes secrete high levels of antibody. This indicates that antibody production in response to protein antigens requires T cell–B cell contact, but the nature of the putative signal induced by such contact is unknown. One hypothesis is that the class II MHC molecules on the B cells transduce activating signals as a result of their interaction with T cell receptors. Cognate interactions appear to be necessary for the growth and differentiation of resting B lymphocytes, whereas B cells that have been recently activated by antigen or polyclonal activators may respond maximally to cytokines alone.

In summary, one can envision the following sequence of events leading to antibody production in response to thymus-dependent antigens (Fig. 9–6):

1. After an antigen enters an individual, it may trigger immune responses at the site of entry as well as in adjacent peripheral lymphoid tissues such as lymph nodes and spleen. In an unimmunized individual, macrophages and/or dendritic cells may be necessary for initiating stimulation of helper T cells by presenting antigens and secreting cytokines like IL–1

and IL–6. The requirement for macrophages explains why primary antibody responses to proteins require immunization with quite large amounts of antigens with adjuvants that recruit and activate macrophages. Once clones of antigen-specific B cells are expanded, they may assume much of the function of antigen presentation. This is especially so in previously immunized individuals and may explain why secondary antibody responses can be induced by lower doses of antigens administered without adjuvants.

2. At the same time as antigen is being presented to initiate helper T cell activation, the antigen activates specific B cells and stimulates their entry into the cell cycle. The recognition of antigen by specific B and helper T lymphocytes is the **cognitive phase** of the humoral immune response.

3. The helper T cells then deliver contact-mediated signals to the B cells and secrete cytokines, which induce the growth and differentiation of B cells. This is the **activation phase** of the response. Cytokines maximally stimulate the antigen-presenting B cells, which are in the closest proximity to the helper

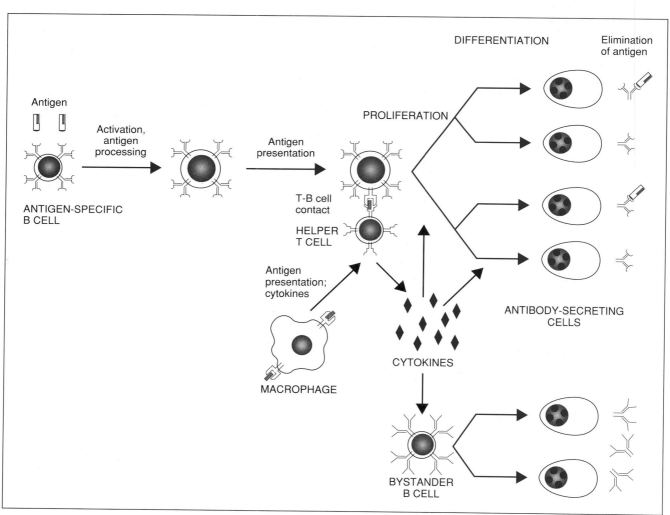

FIGURE 9–6. Cellular interactions in humoral immune responses to protein antigens. *Helper T cells, cytokines, and accessory cells, such as macrophages, act at different stages in humoral immune responses.*

T cells and have become most responsive to T cell–derived signals as a result of their prior encounter with antigen. This leads to the production of antibody specific for the antigen. Cytokines may also stimulate bystander B cells to variable degrees, and this may be responsible for the production of Ig that is not specific for the antigen.

4. Some antigen-stimulated B cells differentiate into antibody-secreting cells, which develop at the sites of antigen exposure and in lymphoid tissues, do not circulate, and secrete antibodies which specifically bind the antigen to initiate the **effector phase** of the response.

5. Other progeny of antigen-stimulated B cells become long-lived memory cells, which may be produced in the germinal centers of lymphoid follicles and are able to recirculate between the blood, lymph, and lymphoid organs. The mechanisms that lead to the development of B cells into memory cells or into antibody secreting cells are not yet known.

The characteristics of antibody responses to thymus-dependent protein antigens are determined by three principal factors:

1. *Type of responding B cells.* Resting, or previously unstimulated, B cells require contact with helper T cells, whereas recently stimulated B cells may be fully responsive to cytokines alone. Memory B cells, whose membrane Ig molecules are of high affinity, may respond to lower concentrations of antigens than resting cells.

2. *Production of cytokines.* The relative proportions of different cytokines at the site of B and T cell interactions influence the nature and magnitude of the antibody response, because various cytokines have selective effects on different phases of B cell growth and differentiation. In addition, different cytokines may synergize with or inhibit one another's actions.

3. *Nature of the antigenic stimulus.* Different antigens and conditions of antigen exposure stimulate helper T cells to varying degrees and may also preferentially induce the production of distinct cytokines.

The type and amount of antigen also influence the extent to which B cell responses are dependent on contact with helper T cells or secreted cytokines.

THYMUS-INDEPENDENT ANTIGENS

The requirement for helper T cells explains why thymus-dependent protein antigens do not induce antibody responses in T cell–deficient animals, such as congenitally athymic (nude) or neonatally thymectomized mice. In contrast, many antigens stimulate antibody production in athymic mice, and these antigens are termed **thymus-independent** (TI). Their properties and the features of the antibody responses they induce are summarized in Table 9–5. TI antigens have been further subdivided into two groups according to their relative independence from T cells and their physicochemical properties.

TI–1 antigens are completely T cell–independent, and most are polyclonal activators of B cells at high concentrations, meaning that they stimulate the proliferation and differentiation of most or all B cells irrespective of antigenic specificity. The best example of a TI–1 antigen is lipopolysaccharide (LPS, or endotoxin), which is a component of the cell walls of several gram-negative bacteria. In mice, LPS at high concentrations (such as $10~\mu g/ml$ or more *in vitro*) stimulates many clones of B cells without binding to their membrane Ig. This indicates that responses to LPS are neither dependent on nor mediated by B cell activation via antigen receptors. At hundred-fold or thousand-fold lower concentrations, however, LPS binds to and stimulates specific B cells only, and this is why LPS, and other TI–1 antigens capable of inducing polyclonal responses, are called "antigens." The activation of B cells by LPS also does not involve known cytokines. It is postulated that a portion of the LPS molecule itself possesses the ability to directly stimulate B cells and thus bypasses the requirement for helper T cells and their cytokines. This may explain both the polyclonal activating ability and T cell

TABLE 9–5. Properties of Thymus-Dependent and Thymus-Independent Antigens

Properties	Thymus-Dependent	Thymus-Independent	
		TI–1	TI–2
Prototypes	Proteins	Lipopolysaccharide, *Brucella abortus*	Polymeric antigens, especially polysaccharides
Antibody Response in			
Athymic mice	No	Yes	Yes
T cell–depleted cultures	No	Yes	No or reduced
Features of Antibody Response			
Isotype switching	Yes	No	No (usually)
Affinity maturation	Yes	No	No
Secondary response (memory B cells)	Yes	No	No
Polyclonal B Cell Activation	No	Yes	No
Ability to Induce Delayed Type Hypersensitivity	Yes	No	No

independence of LPS and other TI-1 antigens. Neither the nature of this stimulatory component of LPS nor the identity of the B cell receptor responsible for the polyclonal activation induced by any TI-1 antigen is known. As one would expect, B cell responses to TI-1 antigens show features that reflect the absence of helper T cells or T cell-derived cytokines. Thus, LPS by itself induces B cell proliferation and high levels of IgM and IgG3 secretion in mice, but not switching to other isotypes. Interestingly, μ and $\gamma3$ constant regions genes are two of the most proximal, i.e., closest to the rearranged VDJ complex, in the mouse heavy chain locus (see Chapter 4). Therefore, LPS may be able to stimulate transcription of these proximal C_H genes, but switching to more 3′ C_H genes requires cytokines such as IL-4 and IFN-γ (see Table 9-4). Since TI-1 antigens do not activate helper T cells, they also fail to induce affinity maturation or memory B cells.

In contrast to TI-1 antigens, which show no demonstrable requirement for T cells, **TI-2 antigens** do not stimulate antibody responses *in vitro* if T cells are rigorously removed from the responding lymphocytes. (Such antigens were called "thymus- or T cell-independent" because they do induce specific antibodies in athymic mice, for reasons that are not well understood.) Most TI-2 antigens are polysaccharides composed of multiple identical antigenic epitopes; examples include dextrans, pneumococcal polysaccharide, and ficoll. Such multivalent antigens may induce maximal cross-linking of membrane Ig on specific B cells, leading to activation without a requirement for cognate T cell help. B cell activation by TI-2 antigens is the one situation in which membrane Ig-mediated signal transduction may be critical for subsequent responses of the cells. TI-2 antigens stimulate only specific B cells and do not function as polyclonal activators. Since polysaccharides cannot be processed and presented to MHC-restricted helper T cells, they cannot be recognized by and stimulate specific helper T cells. Nevertheless, as stated above, TI-2 antigens require small numbers of T cells for generating antibody responses. This may be because cytokines are required for B cell responses to TI-2 antigens, but neither the nature of these cytokines nor the mechanism(s) leading to their production is completely understood. Antibody responses to most TI-2 antigens, like those to TI-1 antigens, consist largely of IgM antibodies of low affinity and do not show significant switching to other isotypes, affinity maturation or memory. However, some TI-2 antigens do induce Ig isotypes other than IgM, probably because these antigens stimulate cytokine production. For instance, in man the dominant antibody class induced by pneumococcal capsular polysaccharide is IgG2.

The practical importance of TI antigens is that many bacterial cell wall polysaccharides belong to this category, and humoral immunity is the major mechanism of host defense against such bacterial infections. For this reason, T cell-deficient individuals are susceptible to lethal infection by many microbes but may show normal resistance to infections by some bacteria, such as pyogenic cocci and gram-negative bacilli, which have polysaccharide-rich cell walls. Antibody responses to TI antigens may occur at particular anatomic sites in lymphoid tissues. Macrophages located in the marginal zones of lymphoid follicles in the spleen are particularly efficient at trapping TI antigens, such as polysaccharides, when these are injected intravenously. Such antigens may persist for prolonged periods on the surfaces of marginal zone macrophages, where they are recognized by specific B cells. This may be the reason why splenectomized individuals have a striking and selective susceptibility to infection by encapsulated bacteria like the pneumococcus, as a result of deficient antibody responses to capsular polysaccharides.

ROLE OF ACCESSORY CELLS IN ANTIBODY RESPONSES

One of the first experiments suggesting the requirement for accessory cells in the responses of lymphocytes to antigens demonstrated that if spleen cells from unimmunized mice were depleted of adherent cells, they would not secrete antibody when stimulated by a T-cell dependent antigen, sheep red blood cells. Responsiveness was restored by the addition of non-lymphoid cells such as macrophages, or, as shown later, by dendritic cells.

Macrophages and other accessory cells can perform various functions in the induction of humoral immunity:

1. *They might be necessary for presenting antigens to helper T lymphocytes,* thereby inducing both cytokine secretion by and clonal proliferation of the T cells. As discussed above, this is probably most important for primary antibody responses, because in secondary responses the expanded clones of antigen-specific B lymphocytes are available for antigen presentation to T cells. There is no evidence that B lymphocytes themselves need to recognize antigens presented by accessory cells, although this may occur *in vivo* with polysaccharides, which bind to marginal zone macrophages, and in secondary responses when follicular dendritic cells bind large amounts of opsonized antigens.

2. *They secrete cytokines,* which induce the proliferation of both B and T lymphocytes. These cytokines include IL-1, TNF, and IL-6. IL-1 is known to enhance the proliferation of helper T lymphocytes; for this reason, it is likely to be most important in primary responses, when the number of specific T cells is small and needs to be expanded. In addition, IL-1 and TNF may directly stimulate B cell proliferation and IL-6 is a growth and differentiation factor for B cells.

Another accessory cell type that is believed to be important in humoral immunity, particularly in secondary antibody responses, is the **follicular dendritic cell,** which resides in the germinal centers of lymphoid follicles in the spleen and lymph nodes (and is not the same as the "dendritic cell" mentioned above). Follicular dendritic cells express high levels of Fc receptors, do not express class II MHC molecules, and are not actively phagocytic. It is thought that as an antibody response develops, immune complexes are formed and deposited on the surfaces of follicular dendritic cells. Antigen fragments may be released slowly over long periods, providing a continuous source of antigen for a low-level stimulation of B cells. This may be important for maintaining a measurable titer of circulating antibodies even against microbes that were encountered in the past. Furthermore, memory B cells, which were generated by primary immunization, either reside in germinal centers or can enter lymphoid follicles during their recirculation. These memory cells may recognize antigens on the surfaces of follicular dendritic cells, leading to secondary antibody responses.

Phenotypic Markers and Functional Surface Molecules on B Lymphocytes

In addition to Ig and class II MHC molecules, whose functions in B cell activation have been discussed in detail, B lymphocytes express a variety of cell surface proteins of immunologic significance. These have been identified by numerous techniques, the most useful of which is the production of monoclonal antibodies against B cells. Most of the cell surface molecules detected by monoclonal antibodies are not unique to B lymphocytes and can be expressed on other hematopoietic cell types. Examples of some surface molecules present on human and mouse B cells are listed in Table 9–6.

TABLE 9–6. Phenotypic Markers of B Lymphocytes

Surface Molecule	Function/Significance
Immunoglobulin (Ig)	Antigen receptor
B220 (CD45R)	Form of leukocyte common antigen; present on all B cells
Complement receptors	
C3b receptor (CR1)(CD35)	?Regulation of B cell responses
C3d receptor (CR2)(CD21)	?Regulation of B cells, receptor for Epstein-Barr virus (human only)
Fc receptors	
Fc receptors for IgG	Negative feedback control of antibody response
Low-affinity Fc receptor for IgE (CD23)	Unknown (induced by interleukin-4)
Class II MHC antigens	Role in helper T cell–B cell interaction
CD5 (Ly-1)	Marker for distinct subset of B cells
CD19 (B4)	Inhibits B cell responses
CD20 (B1)	?Early activation signal for human B cells
CD10 (CALLA)	Marker for acute leukemias
CD9	Marker for acute leukemias

These surface proteins on B cells are important for several reasons:

1. They may be lineage and maturation-specific phenotypic markers for B cells. Combinations of monoclonal antibodies reactive with B lymphocytes form clusters of differentiation that are expressed at different stages of B cell maturation (Fig. 9–7). To date, however, there are few available monoclonal antibodies that definitively distinguish between resting, activated, and memory B lymphocytes, all of which fall into the broad category of "mature B cells." Despite the production of numerous B cell–reactive monoclonal antibodies, the expression of endogenously synthesized membrane Ig is the *sine qua non* of the B lymphocyte and remains the most reliable marker for cells of the B lymphocyte lineage. Recently, a great deal of attention has been given to a small subset of B cells that express CD5 (Ly-1), which was originally identified as a marker for a subset of T lymphocytes. Only 5 to 10 per cent of B cells in the blood and lymphoid organs are CD5+, and these may express a quite limited repertoire of V genes. Surprisingly, virtually all B cell–derived chronic lymphocytic leukemias are CD5+. Moreover, CD5+ B cells spontaneously secrete IgM antibodies that often react with self antigens and these cells may be significantly expanded in autoimmune diseases. Recent work suggests that CD5+ B cells do not develop in the bone marrow, and in mice large numbers of these cells are found as a self-renewing population in the peritoneum. It is, therefore, likely that this small subset of B lymphocytes has unique properties in terms of ontogeny, function, and role in disease.

2. Various surface molecules may function in B cell activation or regulation. Our discussion so far in this chapter has focused on antigen-specific, membrane Ig-mediated B cell activation, but other surface proteins may also play a role in the functional responses of B lymphocytes. Antibodies specific for CD19, CD20, CD23, class II MHC molecules, and type 1 and type 2 complement receptors (CR1 and CR2, respectively) have all been shown to stimulate or inhibit B lymphocyte growth and/or differentiation under different experimental conditions *in vitro*. A low-affinity receptor for IgE, called CD23, is induced on B cells by culture with IL–4 and by infection with the Epstein-Barr virus, which immortalizes human B cells and induces Ig secretion. However, the physiologic function of CD23 is not known. Receptors for the Fc portions of IgG antibodies bind antigen-antibody complexes and inhibit B cell activation. This phenomenon of "antibody feedback" is an important regulatory mechanism that serves to control humoral immune responses (see Chapter 10). The physiologic ligands for most of the other surface proteins are not known, so that it is difficult to define their importance in physiologic pathways of antibody production.

3. Antibodies against surface proteins can be used to localize and treat tumors derived from B lymphocytes. Some CD antigens are expressed at high levels on tumors of B cells, so that monoclonal antibodies specific for these antigens can be used to de-

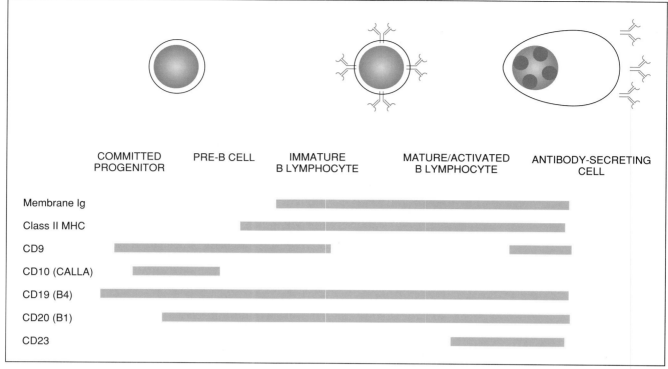

	COMMITTED PROGENITOR	PRE-B CELL	IMMATURE B LYMPHOCYTE	MATURE/ACTIVATED B LYMPHOCYTE	ANTIBODY-SECRETING CELL
Membrane Ig			▓▓▓▓▓	▓▓▓▓▓	▓▓▓▓▓
Class II MHC			▓▓▓▓	▓▓▓▓▓	▓▓▓▓▓
CD9	▓▓▓▓	▓▓▓▓	▓▓		▓▓
CD10 (CALLA)	▓▓				
CD19 (B4)	▓▓▓▓	▓▓▓▓	▓▓▓▓	▓▓▓▓▓	▓▓
CD20 (B1)		▓▓▓	▓▓▓▓	▓▓▓▓▓	
CD23				▓▓▓▓	

FIGURE 9 – 7. Ontogeny of some surface markers of human B lymphocytes. *Different surface molecules are expressed at distinct stages during the maturation and differentiation of B lymphocytes. (Adapted with permission from Zola, H. The surface antigens of human B lymphocytes. Immunology Today 8:308 – 315, 1987.)*

stroy or remove tumor cells. One recent application of such antibodies is in a treatment protocol in which bone marrow is removed from patients with B cell–derived leukemias, treated with antibodies specific for CD9 and CD10 to destroy tumor cells, the patient is given high doses of radiation and/or chemotherapy, and the treated marrow devoid of leukemic cells is injected back to reconstitute the hematopoietic system.

4. Some surface proteins are receptors for cytokines. B cells express high affinity receptors for several cytokines, including IL–1, IL–2, IL–4, IL–5, and IL–6. In general, resting B cells express low numbers of cytokine receptors (a few hundred to 1000 per cell) and expression is enhanced on B cells stimulated via membrane Ig, e.g., with anti-Ig antibody, or by other polyclonal activators.

The advent of hybridoma technology has vastly increased the potential for identifying molecules on B cells that are functionally important. So far, however, these approaches have not proved as fruitful as they have for analyzing the differentiation and functions of T lymphocytes.

SUMMARY

Antibody responses are initiated by the interaction of antigen with specific membrane Ig molecules on B lymphocytes. This interaction stimulates resting B cells to enter the cell cycle, presumably via the production of a variety of intracellular second messengers. In addition, thymus- (or T cell–) dependent protein antigens are processed by the B cells and presented in association with class II MHC molecules to antigen-specific, class II MHC–restricted helper T lymphocytes. The MHC–restricted interaction between B and helper T lymphocytes itself delivers activating signals to resting B cells and also leads to the secretion of various cytokines by the T cells. Different cytokines induce proliferation of B cells, secretion of antibody, heavy chain isotype switching, and other features of the humoral immune response to protein antigens. Accessory cells like macrophages may play a critical role, particularly in primary antibody responses, by presenting antigens to T cells and by secreting cytokines that promote the expansion and differentiation of both B and T lymphocytes.

Thymus-independent antigens induce antibody responses without the participation of antigen-specific helper T cells. Some TI antigens, called TI–1, are polyclonal activators of B lymphocytes and stimulate B cells in the absence of known cytokines by mechanisms that are not defined. Other TI antigens, called TI–2, are usually polymeric polysaccharides that efficiently cross-link membrane Ig on B cells and may require small numbers of T cells (which are not antigen-specific and presumably provide cytokines) for inducing optimal antibody production by the B cells.

Elucidation of the mechanisms operative in humoral immunity is central to the understanding and potential treatment of disorders associated with excessive or deficient antibody production. In addition, the ability to specifically alter patterns of Ig gene expression by defined external stimuli provides valuable models for analyzing the mechanisms of signal transduction in B lymphocytes, and may lead to paradigms that are applicable to diverse biologic systems.

SELECTED READINGS

Abbas, A. K. A reassessment of the mechanisms of antigen-specific T cell–dependent B cell activation. Immunology Today 9:89–94, 1988.

Cambier, J. C., and J. T. Ransom. Molecular mechanisms of transmembrane signaling in B lymphocytes. Annual Review of Immunology 5:175–199, 1987.

Chesnut, R. W., and H. M. Grey. Antigen presentation by B cells and its significance in T-B interactions. Advances in Immunology 39:51–94, 1986.

Finkelman, F. D., J. Holmes, I. M. Katona, J. F. Urban, M. P. Beckmann, L. S. Park, K. A. Schooley, R. L. Coffman, T. R. Mosmann, and W. E. Paul. Lymphokine control of in vivo immunoglobulin isotype selection. Annual Review of Immunology 8:303–333, 1990.

deFranco, A. L. Molecular aspects of B-lymphocyte activation. Annual Review of Cell Biology 3:143–178, 1987.

Hayakawa, K., and R. R. Hardy. Normal, autoimmune, and malignant CD5+ B cells: the Ly-1 B lineage. Annual Review of Immunology 6:197–218, 1988.

Jelinek, D. F., and P. E. Lipsky. Regulation of human B lymphocyte activation, proliferation and differentiation. Advances in Immunology 40:1–60, 1987.

Kishimoto, T., and T. Hirano. Molecular regulation of B lymphocyte response. Annual Review of Immunology 6:485–512, 1988.

Lanzavecchia, A. Receptor-mediated antigen uptake and its effect on antigen presentation to class II MHC-restricted T lymphocytes. Annual Review of Immunology 8:773–793, 1990.

Mosmann, T. R., and R. L. Coffman. Heterogeneity of cytokine secretion patterns and functions of helper T cells. Advances in Immunology 46:111–147, 1989.

Snapper, C. M., and W. E. Paul. Interferon-γ and B cell stimulatory factor-1 reciprocally regulate Ig isotype production. Science 236:944–947, 1987.

Vitetta, E. S., R. Fernandez-Botran, C. D. Myers, and V. M. Sanders. Cellular interactions in the humoral immune response. Advances in Immunology 45:1–105, 1989.

CHAPTER TEN

IMMUNOLOGIC TOLERANCE AND THE REGULATION OF IMMUNE RESPONSES

In the previous chapters of this book we have discussed how foreign antigens stimulate T and B lymphocytes, leading to the induction of immune responses. Antigens can also inhibit specific immune responses. In fact, it is possible that the consequence of exposure of the immune system to all antigens and all types of immunization is a balance between stimulation and inhibition. Antigens can be administered in particular physicochemical forms or in ways that preferentially lead to either induction or inhibition of specific immune responses. This ability to manipulate responses to antigens can be exploited clinically to augment or suppress specific immunity, e.g., in pathologic states associated with excessive immunity. This chapter describes the mechanisms by which various antigens inhibit immune responses and the factors that determine the nature and magnitude of responses to different antigens and forms of immunization. This discussion will conclude our description of how the immune system recognizes and responds to antigens, i.e., the cognitive and activation phases of immune responses.

The inhibitory effects of antigens are important in three situations. First, individuals are unresponsive to, or tolerant of, their own antigens because self antigens block the maturation of lymphocytes that they specifically interact with or inhibit the growth and differentiation of self-reactive lymphocytes. Second, some forms of foreign antigens either fail to induce specific immunity or actually inhibit the activation of specific lymphocytes. Third, the suppressive effects of foreign antigens may play a crucial role in the physiologic down-regulation of all normal immune responses, because of which such responses are self-regulated and wane as the antigenic stimulus is eliminated. Elimination of antigen is itself an important mechanism for self-regulation of the immune response. The reason for this is that many of the products of lymphocyte activation, such as antibodies and cytokines, have short half-lives and are secreted only for brief periods after antigenic stimulation. Furthermore, the effector cells that are produced as a result of antigen-induced lymphocyte differentiation are also short-lived and are not self-renewing. Plasma cells are the best example of this. *In addition to antigen elimination, however, the immune system has evolved a number of regulatory mechanisms whose principal function is to prevent uncontrolled immune responses.*

Antigen-induced block in the development, growth, or differentiation of specific lymphocytes is called **immunologic tolerance.** Tolerance results from the interaction of antigen with antigen receptors on lymphocytes under conditions in which the lymphocytes, instead of becoming activated, are killed or rendered unresponsive. (The term immunologic tolerance is also used to refer to antigen-induced inhibition of immune responses in an individual or experimental animal. In this situation, tolerance may be due to tolerance of specific T or B lymphocytes or to other regulatory mechanisms that prevent lymphocyte activation.) The second possible mechanism for inhibiting an immune response is the stimulation of a class of lymphocytes, called **suppressor T cells,** whose principal function is to suppress the activation of specific T and B lymphocytes. In this case, inhibition is mediated not by the antigen itself but by regulatory cells that are induced by the antigen. Third, it has been postulated that when antigens stimulate the expansion of specific lymphocytes or the production of specific antibodies, the immune system mounts a response to the unique or idiotypic determinants of these lymphocytes or antibodies. Such a **network of complementary idiotypes and anti-idiotypes** may serve to block the stimulation of antigen-specific cells. This type of regulation is initiated by antigen but is actually mediated by immune responses against the lymphocytes that first recognized the antigen. Finally, the products of activation of B and T lymphocytes, namely **antibodies** and **cytokines,** respectively, are themselves capable of regulating specific immunity in addition to functioning as the principal effector molecules of lymphocytes.

The following sections of the chapter describe each of these regulatory mechanisms and their possible contributions to self-tolerance, to the maintenance of homeostasis in the immune system, and to the failure of some antigens or immunization conditions to generate immunity.

IMMUNOLOGIC TOLERANCE

Lymphocyte activation and tolerance are the two possible results of lymphocyte recognition of antigens. Antigens that induce tolerance are called **tolerogens,** to be distinguished from **immunogens,** which generate immune responses. Tolerance to self antigens is a fundamental property of the immune system, and its loss leads to autoimmune diseases (see Chapter 18). Normally, all self antigens are tolerogens. Many foreign antigens can be immunogens or tolerogens, depending on their physicochemical form, dose, and route of administration. Exposure of an individual to immunogenic antigens stimulates specific immunity, and for most immunogenic proteins subsequent exposures generate enhanced secondary responses. In contrast, exposure to a tolerogenic antigen not only fails to induce specific immunity but also inhibits lymphocyte activation by subsequent administration of immunogenic forms of the same antigen (Fig. 10–1). *This antigen-induced, immunologically specific inactivation of lymphocytes is the hallmark of all forms of tolerance.* Thus, the mechanisms responsible for inducing and maintaining lymphocyte tolerance are of central importance because they determine how the immune system discriminates between self and non-self and also how the system responds to different forms of foreign antigens. Although operationally one can distinguish between tolerance to self and to foreign antigens, the cellular and biochemical mechanisms responsible for lymphocyte unresponsiveness to all tolerogens may be the same, as we shall discuss later.

The necessity for maintaining self-tolerance was

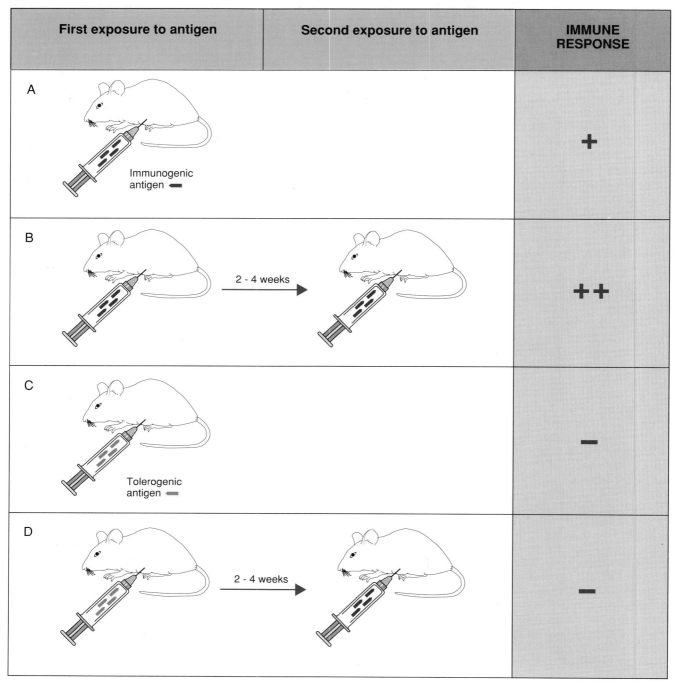

First exposure to antigen	Second exposure to antigen	IMMUNE RESPONSE
A — Immunogenic antigen		+
B — 2 - 4 weeks →		++
C — Tolerogenic antigen		−
D — 2 - 4 weeks →		−

FIGURE 10 – 1. The induction of immunologic tolerance. *An immunogenic antigen stimulates a specific immune response (A) and a stronger secondary response upon subsequent immunization (B). A tolerogenic form of the same antigen does not induce an immune response (C) and prevents the response to subsequent immunization with the immunogenic antigen (D).*

appreciated from the early days of immunology, when the characteristics and specificities of antibody responses to foreign antigens were being defined. The classical studies of Peter Medawar and his colleagues in the 1950s demonstrated, for the first time, that tolerance was an immunologic phenomenon that could be analyzed experimentally. They showed that a mouse of one inbred strain could be made tolerant to the tissue histocompatibility antigens of a different strain by neonatal injection of lymphoid cells from the sec-

ond strain. Once it became an adult, the recipient of the neonatal injection would accept a skin graft from the immunizing strain (Fig. 10 – 2). Moreover, lymphocytes from the recipient would not proliferate when cultured with cells from the donor strain in a mixed leukocyte reaction (see Chapter 16). This induced unresponsiveness to allogeneic major histocompatibility complex (MHC) – encoded molecules was highly specific, since the recipient mouse would reject skin allografts and would respond to stimulator cells

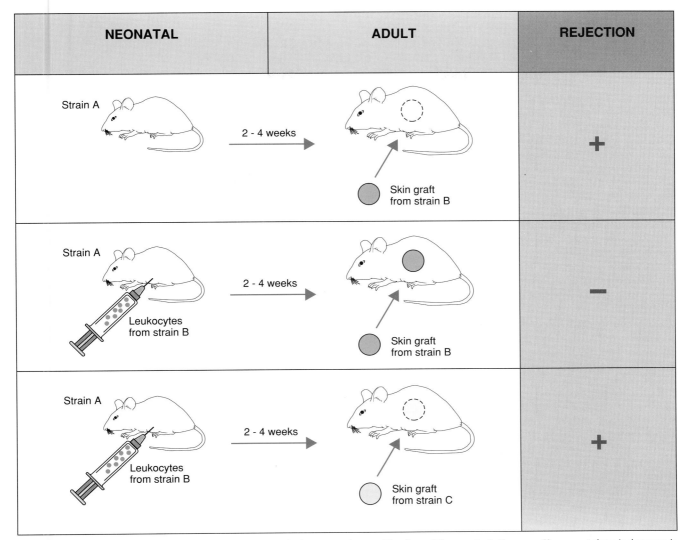

NEONATAL	ADULT	REJECTION

FIGURE 10–2. Neonatal tolerance to allografts. *A normal adult strain A mouse rejects a skin allograft from a strain B mouse. If a neonatal strain A mouse is injected with strain B leukocytes, once the mouse becomes an adult, it fails to reject a skin graft from strain B. This form of tolerance is immunologically specific because the strain A mouse rejects a graft from a strain C donor. In this example, lymphocytes from the neonatally injected strain A mouse will not respond* in vitro *to strain B stimulators (in a mixed leukocyte reaction) but will respond normally to strain C stimulators.*

from all strains that differed from the donor at the MHC locus. Medawar's experiments were also the first to formally demonstrate that although adult animals rejected grafts of foreign cells, exposure of immature (neonatal) animals to foreign antigens, in this case allogeneic MHC molecules, induced long-lived and specific unresponsiveness to these antigens. This form of tolerance, although induced by a single injection of foreign cells, is long-lived probably because some of the injected allogeneic cells survive in the recipient, which is now a "chimera." Thus, immature lymphocytes specific for the donor MHC, which are generated throughout the life of the recipient animal, encounter the persisting donor cells, and this leads to tolerance induction.

Later studies showed that not only cell-associated MHC molecules but also soluble antigens could induce specific tolerance in immature lymphocytes and that certain forms of antigens were tolerogenic

even for mature lymphocytes. Until recently, much of our understanding of self-tolerance was based on experiments done with tolerogenic forms of foreign antigens. As we shall discuss later, molecular techniques and transgenic mice now offer approaches for directly analyzing tolerance to self antigens that are expressed throughout the life of each individual.

General Properties of Immunologic Tolerance

Studies done in a variety of experimental systems have established the following general properties of immunologic tolerance.

1. *Tolerance is immunologically specific,* and, therefore, must be due to the deletion or inactivation of antigen-specific T and/or B lymphocytes. Both lym-

phocyte activation and tolerance are induced by interactions of antigens with the same types of clonally distributed receptors on antigen-specific cells, i.e., membrane immunoglobulin (Ig) on B cells or the $\alpha\beta$ T cell receptor on MHC–restricted T cells. Whether such interactions result in activation or tolerance depends on the maturational stage of the specific lymphocytes and the nature of the antigenic stimulus.

2. *Tolerance to self is learned or acquired.* The potential for autoreactivity exists in all individuals because V genes encoding lymphocyte receptors that might recognize self antigens are present in the germline. Therefore, self-tolerance is induced and maintained by mechanisms that prevent the maturation or stimulation of lymphocyte clones that express receptors for self antigens.

3. *Immature or developing lymphocytes are more susceptible to tolerance induction than are mature or functionally competent cells.* The maintenance of tolerance requires the continuous availability of tolerogenic antigens to interact with immature lymphocytes as they develop from precursors. In fact, during their normal maturation, all lymphocytes may go through a stage at which antigen recognition leads to their death or inactivation. This is, of course, important for maintaining self-tolerance, since potentially self-reactive lymphocyte clones are generated from marrow stem cells for many years in humans and perhaps throughout the life span of each individual. It is also the reason why immunization of neonatal mice, even with foreign antigens, usually leads to unresponsiveness. (Neonatal humans are more immunologically mature than newborn mice, and can be vaccinated shortly after birth.)

4. *Tolerance to foreign antigens is induced even in mature lymphocytes when these cells are exposed to antigens under conditions that are inadequate for activation.* Examples of immunization conditions that favor tolerance induction are mentioned later in the chapter.

Immunologic tolerance in T and B lymphocytes can be induced by two basic mechanisms: (1) the **deletion,** through cell death, of immature lymphocytes that interact with their specific antigens, and (2) the **functional inactivation,** or **anergy,** of lymphocytes that is also induced by encounter with the tolerogen. As we mentioned earlier in this chapter, it is also possible that an individual may not respond to a particular antigen despite the presence of mature, antigen-responsive lymphocytes. In these situations, the growth and differentiation of immunocompetent lymphocytes may be actively inhibited by other mechanisms, such as suppressor T cells. Thus, failure of an individual's immune system to respond to an antigen may be due to any combination of the absence or inactivation of T and/or B lymphocytes and the inhibitory effects of suppressor cells. We will first discuss how T and B lymphocytes are deleted or rendered unresponsive by interacting with tolerogenic antigens; regulation by suppressor cells is discussed later in this chapter.

Mechanisms of T Lymphocyte Tolerance

Tolerance of T lymphocytes is a particularly effective way for maintaining long-lived unresponsiveness to self antigens, for several reasons. First, as we have discussed in previous chapters, class II MHC–restricted helper T cells are critical control elements for all cellular and humoral immune responses. Second, experimental evidence indicates that T cells are rendered unresponsive at very low concentrations of antigens and many self proteins may be present in the circulation and in tissues at low levels.

The available experimental data indicate that tolerance in MHC–restricted T cells may be induced and maintained by both of the mechanisms mentioned previously, *clonal deletion* and *clonal anergy.*

Deletion of self-reactive clones of cytolytic and helper T lymphocytes occurs during the maturation of these cells in the thymus. This process of negative selection results from the specific recognition of MHC–associated protein antigens by developing T cells and has been discussed in detail in Chapter 8. Clonal deletion is the most effective mechanism for inducing T cell tolerance to protein antigens that are present in the thymus. One would predict that antigens present on one's own cells are available in the thymus for interacting with developing T lymphocytes. It is, therefore, not surprising that tolerance to self MHC and other cell surface molecules is induced by clonal deletion of specific T cells in the thymus. What is unexpected is the finding that many other self proteins may be present in the thymus in forms that can be recognized by MHC–restricted T cells. One documented example of such a protein is self hemoglobin in mice. On the other hand, it is also likely that at least some self proteins may never reside in the thymus, so that developing T cells may not have access to these antigens and the specific clones may not be deleted. Therefore, tolerance to these proteins is probably induced in the periphery, after mature T cells have migrated out of the thymus.

The second mechanism of T cell tolerance, the induction of *clonal anergy,* has been demonstrated largely by *in vitro* experiments with cloned lines of antigen-specific class II MHC–restricted, CD4+ T cells. As discussed in Chapter 7, maximal stimulation of CD4+ T cells requires two signals: (1) recognition of class II MHC–associated processed antigens on antigen-presenting cells (APCs), and (2) additional stimuli, collectively called "costimulators," that are provided by the APCs. When such T cells recognize an MHC–associated antigen on APCs that do not produce the necessary costimulators, the T cells survive and even continue to express receptors for the antigen, but they become unresponsive to subsequent stimulation by the same antigen presented by competent APCs such as macrophages and B cells. For example, human CD4+ T cells become unresponsive when they recognize antigens that are processed and presented by other human T cells, which do express

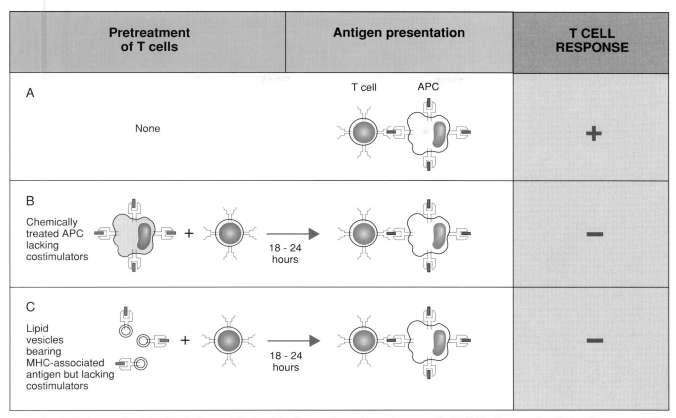

Pretreatment of T cells	Antigen presentation	T CELL RESPONSE
A None	T cell APC	+
B Chemically treated APC lacking costimulators	18 - 24 hours	−
C Lipid vesicles bearing MHC-associated antigen but lacking costimulators	18 - 24 hours	−

FIGURE 10–3. Mechanisms of peripheral T cell tolerance: induction of clonal anergy. A peptide antigen-specific CD4+ T cell responds to that antigen presented by MHC–matched antigen-presenting cells (APCs) (A). Exposure of the T cell to the same peptide presented on chemically treated class II MHC+ APCs (B) or on class II–bearing lipid vesicles (C) inhibits subsequent responses to the antigen presented by competent APCs.

class II MHC molecules but not the obligatory co-stimulators. Similarly, cloned lines of mouse CD4+ T cells specific for known peptides and class II MHC molecules are rendered tolerant when they recognize peptide-MHC complexes presented on synthetic lipid membranes or on APCs that are treated with chemicals that destroy costimulator activities (Fig. 10–3). It is postulated that the same mechanism is responsible for the induction of specific T cell tolerance *in vivo* by the administration of large doses of antigens in aqueous solutions, in the absence of adjuvants. Such antigens may be presented by class II MHC-bearing cells that do not produce costimulators. For instance, a mouse or rat injected with aqueous deaggregated human γ-globulin (HGG) becomes unresponsive to subsequent immunization with aggregated HGG in adjuvant. The likely reason for this is that the deaggregated HGG is presented by APCs lacking costimulators, leading to anergy of HGG–specific CD4+ T cells. Conversely, the administration of protein antigens with adjuvants recruits and activates macrophages, which are competent APCs that do produce costimulators and, therefore, promote T cell activation and prevent tolerance induction. Such results support the hypothesis that the activation of all lymphocytes may require antigen and a second signal, and antigen alone is either nonstimulatory or inhibitory. Self-reactive T cells may also be rendered anergic during their matu-

ration in the thymus, without being deleted. However, the biochemical mechanisms of clonal anergy and the nature and mechanisms of actions of costimulators are largely unknown.

Although T cell tolerance may be the principal mechanism for unresponsiveness to self proteins, it cannot be the mechanism for tolerance to self polysaccharides and lipids because these are not recognized by MHC–restricted T cells. For instance, it has been known for decades that individuals do not make antibodies against their own ABO blood group antigens, which are glycolipids with the ability to stimulate T cell–independent antibody production. Tolerance to such self antigens must be induced directly in B lymphocytes.

Mechanisms of B Lymphocyte Tolerance

As in T lymphocytes, the two principal mechanisms of tolerance induction in B cells are clonal deletion and anergy (Fig. 10–4).

Deletion of antigen-specific B cell clones may occur as B cells arise in the bone marrow and encounter self antigens before they have become functionally competent, perhaps at the stage in their development

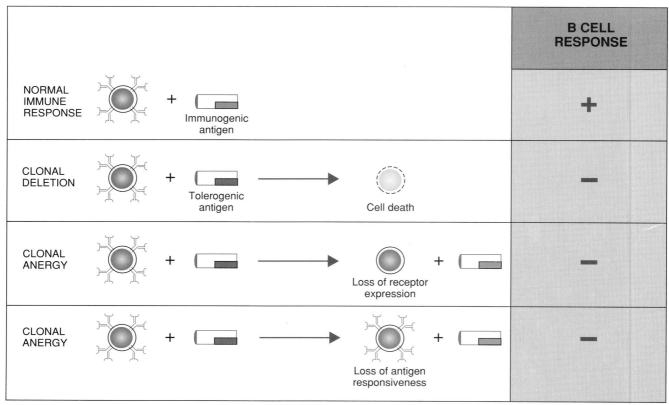

FIGURE 10 – 4. Mechanisms of B lymphocyte tolerance. *A tolerogenic antigen may induce unresponsiveness in the antigen-specific clone of B cells by causing cell death, inhibiting antigen receptor expression, or blocking functional activation. B cell responses are usually measured as antibody production and may require helper T lymphocytes (not shown).*

when they express only the IgM form of membrane receptors for antigens (see Chapter 4, Fig. 4–1). The observation that immature IgM-expressing B cells are tolerance-sensitive whereas mature IgM + IgD-bearing B cells are activated by antigen has led to the postulate that the interaction of antigen with membrane IgM on B cells delivers a lethal or inhibitory signal whereas interaction with IgD is stimulatory. However, to date consistent differences in the biochemical effects of antigen binding to membrane IgM and IgD have not been found.

Clonal deletion of B lymphocytes has been demonstrated in experiments with transgenic mice which express Ig heavy and light chain genes coding for an antibody specific for a class I MHC molecule, the H-2K^k molecule. If these Ig transgenes are expressed in mice of an H-2 haplotype other than H-2^k, most of the peripheral B cells produce the transgenic Ig (endogenous Ig gene rearrangement is blocked by allelic exclusion, as described in Chapter 4). However, if the transgenes are expressed in mice of the H-2^k haplotype, the peripheral lymphoid tissues contain reduced numbers of B cells and none of the surviving B cells produces the transgenic Ig. Thus, the interaction of developing B cells specific for a self MHC molecule with this MHC molecule leads to deletion of the B cells. *However, clonal deletion may play a relatively minor role in B cell tolerance.* This is suggested by

experiments using polyclonal B cell activators, such as lipopolysaccharide, which stimulate virtually all functionally responsive B cells irrespective of their antigenic specificities and without T cell help. Mice injected with lipopolysaccharide produce a variety of antibodies, including autoantibodies that bind to their own cells. This result indicates that many B cells capable of producing antibodies against self antigens may be present in normal animals, implying that they are not deleted but are incapable of being stimulated by the self antigens. The possibility that microbial infections, which cause polyclonal B cell activation, may play a role in autoantibody production and the pathogenesis of autoimmune diseases is discussed in Chapter 18.

When self antigen-specific B cells are present but unresponsive to antigenic stimulation, tolerance may be a result of *clonal anergy* induced by an antigen-receptor interaction. Experimentally, B cells have been shown to become unresponsive to antigenic stimulation by two mechanisms: (1) an antigen-induced block in membrane Ig expression before the cells mature to a stage of functional competence, and (2) functional anergy even with persistent receptor expression (Fig. 10–4). Inhibition of antigen receptor expression (also called clonal abortion) was discovered when the effects of anti-Ig antibody, which are functional analogs of antigens, were examined on mature (adult) and immature (neonatal) mouse B cells. If mature B cells are cultured with anti-Ig antibodies, the membrane Ig molecules are endocytosed and over the next 8 to 24 hours a new set of Ig proteins is synthesized and expressed on the cell surface (see Chapter 9, Fig. 9–3). In contrast, if neonatal B cells, taken from mice that are about a week old, are exposed to the same anti-Ig antibody, the membrane Ig is again endocytosed but new receptor molecules are not produced. Such findings imply that *in vivo,* if immature B cells encounter self or foreign antigens, the cells are not killed but their antigen receptors may be permanently lost and they become unresponsive to these antigens. If, however, these tolerant B cells are stimulated by a polyclonal activator, such as lipopolysaccharide, which functions independently of membrane Ig, they will be induced to secrete antibodies. This may account for the ability of lipopolysaccharide to induce the production of autoantibodies even in normal mice.

Other experiments have shown that if immature or mature B cells are exposed to certain tolerogenic antigens, the cells become anergic to immunogenic forms of these antigens even though receptor expression is not completely abrogated. Among the most potent tolerogens for B cells are antigens containing multiple repeating epitopes, such as polysaccharides. It is speculated that such antigens are effective at cross-linking membrane Ig molecules on B cells, but cannot be processed and presented to helper T cells and, therefore, do not stimulate T cell help. This is again consistent with the two-signal concept of lymphocyte activation, which was mentioned earlier for T cells. Antigen-induced cross-linking of membrane Ig (the first signal) in the absence of T cell help (which is a competent second signal) may have a net inhibitory effect on B lymphocytes.

The importance of clonal anergy as a mechanism of B cell tolerance to self antigens was most clearly demonstrated by experiments using transgenic mice that were first reported in 1988 (Fig. 10–5). In these experiments, two sets of transgenic mice were created, one expressing a transgene encoding a foreign protein, hen egg lysozyme (HEL), and another expressing functionally rearranged Ig heavy chain and light chain genes coding for anti-HEL antibody. The Ig transgenic mice had high serum levels of the anti-HEL antibody, and most of their B cells produced this Ig. The two sets of mice were mated, so that in the F1 offspring the B cells that were producing HEL–specific Ig were exposed from their earliest developmental stage to HEL, which was now in essence a self protein. In these F1 mice, there was no detectable anti-HEL antibody, even after immunization with HEL by itself or conjugated to other proteins. The B cells in the F1 animals expressed HEL–specific membrane Ig, albeit at reduced levels, suggesting that they were not deleted but had been rendered anergic. If the HEL–specific B cells from the F1 transgenic animals were transferred into normal syngeneic recipients that did not contain the HEL transgene, they gradually regained responsiveness to immunization with HEL.

TABLE 10–1. Tolerance in T and B Lymphocytes

	T Lymphocytes	B Lymphocytes
Clonal deletion	Induced in thymus by protein antigens	Induced at unknown sites (bone marrow, periphery?) by proteins and probably non-protein antigens
	Mechanism: high-affinity binding of antigen to immature T cells may lead to cell death (apoptosis)	*Mechanism:* unknown
Clonal anergy	Induced by recognition of MHC–associated protein antigen on APCs lacking co-stimulators	Generally induced by binding of multivalent antigen to immature B cells
	Mechanism: block in T cell activation; normal levels of antigen receptors, CD3, and accessory molecules; biochemical mechanisms unknown	*Mechanisms:* (1) inhibition of membrane Ig expression, or (2) block in B cell activation; biochemical mechanisms unknown
Tolerogenic forms of foreign antigens	Aqueous proteins administered intravenously or orally, without adjuvants	High doses of polysaccharides, polymeric proteins (multiple repeating epitopes) in the absence of helper T cell stimulation
Duration of tolerance	Long-lived	Relatively short-lived
Tolerogenic dose of antigen	Relatively low (may vary with different antigens)	Relatively high

Therefore, clonal anergy in B cells may be short-lived, continuous exposure to antigen is required, and the cells recover if the tolerogen is removed.

It is clear that the mechanisms of tolerance induction in T and B lymphocytes are similar in some respects, but there may also be important differences (Table 10–1). In the final analysis, much remains to be learned about immunologic tolerance. In particular, little is known about the molecular mechanisms of clonal deletion or anergy in lymphocytes or about differences in the biochemical effects of immunogens and tolerogens on specific T and B cells.

SUPPRESSOR T LYMPHOCYTES

Suppressor T cells comprise a class of lymphocytes thought to be distinct from helper and cytolytic T lymphocytes (CTLs), whose function is to inhibit the activation phase of immune responses. The existence of suppressor cells was first demonstrated by Richard Gershon and his associates in the late 1960s, using a rather complicated protocol involving immunizing thymectomized and bone marrow–transplanted mice. In principle, a simpler demonstration of suppressor cell effects is the following (Table

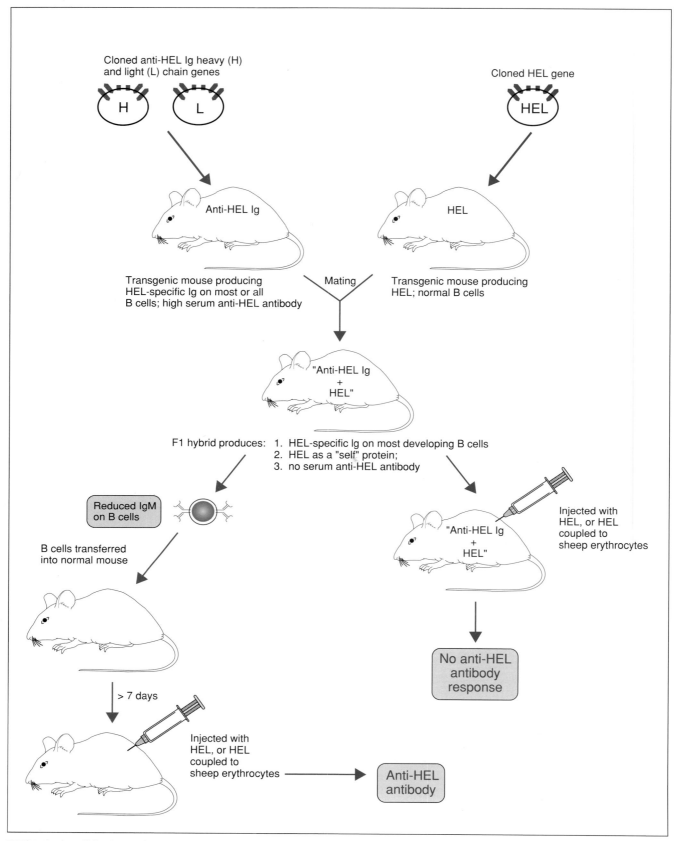

Cloned anti-HEL Ig heavy (H)
and light (L) chain genes

Cloned HEL gene

H   L

HEL

Anti-HEL Ig

HEL

Transgenic mouse producing
HEL-specific Ig on most or all
B cells; high serum anti-HEL antibody

Mating

Transgenic mouse producing
HEL; normal B cells

"Anti-HEL Ig
+
HEL"

F1 hybrid produces: 1. HEL-specific Ig on most developing B cells
                      2. HEL as a "self" protein;
                      3. no serum anti-HEL antibody

Reduced IgM
on B cells

B cells transferred
into normal mouse

"Anti-HEL Ig
+
HEL"

Injected with
HEL, or HEL
coupled to
sheep erythrocytes

No anti-HEL
antibody
response

> 7 days

Injected with
HEL, or HEL
coupled to
sheep erythrocytes

Anti-HEL
antibody

FIGURE 10 – 5. B cell clonal anergy to a "self" antigen in transgenic mice. *A transgenic mouse expressing anti-HEL Ig is bred with another transgenic mouse that produces HEL. In the "double transgenic" F1 hybrid mouse, most B cells express HEL – specific Ig and HEL is a "self" antigen. Such mice do not produce anti-HEL antibody and fail to respond to immunization with HEL or HEL coupled to another antigen, sheep red blood cells (SRBC); in the latter case, unresponsiveness must be due to tolerance of HEL – specific B cells because SRBC – specific T cells can provide help, yet there is no antibody response. Transfer of B cells into normal syngeneic recipients leads to gradual recovery of function. HEL, hen egg lysozyme; Ig, immunoglobulin.*

TABLE 10-2. Identification of Antigen-Specific Suppressor T Cells

Mice Injected with		Antibody Response to	
T Lymphocytes from	Antigen	Antigen X	Antigen Y
None	Antigen X (immunogenic dose)	+	ND
None	Antigen X (suppressive dose)	−	ND
Mice previously given immunogenic dose of antigen X	Antigen X (immunogenic dose)	+	ND
Mice previously given suppressive dose of antigen X	Antigen X (immunogenic dose)	−	ND
Mice previously given suppressive dose of antigen X	Antigen Y (immunogenic dose)	ND	+

Normal mice respond to an immunogenic dose of antigen X but not to a suppressive dose (e.g., high dose of antigen without adjuvant). If T cells from mice given a suppressive dose of antigen X are adoptively transferred into normal syngeneic recipients, the response of the recipients to antigen X but not to antigen Y is inhibited. Thus, the immunosuppressive dose of antigen X induces specific suppressor T cells.

Abbreviation: ND, not done.

10-2). Animals given an antigen in an immunogenic dose and form mount specific immune responses. If the antigen is injected under non-immunogenic conditions, e.g., high doses of aqueous antigen administered intravenously, the animals do not respond and may also be rendered unresponsive to subsequent administration of normally immunogenic antigen. This, of course, is often due to the induction of tolerance in specific lymphocytes. In other situations, however, if the lymphocytes from these unresponsive animals are adoptively transferred into syngeneic recipients, the recipients also fail to respond to the normally immunogenic antigen. This inhibition is immunologically specific because the recipients of the adoptive transfer respond normally to a different antigen. Subsequent studies showed that this form of unresponsiveness, which could be transferred from one individual to another, was mediated by Thy-1+ lymphocytes, which were termed **suppressor T cells.** From such studies evolved the hypothesis that the function of suppressor cells is to inhibit the activation of functionally competent antigen-specific T and/or B lymphocytes.

Suppressor T cells may be important in two situations. First, they may be critical for preventing immune responses to self antigens that are not accessible to immature lymphocytes and therefore cannot induce tolerance. For instance, self proteins that do not reach the thymus cannot induce deletion of potentially self-reactive T cell clones. Second, suppressor cells can inhibit immune responses to foreign antigens. In the 1970s, many experimental systems were used to study suppressor cells and their excessive or deficient function was invoked as the primary basis for a variety of immunologic abnormalities. However, for reasons that are discussed below, progress in our understanding of suppressor T cells has been slow, so that their significance and even their existence is doubted by many investigators.

Studies with cultured human lymphocytes and experimental animals have shown that *suppressor T cells have the following properties:*

1. Suppressor T cells are generally induced by the same immunization conditions that induce clonal anergy of lymphocytes, such as high concentrations of protein antigens or chemically reactive haptens administered without adjuvants or injected intravenously. It has been postulated that such conditions of immunization favor direct interactions of antigens with lymphocytes without the participation of APCs, and suppressor cells were thought to recognize antigens in the absence of MHC molecules.

2. In most experimental systems, the cells that inhibit immune responses are CD8+. Their growth and differentiation may be dependent on CD4+ cells.

3. In mice, different populations of suppressor T cells have been shown to be specific for antigens, such as proteins or haptens, or for the idiotypic determinants of lymphocyte receptors or secreted antibodies (see below). Most studies with human suppressor T lymphocytes have examined the inhibitory effects of CD8+ cells on the responses of polyclonally stimulated B or T cells, and there are few documented examples of antigen-specific or idiotype-specific human suppressor cells. It is, therefore, difficult to draw general conclusions about the immunologic specificity of suppressor cells in humans.

4. The role of the MHC in the development and activation of suppressor T cells is also unclear. Some studies indicate that antigen recognition by suppressor cells, unlike that by most other mature T lymphocytes, is not MHC–restricted, because suppressor cells can bind to native antigens in the absence of APCs or MHC molecules. Some studies in humans have shown that suppressor T cells from one individual can inhibit the activation of lymphocytes from another HLA–disparate individual. Other experiments

done in mice indicated that the stimulation of suppressor T cells may be restricted by a region of the class II MHC that was called "I-J" and thought to be located between the I-A and I-E loci based on analyses of various inbred strains. However, sequencing of the entire mouse class II MHC has conclusively demonstrated that there is no DNA coding for a unique "I-J" molecule at this site, and attempts to demonstrate an "I-J"–encoded cell surface protein have generally failed. The explanation for this apparent artifact remains obscure.

5. The inhibitory effects of suppressor T cells are mediated by secreted proteins. Unlike the cytokines produced by other T lymphocytes, which are not antigen-specific, the suppressor factors secreted by murine suppressor T cells may have the same antigenic or idiotypic specificities as the T cells themselves. This has led to the postulate that suppressor factors are functionally active secreted forms of T lymphocyte receptors, much as secreted and membrane Ig are two forms of the same antigen-specific B lymphocyte product. It is not known how these suppressor factors inhibit immune responses and whether their primary effect is on T or B cells. Recently, several investigators have shown that suppressor cells express CD3–associated T cell receptor $\alpha\beta$ heterodimers and release these proteins in soluble form into culture supernatants. It is possible that soluble receptor molecules bind to MHC–associated antigens on APCs and competitively inhibit the activation of other T cells. However, it is not known whether this occurs *in vivo* or whether secreted T cell receptors play a significant role in the physiologic down-regulation of specific immune responses.

A major problem in the study of suppressor T cells has been that attempts to purify these cells in numbers sufficient for biochemical analyses of receptors and secreted products or to establish stable cloned lines or hybridomas with specific suppressive activity have been largely unsuccessful. As a result, even basic questions, such as the nature of the receptors expressed by suppressor cells, are unresolved. The few suppressor clones and hybridomas that have been established show variable patterns of T cell receptor gene expression and often do not contain functionally rearranged $\alpha\beta$ or $\gamma\delta$ genes. Isolation, biochemical characterization, and molecular cloning of suppressor factors have also not been successful despite considerable effort. It is, therefore, not possible at present to construct a model for the specificity, mode of action, or function of suppressor T cells that fits all the available data.

Despite these concerns, it is likely that some antigens can stimulate lymphocyte populations whose major effect is the down-regulation of specific immune responses. It may be that suppressor T cells are not a unique cell population but actually consist of lymphocytes that can inhibit immune responses in different ways. Like other T lymphocytes, *suppressor cells may recognize antigens or idiotypes in a specific manner, and may function by various non-specific effector mechanisms.* These inhibitory mechanisms could include the following:

1. Suppressor cells may produce an excess of cytokines with inhibitory function. Because cytokines have both stimulatory and inhibitory effects on lymphocytes, the nature and magnitude of the overall immune response are determined by the relative proportions of different cytokines at the site of immune activation. For instance, transforming growth factor-β (TGF-β) is a powerful inhibitor of T and B cell proliferation, and γ-interferon (IFN-γ) inhibits the proliferation of B cells *in vitro*. Therefore, an excess of TGF-β or IFN-γ can inhibit immune responses and cells that secrete large amounts of these cytokines may function as suppressor cells.

2. Suppressor cells can absorb necessary growth and differentiation factors. Mouse T cells stimulated with the lectin concanavalin A (ConA), a potent polyclonal activator, express large numbers of high-affinity receptors for interleukin-2 (IL-2), which is a lymphocyte growth and differentiation factor. ConA-activated T cells function as nonspecific suppressors of a variety of immune responses *in vitro*, presumably by absorbing IL-2 and inhibiting the stimulation of other lymphocytes in the culture. To date, however, there is no demonstrated example of such a phenomenon occurring *in vivo* or in cultures of lymphocytes stimulated with antigens.

3. Suppressor cells may have cytolytic activity. Antigen-specific CD8+ and some CD4+ T lymphocytes can lyse target cells bearing the stimulating antigens in association with MHC molecules (class I and class II, respectively). This cytolysis results from direct cell-cell contact or the secretion of cytokines such as tumor necrosis factor (TNF) and lymphotoxin that lyse other cells (see Chapter 12). It is possible that CTLs can specifically lyse B and helper T cells that express foreign protein antigenic determinants in association with their MHC molecules and, therefore, serve as targets for the CTLs, or nonspecifically destroy lymphocytes that are present at sites of lymphotoxin and TNF production.

4. In addition to the antigen-specific suppressors mentioned above, lymphocytes that inhibit various immune responses nonspecifically, called **natural suppressors,** have been demonstrated in neonatal animals and after total lymphoid irradiation or bone marrow transplantation. These natural suppressors may be related in lineage and function to natural killer (NK) cells (see Chapter 12). Their receptors, mode of induction, and mechanisms of action are incompletely understood. It has, however, been hypothesized that natural suppressors contribute to neonatal self-tolerance and to the immunodeficiency seen following irradiation and in graft-versus-host disease (see Chapter 16).

Such postulated mechanisms for the suppressive effects of certain T lymphocytes largely fit the paradigm wherein the cognitive functions of T cells are antigen-specific but their effector functions are nonspecific. However, this does not explain the published

reports of antigen-specific or idiotype-specific suppressor factors. It is clear that simple, quantitative experimental systems are needed to better analyze the role of suppressor T lymphocytes in the down-regulation of immune responses and the maintenance of tolerance to self antigens.

IDIOTYPIC REGULATION

The third mechanism for antigen-initiated immune regulation, in addition to tolerance and suppressor cells, is based on the concept of idiotypes, which are components of antigen receptors. The specificity of this type of regulation is not for the antigen but for the lymphocyte receptors that recognize the antigen. The idea that cells in an individual can respond to and discriminate between receptors on other similar cells is unique to the immune system because only the immune system is endowed with sufficient diversity to allow such reciprocal recognition. This is a theoretical idea that continues to fascinate immunologists, although there is little formal proof that regulatory mechanisms based on recognition of idiotypes are important for the physiologic control of immune responses or as primary pathogenic mechanisms in immunologic diseases.

Idiotypes and Anti-idiotypic Immune Responses

The concept of idiotypes is based on the fact that antigen receptors on T and B lymphocytes are structurally diverse, containing variable regions that differ among different clones. These receptors are also capable of distinguishing between subtle variations in protein sequences, so that lymphocytes can recognize proteins that are only slightly different from self proteins. It is, therefore, conceivable that if one clone of lymphocytes is expanded during an immune response to a foreign antigen, other lymphocytes might specifically recognize and respond to the variable regions of the antigen receptors on the antigen-stimulated clone. Such receptor-specific lymphocytes may then interact with and alter the function of the receptor-bearing clone. The structures or determinants of antigen receptors that distinguish each clone of lymphocytes from all others are called **idiotypes** (see Box 3–2, Chapter 3). Immune responses specific for idiotypes are called **anti-idiotypic.** Such responses can either augment or inhibit the activation of lymphocytes that produce the idiotypes. Thus, idiotypes and anti-idiotypes may constitute a system of self-regulation that is both stimulated by and acts on immunocompetent lymphocytes and consequently influences immune responses to foreign antigens.

The discovery of idiotypes evolved from studies showing that an antibody can be produced against one Ig molecule that would recognize that Ig but no others, even from the same species and inbred strains

of animals. Most of these anti-idiotypic antibodies specifically recognize the antigen-combining sites of Ig molecules and, therefore, bind only to Ig molecules with a particular antigenic specificity. Combining site-specific anti-idiotypic antibodies can influence immune responses only against that antigen. In contrast, other anti-idiotypic antibodies have been produced that bind to the hypervariable region determinants of Ig molecules that are close to but not within the antigen-combining site. Similar determinants may be present on Ig molecules of different specificities. Therefore, such anti-idiotypes may be induced by one antigen-specific Ig but may bind to immunoglobulins specific for other antigens and may, therefore, regulate immune responses against multiple antigens (Fig. 10–6). These principles, which were first established with secreted antibodies, may apply equally to the variable portions of membrane Ig molecules on B cells and to antigen receptors on T lymphocytes because all such receptors have idiotypes. Moreover, idio-

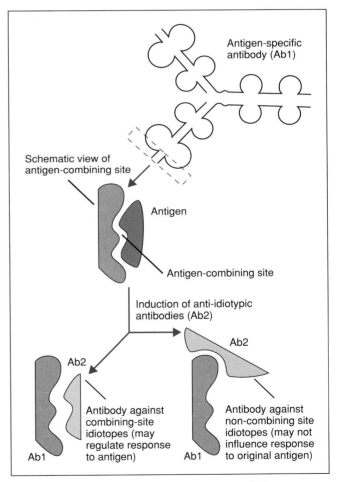

FIGURE 10–6. Production of idiotypes and anti-idiotypic antibodies. *The combining site of an antibody, Ab1, specific for an antigen has a shape complementary to that of the antigen. Anti-idiotypic antibodies (Ab2) against Ab1 may be specific for the combining site of Ab1, in which case they may influence responses to the antigen, or they may be specific for idiotypic determinants of Ab1 that are not part of the combining site.*

types may stimulate the production of antibodies and also of T cells specific for idiotypic determinants. Therefore, in theory, anti-idiotypic immune responses can be of both types, humoral and cell-mediated.

Regulatory Functions of Idiotypic Networks

The potential regulatory role of anti-idiotypic immune responses was most clearly appreciated by Niels Jerne and enunciated in his **network hypothesis** in 1974. Jerne postulated that an antigen stimulates a specific T and/or B cell response, which in turn induces a wave of complementary anti-idiotypic responses (Fig. 10–6). Idiotype-specific antibodies can recognize the original antigen-specific responding lymphocytes and inhibit or augment their activation. Anti-idiotypic T cells may function in the same manner, perhaps by recognizing idiotypic determinants of membrane Ig on B cells that is recycled, processed, and presented in association with MHC molecules by the idiotype-producing B cells themselves. According to Jerne's network hypothesis, a steady state in the immune system is maintained by this network of reciprocal idiotypes and anti-idiotypes. The introduction of antigen perturbs that balance and leads to detectable immune responses.

The analysis of idiotypic regulation has focused largely on two issues: (1) the production of anti-idiotypic antibodies following immunization with foreign antigens, and (2) the effects of anti-idiotypic antibodies on immune responses to foreign antigens. Much of the experimental evidence in support of the regulatory role of idiotypic interactions has come from experimental systems in which the immune response to an antigen is dominated by one or a few clones of responding lymphocytes. In such monoclonal or oligoclonal responses, one or a few antibodies with their unique idiotypes are dominant, so that their regulation can be manipulated and measured experimentally. A good example is the antibody response to phosphorylcholine (PC), which is a component of the cell walls of many bacteria. In BALB/c mice, almost 95 per cent of the antibodies produced in response to PC arise from B cells that express one V gene. Fortuitously, a chemically induced myeloma of BALB/c mice, called TEPC15 (abbreviated to T15) appears to have arisen by neoplastic transformation of a PC–specific B cell clone that expresses the same V gene. In other words, the antibody response of BALB/c mice to PC is dominated by the T15 idiotype. Since large amounts of this monoclonal Ig can be isolated from the myeloma, it is relatively simple to produce anti-idiotypic antibodies and to use these to measure levels of T15 idiotype following immunization with PC, as well as to alter the level of this idiotype following antigen administration. Similar **dominant idiotypes** are seen in immune responses to several other haptens in different inbred strains of mice. During the 1970s, interactions between idiotypes and anti-idiotypes were investigated in many such experimental systems. The potential importance of regulatory idiotypic interactions is supported by several studies, two illustrative examples of which are the following:

1. Injection of anti-T15 antibody into BALB/c mice inhibits the anti-PC antibody response to PC–coupled antigens, presumably by binding to and inhibiting PC–specific B cells, most of which express the T15 idiotype. In other experimental systems, different anti-idiotypic antibodies have been shown to enhance or inhibit responses to antigens. Such results formally demonstrate the ability of anti-idiotypic immunity to regulate immune responses to foreign antigens.

2. Immunization of BALB/c mice with PC–containing antigens leads to production of anti-PC antibody expressing the T15 idiotype, followed some days later by the expansion of B cells specific for the T15 idiotype. As the number of anti-idiotypic B cells increases, the number of cells that secrete PC–specific antibody in the spleen decreases. Such findings demonstrate that lymphocytes producing the idiotype (i.e., antibody against the antigen) as well as cells producing the complementary anti-idiotype can be stimulated in the same animal in response to antigen alone, at least in situations in which only one or a few clones of lymphocytes are responding to the antigen.

Despite the demonstrated potential for regulation mediated by anti-idiotypic immune responses, the actual significance of this mechanism for controlling specific immunity is uncertain, for several reasons. Little is known about the role of idiotypic regulation in responses to multideterminant antigens, which presumably stimulate numerous clones of lymphocytes so that no single idiotype is dominant or even detectable. In such multiclonal responses, it is not possible to determine whether any anti-idiotypic antibodies or T cells are stimulated or whether they are at a level sufficient to mediate regulatory functions. Moreover, administration of some anti-idiotypic antibodies specific for a particular monoclonal Ig may induce or regulate immune responses that are unrelated in specificity to that Ig or to the antigen that initiated its production. This is probably because the anti-idiotype reacts with idiotypic determinants that are located outside antigen-combining sites and are, therefore, present on Ig molecules or antigen receptors of different specificities. In such situations, the effects of idiotypic regulation may be unrelated to the antigen-specific immune response and their significance is unclear. In the final analysis, it has been difficult to establish the physiologic or pathologic role of idiotypes and anti-idiotypic immunity, and it will continue to be so until techniques are developed to measure and isolate antibodies and T cells with complementary idiotypes in conventional immune responses to a variety of antigens.

ANTIBODY FEEDBACK

Antibodies produced in response to an antigen are capable of inhibiting further immune responses to that antigen. For instance, if antigen-specific antibodies are administered to an animal either shortly before immunization with the target antigen or during an ongoing response subsequent antibody production is reduced. This phenomenon, called **antibody feedback**, can down-regulate both humoral and cell-mediated immune responses. Feedback mediated by antibodies is important for ensuring that immune responses are self-limited and decrease in intensity with time after immunization.

This negative feedback function of antibodies is due to several mechanisms that may be operative at the same time:

1. *Antibodies eliminate and neutralize antigens and thereby remove the initiating stimulus for the immune response.* An injected antibody, or an antibody formed during an active response, complexes with the antigen. If the antigen-antibody complexes are formed by IgM or certain subclasses of IgG antibodies, they may subsequently activate the complement system (see Chapter 13). The complexes are avidly bound to and eliminated by Fcγ and/or complement receptor-bearing phagocytes and red blood cells. Clearance of antigens by enhancing their phagocytosis is one of the principal effector functions of antibodies. Antibodies also neutralize the stimulatory capacity of antigens by binding to antigenic determinants and blocking their access to specific membrane Ig on B lymphocytes. This effectively limits B cell activation. For this reason, antibodies that mediate feedback inhibition are also called "blocking antibodies."

2. *Antibodies directly inhibit B lymphocyte activation by binding to Fc receptors on B cells.* Immune complexes composed of an antigen and specific IgG antibody have been shown to inhibit the activation of B lymphocytes specific for that antigen *in vitro* and *in vivo*. Such immune complexes can form in the circulation during a humoral immune response or can be artificially produced *in vitro*. It is thought that immune complex–mediated inhibition results from simultaneous interaction of the antigenic portion of the complex with membrane Ig molecules on specific B cells and of the antibody portion of the complex with Fcγ receptors on the same cells (Fig. 10–7). This can occur only with multideterminant antigens, in which one epitope of the antigen will participate in the formation of the immune complex and another epitope will be available for binding to membrane Ig on specific B cells. An essentially similar phenomenon can be mimicked by exposing B cells to intact anti-Ig antibodies whose combining sites bind to the B cell membrane Ig and Fc "tails" bind to Fc receptors (Fig. 10–7). It is, in fact, known that B cells are stimulated by F(ab′)₂ fragments of anti-Ig antibodies or by intact anti-immunoglobulins that do not bind to Fc receptors. In contrast, intact anti-Ig antibodies that bind simultaneously to membrane Ig and to Fc receptors do not activate the B cells but, in fact, inhibit their responses even to polyclonal activators. The interaction of immune complexes or anti-Ig antibodies with Fc receptors on B cells may inhibit the generation of intracellular second messengers, such as increases in

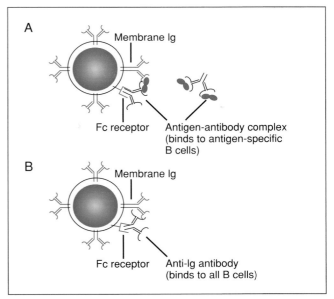

FIGURE 10–7. Antibody feedback: Fc receptor-mediated inhibition of B lymphocytes. *Simultaneous engagement of membrane Ig and Fcγ receptors inhibits B cell activation. This may occur when antigen-antibody complexes bind to antigen-specific B cells* (A), *or in an experimental situation when an anti-Ig antibody binds to the B cell* (B).

phosphatidyl inositol metabolites and intracellular Ca⁺⁺ (see Chapter 9). This leads to a block in the response of the B cells and, consequently, down-regulation of humoral immunity. Thus, the major physiologic function of Fc receptors on B lymphocytes may be their role in antibody-mediated feedback inhibition.

3. *Antigen-antibody complexes may regulate T cell responses.* It has been suggested that antigen-antibody complexes inhibit helper T cell activation and/or induce antigen-specific suppressor T lymphocytes, although there is little definitive evidence to support either mechanism. Some human peripheral blood T lymphocytes express Fc receptors specific for IgM or IgG antibody. Moreover, Fc receptors specific for different Ig isotypes can be induced on mouse and human T cells by exposing them to high concentrations of that isotype *in vivo* or *in vitro*. Therefore, the potential exists for antibodies or immune complexes to interact with T lymphocytes, although the functions of Fc receptor-bearing T cells in immune responses remain incompletely defined.

4. *Antibodies may induce or perturb regulatory idiotypic networks.* As discussed above, antibodies can trigger complementary anti-idiotypic responses, which may regulate both humoral and cell-mediated immunity.

5. *Antigen-antibody complexes may alter cytokine cascades.* For instance, macrophages exposed to immune complexes produce an IL–1 receptor antagonist that competitively inhibits binding of IL–1 to its receptor (see Chapter 11).

Antibody feedback is an excellent example of self-regulation because the effector molecules produced by the humoral immune response themselves serve to down-regulate the response. A practical application of antibody feedback is in the prevention of **Rh disease,** which remains one of the most dramatic examples of successful immunologic intervention for a serious disorder. Rh disease affects infants born of mothers who do not express Rh blood group antigens and fathers who do. The erythrocytes of such a fetus are Rh-positive because of inheritance of the paternal Rh genes. Fetal blood enters the maternal circulation in small amounts during gestation and in substantial quantities during the delivery itself. The immune system of the Rh-negative mother recognizes the fetal Rh as a foreign antigen. Therefore, the mother makes increasing amounts of anti-Rh antibodies with each successive pregnancy. During pregnancy these maternal antibodies cross the placenta, enter the fetal circulation, bind to the fetal erythrocytes, and cause hemolysis, which increases in severity with each pregnancy and can lead to fetal death. In order to prevent this disease when an Rh incompatibility between the mother and the father is detected, the mother is injected with a large dose of an anti-Rh antibody immediately after each delivery. This antibody presumably binds to fetal Rh$^+$ cells, inhibits the maternal immune response to fetal Rh antigens that are encountered at each delivery, and completely prevents the disease from developing.

REGULATORY EFFECTS OF CYTOKINES

In addition to immune regulation mediated by the products of B cells, cytokines produced by T lymphocytes and accessory cells exert both stimulatory and inhibitory effects on immune responses. These effects are generally not antigen-specific. The **stimulatory functions** of cytokines frequently generate amplification loops that enable the small number of lymphocytes specific for any one antigen to recruit the multiple effector mechanisms required to eliminate that antigen. Cytokine cascades, in which one cytokine enhances the production of or functional responses to others, are described in Chapter 11. Among the most striking examples of cytokine-mediated amplification of immune responses are the bidirectional interactions between T lymphocytes and macrophages. For instance, CD4$^+$ T cells secrete IFN$-\gamma$, which enhances the expression of class II MHC molecules on mononuclear phagocytes. Since these T cells recognize foreign antigens in association with class II MHC products, increased MHC gene expression makes the macrophages better APCs and promotes T cell activation (see Fig. 6–4, Chapter 6). Interleukin-4 (IL–4), secreted by CD4$^+$ T cells, augments class II MHC gene expression in B cells and may similarly enhance the avidity of antigen-specific, MHC restricted T cell–B cell interactions. Some class I MHC–restricted CTLs secrete IFN$-\gamma$, lymphotoxin, and tumor necrosis factor (TNF), all of which stimulate class I MHC gene

expression in target cells and enhance CTL–target interactions.

Cytokines also have profound **inhibitory effects** that might serve to regulate immune responses. The reciprocal antagonistic effects of IFN$-\gamma$ and IL–4 on murine B cells were described in Chapter 9. TGF$-\beta$, which is produced by many cell types, including T lymphocytes, is a potent immunosuppressive factor. Such phenomena are being appreciated more and more as immunologists begin to analyze the regulatory functions of cytokines.

FACTORS THAT DETERMINE THE NATURE AND MAGNITUDE OF IMMUNE RESPONSES

Exposure of the immune system to foreign antigens sets into motion the series of events that lead to lymphocyte activation and the generation of humoral and cell-mediated immunity. Different antigens and conditions of immunization lead to responses that vary both quantitatively and qualitatively. For instance, different antigens preferentially stimulate the production of antibodies of various heavy chain isotypes or generate CTLs or other effectors of cell-mediated immunity. Such variability is important because it enables the immune system to protect an individual from the many distinct types of microbes present in the environment. We now know that the development of specific immunity is regulated by many different factors, whose functional effects have the following general features:

1. *The magnitude of an immune response to an antigen is determined by a balance between lymphocyte activation and tolerance induced by that antigen.* In fact, as we discussed earlier in this chapter, even the same antigen can be administered in ways that preferentially stimulate lymphocyte growth and differentiation or inactivate lymphocytes and induce functional unresponsiveness.

2. *The nature of an immune response to an antigen is determined by the specificities and functional classes of lymphocytes that are activated by that antigen.* In particular, since CD4$^+$ helper T lymphocytes play pivotal roles in the generation of both humoral and cell-mediated immunity, these cells are key determinants of the type of immune response. Different subpopulations of helper T cells may produce different cytokines, and thus stimulate distinct types of immune responses. The principal factors that determine which lymphocyte classes respond to an antigen and how they respond are: the characteristics of the antigen, the accessory cells that participate in lymphocyte stimulation, and the repertoires of antigen-specific cells that are available to recognize the antigen.

3. *Different regulatory mechanisms may act at the cognitive, activation, and effector phases of immune responses.* Antigen recognition is determined largely by the repertoires of specific lymphocytes present in

TABLE 10-3. Factors That Determine the Nature and Magnitude of Immune Responses

	Factors That Favor	
	Stimulation of Immune Responses	Inhibition or Lack of Immune Responses
COGNITIVE PHASE		
Lymphocyte repertoire	Diversity of lymphocyte receptors for foreign antigens	Deletion of self-reactive lymphocytes
Antigen presentation	Presence of MHC molecules capable of binding processed antigens	Absence of MHC molecules capable of binding certain antigenic determinants (Ir gene effect)
INDUCTION AND ACTIVATION PHASE		
Features of antigen		
Nature	Immunogenic forms	Tolerogenic forms
Amount	Optimal doses vary for different antigens	High doses favor tolerance
Portal of entry	Subcutaneous, intradermal	Intravenous, oral
Accessory cells	Recruitment and activation by adjuvants	Antigens without adjuvants are non-immunogenic or tolerogenic
Antigen-specific T cells	Helper T cells	Suppressor T cells
Anti-idiotypic immune responses	Can be stimulating or inhibitory	Can be stimulating or inhibitory
Antibodies	Enhance antigen uptake and presentation by macrophages	Antibody feedback
Cytokines	Positive amplification loops	Antagonistic effects of different cytokines; immunosuppressive effects

each individual and, for MHC-restricted T lymphocytes, by the participation of APCs. Lymphocyte activation is also influenced by accessory cells and is probably the principal stage at which regulatory mechanisms such as suppressor T cells and idiotypic networks function to down-regulate immunity. Much less is known about the regulation of the effector phase of immune responses. It may be that once effector cells are generated, their brief life spans are the principal reason why their activities are short-lived and self-regulated.

Understanding the regulation of immune responses is important not only because of its role in physiologic immunity but also for the design of protective vaccines and the therapy of diseases associated with deficient or excessive immunity. In the next section of the chapter, we discuss how antigens, accessory cells, and responding lymphocytes may contribute to the evolution of various immune responses (Table 10-3). Although each of these factors is considered individually, it should be kept in mind that antigens, accessory cells, and lymphocytes influence one another in multiple ways and are not separable in the induction or regulation of immune responses.

The Role of Antigen

Antigens are the obligatory first signals for lymphocyte activation. The nature of the antigen has a significant influence on the type and magnitude of the immune response that develops. These regulatory effects are of many different types:

1. *Chemically different antigens stimulate different types of immune responses.* Whereas protein antigens induce both humoral and cell-mediated immunity, polysaccharides and lipids are incapable of MHC-associated presentation, so that they fail to stimulate MHC-restricted T cells and to induce cell-mediated immune responses. Antibody responses to polysaccharides and lipids are typically T cell-independent and consist largely of low-affinity IgM antibodies (see Chapter 9). Proteins, on the other hand, stimulate isotype switching, affinity maturation, and the generation of memory B cells. Thus, encapsulated bacteria, whose principal immunogens are capsular polysaccharides, usually stimulate low-affinity IgM and some IgG antibodies, and immunity against these microbes is short-lived. In contrast, the protein antigens of some bacteria and most viruses induce strong humoral and cell-mediated immunity and long-lived immunologic memory. This is the reason why individuals who are naturally infected with or actively vaccinated against many viruses remain resistant for many years, and often for life.

2. *The amount of antigen to which an individual is exposed influences the magnitude of the immune response generated.* Optimally immunogenic doses vary, depending on the antigen. In general, however, very large doses or repeated administration of small amounts of antigens are often inhibitory. Large amounts of polysaccharide and protein antigens composed of multiple identical determinants tend to induce tolerance in specific B lymphocytes and thus inhibit antibody production. This may be the reason why patients who have fulminant bacterial infections are sometimes unresponsive, or anergic, to the particular infectious microbe.

3. *The immune response to an antigen varies according to the portal of entry of that antigen.* Antigens that are administered subcutaneously or intradermally are usually immunogenic, whereas large amounts of antigens administered intravenously or orally often induce specific unresponsiveness. Such unresponsiveness has been attributed to tolerance induction in T and/or B lymphocytes or to the stimulation of specific suppressor T cells.

It has also been observed that individuals vary in their responsiveness to different foreign antigenic determinants. Unresponsiveness may be due to the absence of mature antigen-specific lymphocytes. Alternatively, individuals lacking MHC molecules capable of binding a foreign antigenic epitope cannot present this epitope to T cells, so that an immune response may not be induced against this epitope even if specific T cells are present.

The Role of Accessory Cells

As we discussed in Chapters 6 and 7, accessory cells such as macrophages, B lymphocytes, and dendritic cells are essential for the induction of T cell–dependent immune responses. Accessory cells present antigens to MHC–restricted T cells and produce membrane-associated and secreted costimulators that enhance the proliferation and differentiation of both T and B lymphocytes. *It follows, therefore, that the presence of competent accessory cells will stimulate T cell–dependent immune responses and that their absence will lead to deficient responses or tolerance induction.* Because adjuvants recruit and activate macrophages at the sites of antigen administration, the administration of protein antigens with adjuvants promotes cell-mediated immunity and T cell–dependent antibody production. Vaccines are most effective for generating systemic immunity when administered subcutaneously or intradermally together with adjuvants. Some microorganisms contain adjuvants in their cell walls that influence the type and strength of specific immune responses that these microbes induce. For instance, the cell walls of mycobacteria contain muramyl dipeptide, which is a potent adjuvant and is at least partly responsible for the propensity of mycobacteria to stimulate strong T cell–mediated immune responses.

Accessory cells may influence the development of immune responses by many other mechanisms. The role of MHC alleles expressed by APCs in the induction of T cell responses has been described earlier. It is also possible that even though all the accessory cells in an individual express the relevant MHC allele(s), some antigens are processed and presented optimally by B cells and others by macrophages. In these cases, the magnitude of the immune response will depend on the relative numbers of B cells and macrophages that are present at the site of antigen administration or in adjacent lymphoid organs. Different APCs may also process the same endocytosed antigen in distinct ways, leading to the expression of different MHC–associated peptide epitopes. As a result, the type of APCs involved in initiating T cell activation may influence the fine specificity of the response to a multideterminant protein antigen. To date, however, there are no clearly documented examples of variations in APC function leading to variations in the specificity of immune responses. Finally, various subpopulations of T cells may preferentially respond to antigens presented by different accessory cells. Examples of these are mentioned below.

The Types of Responding Lymphocytes

Under most conditions of antigen exposure, protein antigens induce both humoral and cell-mediated immunity, albeit to different extents. However, it is also known that the nature of the immune response to various immunizations, which reflects the profile of antigen-specific lymphocytes that are stimulated, may differ significantly. *This is because lymphocytes, particularly T cells, consist of subpopulations that differ in their function and in responses to different antigens and accessory cells.* For instance, as discussed in Chapter 6, in virally infected cells the endogenously synthesized viral antigens usually bind to class I MHC molecules and stimulate $CD8^+$, class I MHC–restricted CTLs. In contrast, extracellular microbial antigens are endocytosed by APCs, processed, and associated preferentially with class II MHC molecules and, therefore, activate mostly $CD4^+$ class II MHC–restricted helper cells. This leads to antibody production and macrophage activation but usually does not generate potent CTLs.

Even within the population of helper T cells, subsets that produce functionally distinct cytokines may be preferentially expanded by different antigens or immunization conditions. Thus, in some situations the helper T cells that are maximally activated secrete cytokines that stimulate cell-mediated immunity, whereas in other cases the T cells may produce cytokines that induce B cell growth and differentiation, giving rise to humoral immune responses. We have mentioned in Chapter 9 that mouse $CD4^+$ helper T cell clones can indeed be divided into subsets that secrete either IL–2 and IFN–γ and stimulate cell-mediated immunity or IL–4, IL–5, and IL–6 and are particularly efficient helpers for antibody production. It is postulated that preferential activation of such subsets may be responsible for the distinct clinicopathologic features of some infectious diseases. For instance, the granulomatous inflammation seen in mycobacterial infections is presumably due to stimulation of Th1-like cells and production of IFN–γ and TNF. In contrast, helminthic parasites may preferentially activate T cells of the Th2 type that produce IL–4, which induces high levels of IgE antibody, and IL–5, which stimulates eosinophilia. Experimentally, skin contact with chemically reactive forms of haptens preferentially induces cell-mediated immunity, whereas subcutaneous injection of the same haptens coupled to protein carriers and given with adjuvants stimulates strong antibody production. In all these situations, differences in cytokine production by T cells may lead to different immune responses induced by immunization. It is possible that the nature of the APCs or costimulators may determine which T cells are preferentially expanded and what cytokines they produce. Studies to test these hypotheses have not yet provided conclusive results.

SUMMARY

The nature and magnitude of all immune responses are determined by the repertoires of antigen-specific lymphocytes that exist prior to antigen exposure and by mechanisms that regulate the induction and extent of lymphocyte growth and differentiation.

Normal individuals contain immunocompetent lymphocytes that recognize and respond to foreign but not self antigens. The diversity of this repertoire for foreign antigens is created by the expression of genes encoding antigen receptors. Tolerance to self antigens is induced and maintained by two basic mechanisms: deletion of self-reactive clones of lymphocytes, and the induction of a state of anergy by encounter of lymphocytes with self antigens. It is possible that potentially self-reactive cells that escape deletion and are not rendered anergic may be prevented from responding to self antigens by other lymphocytes, called suppressor cells, but suppressor cells specific for self antigens have not yet been identified. Many of the mechanisms that induce self-tolerance may also be responsible for the induction of unresponsiveness to certain foreign antigens administered under conditions that favor tolerance and not immunity.

Factors that influence the induction of specific immunity include the type and amount of antigen, its portal of entry, and the participation of accessory cells in the immune response. These factors may determine what types of lymphocytes are stimulated and may influence the balance between lymphocyte activation and tolerance. Finally, ongoing immune responses are regulated by a variety of mechanisms generated during the response itself. These include the induction of suppressor T lymphocytes, complementary idiotypic interactions, feedback inhibition mediated by secreted antibodies, and cytokines that have both stimulatory and inhibitory effects on lymphocyte activation. Such regulatory interactions are incompletely understood at present, largely because regulation often has to be studied in intact individuals and involves multiple bidirectional communications between the cells and molecules of the immune system. Despite this complexity, detailed analysis of immune regulation is one of the major challenges facing immunologists, because of its obvious importance in normal and disordered immune responses.

SELECTED READINGS

Asherson, G. L., V. Colizzi, and M. Zembala. An overview of T-suppressor cell circuits. Annual Review of Immunology 4:37–68, 1986.
Batchelor, J. R., G. Lombardi, and R. I. Lechler. Speculations on the specificity of suppression. Immunology Today 10:37–40, 1989.
Billingham, R. E., L. Brent, and P. B. Medawar. "Actively acquired tolerance" of foreign cells. Nature 172:603–606, 1953.
Burkly, L. C., D. Lo, and R. A. Flavell. Tolerance in transgenic mice expressing major histocompatibility molecules extrathymically on pancreatic cells. Science 248:1364–1368, 1990.
Goodnow, C. C., S. Adelstein, and A. Basten. The need for central and peripheral tolerance in the B cell repertoire. Science 248:1373–1379, 1990.
Goodnow, C. C., J. Crosbie, S. Adelstein, T. B. Lavoie, S. J. Smith-Gill, R. A. Brink, H. Pritchard-Briscoe, J. S. Witherspoon, R. H. Loblay, K. Raphael, R. J. Trent, and A. Basten. Altered immunoglobulin expression and functional silencing of self-reactive B lymphocytes in transgenic mice. Nature 334:676–682, 1988.
Jerne, N. K. Towards a network theory of the immune system. Annals of Immunology (Institute Pasteur) 125C:373–389, 1974.
Miller, J. F. A. P., G. Morahan, and J. Allison. Immunological tolerance: new approaches using transgenic mice. Immunology Today 10:53–57, 1989.
Nemazee, D. A., and K. Burki. Clonal deletion of B lymphocytes in a transgenic mouse bearing anti-MHC class I antibody genes. Nature 337:562–566, 1989.
Nossal, G. J. V. Immunologic tolerance and the collaboration between antigen and lymphokines in lymphocyte signaling. Science 245:145–153, 1989.
Rajewsky, K., and T. Takemori. Genetics, expression and functions of idiotypes. Annual Review of Immunology 1:569–607, 1983.
Schwartz, R. H. A cell culture model for T lymphocyte clonal anergy. Science 248:1349–1356, 1990.

EFFECTOR MECHANISMS OF IMMUNE RESPONSES

The physiologic function of all specific immune responses is to eliminate the initiating antigen. The mechanisms by which specific lymphocytes recognize and respond to foreign antigens, i.e., the cognitive and activation phases of immune responses, were discussed in Section II. Section III describes the effector mechanisms that are recruited and stimulated by antigen-activated lymphocytes. In Chapter 11 we describe cytokines that are produced by T lymphocytes and by some non-lymphoid cells. These molecules are soluble mediators of cell-mediated immunity as well as non-immune inflammatory reactions. Chapter 12 presents the effector cells of cell-mediated immunity, including cytolytic T lymphocytes, natural killer cells, and macrophages, which function as the primary defense mechanisms against intracellular microbes. Chapter 13 deals with the complement system, one of the major effector mechanisms of the humoral immune response. Chapter 14 discusses a special reaction associated with humoral immunity, namely immediate hypersensitivity, which is due to the production of IgE antibody and the activation of mast cells and basophils.

CYTOKINES

In chapter 1 we introduced the concept that defense against foreign organisms, such as viruses or bacteria, is mediated by natural (or innate) and by specific (or acquired) immunity. The effector phases of both natural and specific immunity are in large part mediated by protein hormones called **cytokines**. In natural immunity, the effector cytokines are mostly produced by mononuclear phagocytes and are therefore often called **monokines**. Although monokines can be elicited directly by microbes, they also can be secreted by mononuclear phagocytes in response to antigen stimulated T cells, i.e., as part of specific immunity. In addition to mediating some of the effector functions of mononuclear phagocytes, monokines play important roles as costimulators of lymphocyte activation, thus providing amplification mechanisms for specific immune responses. Most cytokines in specific immunity are produced by activated T lymphocytes, and such molecules are commonly called **lymphokines.** T cells produce several cytokines that serve primarily to regulate the activation, growth, and differentiation of various lymphocyte populations. Other T cell–derived cytokines function principally to activate and regulate inflammatory cells, such as mononuclear phagocytes, neutrophils, and eosinophils. Thus, these T cell–derived cytokines are the effector molecules of cell-mediated immunity and are also responsible for communications between the cells of the immune and inflammatory systems. Finally, both lymphocytes and mononuclear phagocytes produce other cytokines, collectively called **colony-stimulating factors** (CSFs), which stimulate the growth and differentiation of immature leukocytes in the bone marrow, providing a source of additional inflammatory cells.

In this chapter, we discuss the structure, production, and biologic actions of cytokines. Before describing the specific molecules, we will begin with a brief historical overview of cytokine research and with a review of the general properties shared by cytokines that allow us to consider them as a group.

Discovery and Characterization of Cytokines

The discovery of particular cytokines can often be traced to investigations of infectious disease or of antigen-induced immune responses. Early studies of cytokines, extending from about 1950 to 1970, largely involved the description of numerous protein factors produced by different cells that mediated particular functions in particular bioassays. It was in this era, for example, that anti-viral interferons, fever-producing pyrogens, and macrophage-activating factors were discovered. The second phase of cytokine research, encompassing roughly the 1970s, involved the partial purification and characterization of many individual

cytokines as well as production of specific neutralizing antisera. In this period, it was first appreciated that diverse cytokine-mediated effects being studied by different investigators were often mediated by the same molecules. For example, gamma interferon (IFN–γ) was discovered by virologists as a T cell–derived anti-viral protein and independently discovered by immunologists as a T cell–derived activator of macrophage functions. Similarly, interleukin-1 (IL–1) was discovered as an endogenous mediator of fever (a pyrogen) produced in response to bacterial infections and was discovered by immunologists as a costimulator of T cell activation. An important hypothesis generated at this time was that cytokines were principally synthesized by leukocytes and primarily acted on (other) leukocytes, and thus could be called **interleukins** (ILs). For example, a macrophage-derived costimulator activity for T cells was designated interleukin-1 and a T cell–derived T cell growth factor was called interleukin-2. However, preparations of cytokines available in the 1970s were often impure and many of the available anti-cytokine antibodies were not absolutely specific for one cytokine. These methodological limitations prevented firm identification of the active factors as the same or distinct molecules.

The golden age of cytokine research began in the 1980s. It has been characterized by the molecular cloning and expression of individual cytokine molecules and by the production of completely specific, often monoclonal, neutralizing antibodies. These reagents allowed definitive identification of the structure and properties of individual cytokine molecules. The 1980s were more than a culmination of the early work because, in addition, many new cytokines were discovered and many previously unexpected properties of known cytokines were revealed. As a result of these studies, there is now a wealth of information about the sources and biological activities of particular cytokines.

There are two continuing challenges in cytokine research. First, although much has been learned about the effects of cytokines *in vitro*, it is still largely unknown which biological actions of a particular cytokine are important *in vivo* and which effects are necessary for a particular biological response to occur. Experiments designed to answer these questions are in progress using recombinant cytokine molecules, transgenic animals expressing cytokine genes, and neutralizing antibodies as specific inhibitors of responses. Second, the availability of recombinant cytokines and specific neutralizing antibodies has opened the possibility for clinicians to modify immune responses in predictable fashion to influence the course of a disease. The task is to discover the most efficacious ways to use these **biological response modifiers** to achieve a desired outcome. Some of these clinical uses of cytokines and their antagonists will be discussed in subsequent chapters on immunologic diseases, transplantation, and tumor immunity.

GENERAL PROPERTIES OF CYTOKINES

Although cytokines are a diverse group of proteins, there are a number of properties shared by these molecules:

1. *Cytokines are produced during the effector phases of natural and specific immunity and serve to mediate and regulate immune and inflammatory responses.* In natural immunity, microbial products, such as lipopolysaccharide (LPS), directly stimulate mononuclear phagocytes to secrete their cytokines. In contrast, T cell–derived cytokines are elicited primarily in response to specific recognition of foreign antigens. However, these distinctions are not absolute because cytokines produced by one cell type often regulate the synthesis of cytokines by other cells.

2. *Cytokine secretion is a brief, self-limited event.* In general, cytokines are not stored as pre-formed molecules and their synthesis is initiated by new gene transcription. Such transcriptional activation is usually transient, and cytokine messenger RNA (mRNA) molecules are unstable. The combination of a short period of transcription and a short-lived mRNA transcript ensures that cytokine synthesis is transient. Once synthesized, cytokines are rapidly secreted, resulting in a burst of cytokine release as needed.

3. *Many individual cytokines are produced by multiple diverse cell types.* To emphasize that the cellular source of these molecules is usually not a distinguishing characteristic, investigators are increasingly adopting the convention followed in this book, namely to refer to these molecules collectively as cytokines rather than as lymphokines or monokines, regardless of their cellular source in a particular experiment.

4. *Cytokines not only are produced by different cell types but also act upon many different cell types.* This property is called **pleiotropism.** The earlier view that cytokines are primarily molecules produced by leukocytes that act particularly on leukocytes ("interleukins") is now considered too restricted a concept.

5. *Cytokine actions are often redundant.* Many functions originally attributed to one cytokine have proved to be shared properties of several different cytokines.

6. *Cytokines often influence the synthesis of other cytokines,* leading to cascades in which a second or third cytokine may mediate the biologic actions of the first cytokine. The ability of one cytokine to enhance or suppress the production of others may provide important positive and negative regulatory mechanisms for immune and inflammatory responses.

7. *Cytokines often influence the action of other cytokines.* Two cytokines may interact to antagonize each other's action, to produce additive effects, or, in some cases, to produce greater than anticipated or even unique effects, a kind of interaction commonly referred to as synergy.

8. *Cytokines, like other polypeptide hormones, initiate their action by binding to specific receptors on the surface of target cells.* The relevant target cells may be the same cell that secretes the cytokine (**autocrine** action), a nearby cell (**paracrine** action), or, like true hormones, a distant cell stimulated via cytokines secreted into the circulation (**endocrine** action). Receptors for cytokines often show very high affinities for their ligands, with dissociation constants (K_d) in the range of 10^{-10} to 10^{-12} M. (For comparison, recall that antibodies typically bind antigens with a K_d of 10^{-7} M to 10^{-11} M and the MHC molecules bind peptides with a K_d of only about 10^{-6} M.) As a consequence, only very small quantities of a cytokine need be produced to elicit a biologic effect.

9. *The expression of many cytokine receptors is regulated by specific signals.* These signals may be other cytokines, or they may be the cytokine that binds to the receptor, permitting positive amplification or negative feedback.

10. *Most cellular responses to cytokines are slow, occurring over a period of hours, and require new mRNA and protein synthesis.* The mechanism by which cytokine binding to cell surface receptors stimulates transcription is still not completely known. Some recent studies have identified nucleotide sequences in the 5′ flanking regions of genes whose transcription is activated by cytokine action. It is presumed that cytokines stimulate the production or binding of specific nuclear regulatory factors to these target sequences, and such binding, in turn, causes transcription.

11. *For many target cells, cytokines act as regulators of cell division, i.e., as growth factors.* Some immunologists now feel that cytokines should be categorized with epithelial and mesenchymal cell growth factors into a larger functional group of polypeptide regulatory molecules. However, we will continue to distinguish those molecules whose primary actions are as mediators of host defense (i.e., cytokines) from those molecules whose primary role resides in tissue repair (i.e., the epithelial and mesenchymal cell polypeptide growth factors).

FUNCTIONS OF CYTOKINES

We have organized our discussion of specific cytokines into four broad categories of function: (1) *mediators of natural immunity,* which are elicited by infectious agents from mononuclear phagocytes; (2) *regulators of lymphocyte activation, growth, and differentiation,* which are elicited in response to specific antigen recognition by T lymphocytes; (3) *activators of nonspecific inflammatory cells,* which are also elicited in response to specific antigen recognition by T lymphocytes; and (4) *stimulators of immature leukocyte growth and differentiation,* which are produced by both stimulated lymphocytes and other cells. This classification is based on what appear to be the principal biologic actions of a particular cytokine, although, as we shall see, many cytokines may function in more than one of these categories.

Cytokines That Mediate Natural Immunity

The cytokines that mediate natural immunity include those that protect against viral infection and those that initiate inflammatory reactions that protect against bacteria. The cytokines discussed here are summarized in Table 11–1.

TYPE I INTERFERON

Type I interferons (IFNs) comprise two serologically distinct groups of proteins. The first group, collectively called IFN–α, is a family of about 20 structurally related polypeptides of approximately 18 kD, each encoded by a separate gene. Natural IFN–α preparations are usually a mixture of these molecules and neutralizing sera react with all members of the IFN–α family. The major cell source for production of IFN–α is the mononuclear phagocyte, and IFN–α is sometimes called **leukocyte interferon.** The second serological group of type I IFN consists of a single gene product, a 20 kD glycoprotein called IFN–β. The usual cell source for isolation of IFN–β is the cultured fibroblast, and IFN–β is sometimes called **fibroblast interferon.** However, many cells make both IFN–α

and IFN–β. The most potent natural signal that elicits type I IFN synthesis is viral infection. Experimentally, production of type I IFN is commonly elicited by synthetic double-stranded RNA molecules, which may mimic a signal produced during viral replication. Both IFN–α and IFN–β are also secreted during immune responses to antigens. In this case, antigen-activated T cells stimulate mononuclear phagocytes to synthesize IFN. IFN–α and IFN–β show little structural similarity to each other. Nevertheless, all type I IFN molecules bind to the same cell surface receptor and appear to induce an identical series of cellular responses.

There are four principal biologic actions of type I IFN:

1. *Type I IFN inhibits viral replication.* IFN causes cells to synthesize a number of enzymes, such as 2′-5′ oligoadenylate synthetase, that collectively interfere with replication of viral RNA or DNA. The anti-viral action of type I IFN is primarily paracrine, in that a virally infected cell secretes IFN to protect neighboring cells not yet infected. A cell that has responded to IFN and is resistant to viral infection is said to be in an **anti-viral state.**

2. *Type I IFN inhibits cell proliferation.* This may be due to induction of the same enzymes that inhibit viral replication but also may involve other enzymes that prevent amino acid synthesis, especially of essential amino acids such as tryptophan. Although the mechanisms may be partly different, the anti-viral ef-

TABLE 11–1. Mediators of Natural Immunity

Cytokine	Number of Genes	Polypeptide Size	Cell Source	Cell Target	Primary Effects on Each Target
Type I IFN	~20 IFN–α; 1 IFN–β	18 kD (monomer)	Mononuclear phagocyte, other (α); fibroblast, other (β)	All	Anti-viral, antiproliferative, increased class I MHC expression
				NK cell	Activation
Tumor necrosis factor	1	17 kD (homotrimer)	Mononuclear phagocyte, T cell	Neutrophil	Activation (inflammation)
				Endothelial cell	Activation (inflammation, coagulation)
				Hypothalamus	Fever
				Liver	Acute phase reactants (serum amyloid A protein)
				Muscle, Fat	Catabolism (cachexia)
				T cell, B cell	Costimulator
Interleukin-1	2 (IL–1α, IL–1β)	17 kD (monomer)	Mononuclear phagocyte, other	T cell, B cell	Costimulator
				Endothelial cell	Activation (inflammation, coagulation)
				Hypothalamus	Fever
				Liver	Acute phase reactants (serum amyloid A protein)
				Muscle, fat	Catabolism (cachexia)
Interleukin-6	1	26 kD (monomer)	Mononuclear phagocyte, endothelial cell, T cell	T cell, B cell	Costimulator
				Mature B cell	Growth
				Liver	Acute phase reactants (fibrinogen)
Low molecular weight inflammatory cytokines	20+ related genes	8–10 kD (monomer or dimer)	Mononuclear phagocyte, endothelial cell; fibroblast; T cell; platelet	Leukocytes	Leukocyte chemotaxis and activation

Abbreviations: MHC, major histocompatibility complex; NK, natural killer; kD, kilodalton; IFN, interferon; IL, interleukin.

fects and the antiproliferative effects of IFN cannot be uncoupled. It has been proposed that IFN–β is a physiologic inhibitor of normal cell growth.

3. *Type I IFN increases the lytic potential of natural killer (NK) cells.* As will be discussed in Chapter 12, a major function of NK cells is to kill virally infected cells.

4. *Type I IFN modulates MHC molecule expression.* In general, type I IFN increases expression of class I MHC molecules and profoundly inhibits class II MHC molecule expression. Because most cytolytic T lymphocytes (CTLs) recognize foreign antigens bound to class I MHC molecules, type I IFN boosts the effector phase of cell-mediated immune responses by enhancing the efficiency of CTL-mediated killing. At the same time, type I IFN may inhibit the cognitive phase of immune responses, by preventing the activation of class II MHC–restricted helper T lymphocytes.

Thus, three of the principal activities of type I IFN, namely the induction of the anti-viral state, the activation of NK cell lytic functions, and the increase in class I MHC molecule expression on virally infected cells, all act in concert to eradicate viral infections.

TUMOR NECROSIS FACTOR

Tumor necrosis factor (TNF) *is the principal mediator of the host response to gram-negative bacteria* and may also play a role in the response to other infectious organisms. The active components of gram-negative bacteria are **lipopolysaccharide** (LPS) molecules (also called **endotoxin**) derived from the bacterial cell wall. TNF was originally identified (and was so named) as a mediator of tumor necrosis present in the serum of animals treated with LPS (see Chapter 17). At low concentrations, LPS stimulates the functions of mononuclear phagocytes and acts as a polyclonal activator of B cells (see Chapters 9 and 12), host responses that contribute to elimination of the invading bacteria. However, high concentrations of LPS cause tissue injury, disseminated (widespread) intravascular coagulation (DIC), and shock, often resulting in death. The Shwartzman reaction is an experimental model for studying the pathologic effects of LPS (Box 11–1). It is now clear that TNF is one of the principal mediators of these effects of LPS.

The major cellular source of TNF is the LPS-activated mononuclear phagocyte, although antigen-stimulated T cells, activated NK cells, and activated mast cells can also secrete this protein. IFN–γ, produced by T cells, augments TNF synthesis by LPS-stimulated mononuclear phagocytes. Thus, TNF is a mediator of both natural and acquired immunity and an important link between specific immune responses and acute inflammation. In the mononuclear phagocyte, TNF is initially synthesized as a nonglycosylated transmembrane protein of approximately 25 kD. The orientation of membrane TNF is unusual, in that the amino terminus is intracellular, the transmembrane segment is near the amino terminus, and the carboxy terminus is extracellular. A 17 kD fragment, including the carboxy terminus, is proteolytically cleaved off the plasma membrane of the mononuclear phagocyte to produce the "secreted" form, which circulates as a stable homotrimer of 51 kD.

TNF actions are initiated by binding of the soluble trimer to cell surface receptors. The sequence of the TNF receptor has recently been determined by molecular cloning and appears structurally related to the receptor for nerve growth factor but not to other cytokine receptors. The affinity of TNF for its receptor

BOX 11–1. THE SHWARTZMAN REACTION

The mechanism of LPS-mediated tissue injury was investigated by Shwartzman, who found that two intravenous injections of a sublethal quantity of LPS, administered 24 hours apart, would cause DIC in the rabbit. This is called the **systemic Shwartzman reaction** and is due to widespread intravascular thrombus formation on the surfaces of endothelial cells. If the first LPS injection is given intradermally, the second intravenous injection causes hemorrhagic necrosis of skin exclusively at the intradermal injection site (see Figure). In this **localized Shwartzman reaction,** tissue injury is caused by activated neutrophils and by inadequate perfusion of the tissue. The inadequate tissue perfusion results from local intravascular coagulation (fibrin formation) and from cellular plugging of the microcirculation by neutrophils and platelets. Recent studies have shown that TNF can in large part substitute for LPS in eliciting both the local Shwartzman reaction and the systemic toxicity of LPS. Moreover, neutralizing antibody to TNF affords protection against both the injurious and the lethal effects of LPS. Thus TNF is thought to be an obligatory mediator of LPS-induced tissue injury.

The Shwartzman reaction is an exaggerated form of a host response to microbes, which, under less extreme physiologic conditions, functions primarily to eliminate microbes and limit their spread. Although TNF is now known to be one of the principal cytokines involved in such host responses as noted in the text, TNF was first identified as a factor present in the plasma of LPS-treated animals that could cause hemorrhagic necrosis of tumors. Some of the anti-tumor action of TNF is mediated by direct tumor cell lysis, a process not well understood but believed to involve TNF binding to surface receptors on tumor cells, thereby initiating phospholipase activation and perhaps free radical-mediated cell injury. Mostly, however, TNF induces tumor necrosis by causing a local Shwartzman-like reaction to occur in the tumor vascular bed. The basis for the selective effect on tumor blood vessels is not known, but tumor cells appear to release factors that increase the sensitivity of endothelial cells to TNF.

Continued

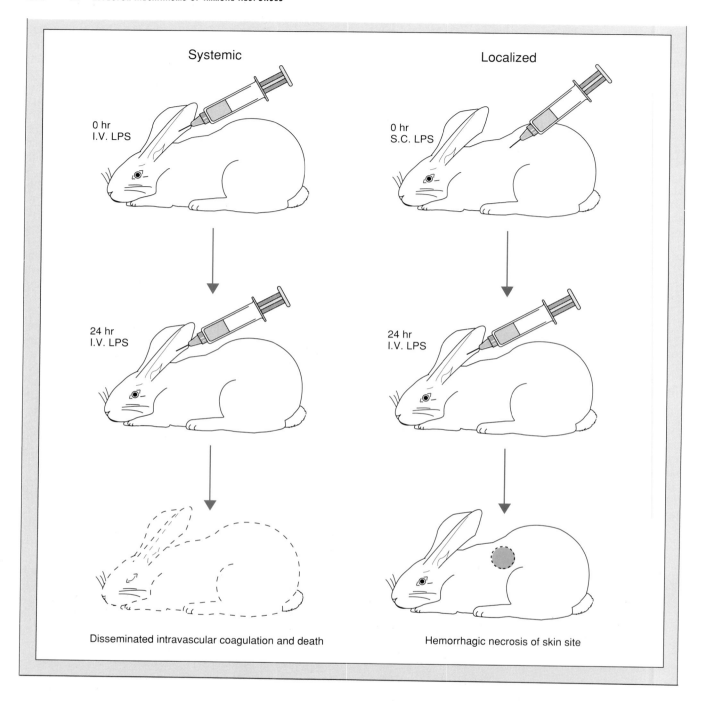

Systemic

0 hr
I.V. LPS

24 hr
I.V. LPS

Disseminated intravascular coagulation and death

Localized

0 hr
S.C. LPS

24 hr
I.V. LPS

Hemorrhagic necrosis of skin site

is unusually low for a cytokine, the K_d being only approximately 10^{-9} M. However, TNF is synthesized in very large quantities and can easily saturate its receptors. TNF receptors are present on almost all cell types examined.

The biologic actions of TNF, like those of LPS, are best understood as a function of quantity. *At low concentrations, i.e., at approximately 10^{-9} M, TNF acts locally as a paracrine and autocrine regulator of leukocytes and endothelial cells.* The principal biologic actions of TNF at low concentrations are the following:

1. TNF causes vascular endothelial cells to become adhesive for leukocytes, initially for neutrophils and subsequently for monocytes and lymphocytes. TNF also acts on neutrophils to increase their adhesiveness for endothelial cells. These actions contribute to accumulation of leukocytes at local sites of inflammation (see Chapter 12).

2. TNF activates inflammatory leukocytes to kill microbes. TNF is especially potent at activating neutrophils but also affects eosinophils and mononuclear phagocytes.

3. TNF stimulates mononuclear phagocytes and

other cell types to produce cytokines, including IL–1, IL–6, TNF itself, and low molecular weight inflammatory cytokines of the IL–8 family.

4. TNF may function as a costimulator for T cell activation and stimulates antibody production by B cells. However, two other mononuclear phagocyte–derived cytokines, IL–1 and IL–6, are more potent than TNF at mediating these effects.

5. TNF induces synthesis of CSFs by vascular endothelial cells and fibroblasts.

6. TNF exerts an interferon-like protective effect against viruses and augments expression of class I MHC molecules, potentiating CTL–mediated lysis of virally infected cells.

These effects of TNF are critical for inflammatory responses to microbes. If inadequate quantities of TNF are present, e.g., in animals treated with neutralizing anti-TNF antibodies, a consequence may be a failure to contain infections.

If the stimulus for TNF production is sufficiently strong, greater quantities of the cytokine are produced. In this setting, TNF enters the blood stream, where it can act as an endocrine hormone. *The principal systemic actions of TNF in physiologic host responses to infections are the following:*

1. TNF is an *endogenous pyrogen* which acts on cells in hypothalamic regulatory regions of the brain to induce fever. It shares this property with IL–1, and both cytokines are found in the serum of animals or people exposed to LPS, which functions as an exogenous pyrogen. Fever production in response to TNF or IL–1 is mediated by increased synthesis of prostaglandins by cytokine-stimulated hypothalamic cells. Prostaglandin synthesis inhibitors, such as aspirin, reduce fever by blocking this action of TNF or IL–1.

2. TNF acts on mononuclear phagocytes and

perhaps vascular endothelial cells to stimulate secretion of IL–1 and IL–6 into the circulation (Fig. 11–1). This is one example of a cascade of cytokines that share many biologic activities.

3. TNF acts on hepatocytes to increase synthesis of certain serum proteins, such as serum amyloid A protein. The spectrum of hepatocyte proteins induced by TNF is identical to that induced by IL–1 but differs from that induced by IL–6 (described below). The combination of hepatocyte–derived plasma proteins induced by TNF or IL–1 plus those induced by IL–6 constitutes the **acute phase response** to inflammatory stimuli. Although the physiologic role of the acute phase response is not fully known, it is thought to enhance the efficacy of nonspecific immunity (Box 11–2).

4. TNF activates the coagulation system, primarily by altering the balance of the procoagulant and anticoagulant activities of vascular endothelium.

5. TNF suppresses bone marrow stem cell division. Chronic administration of TNF may lead to lymphopenia and immunodeficiency.

6. Long-term systemic administration of TNF to experimental animals causes the metabolic alterations of cachexia, a state characterized by wasting of muscle and fat cells. The cachexia is produced partly by TNF–induced appetite suppression and partly by TNF–mediated suppression of the synthesis of lipoprotein lipase, an enzyme needed to release fatty acids from circulating lipoproteins so that they can be utilized by the tissues. Although TNF by itself can produce cachexia in experimental animals, other cytokines, such as IL–1, may also contribute to the cachectic state accompanying certain diseases such as cancer.

The combination of fever, elevated IL–6 levels, elevated acute phase reactants, bone marrow sup-

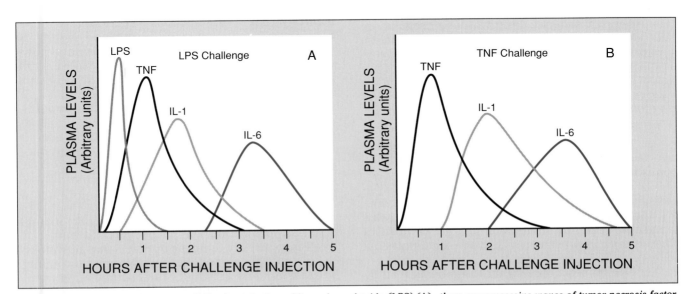

FIGURE 11–1. Cytokine cascades in sepsis. *Following injection of lipopolysaccharide (LPS) (A), there are successive waves of tumor necrosis factor (TNF), IL–1, and IL–6 detectable in plasma. Injection of TNF (B) produces successive waves of IL–1 and IL–6. In the presence of antibody to TNF, LPS–induced plasma elevations of IL–1 and IL–6 are inhibited, and in the presence of antibody to IL–1, plasma elevations of IL–6 are inhibited. These data suggest that there are ordered cascades of cytokine production: LPS induces TNF, which induces IL–1, which induces IL–6 synthesis.*

BOX 11-2.   THE ACUTE PHASE RESPONSE

The acute phase response consists of a rapid adjustment of plasma protein composition in response to injurious stimuli, including infection, burns, trauma, and neoplasia. Several different plasma proteins rise in concentration, whereas others fall. Among the proteins whose levels increase are C-reactive protein, which functions as a nonspecific opsonin to augment phagocytosis of bacteria; α_2 macroglobulin and other anti-proteinases; the clotting protein fibrinogen; and serum amyloid A protein, a molecule of uncertain function. Albumin and transferrin, the iron transport protein, decline. Most of these changes in plasma concentrations can be directly attributed to alterations in the levels of synthesis of these plasma proteins by hepatocytes. Experiments using whole animals, liver slices, cultured hepatocytes, or hepatocyte-derived tumor cell lines have revealed that these changes in biosynthesis are caused by alterations in gene transcription regulated primarily by IL-6, often in conjunction with IL-1 and TNF.

The precise function of the acute phase response is largely unknown. The increases in opsonizing proteins and anti-proteinases are believed to aid natural immunity and protect against tissue injury, respectively. Elevation in fibrinogen, caused by IL-6, is of uncertain benefit but has had major impact on clinical medicine. Specifically, elevated levels of fibrinogen can cause red blood cells to form stacks (rouleaux). When blood is collected and allowed to stand at unit gravity, rouleaux sediment more rapidly than individual red blood cells. Rouleaux in venous blood may sediment before the red blood cells are fully oxygenated, leading

to a dark mass at the bottom of the container. In ancient times, this mass of dark, deoxygenated red blood cells was called "black bile," and ancient and medieval physicians would perform bleeding of patients to remove this "sickly humor." In modern times, the realization that the more rapid red blood cell sedimentation reflected the presence of illness, rather than representing its cause, allowed measure of the **erythrocyte sedimentation rate** to become a useful diagnostic test for the presence of the acute phase response. In the past few years, more specific measures of the acute phase response, for example, of C-reactive protein or of IL-6, have now largely supplanted this useful tool.

Although the acute phase response is characterized by rapid onset, it can persist in the setting of chronic inflammation. In some patients with chronic inflammatory disease (e.g., rheumatoid arthritis; see Chapter 17), persistent elevations of serum amyloid A protein may lead to deposition of this protein in the interstitium of tissues. Such deposited protein, in the form of fibrils rich in β-pleated sheet structure, can interfere with normal organ function (e.g., myocardial contraction, glomerular filtration). Such patients are said to have developed "amyloidosis" because such protein deposits stain with acidic iodine, a reaction originally developed for amylose or animal starch. Similar fibrils can develop in other settings (e.g., multiple myeloma, Alzheimer's disease, or endocrine cell tumors); however, in these cases, the protein fibrils are not of serum amyloid A protein origin and are unrelated to the acute phase response.

---

pression, and activation of coagulation has been noted in patients treated with intravenous TNF for cancer chemotherapy.

In the setting of gram-negative bacterial sepsis, massive quantities of TNF are produced, and serum concentrations of TNF can transiently exceed 10^{-7} M. Animals producing this much TNF die of circulatory collapse and disseminated intravascular coagulation. Neutralizing antibodies to TNF can prevent mortality, implicating this cytokine as a critical mediator of septic or endotoxin shock (Fig. 11-2). Moreover, infusion of high levels of TNF is by itself lethal, producing a shocklike syndrome. *Several specific actions of TNF may contribute to its lethal effects at extremely high concentrations.*

1. TNF reduces tissue perfusion by depressing myocardial contractility. The mechanism of this action is not yet known.

2. TNF further reduces blood pressure and tissue perfusion by relaxing vascular smooth muscle tone. TNF may act directly on smooth muscle cells and also can act indirectly by stimulating production of vasodilators, such as prostacyclin, by vascular endothelial cells.

3. TNF causes intravascular thrombosis, leading to reduced tissue perfusion. This is due to a combination of endothelial alterations, which promote coagulation, and activation of neutrophils leading to vascular plugging by these cells. These TNF-mediated

actions account for many of the effects of LPS seen in the local Shwartzman reaction.

4. TNF causes severe metabolic disturbances, such as a fall in blood glucose concentrations to levels that are incompatible with life.

Many of the biologic actions of TNF are augmented by IFN-γ. In some cells that are targets of TNF effects, this interaction may be explained by IFN-γ-stimulated increases in TNF receptor numbers. However, in many cases, IFN-γ enhancement of TNF activity is noted without any effect on TNF binding. The full significance of this interaction is not clear, but activated T cells often secrete TNF and IFN-γ coordinately. Coordinate secretion of these two cytokines may provide a means of locally enhancing the actions of TNF without requiring concentrations that produce systemic toxicity.

INTERLEUKIN-1

Interleukin-1 was first defined as a polypeptide derived from mononuclear phagocytes that enhanced T cell responses to antigens or polyclonal activators, i.e., as a costimulator of T cell activation. A convenient bioassay for this activity is the costimulation (with concanavalin A or phytohemagglutinin) of murine thymocyte proliferation. It is now appreciated that this assay is not specific for IL-1 and may also detect IL-6 or TNF. Although IL-1 was discovered as a co-

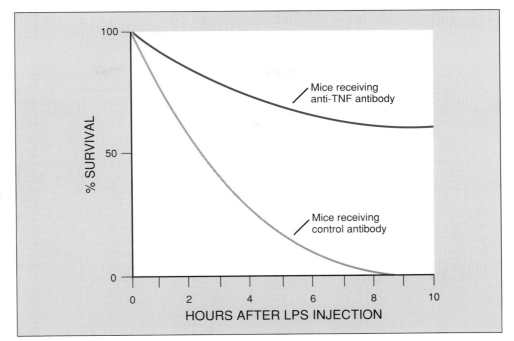

FIGURE 11-2. Tumor necrosis factor (TNF) mediates septic shock. *Antibody to TNF can significantly reduce mortality associated with gram-negative sepsis or injection of lethal concentrations of lipopolysaccharide (LPS).*

stimulator of T cells, *it is now clear that a principal function of IL-1, similar to TNF, is as a mediator of the host inflammatory response in natural immunity.*

The major cellular source of IL-1, like that of TNF, is the activated mononuclear phagocyte. IL-1 production by mononuclear phagocytes can be triggered by bacterial products such as LPS, by macrophage-derived cytokines such as TNF or IL-1 itself, and by contact with CD4+ T cells. Like TNF, IL-1 can be found in the circulation following gram-negative bacterial sepsis, where it can act as an endocrine hormone (see Fig. 11-1). IL-1 synthesis differs from that of TNF in two important regards. First, T cells are more effective than LPS at eliciting synthesis of IL-1 by mononuclear phagocytes. Second, IL-1 is made by many diverse cell types, such as epithelial and endothelial cells, providing potential local sources of IL-1 in the absence of macrophage-rich infiltrates.

Biochemical purification of IL-1 secreted by mononuclear phagocytes revealed that the biologic activity of this cytokine actually resided in two major polypeptide species, each approximately 17 kD but with distinct isoelectric points of 5.0 and 7.0. It is now known that these two forms, called IL-1α and IL-1β, respectively, are products of two different genes. The two forms of IL-1 show less than 30 per cent structural homology to each other, but both species bind to the same cell surface receptors and their biologic activities are essentially identical.

Both IL-1 polypeptides are synthesized as approximately 33 kD precursors that are proteolytically cleaved to generate the mature 17 kD proteins. The 33 kD IL-1α precursor is biologically active, but IL-1β must be processed to the 17 kD form before it can exert biologic effects. The complete amino acid sequence of both IL-1 species presents a theoretical

problem: unlike conventionally secreted proteins, neither IL-1 polypeptide has a hydrophobic leader sequence to target the nascent polypeptide to the endoplasmic reticulum, and both proteins appear to be synthesized as cytoplasmic proteins. It is therefore unknown how these molecules are secreted. Furthermore, IL-1α may be isolated with the plasma membrane of the cell that synthesizes it, exerting biologic activity in a membrane-associated form. However, no structural feature of IL-1α has been identified to explain membrane association. Most of the IL-1 activity found in the circulation is IL-1β.

IL-1 receptors are present on almost all cell types examined. A gene encoding a lymphocyte receptor for IL-1 has been cloned from a T cell line. This IL-1 receptor contains immunoglobulin (Ig)-like domains and is thus a member of the Ig gene superfamily (Box 11-3). It has slightly higher affinity for IL-1β than for IL-1α. B cells express a different receptor that has a higher affinity for IL-1α than IL-1β.

The mechanism of IL-1 action after it binds to its receptor is unclear. In some cell lines, IL-1 activates adenylate cyclase, causing an elevation in cellular cyclic adenosine monophosphate (cAMP) and consequent activation of protein kinase A. In other cells, IL-1 induces various nuclear factors that function as transcriptional activators of cellular genes. In one T cell tumor line, IL-1 can augment IL-2 gene transcription by causing synthesis of the c-Jun subunit of transcription factor AP-1 (see Chapter 7). It has not yet been possible to establish any of these pathways or any other second messenger system as essential for the biologic effects of IL-1 in most cell types examined. IL-1 taken up by target cells resists biochemical degradation and can be found associated with the cell nucleus. It has been speculated that such intranuclear

BOX 11-3. CYTOKINE RECEPTOR FAMILIES

The genes encoding many receptors for cytokines have been cloned, sequenced, and, by transfection into receptor-negative cells, shown to confer the ability to bind and/or respond to the relevant cytokine. Based on nucleotide sequences, most of the receptors for the known cytokines can be divided into two families. Receptors for IL-1, monocyte-macrophage colony-stimulating factor (M-CSF, also called CSF-1), and platelet-derived growth factor (PDGF) have extracellular Ig-like domains. Therefore, they are members of the **Ig gene superfamily.** Many of the other cytokine receptors have conserved features, because of which they are classified as members of a newly discovered **cytokine receptor family** (see Figure). The extracellular domains of these receptor proteins contain four cysteine residues at the same location and a tryptophan-serine-X-tryptophan-serine (trp-ser-X-trp-ser) motif in the region just external to the plasma membrane. The functional signifiance of these conserved features is unknown, but they do suggest a common evolutionary origin. The

trp-ser-X-trp-ser motif is also found in some proteins of the complement system, but these proteins do not function as cytokines. In the IL-6 receptor, the approximately 90 amino acid residues at the amino terminus form an Ig-like domain, so that this receptor can be classified as a member of both families. The IFN-γ and TNF receptors appear to be structurally unrelated to both these protein families.

This impressive structural information has not yet provided any clues about the mechanisms by which cytokines mediate their biologic effects. The cytoplasmic domain of the M-CSF receptor is homologous to a tyrosine kinase, but all the other cytokine receptors defined to date do not contain kinase domains. It is possible that the receptors provide specific ligand binding, but cytokine generated signals are transduced by other, associated proteins. In fact, the IL-6 receptor is non-covalently attached to a 130 kD glycoprotein that does not bind IL-6 but is required for the biologic effects of this cytokine.

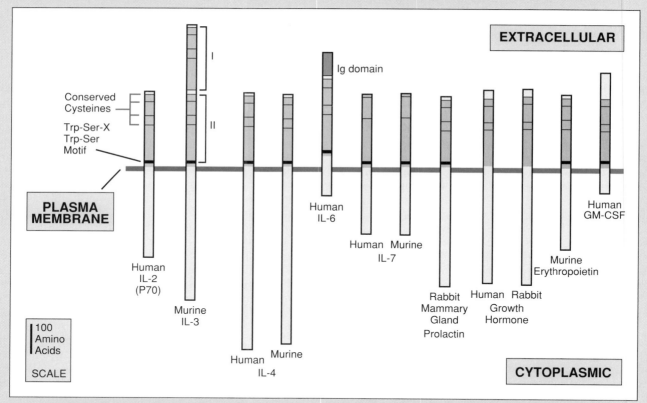

(Modified with permission from: Cosman, D., S. D. Lyman, R. L. Idzerda, M. P. Beckmann, L. S. Park, R. G. Goodwin, and C. J. March. A new cytokine receptor superfamily. Trends in Biochemical Sciences 15:265–269, 1990.)

IL-1 or its activated receptor may directly stimulate gene transcription. In many cell types, IL-1 causes synthesis of enzymes that produce prostaglandins. The increased levels of prostaglandins mediate some of the actions of IL-1, such as fever.

When locally produced at low concentrations the predominant effects of IL-1 are probably immunoregulatory:

1. *IL-1 functions together with polyclonal activators to enhance the proliferation of CD4+ T cells and the growth and differentiation of B cells.* IL-1 is one of the few known soluble costimulators for T cell activation, providing a mechanism by which microbes that activate mononuclear phagocytes indirectly augment specific immune responses. In several T cell tumor lines, a demonstrated effect of IL-1 is to stimulate the tran-

scription of the IL-2 gene. Surprisingly, many mouse T cell clones that synthesize IL-2 in response to antigen do not appear to have IL-1 receptors and most murine T cell clones that do have IL-1 receptors appear to produce IL-4 but not IL-2. Thus, IL-1 may function as a costimulator for only some T cells.

2. *IL-1 stimulates a variety of cells that function as effectors of immune and inflammatory responses.* Specifically, IL-1 acts on mononuclear phagocytes and vascular endothelium to increase further synthesis of IL-1 and induce synthesis of IL-6. It also shares many of the inflammatory properties of TNF. For example, IL-1 acts on endothelial cells to promote coagulation and leukocyte adhesion. IL-1 does not directly activate inflammatory leukocytes, such as neutrophils, but it causes mononuclear phagocytes and endothelial cells to synthesize low molecular weight inflammatory cytokines of the IL-8 family that do activate leukocytes (see below).

When secreted in larger quantities, IL-1 enters the blood stream and exerts endocrine effects. *Systemic IL-1 shares with TNF the ability to cause fever, to induce synthesis of acute phase plasma proteins by the liver, and to initiate metabolic wasting (cachexia).*

It was initially very surprising to note the extensive similarities of IL-1 actions with those of TNF, a striking example of the redundancy of cytokine effects. However, there are several important differences between these cytokines. First, IL-1 does not produce tissue injury by itself, although it is secreted in response to LPS and can potentiate tissue injury caused by TNF. Moreover, even at very high systemic concentrations, IL-1 is not lethal. Second, although IL-1 mimics many of the inflammatory and procoagulant properties of TNF, IL-1 cannot replace TNF as a mediator of the Shwartzman reaction and does not cause hemorrhagic necrosis of tumors. Third, most tumor cell lines are not directly lysed by IL-1 *in vitro*. Fourth, IL-1 does not share with TNF an ability to increase expression of MHC molecules. Fifth, IL-1 potentiates rather than suppresses the actions of CSFs on bone marrow cells. Finally, IL-1 appears to be more potent than TNF as a costimulator for increasing T cell responses.

IL-1 is the only cytokine to date for which **naturally occurring inhibitors** have been described. The best defined of these is produced by human mononuclear phagocytes activated by antigen-antibody complexes. It is structurally homologous to IL-1 and binds to IL-1 receptors but is biologically inactive, so that it functions as a competitive inhibitor of IL-1. Such inhibitory molecules may be endogenous regulators of cytokine action. It may also be possible to use cytokine inhibitors as biological response modifiers in disease states that are caused by excessive or unregulated cytokine production.

INTERLEUKIN-6

Interleukin-6 (IL-6) is a cytokine of approximately 26 kD that is synthesized by mononuclear phagocytes, vascular endothelial cells, fibroblasts, and other cells in response to IL-1 and, to a lesser extent, TNF. It is also made by some activated T cells. IL-6 can be detected in the circulation following gram-negative bacterial infection or TNF infusion and appears to be secreted in response to TNF or IL-1 rather than LPS itself (Fig. 11-1). IL-6 does not cause vascular thrombosis or the tissue injury that is seen in response to LPS or TNF.

The IL-6 receptor belongs to a recently described family of cytokine receptor proteins (Box 11-3). This receptor also contains one Ig-like domain and is thus a member of the Ig gene superfamily as well. Many of the other cytokine receptors that have been molecularly cloned belong to one of these gene families.

The two best described actions of IL-6 are on hepatocytes and B cells:

1. *Interleukin-6 causes hepatocytes to synthesize several plasma proteins, such as fibrinogen, that contribute to the acute phase response* (Box 11-2). The pattern of hepatocyte-derived plasma proteins induced by IL-6 is unique and complements those induced by IL-1 and TNF.

2. *Interleukin-6 serves as the principal growth factor for activated B cells late in the sequence of B cell differentiation.* IL-6 similarly acts as a growth factor for many malignant plasma cells (plasmacytomas or myelomas), and many plasmacytoma cells that grow autonomously actually secrete IL-6 as an autocrine growth factor. Moreover, IL-6 can promote the growth of somatic cell hybrids produced by fusing normal B cells with plasmacytoma cells, i.e., the "hybridomas" that produce monoclonal antibodies (Box 3-1, Chapter 3). Transgenic mice that overexpress the IL-6 gene develop massive polyclonal proliferation of plasma cells.

In addition to these well described actions, IL-6 can serve as a costimulator of T cells and of thymocytes. IL-6 also acts as a cofactor with other cytokines for the growth of early bone marrow hematopoietic stem cells. Finally, it should be noted that one of the first activities ascribed to IL-6, that of an interferon, has not been confirmed using recombinant preparations of IL-6, and the alternative name of IFN-β_2 for this cytokine is best discarded.

LOW MOLECULAR WEIGHT INFLAMMATORY CYTOKINES: THE INTERLEUKIN-8 FAMILY

A recent discovery in the cytokine field is the existence of a large family of structurally homologous cytokines, approximately 8 to 10 kD in size. All of these molecules contain two internal disulfide loops. Some investigators separate these factors into two subfamilies, based on whether the two central cysteine residues are immediately adjacent or separated by one amino acid. These structural differences do not correlate with function.

Members of this family of cytokines are derived from three cellular sources: (1) antigen-activated T cells; (2) LPS-activated or cytokine-activated mononuclear phagocytes, endothelial cells, fibroblasts or epithelial cells; and (3) platelets. Almost all members of this family have been shown to cause inflammation by stimulating leukocytes. The best characterized of the inflammatory cytokines is interleukin-8 (IL–8). It is produced by mononuclear phagocytes and other cells that are stimulated by LPS or by cytokines such as TNF and IL–1. IL–8 is an activating and chemotactic factor for neutrophils and, to a lesser extent, for eosinophils, basophils, and lymphocytes. Another member of the family, called monocyte chemotactic protein–1 (MCP–1), appears to be specific for mononuclear phagocytes. Injection of IL–8 or MCP–1 into the tissues of animals produces inflammatory reactions. It is now believed that the neutrophil activation induced by TNF and IL–1 is largely due to the secretion of IL–8 and related proteins that is stimulated by TNF and IL–1. *Thus, IL–8 and related cytokines may serve as the principal secondary mediators of inflammation.*

Cytokines That Regulate Lymphocyte Activation, Growth, and Differentiation

Some cytokines are produced principally by antigen-activated T lymphocytes, most commonly of the CD4+ subset. Such T cells provide help for both cell-mediated and humoral immune response, in large part through the secretion of cytokines. The cytokines that act primarily to regulate lymphocytes themselves are interleukin-2, interleukin-4, and transforming growth factor–β (TGF–β). The properties of the cytokines discussed in this section are listed in Table 11–2.

Interleukin-2

Interleukin-2 (IL–2), originally called **T cell growth factor** *(TCGF), is the principal cytokine responsible for progression of T lymphocytes from the G1 to S phase of the cell cycle.* IL–2 is produced by CD4+ T cells, and in lesser quantities by CD8+ T cells. IL–2 acts on the same cells that produce it; i.e., it functions as an **autocrine growth factor.** IL–2 also acts on nearby T lymphocytes, including both CD4+ and CD8+ cells, and is also therefore a **paracrine growth factor.** During physiologic immune responses, IL–2 does not circulate in the blood to act at a distance and thus it is not considered to be an endocrine growth factor.

Secreted IL–2 is a 14 to 17 kD glycoprotein encoded by a single gene on chromosome 4 in humans. The size heterogeneity of the mature protein is due to variable extents of glycosylation of an approximately 130 amino acid residue polypeptide. Normally, IL–2 is transcribed, synthesized, and secreted by T cells only upon activation by antigens. IL–2 synthesis is usually transient, with an early peak of secretion occurring about 4 hours after activation. The mechanisms of transcriptional regulation of IL–2 synthesis have been described in Chapter 7.

The principal actions of IL–2 are on lymphocytes:

1. *Interleukin-2 is the major autocrine growth factor for T lymphocytes, and the quantity of IL–2 synthesized by activated CD4+ T cells is an important determinant of the magnitude of immune responses.* In addition to its effects on T cell growth, IL–2 can stimulate a second round of IL–2 synthesis from the activated T cells, with peak secretion occurring at about 24 hours after initial activation. IL–2 also stimulates synthesis of other T cell–derived cytokines such as IFN–γ and lymphotoxin (LT). Failure to synthesize adequate quantities of IL–2 has been described as a cause of antigen-specific T cell anergy.

The action of IL–2 on T cells is mediated by binding to IL–2 receptor proteins. This system is perhaps the best understood of all cytokine receptors. Two distinct cell surface proteins on T cells bind IL–2. The first to be identified is a 55 kD polypeptide (p55) that appears upon T cell activation and is therefore called Tac (for T activation) antigen. The Tac polypeptide, or p55, binds IL–2 with a K_d of approximately 10^{-8} M. Binding of IL–2 to cells expressing only p55 does not

TABLE 11–2. Mediators of Lymphocyte Activation, Growth, and Differentiation

Cytokine	Number of Genes	Polypeptide Size	Cell Source	Cell Target	Primary Effects on Each Target
Interleukin-2	1	14–17 kD (monomer)	T cells	T cell	Growth; cytokine production
				NK cell	Growth, activation
				B cell	Growth, antibody synthesis
Interleukin-4	1	20 kD (monomer)	CD4+ T cell	T cell	Growth
				B cell	Activation and growth; isotype switching to IgE
				Mononuclear phagocyte, B cell	FcϵRIIb expression
Transforming growth factor–β	2	14 kD (homodimer or heterodimer)	T cells, mononuclear phagocyte, other	T cell	Inhibit activation and proliferation
				Mononuclear phagocyte	Inhibit activation
				Other cell types	Growth regulation

Abbreviations: NK, natural killer; kD, kilodalton; Ig, immunoglobulin; Fc, fragment.

lead to any detectable biological response. The second IL–2 binding protein is about 70 to 75 kD (called variously p70 or p75) and is also a member of the cytokine receptor family (Box 11–3). The affinity of binding of IL–2 to this receptor is higher than to p55, with a K_d of approximately 10^{-9} M. IL–2 causes growth of cells expressing only p70, with half maximal growth stimulation occurring at the same concentration of IL–2 that produces half maximal binding. Cells that express both p55 and p70 can bind IL–2 much more tightly, with a K_d of approximately 10^{-11} M. Growth stimulation of such cells occurs at a similarly low IL–2 concentration. Both IL–2 binding and growth stimulation can be blocked by antibodies to either p55 or p70. These observations have been interpreted to mean that *p55 forms a complex with p70, increasing the affinity of the p70 receptor for IL–2 and thereby allowing a growth signal to be delivered at significantly lower IL–2 concentrations.* It is believed that IL–2 first binds rapidly to p55, and this facilitates association with p70. As depicted in Figure 11–3, resting T cells express p70 but not p55 and can be stimulated only by high levels of IL–2. Upon antigen receptor-mediated T cell activation, p55 is rapidly ex-

pressed, thereby reducing the concentration of IL–2 needed for growth stimulation. In fact, IL–2 itself can further increase p55 synthesis. Although much is known about the interaction of IL–2 with its receptor, the intracellular signals produced by cytokine binding have not been identified. To date, there is no evidence for involvement of intracellular Ca^{++}, protein kinase A, or protein kinase C in the mediation of IL–2 effects. Recent evidence suggests that a third polypeptide may be involved in transducing signals generated by binding of IL–2.

2. *IL–2 stimulates the growth of NK cells and enhances their cytolytic function,* producing so-called lymphokine-activated killer (LAK) cells (see Chapter 12). NK cells, like resting T cells, express p70 and can be stimulated by high levels of IL–2. NK cells, however, do not express p55 and therefore do not reduce their requirement for IL–2, even after activation. Thus, only high concentrations of IL–2 will lead to LAK cell formation. Experimentally, LAK cells are usually generated *in vitro* and their role in physiologic immune responses *in vivo* is unknown.

3. *IL–2 acts on human B cells both as a growth factor and as a stimulus for antibody synthesis.* It does

FIGURE 11–3. IL–2 receptors. *The high-affinity IL–2 receptor (IL–2R) is composed of a complex of two separate polypeptides (p70 and p55) which interact to bind IL–2 with high affinity. Resting T cells express only p70, which binds IL–2 with lower affinity. T cell activation by antigen and an antigen-presenting cell (APC) leads to p55 synthesis and expression, thereby increasing the affinity of the p70 receptor and allowing growth stimulation at physiological IL–2 concentrations. IL–2, produced by the activated T cell, further increases p55 expression and stimulates IL–2 synthesis, providing a positive amplification system.*

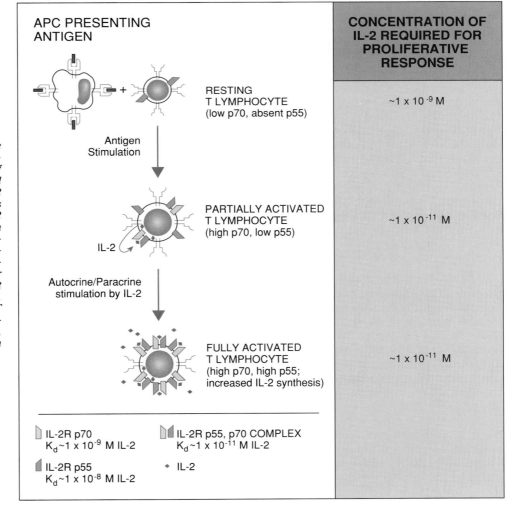

APC PRESENTING ANTIGEN

	CONCENTRATION OF IL-2 REQUIRED FOR PROLIFERATIVE RESPONSE
RESTING T LYMPHOCYTE (low p70, absent p55)	~1 x 10^{-9} M
PARTIALLY ACTIVATED T LYMPHOCYTE (high p70, low p55)	~1 x 10^{-11} M
FULLY ACTIVATED T LYMPHOCYTE (high p70, high p55; increased IL-2 synthesis)	~1 x 10^{-11} M

Antigen Stimulation

IL-2

Autocrine/Paracrine stimulation by IL-2

IL-2R p70
K_d~1 x 10^{-9} M IL-2

IL-2R p55
K_d~1 x 10^{-8} M IL-2

IL-2R p55, p70 COMPLEX
K_d~1 x 10^{-11} M IL-2

IL-2

not appear to cause isotype switching. These activities of IL–2 are discussed more fully in Chapter 9.

Actions of IL–2 on other cell populations are less well established. IL–2 receptor proteins have been detected on mononuclear phagocytes. However, a specific IL–2 function in this cell type has not been described. IL–2 may also act on immature bone marrow cells, perhaps to increase responsiveness to other cytokines. Finally, IL–2 may be a growth factor for immature T cells in the thymus.

Chronic T cell stimulation leads to shedding of IL–2 receptors. Shed receptor proteins may bind free IL–2, preventing its interaction with cells. Clinically, an increased level of shed p55 in the serum is a marker of strong antigenic stimulation, e.g., acute rejection of a transplanted organ. Infection of T cells by human T lymphotrophic virus–1 (HTLV–1) activates p55 synthesis and also leads to shed p55 in the serum.

INTERLEUKIN-4

Interleukin-4 (IL–4) was initially identified as a helper T cell–derived cytokine of approximately 20 kD that stimulated the proliferation of resting mouse B cells in the presence of anti-Ig antibody, an analog of antigen (see Chapter 9). Purified IL–4 also causes enlargement of resting B cells and increased expression of class II MHC molecules. In accordance with these activities, IL–4 was initially called B cell stimulatory factor–1. Although CD4$^+$ T cells are the major source of IL–4, it may also be produced by activated mast cells.

The genes encoding the human and mouse IL–4 receptors have been cloned and sequenced. Based on this sequence, the IL–4 receptor is included as a member of the cytokine receptor family (Box 11–3). Messenger RNA for the receptor is present in a wide variety of cell types. Interestingly, in many cells, including lymphocytes, 5 to 10 per cent of this mRNA encodes a secreted form of the receptor, lacking membrane and cytoplasmic segments. The biologic function of this soluble receptor is unknown.

To date, most of the effects of IL–4 have been studied in mice, in which IL–4 has been shown to have important effects on four main cell types:

1. *IL–4 is a growth and differentiation factor for B lymphocytes* and may be necessary for both proliferation of and antibody secretion by B cells in response to protein antigens. *IL–4 is also the only known switch factor for IgE production.* These functions of IL–4 in humoral immunity were discussed in more detail in Chapter 9. Transgenic mice that overexpress an IL–4 gene show increased levels of serum IgE antibody.

2. *IL–4 is an autocrine growth factor for a subset of cloned CD4$^+$ T cells* that secrete IL–4, IL–5, and IL–6, in contrast to the majority of clones which produce IL–2, IFN–γ, and lymphotoxin. The possible functional significance of these subsets was discussed in Chapters 9 and 10. Most human T cell clones examined to date produce either IL–2 or both IL–2 and IL–4, and resting T cells in all species may also be capable of producing multiple cytokines. Therefore, the existence of IL–2 and IL–4 producing T cells may be unique to some species and stages of T cell maturation. Like IL–2, IL–4 may stimulate the growth of developing T cells in the thymus.

3. *IL–4 is a growth factor for mast cells* and synergizes with interleukin-3 (IL–3) in stimulating mast cell proliferation.

4. *IL–4 is also a macrophage activating factor,* but its effects on mononuclear phagocytes are much less potent than the effects of IFN–γ. In some cases, IL–4 may antagonize IFN–γ mediated activation of macrophages and inhibit production of IL–1 and TNF.

Human IL–4 has also been molecularly cloned and the recombinant cytokine produced. As in the mouse, IL–4 in humans is produced by CD4$^+$ T cells. However, in humans, IL–4 has not been found to be a growth factor for B cells or mast cells, is not produced exclusively by a significant subset of T cell clones, and may not be a macrophage-activating factor. The one biologic activity of IL–4 shared in both species is the ability of IL–4 to induce switching of B cells to IgE production. Since IgE is the principal mediator of immediate hypersensitivity (allergic) reactions (see Chapter 14), enhanced production of or responsiveness to IL–4 may play an important role in allergies. IL–4 also induces human B cells and macrophages to express CD23, a low-affinity receptor for the Fc portion of IgE, but the function of this receptor is not yet known.

Recent evidence has suggested that IL–4 may also contribute to cell-mediated immunity. Specifically, IL–4 can cause endothelial cells to bind lymphocytes and monocytes. IL–4 also activates CTL functions. However, mouse T cell clones that secrete IL–4, but not IL–2 or IFN–γ, are unable to adoptively transfer cell-mediated immunity.

TRANSFORMING GROWTH FACTOR–β

The original description of transforming growth factor–β was made in the field of tumor biology. It was noted that certain tumors produced activities, called transforming growth factor, that would allow normal cell types to grow in soft agar, a characteristic of malignant ("transformed") cells. Subsequently, it was found that growth stimulation was caused by one polypeptide, called TGF–α, but that survival in soft agar required a second factor, called TGF–β. TGF–α is a polypeptide growth factor for epithelial and mesenchymal cells and will not be discussed further. TGF–β is a dimeric protein of approximately 28 kD. The two 14 kD subunits can be identical or closely related polypeptides, depending on the cell source. TGF–β is synthesized by almost all cells in culture, although it is normally secreted in a latent form that must be activated by proteases. Both antigen-activated T cells and LPS–activated mononuclear phagocytes secrete biologically active TGF–β.

The actions of TGF–β are highly pleiotropic. TGF–β inhibits the growth of many cell types and stimulates the growth of others. Often, TGF-β can either inhibit or stimulate growth of the same cell type, depending upon culture conditions such as degree of confluence. TGF-β causes synthesis of extracellular matrix proteins, such as collagens, and of cellular receptors for matrix proteins. (The ability of TGF-β to induce extracellular matrix probably underlies its ability to promote cell growth in soft agar.) *In vivo*, TGF-β causes the growth of new blood vessels, a process called angiogenesis.

As a cytokine, TGF-β is potentially important because it antagonizes many responses of lymphocytes. For example, TGF-β inhibits T cell proliferation to polyclonal mitogens or in mixed leukocyte reactions (see Chapter 16) and inhibits maturation of CTLs. It can also inhibit macrophage activation. TGF-β also acts on non-immune effector cells, such as polymorphonuclear leukocytes and endothelial cells, again largely to counteract the effects of pro-inflammatory cytokines. In this sense, TGF-β is an "anti-cytokine" and may be a signal for shutting off immune responses. Signals that cause T cells to synthesize TGF-β may cause them to behave as suppressor cells (see Chapter 10). *In vivo,* certain tumors may escape an immune response by secreting large quantities of TGF-β.

Although TGF-β is largely a negative regulator of immunity, it may have some positive effects as well. For example, in mice, TGF-β has been shown to switch B cells to the IgA isotype and it may therefore be important in the generation of mucosal immune responses that are mediated by IgA.

Cytokines That Activate Inflammatory Cells

We will now discuss a group of cytokines derived principally from antigen-activated CD4+ and CD8+ T lymphocytes that serve primarily to activate the functions of nonspecific effector cells. Thus, these cytokines mediate the effector phase of cell-mediated immune responses. The molecules described in this section are summarized in Table 11-3.

IMMUNE OR GAMMA INTERFERON

Gamma interferon (IFN-γ), also called immune or type II interferon, is a homodimeric glycoprotein containing approximately 21 to 24 kD subunits. The size variation of the subunit is caused by variable degrees of glycosylation, but each subunit contains an identical 18 kD polypeptide encoded by the same gene. IFN-γ is produced both by IL-2 secreting CD4+ helper T cells and by nearly all CD8+ T cells. Transcription is directly initiated as a consequence of antigen activation and is enhanced by IL-2. IFN-γ has been detected in profoundly T cell-deficient animals, and the presumed source in this setting is NK cells; however, NK cells appear to be a minor source of IFN-γ in normal individuals.

As its name implies, IFN-γ shares many activities with type I IFN. Specifically, IFN-γ induces an antiviral state and is antiproliferative. However, IFN-γ binds to a unique cell surface receptor, different from that utilized by type I IFN. The IFN-γ receptor is not related structurally to the other receptor families described earlier. More importantly, IFN-γ has several properties related to immunoregulation that separate it functionally from type I IFN.

1. *IFN-γ is a potent activator of mononuclear phagocytes.* It directly induces synthesis of the enzymes that mediate the respiratory burst, allowing macrophages to kill phagocytosed microbes. Along with second signals, such as LPS and perhaps TNF, it allows macrophages to kill tumor cells. Cytokines that cause such functional changes in mononuclear phagocytes have been called **macrophage-activating factors** (MAFs). *IFN-γ is the principal MAF and provides the means by which T cells activate macrophages.* Other MAFs include GM-CSF and, to a lesser extent, IL-1, TNF, and, in the mouse, IL-4. Macrophage activation is described in more detail in Chapter 12. It is worth noting here that macrophage activation actually in-

TABLE 11-3. Mediators of Effector Cell Activation

Cytokine	Number of Genes	Polypeptide Size	Cell Source	Cell Target	Primary Effects on Each Target
Gamma interferon	1	21-24 kD (homodimer)	T cell, NK cell	Mononuclear phagocyte	Activation
				Endothelial cell	Activation
				NK cell	Activation
				All	Increased class I and class II MHC molecules
Lymphotoxin	1	24 kD (homotrimer)	T cell	Neutrophil	Activation
				Endothelial cell	Activation
Interleukin-5	1	20 kD (monomer)	T cell	Eosinophil	Activation
				B cell	Growth and activation
Migration inhibition factor	?	?	T cell	Mononuclear phagocyte	Conversion from motile to immotile state

Abbreviations: NK, natural killer; kD, kilodalton; MHC, major histocompatibility complex.

volves several different responses, and macrophages are said to be activated when they perform a particular function being assayed. For example, IFN – γ fully activates macrophages to kill phagocytosed microbes but only partly activates macrophages to kill tumor cells.

2. *IFN – γ increases class I MHC molecule expression and, in contrast to type I IFN, also causes a wide variety of cell types to express class II MHC molecules.* Thus, IFN – γ amplifies the cognitive phase of the immune response by promoting the activation of class II – restricted CD4+ helper T cells. *In vivo*, IFN – γ can enhance both cellular and humoral immune responses through these actions at the cognitive phase.

3. *IFN – γ acts directly on T and B lymphocytes to promote differentiation.* It is one of the factors that promotes CTL maturation and also stimulates B cell secretion of antibody. In mice, it causes B cell switching to the Ig2a isotype. IFN – γ is not a growth factor for lymphocytes and often inhibits proliferation of lymphocytes, particularly B cells. In mice, IFN – γ can antagonize IL – 4 mediated effects, such as isotype switching to IgE.

4. *IFN – γ activates neutrophils,* upregulating their respiratory burst. It is a less potent activator of neutrophils than TNF or lymphotoxin.

5. *IFN – γ is a potent activator of NK cells,* more so than type I IFN.

6. *IFN – γ is an activator of vascular endothelial cells,* promoting CD4+ T lymphocyte adhesion and morphologic alterations that facilitate lymphocyte extravasation. As mentioned earlier, IFN – γ also potentiates many of the actions of TNF on endothelial cells.

LYMPHOTOXIN

Lymphotoxin is a 21 to 24 kD glycoprotein that is approximately 30 per cent homologous to TNF and competes with TNF for binding to the same cell surface receptors. In humans, LT and TNF genes are located in tandem within the MHC on chromosome 6 (see Chapter 5). LT is produced exclusively by activated T lymphocytes and is often produced coordinately with IFN – γ by such cells. Human LT, unlike TNF, contains one or two N-linked oligosaccharides (accounting for the variability in molecular sizes). In further contrast to TNF, LT is synthesized as a true secretory protein without a membrane-spanning region.

Most studies have found little difference between the biologic effects of TNF and LT, consistent with their binding to the same receptor. The most important distinction between these cytokines appears to be that LT is exclusively synthesized by T cells, whereas TNF, although made by T cells, is predominantly derived from mononuclear phagocytes. In general, the quantities of LT synthesized by T cells are much less than the amounts of TNF made by LPS – stimulated mononuclear phagocytes and LT is not readily detected in the circulation. Therefore, LT is usually a locally acting paracrine factor and not a mediator of systemic injury. Although neither TNF nor LT is toxic for normal (non-neoplastic) cells, both

factors may contribute to CTL – mediated lysis of target cells (see Chapter 12). Like TNF, LT is a potent activator of neutrophils and thus provides lymphocytes with a means of regulating acute inflammatory reactions. It is more potent than IFN – γ as an activator of neutrophils and the actions of LT are enhanced by IFN – γ. LT is also an activator of vascular endothelial cells, causing increased leukocyte adhesion, cytokine production, and morphologic changes that facilitate leukocyte extravasation. These effects, like those of TNF, are also enhanced by IFN – γ.

INTERLEUKIN-5

Interleukin-5 (IL – 5) is a cytokine of approximately 20 kD produced by certain activated CD4+ T cells and by activated mast cells. IL – 5 acts as a costimulator for the growth of antigen-activated mouse B cells and was previously called either B cell growth factor 2 or T cell replacing factor. IL – 5 may function synergistically with other cytokines, such as IL – 2 and IL – 4, to stimulate the growth and differentiation of B cells. IL – 5 has also been found to act on more mature B cells to cause increased synthesis of immunoglobulin, especially of IgA. These actions are discussed in greater detail in Chapter 9.

An important action of IL – 5 is its ability to stimulate the growth and differentiation of eosinophils and to activate mature eosinophils in such a way that they can kill helminths. In mice, neutralizing antibodies to IL – 5 inhibit the eosinophilia seen in response to helminthic infection. Thus, IL – 5 provides a means by which T cells can regulate eosinophil-mediated inflammation.

MIGRATION INHIBITION FACTOR

We conclude our discussion of cytokines that regulate effector cells by considering the issue of migration inhibitor factor (MIF). One early view of cell mediated immune reactions proposed that mononuclear phagocyte accumulation in tissues depended on the retention of such cells in response to locally produced cytokines that inhibit motility. It now seems more likely that retention of leukocytes in the tissues is controlled primarily by expression of specific receptors for extracellular matrix molecules, such as integrins (see Box 7 – 4, Chapter 7). Nevertheless, one of the first cytokine activities identified was one that inhibited macrophage motility *in vitro*, called migration inhibition factor. MIF has still not been identified as a unique cytokine, although some recently cloned molecules appear to demonstrate MIF activity. At present, both the biochemical identity and biologic significance of MIF remain largely undefined.

Cytokines That Stimulate Hematopoiesis

Several of the cytokines generated during both natural immunity and antigen-induced specific immune responses have potent stimulatory effects on the growth and differentiation of bone marrow progenitor cells. Thus, immune and inflammatory reactions, which consume leukocytes, may also elicit production of new leukocytes to replace inflammatory cells. All of the various mature leukocyte cell populations arise as a consequence of progressive expansion and irreversible differentiation of the progeny of self-renewing stem cells. Maturation of a leukocyte involves commitment to a particular lineage and occurs concomitantly with loss of ability to develop into other mature cell types. This process has been depicted as a simple tree (see Fig. 2–8, Chapter 2). The cytokines that stimulate expansion and differentiation of bone marrow progenitor cells are collectively called **colony-stimulating factors** (CSFs) because they are often assayed by their ability to stimulate the formation of cell colonies in bone marrow cultures. These colonies of cells mature during the *in vitro* assay, acquiring characteristics of specific cell lineages (e.g., granulocytes, mononuclear phagocytes). Different CSFs act on bone marrow cells at different stages of maturation and preferentially promote development of colonies of different lineages. The names assigned to CSFs reflect the types of colonies that arise in these assays.

Some of the actions of CSFs are influenced by other cytokines. For example, TNF, LT, IFN-γ, and TGF-β all inhibit growth of bone marrow progenitor cells. In contrast, IL–1 and IL–6 enhance responses to CSFs. In general, cytokines are thought both to be necessary for normal marrow function and to provide a means of fine tuning function in response to stimulation. Some of the specific CSFs are listed in Table 11–4.

INTERLEUKIN-3

Interleukin-3 (IL–3) also known as **multilineage colony-stimulating factor,** is a 20 to 26 kD product of CD4+ T cells that acts on the most immature marrow progenitors and promotes the expansion of cells that differentiate into all known mature cell types. In mice, IL–3 also promotes the growth and development of mast cells from bone marrow–derived progenitors, an action enhanced by IL–4. In the mouse, IL–3 is produced both by CD4+ helper T cell clones that secrete IL–2 and by those that secrete IL–4. Human IL–3 has been identified by the complementary DNA (cDNA) cloning of a molecule homologous to mouse IL–3. Although IL–3 is made by some human T cell clones, it has been harder to establish a role for this cytokine in experimental systems of hematopoiesis in humans. In fact, many actions attributed to murine IL–3 appear to be performed by human granulocyte-macrophage CSF (see below). It is not known whether these experimental results reflect differences in species or in experimental conditions.

GRANULOCYTE-MACROPHAGE COLONY-STIMULATING FACTOR

Granulocyte-macrophage colony-stimulating factor (GM–CSF) is a 22 kD glycoprotein made by activated T cells and by activated mononuclear phagocytes, vascular endothelial cells, and fibroblasts. GM–CSF in the mouse acts primarily on bone marrow progenitors already committed to develop into leukocytes and thus presumably acts on a more differentiated population than IL–3. In human systems, however, GM–CSF also promotes growth of cells not yet committed to form leukocytes (e.g., platelets and progenitors of red blood cells), replacing IL–3. GM–CSF also activates mature leukocytes. For example, it mimics some of the actions of IFN-γ as an activator of macrophages, although it is usually less potent.

GM–CSF is not detected in the circulation and

TABLE 11–4. Mediators of Immature Leukocyte Growth and Differentiation

Cytokine	Number of Genes	Polypeptide Size	Cell Source	Cell Target	Primary Effects on Each Target
Interleukin-3	1	20–26 kD (monomer)	T cell	Immature progenitor	Growth and differentiation to all cell lines
Granulocyte-macrophage CSF	1	22 kD (monomer)	T cell, mononuclear phagocyte, endothelial cell, fibroblast	Immature progenitor / Committed progenitor / Mononuclear phagocyte	Growth and differentiation to all cell lines / Differentiation to granulocytes and mononuclear phagocytes / Activation
Macrophage CSF	1	40 kD (dimer)	Mononuclear phagocyte, endothelial cell, fibroblast	Committed progenitor	Differentiation to mononuclear phagocytes
Granulocyte CSF	1	19 kD (monomer)	Mononuclear phagocyte, endothelial cell, fibroblast	Committed progenitor	Differentiation to granulocytes
Interleukin-7	1	25 kD (monomer)	Fibroblast, bone marrow stromal cells	Immature progenitor	Growth and differentiation to B lymphocytes

Abbreviations: CSF, colony-stimulating factor; kD, kilodalton.

presumably acts locally at sites of production. Thus, in peripheral tissues T cell and macrophage derived GM–CSF may function mainly to activate mature leukocytes at sites of immune inflammatory responses, whereas hematopoietic effects may be mediated by GM–CSF produced by T cells, endothelial cells, or stromal fibroblasts in the bone marrow.

MONOCYTE-MACROPHAGE COLONY-STIMULATING FACTOR

Monocyte-macrophage colony-stimulating factor (M-CSF), also called CSF–1, is made by macrophages and by endothelial cells and fibroblasts. The secreted polypeptide is approximately 40 kD and forms a stable dimer. M-CSF acts primarily on those progenitors that are already committed to develop into monocytes and are presumably more mature than the targets for GM–CSF. Like GM–CSF, M-CSF does not circulate and the major colony-stimulating effect may be derived from local production within the marrow cavity.

M-CSF is one of the few cytokines whose mechanism of action is partly understood. This is because the M-CSF receptor has been identified as a tyrosine kinase. Interestingly, the M-CSF receptor was first identified as the normal cellular counterpart of a viral oncogene, called *v-fms*.

GRANULOCYTE COLONY-STIMULATING FACTOR

Granulocyte colony-stimulating factor (G-CSF) is made by the same cells that make GM-CSF. The secreted polypeptide is approximately 19 kD. In contrast to other CSFs, G-CSF does normally circulate. It acts primarily on marrow progenitors already committed to develop into granulocytes, again a more mature population than that responsive to GM–CSF. Because G-CSF can act at a distance, neutrophil maturation and release from bone marrow are highly influenced by inflammatory reactions occurring in the periphery, outside the marrow.

INTERLEUKIN-7

Interleukin 7 (IL–7) is a recently described cytokine secreted by marrow stromal cells that acts on hematopoietic progenitors committed to the B lymphocyte lineage. Most models of hematopoiesis suggest that lymphocyte progenitors differentiate from common stem cells very early in maturation, so that IL–7 is probably acting on cells at the same level of development as IL–3 or GM–CSF. Recent studies suggest that IL–7 may also stimulate the growth and maturation of immature CD4⁻CD8⁻ T cell precursors in the thymus. However, this is based on *in vitro* experiments, and the cellular source of IL–7 in the thymus is not known. Transgenic mice that overexpress IL–7 show markedly increased numbers of pre–B cells in the bone marrow and peripheral lymphoid tissues and variable increases in immature T cells in the thymus.

The list of molecularly defined cytokines continues to grow. IL–9 is a 30 to 40-kD protein that supports the growth of some T cell lines and of bone marrow–derived mast cell progenitors. It may also stimulate development of other lineages from marrow-derived precursors. However, it is not known whether IL–9 has an effect on normal lymphocytes (other than cell lines) or if it plays a role in the regulation of immune responses or hematopoiesis *in vivo*.

IL–10 is a ~20 kD protein that was originally identified as a product of IL–4–secreting (Th2) murine T cell clones. It is now thought to be produced also by B lymphocytes and some stromal cells. IL–10 inhibits the production of IFN–γ by T cells and by natural killer cells and the production of IL–2 by T cells. Thus, IL–10 may function to reduce activation of Th1-like cells and cause a relative increase in the expansion of Th2 cells. It may play this role in parasitic infections, in which IL–4–stimulated IgE secretion and IL–5–mediated eosinophilia (both being typical responses elicited by Th2 cells) are prominent. Interestingly, the Epstein-Barr virus genome contains a gene homologous to IL–10 whose protein product has the same biologic activities. This raises the interesting possibility that pathogenic microbes may have "picked up" host genes whose products function to inhibit microbial immunity. The mechanism of action of IL–10 is not well understood. Its effects on T cells may be due to a direct effect on antigen-presenting cells rather than on the T cells themselves.

IL–11 is a ~20 kD cytokine produced by bone marrow stromal cells, especially after activation (which may be achieved experimentally by pharmacologic agents such as phorbol esters). IL–11 stimulates megakaryopoiesis and may prove to be of therapeutic benefit in patients with platelet deficiencies. It also enhances the development of macrophages and perhaps other cell lineages from marrow precursors.

SUMMARY

Cytokines are a family of protein mediators of both natural and acquired immunity. The same cytokines are often made by many cell types and individual cytokines often act on many cell types. The actions of different cytokines are often redundant and influence the action of other cytokines. In general, cytokines are synthesized in response to inflammatory or antigenic stimuli and act locally, in an autocrine or paracrine fashion, by binding to high affinity receptors on target cells. Certain cytokines may be produced in sufficient quantity to circulate and exert endocrine actions. For many cell types, cytokines serve as growth factors.

We have classified cytokines into four groups, according to their principal actions:

The first group consists of those cytokines that mediate natural immunity and includes the anti-viral type I interferons and the pro-inflammatory cytokines — tumor necrosis factor, interleukin-1, interleukin-6 and members of the newly described family of low molecular weight inflammatory cytokines. The predominant cellular source of these molecules is mononuclear phagocytes.

The second group of cytokines is derived largely from antigen-stimulated CD4[+] T lymphocytes and serves to regulate the activation, growth, and differentiation of B and T cells. This group includes interleukin-2, the principal T cell growth factor; interleukin-4, the major regulator of IgE synthesis; and transforming growth factor–β, which inhibits lymphocyte responses.

The third group of cytokines, produced by antigen-activated CD4[+] and CD8[+] T lymphocytes, serves to activate inflammatory leukocytes and places these effector cells under T cell regulation. This group includes γ-interferon, the principal activator of mononuclear phagocytes; lymphotoxin, an activator of neutrophils; and interleukin-5, an activator of eosinophils.

The fourth group, collectively called colony-stimulating factors, consists of cytokines derived from both nonspecific effector cells and T cells, which stimulate the growth of bone marrow cells, thereby providing a source of additional inflammatory leukocytes.

Thus, cytokines serve many functions that are critical to host defense against pathogens and provide links between specific and natural immunity. Cytokines also regulate the magnitude and nature of immune responses by influencing the growth and differentiation of lymphocytes. Finally, cytokines provide important amplification mechanisms that enable small numbers of lymphocytes specific for any one antigen to activate a variety of effector mechanisms to eliminate the antigen. Excessive production or actions of cytokines can lead to tissue injury and even death. The administration of cytokines or their inhibitors is a potential approach for modifying biologic responses associated with disease.

SELECTED READINGS

Arai, K., F. Lee, A. Miyajima, S. Miyatake, N. Arai, and T. Yokota. Cytokines: coordinators of immune and inflammatory responses. Annual Review of Biochemistry 59:783–836, 1990.

Balkwill, F. R., and F. Burke. The cytokine network. Immunology Today 10:299–304, 1989.

Beutler, B., and A. Cerami. The biology of cachectin-TNF: a primary mediator of the host response. Annual Review of Immunology 7:625–655, 1988.

DeMaeyer, E., and J. DeMaeyer-Guignard. Interferons and Other Regulatory Cytokines. New York, John Wiley & Sons, 1988.

diGiovine, F. S., and G. W. Duff. Interleukin 1: the first interleukin. Immunology Today 11:13–20, 1990.

Matsushima, K., and J. J. Oppenheim. Interleukin 8 and MCAF: novel inflammatory cytokines inducible by IL-1 and TNF. Cytokine 1:2–13, 1989.

Nicola, N. A. Hematopoietic cell growth factors and their receptors. Annual Review of Biochemistry 58:45–77, 1989.

Paul, N. L., and N. H. Ruddle. Lymphotoxin. Annual Review of Immunology 6:407–438, 1987.

Paul, W. E., and J. Ohara. B-cell stimulatory factor–1/interleukin 4. Annual Review of Immunology 5:429–460, 1987.

Reeves, R., and N.S. Magnuson. Mechanisms regulating transient expression of mammalian cytokine genes and cellular oncogenes. Progress in Nucleic Acid Research and Molecular Biology 38:241–282, 1990.

Roberts, A. B., and M. B. Sporn. Transforming growth factor. Advances in Cancer Research 51:107–145, 1988.

Sanderson, C. J., H. D. Campbell, and I. G. Young. Molecular and cellular biology of eosinophil differentiation factor (interleukin-5) and its effects on human and mouse B cells. Immunological Reviews 102:29–50, 1988.

Smith, K. A. Interleukin-2: Inception, impact and implications. Science 240:1169–1176, 1988.

Smith, K. A. The interleukin 2 receptor. Annual Review of Cell Biology 5:397–425, 1989.

van Snick, J. Interleukin-6: an overview. Annual Review of Immunology 8:253–278, 1990.

CHAPTER TWELVE

EFFECTOR CELLS OF CELL-MEDIATED IMMUNITY

Historically, specific immunity has been divided into *humoral immunity,* which can be adoptively transferred from an immunized donor to a naive host by antibodies in the absence of cells, and *cell-mediated immunity,* which can be adoptively transferred only by viable T lymphocytes. This classification, first evident through adoptive transfer experiments, is actually quite general because it is based upon fundamental differences among various effector mechanisms in the immune system. The effector phase of the immune response is initiated and targeted by specific antigen recognition. *In humoral immunity, specific recognition of antigen in the effector phase is mediated by the binding of secreted antibody molecules to antigen.* Antibody is thus sufficient to adoptively transfer humoral immunity. *In cell-mediated immunity, in contrast, the effector phase, as well as the cognitive phase, is initiated through specific antigen recognition by T cells.*

In some forms of cell-mediated immunity, antigen-specific T cells directly perform the effector function, as when cytolytic T lymphocytes (CTLs) lyse specific target cells; in others, antigen-activated T cells secrete cytokines that recruit and activate effector cells that are not specific for the antigen, such as macrophages and natural killer (NK) cells. When the effector cells are nonspecific, antigen specificity is conferred by proximity to the antigen stimulated T cells. T cells can recognize and respond to foreign antigen only when it is presented in a complex with a self major histocompatibility complex (MHC) molecule on the surface of an appropriate antigen-presenting cell (APC) or target cell. *Therefore, cell-mediated immunity is directed at or near cells that bear foreign antigens on their surface and cell-mediated immune reactions are physiologically most important for eradicating microbes or viruses that live intracellularly, i.e., within APCs.* Indeed, the original description of cell-mediated immunity was the adoptive transfer of protection against *Listeria monocytogenes,* an intracellular bacterium (see Chapter 15). Cell-mediated immune reactions may also be important for elimination of cells that express foreign MHC molecules, as in an allograft (see Chapter 16) or express tumor-specific antigens as in a malignant tumor (see Chapter 17).

Different types of cell-mediated immune reactions may result from T cell recognition of antigen.

1. In **delayed type hypersensitivity** (DTH), antigen-activated CD4$^+$ T cells secrete cytokines, which have several effects. Some cytokines activate venular endothelial cells to recruit monocytes from the blood at the site of antigen challenge. Other cytokines convert the monocytes into activated macrophages which serve to eliminate the antigen.

2. In **CTL responses** to viral infections or organ transplants, antigen-activated CD8$^+$ T cells differentiate into functional CTLs, which lyse target cells expressing specific antigen-MHC complexes. This process of differentiation often requires "help" in the form of cytokines secreted by antigen-activated CD4$^+$ T cells.

3. In graft-versus-host disease (see Chapter 16), **natural killer (NK) cells,** stimulated by cytokines

from antigen-activated CD4$^+$ T cells, differentiate into **lymphokine-activated killer (LAK) cells,** which nonspecifically lyse target cells.

This chapter begins with a discussion of the T cells that regulate cell-mediated immune reactions and then considers the various effector cell populations that are involved in each of these distinct reaction patterns.

CD4$^+$ T Lymphocytes and the Initiation of Cell-Mediated Immune Reactions

CD4$^+$ T cells initiate specific immunity, both cell-mediated and humoral, by recognizing portions of protein antigens (peptides) bound to self class II MHC molecules on the surface of APC. Upon activation by specific antigen, these T cells secrete cytokines, many of which act on other cell populations involved in host defense. For example, tumor necrosis factor (TNF) and lymphotoxin (LT) activate neutrophils and vascular endothelial cells; interleukin-5 (IL-5) activates eosinophils; γ-interferon (IFN-γ) activates mononuclear phagocytes; and interleukin-2 (IL-2) activates NK cells as well as both T and B lymphocytes. *By means of cytokine secretion, CD4$^+$ T cells stimulate the function and focus the activity of nonspecific effector cells of natural immunity, thereby converting these cells into agents of specific immunity.* Indeed, the first function of T cells in the evolutionary development of specific immunity may well have been to augment and direct the effector mechanisms of natural immunity. As antigen-specific effector cells, such as CTLs and B lymphocytes, evolved the general pattern of CD4$^+$ T cell function remained the same: through the secretion of cytokines, such as IL-2 and IL-4, CD4$^+$ cells provide "help" necessary for the activation of other lymphocytes.

The multitude of cytokines produced by antigen-activated CD4$^+$ T cells, each with distinct but overlapping sets of cellular targets, raises the question of how particular antigens elicit particular types of immune reactions. CD4$^+$ T cells may produce different quantities or types of cytokines, depending on their activation conditions, or may consist of subsets that secrete distinct cytokines. Alternatively, each CD4$^+$ T cell may produce multiple cytokines but influences different effector cell types (e.g., B cells or macrophages or CTLs), depending on which of these cell types is in close proximity to the site of CD4$^+$ T cell activation.

Delayed Type Hypersensitivity and Its Effector Cells

Delayed type hypersensitivity is a form of cell-mediated immunity in which the ultimate effector cell is the activated **mononuclear phagocyte (macrophage).** This type of cell-mediated immunity is the primary defense mechanism against intracellular bacteria, such as *Listeria monocytogenes* and mycobacteria. The same reaction can be elicited by soluble protein antigens and by chemically reactive haptens. The classical animal model of DTH is the response of an immunized guinea pig to antigen applied by "skin painting" or introduced by intradermal injection.

Such reactions may be induced in humans by contact sensitization with chemicals and environmental antigens or by intradermal injection of microbial antigens in individuals immunized by prior infection (Fig. 12–1). For example, purified protein derivative (PPD), a protein prepared from *Mycobacterium tuberculosis*, will elicit a DTH response when injected into

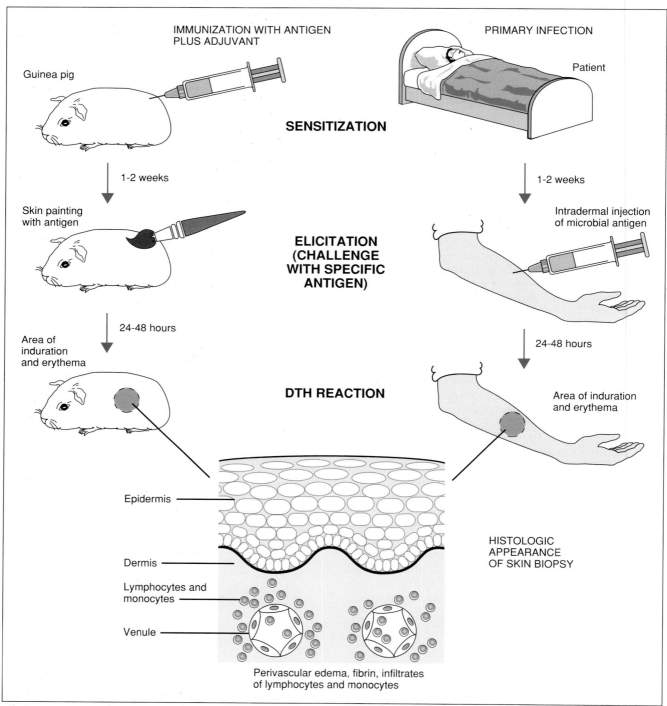

FIGURE 12 – 1. Sensitization for and elicitation of a delayed type hypersensitivity (DTH) reaction. *A guinea pig is sensitized experimentally by injection of antigen or by skin painting with antigen (not shown); in humans, sensitization occurs through infection or by vaccination (not shown). In these two species, subsequent challenge of sensitized individuals with specific antigens then elicits histologically similar DTH reactions.*

individuals who have recovered from primary tuberculosis or who have been vaccinated against tuberculosis. The characteristic response of DTH evolves over 24 to 48 hours. About 4 hours after injection of antigen, neutrophils accumulate around the post-capillary venules at the injection site. The neutrophil infiltrate rapidly subsides, and by about 12 hours the injection site becomes infiltrated by T cells and blood monocytes, also organized in a perivenular distribution (Fig. 12–2). The endothelial cells lining these venules become plump, show increased biosynthetic organelles, and become leaky to plasma macromolecules. Fibrinogen escapes from the blood vessels into the surrounding tissues, where it is converted into fibrin. The deposition of fibrin and, to a lesser extent, accumulation of T cells and monocytes within the extravascular tissue space around the injection site cause the tissue to swell and become hard ("indurated"). Induration, the hallmark of DTH, is detectable by about 18 hours after injection of antigen and is maximal by 24 to 48 hours. The lag in the onset of palpable induration is the reason for calling the response delayed type.

Although experimental DTH was first described in guinea pigs, DTH–like reactions may be elicited in other animals such as mice or rats. Histologically, these murine reactions differ from DTH responses in guinea pig or man in that the inflammatory infiltrate at 18 to 24 hours shows a paucity of T cells and activated macrophages but rather consists largely of neutrophils. The basis of this difference is not known, but may reside in the inflammatory functions of vascular endothelium or species differences in the production or effects of cytokines. Nevertheless, in all species examined, DTH reactions to most protein antigens may be adoptively transferred by antigen-sensitized CD4+ T cells. Recent studies indicate that CD8+ T cells are also capable of adoptively transferring DTH–like reactions. In fact, intracellular viruses tend to stimulate strong CD8+ T cell responses, and these cells are important sources of IFN–γ, the principal cytokine involved in DTH. Therefore, DTH reactions against viral antigens may be mediated largely by CD8+ T cells and against injected proteins or extracellular antigens by CD4+ cells.

In clinical practice, loss of DTH responses to uni-

FIGURE 12–2. Morphology of a DTH reaction.
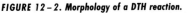
A. *Low-power photomicrograph depicting mononuclear cell infiltrates surrounding venules (V) in human skin in a reaction to foreign antigen. (Reproduced with permission from Dvorak, H. F., and M. C. Mihm, Jr. Basophilic leukocytes in allergic contact dermatitis. Journal of Experimental Medicine 135:235-254, 1972. Copyright permission of the Rockefeller University Press, New York.)*
B. *High-power photomicrograph showing morphologically altered venular endothelium (E) in the midst of the inflammatory infiltrates. (Reproduced with permission from Dvorak, H. F., S. J. Galli, and A. M. Dvorak. Expression of cell mediated hypersensitivity in vivo: recent advances. International Review of Experimental Pathology 21:119-194, 1980.)*

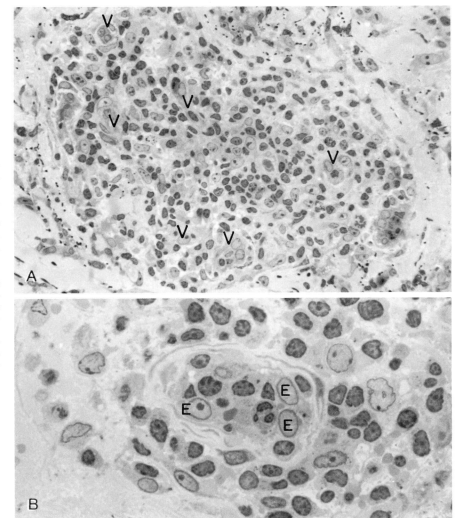

versally encountered antigens (e.g., candidal antigens) is an indication of deficient T cell function, a condition known as **anergy.** (This general loss of immune responsiveness should be distinguished from "clonal anergy," a mechanism for providing tolerance to specific antigens, discussed in Chapter 10.) Anergic individuals are extremely susceptible to infection by microorganisms that are normally resisted by cell-mediated immunity such as mycobacteria and fungi.

DTH reactions, like other types of specific immunity, consist of three sequential processes:

1. The *cognitive phase,* in which CD4+ and sometimes CD8+ T cells recognize foreign protein antigens presented on the surface of APCs.

2. The *activation phase,* in which the T cells secrete cytokines and proliferate.

3. The *effector phase.* In DTH, the effector phase can be further subdivided into two steps: (a) **inflammation,** in which vascular endothelial cells, activated by cytokines, recruit circulating leukocytes into the tissues at the local site of antigen challenge; and (b) **resolution,** in which macrophages, activated by cytokines, act to eliminate the foreign antigen (Fig. 12-3).

These stages will be discussed in the context of the cell type central to each step of the process.

Antigen-Presenting Cells and the Cognitive and Activation Phases of Delayed Type Hypersensitivity

The identity of the APCs which present antigens to CD4+ T cells and thus initiate DTH is uncertain. Several candidate APCs have been proposed in skin (Fig. 12-4).

1. *Specialized resident APCs, such as Langerhans cells in the epidermis,* could carry antigen from the portal of entry (e.g., the skin) to the draining lymph nodes, where contact with antigen-specific T cells is more likely to occur. Activated T cells both expand in number and increase their ability to cross endothelial barriers. Both changes could serve to enhance the likelihood of encounter with antigen at the peripheral site. Langerhans cells are likely to present antigen for initial immunization, but this process is probably too slow to account for DTH reactions in sensitized individuals.

2. *Macrophages,* resident in the dermis, could present antigen to those T cells that coincidentally exit the blood stream at the site of exposure to foreign antigen. If these macrophages are also stimulated by a

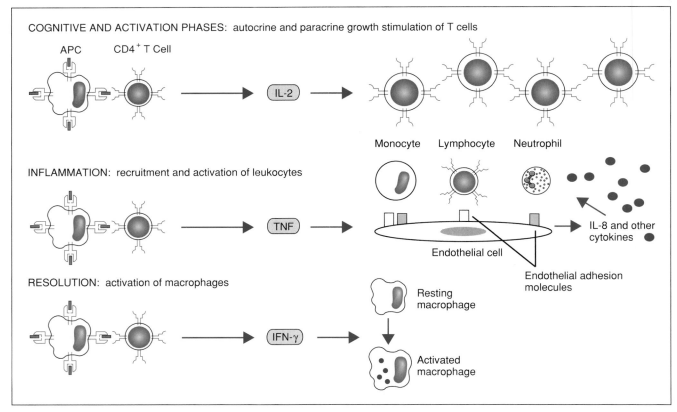

FIGURE 12 – 3. Stages of a DTH reaction. *DTH reactions are initiated by T cell recognition of an MHC – associated antigen on an antigen-presenting cell (APC); in the example shown, this is a class II – associated antigen recognized by a CD4+ T cell, but a CD8+ T cell is capable of inducing a similar reaction. Different cytokines secreted by the T cell in response to antigen recognition play predominant roles in different phases of the reaction, as shown. Other cytokines that are not shown may play auxiliary roles.*

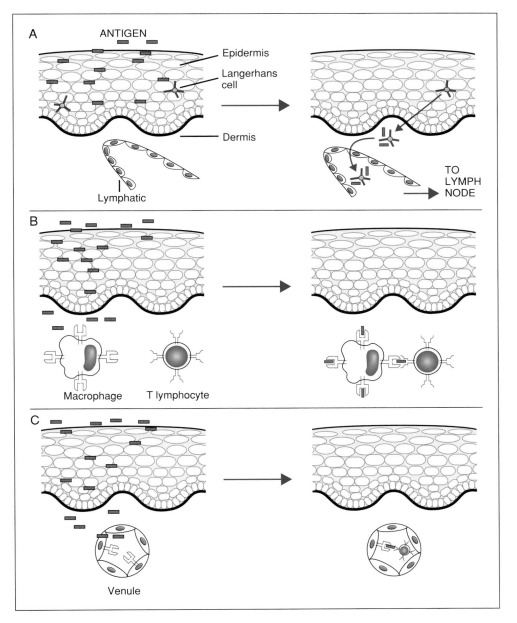

FIGURE 12-4. Antigen-presenting cells (APCs) for initiating DTH reactions. *Three different cell types have been proposed as APCs to initiate DTH reactions in the skin: epidermal Langerhans cells* (A), *dermal macrophages* (B), *and venular endothelial cells* (C). *In humans, antigen presentation by Langerhans cells probably initiates sensitization whereas antigen presentation by endothelial cells probably initiates DTH reactions upon subsequent challenge. Note that Langerhans cells* (A) *bear class II MHC–associated processed antigen on their surface (not shown).*

Labels within figure: ANTIGEN, Epidermis, Langerhans cell, Dermis, Lymphatic, TO LYMPH NODE (A); Macrophage, T lymphocyte (B); Venule (C).

bacterial product, such as lipopolysaccharide (LPS) or the mycobacterial cell wall product, muramyl dipeptide, they may secrete TNF and interleukin-1 (IL–1), which through their actions on venular endothelial cells (see below) can nonspecifically recruit T cells into the site. This would increase the likelihood of T cells encountering the antigen. Once the first CD4+ T cell is stimulated, it can also produce TNF, further increasing the likelihood of other antigen-specific T cells joining the reaction. This amplification mechanism may be critical for the development of DTH.

3. *Endothelial cells* lining the post-capillary venules could present antigen on the luminal surface of the blood vessel. Venular endothelial cells in humans and some other species such as baboons and dogs express class II MHC molecules *in situ* and demonstrate T cell costimulatory activities *in vitro*. In other species, such as guinea pig, endothelial cells are induced to express class II MHC molecules as one of the earliest events in DTH reactions. In certain other species, notably the rat, endothelial cells rarely express class II MHC molecules *in situ* and are unlikely to present extracellular antigens. For DTH reactions to viral antigens that are mediated by CD8+ T cells, endothelial cells may present antigens in association with class I MHC molecules.

These models are not exclusive, and no single APC type may be responsible for initiating DTH in all species, in all tissues, and to all antigens.

Once activated by an appropriate APC, the T cells that mediate DTH do so by secretion of cytokines. Four cytokine-mediated effects appear most important for development of the characteristic inflammatory reaction (see Fig. 12 – 3).

1. IL – 2 causes autocrine and paracrine proliferation of antigen activated T cells. Higher concentrations of IL – 2 can also stimulate bystander T cells not specific for the antigen. Indeed, by the time lymphocytic infiltrate becomes pronounced, more than 90 per cent of the activated T cells present at the site of antigen challenge are not specific for the eliciting antigen. In addition to its effects of proliferation, IL – 2 augments synthesis of cytokines by CD4$^+$ T cells, including IL – 2 itself, IFN – γ, and TNF. Lymphotoxin is also produced and, at later times, may be secreted in greater quantities than TNF.

2. IFN – γ acts on APCs, such as endothelium or macrophages, to increase class II MHC molecule expression, increasing the efficiency of antigen presentation to CD4$^+$ T cells at the local site. This is another important amplification mechanism for the induction of DTH.

3. TNF and LT act on venular endothelial cells to augment their capacities to bind and activate leukocytes, leading to inflammation. IFN – γ and IL – 4 may have similar actions on endothelial cells.

4. IFN – γ acts on monocytes infiltrating the inflammatory site to activate their capacity to eliminate antigen. Because IFN – γ is the most potent macrophage-activating cytokine in all species examined, it is the most important mediator of DTH.

Venular Endothelial Cells and Inflammation

Venular endothelial cells at sites of antigen administration may play two roles in the DTH reaction. First, as discussed above, venular endothelial cells may act as APCs to initiate T cell activation. Second, *venular endothelial cells regulate the infiltration of leukocytes into the inflammatory reaction.*

In the past, two alternative mechanisms have been proposed to explain the recruitment of leukocytes from the blood into the tissues (Fig. 12 – 5).

1. Antigen-activated T cells and other leukocytes in the tissue release leukocyte-attracting factors, such as members of the interleukin-8 (IL – 8) family (see Chapter 11). Circulating leukocytes sense these molecules in the blood stream and then migrate along a gradient of increasing concentration (chemotaxis) to the tissue source, e.g., the activated T cell. Chemotaxis has largely fallen into disfavor as an explanation for inflammation because leukocytes do not simply follow gradients across capillary beds but, rather, exclusively migrate through post-capillary venules. Moreover, it is not clear that a gradient of a soluble mediator can be maintained in the blood stream.

2. An alternative explanation emphasizes a primary role of the venular endothelial cell as the regulator of leukocytic extravasation. It has been proposed

that under the influence of TNF and other cytokines, venular endothelial cells perform four functions that contribute to inflammation:

a. By production of vasodilator substances such as prostacyclin (PGI$_2$), venular endothelial cells cause increased blood flow and optimize delivery of leukocytes at the site of inflammation. TNF increases the expression of enzymes in endothelial cells that synthesize prostacyclin.

b. By expression of new or increased levels of certain surface proteins, endothelial cells become adhesive for leukocytes. In this adhesive state, a random encounter of a circulating leukocyte with a venular endothelial cell will result in an increase in the residence time of leukocytes on the venular surface. As has been shown for lymphocyte diapedesis across high endothelial venules in organized lymphoid tissues (see Chapter 2), such increased residence time can serve to increase the likelihood of extravasation. Several leukocyte adhesion molecules on vascular endothelium are induced in peripheral tissues in response to cytokines. Soon after exposure to TNF, endothelial cells express **endothelial leukocyte adhesion molecule – 1** (ELAM – 1), an adhesive molecule structurally homologous to the lymphocyte homing receptor recognized by the MEL – 14 antibody (see Chapter 2, Box 2 – 2). ELAM – 1 selectively binds neutrophils, although the structure on the neutrophil recognized by ELAM – 1 is as yet unknown. At later times, ELAM – 1 expression declines and endothelial cells instead express **intercellular adhesion molecule – 1** (ICAM – 1) and **vascular cell adhesion molecule – 1** (VCAM – 1). As discussed in Chapters 2 and 7, ICAM – 1 is a ligand for the lymphocyte function – associated antigen – 1 (LFA – 1) integrin molecule on leukocytes. VCAM – 1, a member of the Ig gene superfamily that binds monocytes and lymphocytes, is a ligand for VLA – 4, a different integrin which also functions as a homing receptor for lymphocytes migrating to Peyer's patch. *These sequential changes in the endothelial cell surface are caused by TNF and lead to sequential adhesion, first of neutrophils and then of lymphocytes and monocytes.*

c. TNF causes endothelial cells to secrete low molecular weight inflammatory cytokines, such as IL – 8 and monocyte chemotactic protein – 1 (MCP – 1), that cause increased mobility of leukocytes. These cytokines may preferentially act on leukocytes that are bound to the endothelial cells, thus stimulating their extravasation.

d. TNF, acting in concert with IFN – γ, causes endothelial cells to undergo shape changes and basement membrane remodeling that favor leakage of macromolecules and extravasation of cells. Leakage of plasma macromolecules, especially fibrinogen, is the basis of induration. Plasma leakage also serves to reduce the shear force imparted by flowing blood, thereby favoring leukocyte attachment to endothelium.

In the endothelial-based model of inflammation, chemotactic molecules such as IL – 8 and MCP – 1 are

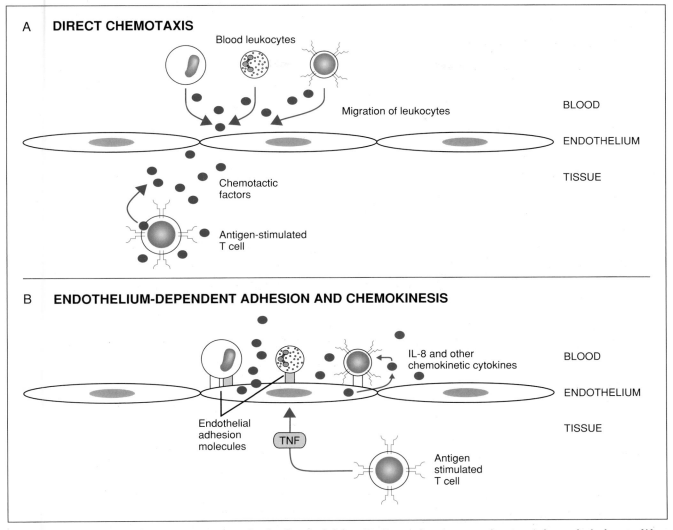

FIGURE 12 – 5. Mechanisms of leukocyte recruitment in DTH: roles of T cells and endothelium. *T cells may directly secrete chemotactic factors for leukocytes (A) or they may secrete cytokines (e.g., tumor necrosis factor) that increase expression of endothelial-leukocyte adhesion molecules and stimulate secretion of endothelial cell – derived cytokines (e.g., IL – 8) that enhance leukocyte migration (B). Recent data favor the more active role of vascular endothelium (B).*

still presumed to participate as important mediators of inflammation, acting primarily as stimulators of extravasation by those leukocytes that are marginated on the surface of the venule. However, the endothelial cells themselves rather than antigen-activated T cells may be the principal source of the relevant chemoattractants, and the initial actions of these cytokines may be to stimulate cell migration (chemokinesis) rather than migration along a chemical gradient.

Once leukocytes enter the tissues, they may die in a few days (especially characteristic of neutrophils), may become activated (especially characteristic of T cells and monocytes), or may leave, probably through lymphatic vessels. The molecules controlling these processes are not yet defined. It seems likely that leukocytes may remain at the site of inflammation because cell activation increases the expression of receptors for extracellular matrix molecules. The

members of the $\beta 1$ integrin family (see Chapter 7, Box 7 – 4) are particularly important. VLA – 4 and VLA – 5 allow leukocytes to bind to fibronectin and VLA – 6 mediates attachment to laminin.

Activated Macrophages and Resolution of Delayed Type Hypersensitivity

Once blood monocytes leave the circulation and enter the extravascular tissues at sites of DTH reactions, they differentiate into macrophages, which are the ultimate effector cells of these reactions. The macrophages function to eliminate microorganisms and other sources of antigen. The differentiation of monocytes into effector cells is called **macrophage activation.**

The activation of macrophages is not a single process. A macrophage is considered to be activated if it performs a function measured in a specific assay, e.g., killing a microbe. In other assays, e.g., initiating blood coagulation or killing a tumor cell, the same macrophage may appear to be unactivated. Because such functional assays are biologically complex, it is preferable to divide the process of activation into more simple components. The unstimulated blood monocyte is usually considered to be at rest. *Activation consists of quantitative alterations in the expression of various gene products (proteins) that endow the activated macrophage with the capacity to perform some function that cannot be performed by the resting monocyte.* In general, macrophage activation thus results from new or increased gene transcription. For example, activation may consist of increasing expression of a cytochrome enzyme that catalyzes the generation of active oxygen species. By expressing this enzyme, the activated macrophage has acquired increased capacity to generate active oxygen. As a consequence of this capacity, the activated macrophage may be able to perform a function, e.g., killing of phagocytosed bacteria, that cannot be performed by the resting monocyte. The agents that cause gene transcription and thus macrophage activation are soluble cytokines, bacterial products (e.g., LPS), and extracellular matrix molecules. The best described macrophage-activating factor is the cytokine IFN-γ. However, IFN-γ is not the only cytokine that can activate macrophages, and IFN-γ does not activate all possible capacities of the macrophage. Some specific examples of the functions of activated macrophages follow:

1. *Activated macrophages kill microorganisms.* Killing of bacteria by macrophages involves phagocytosis and generation of active oxygen species. Cytokines such as IFN-γ augment both endocytosis and phagocytosis by monocytes. Phagocytosis of specific particles can be further enhanced by opsonizing bacteria, that is, coating the bacteria with specific IgG molecules or complement components (see Chapters 3 and 13). IFN-γ causes macrophages to increase expression of high-affinity receptors for the Fc portion of IgG, promoting uptake of opsonized bacteria. Once in the cell, macrophages kill bacteria by generating active oxygen species. IFN-γ induces transcription of the gene encoding the enzyme that generates active oxygen. *IFN-γ is thus sufficient to fully activate macrophages for killing of microorganisms.*

2. *Activated macrophages stimulate acute inflammation, often through secretion of short-lived inflammatory mediators.* Many of these mediators, such as platelet-activating factor (PAF), prostaglandins, and leukotrienes, are lipids. Some are synthesized by macrophages themselves and others are generated from plasma molecules in response to enzymes and related molecules secreted by the macrophages. For example, macrophages produce a protein called tissue factor, which can initiate the extrinsic clotting cascade; thrombin, a blood protease activated during the clot-

ting cascade, causes neutrophils and endothelial cells to synthesize PAF. Treatment with cytokines, such as IFN-γ, enhances the biosynthetic capacities of the macrophage to generate mediators such as tissue factor. The collective action of these macrophage-derived mediators is to produce local inflammation. The inflammatory reaction that results is rich in neutrophils and serves to contain and destroy infectious organisms and to get rid of injured tissue. Thus, the activated macrophage acts as an endogenous surgeon to cauterize the wound, leading to elimination of antigen and resolution of the DTH reaction.

3. *Activated macrophages become more efficient APCs.* A significant part of the enhanced antigen-presenting capacity may be attributed to increased surface expression of class II MHC molecules. IFN-γ is the best known activator of the transcription of class II MHC genes, but in macrophages both IL-4 and granulocyte-macrophage colony-stimulating factor (GM-CSF) may also have some effect. It is also likely that costimulator functions are enhanced in activated macrophages. IL-1 and TNF both act on macrophages to increase synthesis of IL-1, TNF, and IL-6, cytokines that augment T cell activation. Activated macrophages also express increased levels of cell surface ligands, such as ICAM-1 and LFA-3, that interact with T cell accessory molecules LFA-1 and CD2, respectively (see Chapter 7).

4. *Activated macrophage products, such as cytokines and growth factors, progressively modify the local tissue environment, initially leading to destruction of tissue and later causing replacement by connective tissue.* IFN-γ facilitates synthesis of cytokines by macrophages but is not sufficient to completely activate these functions. Often, a microorganism can supply a necessary second signal for cytokine synthesis, such as LPS from a bacterial cell wall. Other T cell-derived cytokines can substitute for LPS and work with IFN-γ to stimulate macrophages to secrete cytokines. The effects of macrophage-derived cytokines and growth factors occur in two phases. Acutely, TNF, IL-1, and possibly IL-6 augment cell-mediated immune reactions through their actions on T cells, on inflammatory leukocytes, and on endothelial cells. Thus, cytokines act in concert with the inflammatory mediators described above to cause local tissue destruction. Chronically, these same cytokines also stimulate fibroblast proliferation and collagen production. These slow actions of cytokines are augmented by the actions of macrophage-derived polypeptide growth factors. Platelet-derived growth factor, produced by activated macrophages, is a potent stimulator of fibroblast proliferation, whereas macrophage-derived transforming growth factor-β (TGF-β) augments collagen synthesis. Macrophage secretion of fibroblast growth factor causes endothelial cell migration and proliferation, leading to new blood vessel formation (**angiogenesis**). The consequence of these slow actions of cytokines and growth factors is that prolonged activation of macrophages in a tissue, e.g., in the setting of chronic antigenic stimulation, leads to replacement of differentiated tissues by fibrous tissue, a process called **fibrosis.** *Fibrosis is the outcome of*

chronic DTH, when elimination of antigen and rapid resolution are unsuccessful.

5. *Activated macrophages kill tumor cells.* Although the activated macrophage is usually thought of as an effector of host defense against infectious organisms, tumor biologists have observed that activated macrophages also selectively kill malignant cells. This phenomenon is discussed in greater detail in Chapter 17. Suffice it to say here that much of the antitumor effect of activated macrophages may be attributed to the ability of TNF, produced by these cells, to cause tumor cell death. A second anti-tumor mechanism may involve generation of toxic metabolites such as nitric oxide.

In chronic DTH reactions, activated macrophages themselves undergo changes. Such macrophages develop increased cytoplasm and cytoplasmic organelles. In standard histologic sections stained with hematoxylin and eosin, activated macrophages may resemble skin epithelial cells and have therefore been called "epithelioid." Sometimes, these macrophages can fuse to form multinucleate giant cells. Individual clusters of activated macrophages, often focused about particulate sources of antigen such as *Mycobacterium,* produce palpable nodules of inflammatory tissue called **granulomas** (i.e., granular masses) (Fig. 12–6). Granulomatous inflammation is a characteristic response to some persistent microbes, such as *Mycobacterium tuberculosis,* and simply represents a form of chronic DTH. Experimentally, granulomas can be elicited by attaching soluble protein antigens to undigestible latex beads so they are particulate and persistent in tissues.

In summary, acute DTH is a form of cell-mediated immunity in which the presumed sequence of events is that CD4+ T cells recognize soluble protein antigens or CD8+ T cells recognize intracellular microbe-derived antigens and respond by secreting cytokines. Some of these cytokines, especially TNF, activate vascular endothelial cells lining nearby post-capillary venules. The endothelial cells function in turn to recruit circulating neutrophils and then lymphocytes and monocytes into the tissue site. Other cytokines, especially IFN–γ, then activate the recruited monocytes into macrophages, which function to eliminate the antigen. If antigenic stimulation persists, the macrophages become chronically activated and secrete additional cytokines and growth factors that cause the original tissue to be replaced by fibrous tissue. In early DTH, the inflammatory infiltrates are rich in CD4+ T cells with phenotypic characteristics of activated cells (e.g., increased expression of the p55 subunit of the IL–2 receptor) and activated macrophages (expressing elevated levels of class II MHC molecules and receptors for the Fc portion of IgG molecules). These cells are clustered about plump, activated venular endothelial cells (expressing elevated levels of ELAM–1, ICAM–1, VCAM–1, and MHC molecules). At later times, in chronic DTH, clusters of epithelioid macrophages and giant cells are associated with increased numbers of fibroblasts and new blood vessels.

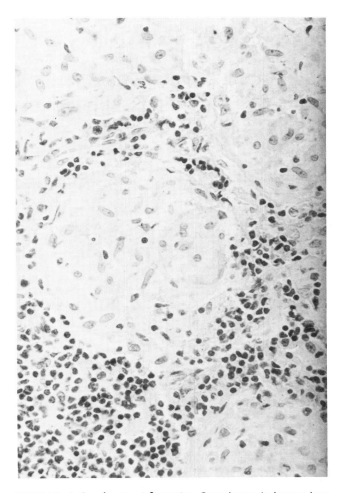

FIGURE 12–6. Granulomatous inflammation. *Granulomas in human lung, showing T cells surrounding nodular collections of activated macrophages. (Courtesy of Dr. Carol Farver, Department of Pathology, Brigham and Women's Hospital, Boston.)*

CYTOLYTIC T LYMPHOCYTES

Cytolytic T lymphocytes are a subset of T cells that kill target cells expressing specific antigen. CTLs appear to be important effector cells in three settings: viral infection, acute allograft rejection, and rejection of tumors. Each of these processes is discussed in more detail in Section IV. In this chapter, we focus upon the characteristics of CTLs and their mechanisms of action.

The majority of CTLs express the CD8 molecule and specifically recognize foreign peptides derived from intracellularly synthesized antigens associated with self class I MHC molecules. Rare CTLs express the CD4 molecule and recognize peptides associated with class II molecules. As discussed in Chapter 8, the T cell antigen receptor genes utilized by CD8+ CTLs are indistinguishable from those utilized by CD4+ helper T cells. The preference of CD8+ T cells for class I MHC molecules is instead related to the direct binding of CD8 to nonpolymorphic regions of the class I

MHC molecule. Like helper T cells, CTLs undergo maturation and selection in the thymus.

Development and Differentiation of Functional CTLs

CTLs are not fully differentiated when they exit the thymus. Although they express functional $\alpha\beta$ T cell receptor molecules and recognize antigen, they cannot lyse target cells. Indeed, very few, if any, functional CTLs specific for an allograft can be detected in the blood of a potential allograft recipient prior to transplantation (see Chapter 16). However, if T lymphocytes are cultured with leukocytes from the donor of an allograft, i.e., in a mixed leukocyte reaction (see Chapter 16), graft specific CD8+ CTLs can be detected in the culture after 7 to 10 days. Similarly, if T cells from a virus-infected individual are stimulated with virus-infected syngeneic cells *in vitro,* virus-specific self MHC-restricted CD8+ CTLs are detected within 5 to 10 days. The appearance of functional CTLs depends upon a process of differentiation.

The principal features of CTL differentiation are the following:

1. *CTLs develop or differentiate from "pre-CTLs."* Pre-CTLs are T cells that are committed to the CTL lineage, have undergone thymic maturation, and are already specific for a particular foreign antigen. These cells express CD3–associated $\alpha\beta$ T cell receptors (TCRs) and CD8, but they lack cytolytic function.

2. *Pre-CTLs do not require a special microenvironment for differentiation.* Pre-CTLs are normally present at low frequency in the blood and peripheral lymphoid tissues and can be detected by stimulating differentiation *in vitro* before assessing cytolytic function.

3. *Differentiation of pre-CTL to functional CTL requires at least two separate kinds of signals: the first is specific recognition of antigen on a target cell, and the second is usually provided by CD4+ T cell–derived cytokines* (Fig. 12–7). Antigen binding to pre-CTL makes these cells responsive to subsequent stimulation by cytokines. Part of this process is understood. The acquisition of responsiveness to IL–2, one of the cytokine signals provided by CD4+ T cells, depends on synthesis of the p55 subunit of the IL–2 receptor, and expression of p55 can be induced by binding of antigen to the CTL antigen receptor (see Chapter 11, Fig. 11–3). IL–2 is necessary but insufficient for development of functional CTLs from pre-CTLs. Several other cytokines, including IL–4, IFN–γ, and IL–6, have been shown to function as CTL differentiation factors in various experimental situations. As discussed in Chapters 7 and 9, the two-signal model of lymphocyte activation also applies to helper T cells and B cells.

The involvement of CD4+ T cell–derived cytokines in CTL differentiation implies that both CD8+ T cells (the pre-CTLs) and CD4+ T cells (the source of the cytokines) must be stimulated by antigen to obtain optimal generation of functional CTLs. Therefore,

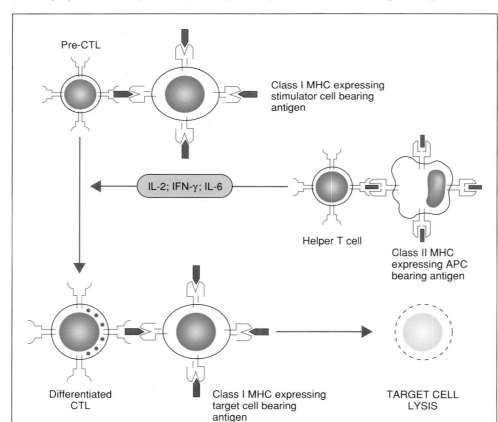

FIGURE 12–7. Stimuli for the differentiation of cytolytic T lymphocytes (CTLs). In order to differentiate into fully functional CTLs, CD8+ pre-CTLs require two signals: recognition of class I MHC–associated antigen on a stimulator cell, and cytokines provided by CD4+ helper T cells.

Pre-CTL

Class I MHC expressing stimulator cell bearing antigen

IL-2; IFN-γ; IL-6

Helper T cell

Class II MHC expressing APC bearing antigen

Differentiated CTL

Class I MHC expressing target cell bearing antigen

TARGET CELL LYSIS

maximal CTL responses depend upon antigen presentation utilizing both class I and class II MHC molecules, and CTLs are not efficiently generated if class II–bearing APCs are absent from the cultures.

Functions of CTLs

The function of differentiated CTLs is to lyse (i.e., kill) target cells. Differentiation from pre-CTLs involves the acquisition of the machinery to perform cell lysis. Two parallel sets of changes occur during this process. First, CTLs develop specific membrane-bound cytoplasmic granules. These granules contain several macromolecules, including a membrane pore-forming protein called **perforin** or **cytolysin;** a series of enzymes that contain reactive serines in their active site (commonly called "serine esterases"); protein toxins, which are either identical or structurally related to LT; and proteoglycans. Second, CTLs develop the capacity to transcribe and secrete cytokines and other proteins upon activation, most specifically IFN–γ, LT, and, to a lesser degree, IL–2. (Although functional CTLs secrete cytokines, they appear incapable of producing sufficient quantities or types of cytokines to cause pre-CTLs to differentiate. This is why CD4+ helper cells are necessary for CTL differentiation.) As discussed below, both granule contents and secreted cytokines may be directly involved in CTL–mediated lysis.

Mechanisms of CTL–Mediated Lysis

There are several key features of CTL–mediated lysis.

1. *CTL killing is antigen-specific.* Only target cells that bear the same class I MHC–associated antigen that triggered pre-CTL differentiation can be killed by an individual CTL.

2. *CTL killing requires cell contact.* This requirement arises from the need of CTLs to be triggered by recognition of a target antigen associated with a cell surface MHC molecule. CTLs kill only those cells to which they attach, and bystander cells are not injured. This is because the lytic mechanisms of CLTs are directed toward the point of contact of the TCR molecule with antigen.

3. *CTLs themselves are not injured during lysis of target cells.* Moreover, each individual CTL is capable of sequentially killing multiple target cells. The mechanisms that protect CTLs from lysis are, as will be discussed below, not fully understood.

The process of CTL–mediated lysis consists of five steps (Fig. 12–8);

1. *Recognition of antigen and conjugate formation.* The CTL binds to the target cell using its specific antigen receptor and other accessory molecules, such as CD8, CD2, and LFA–1. Target cell recognition, there-

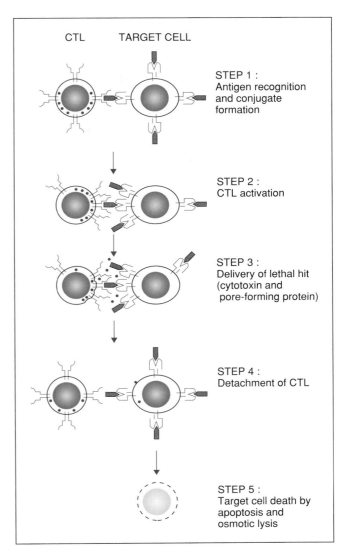

FIGURE 12 – 8. Steps in cytolytic T lymphocyte (CTL) – mediated lysis of target cells. *Note that conjugate formation (step 1) also requires interactions between CTL accessory molecules (LFA – 1, CD8) on the CTLs and their specific ligands on the target cell; these are not shown (see Figure 7 – 7, Chapter 7).*

fore, involves class I MHC molecules (the ligand for CD8), complexed to specific peptide (the complex serving as the ligand for the TCR), LFA – 3 (the ligand for CD2), and ICAM – 1 or ICAM – 2 (the ligand for LFA – 1). It may be that transient conjugate formation can occur via CD2 and LFA – 1 mediated adhesion in the absence of or prior to specific antigen recognition, or that antigen recognition may enhance the ability to form conjugates by augmenting the binding function of the adhesion molecules. CTL – mediated killing of target cells that do not express ICAM – 1 or LFA – 3 is very inefficient.

2. *Activation of the CTL.* The CTL is activated by cross-linking of its antigen receptor. Cross-linking or clustering of TCR:CD3 complexes on CTLs may be a simple consequence of multivalent recognition of MHC – peptide complexes on the target cell. The intracellular signals generated by the TCR may be aug-

mented by signals delivered through the various accessory molecules. The process of CTL activation is thus entirely analogous to the activation of helper T cells described in Chapter 7.

3. *Delivery of a "lethal hit" by the activated CTL to its conjugated target* (see below).

4. *Release of the CTL.* The CTL is released from its target cell, a process that may be facilitated by decreases in the affinity of accessory molecules for their ligands.

5. *Programmed death of the target cell as a consequence of receiving a lethal hit.*

Delivery of the lethal hit appears to occur by two parallel mechanisms, either one of which is adequate for target cell lysis: *In the first mechanism, CTLs focus and then secrete (exocytose) the contents of some of their cytoplasmic granules in the areas of contact with their target cells.* Focusing of the granules is initiated by clustering of TCR:CD3 molecules and involves the cytoskeleton. The microtubule organizing center of the CTL is moved to the area of the cytoplasm near the contact with the target cell, and granules are clustered in this same region. As a consequence of granule content exocytosis, the pore-forming protein, present as a monomer in the granule, comes in contact with extracellular concentrations of calcium (typically 1 to 2 mM) and undergoes polymerization. Polymerization of the pore-forming protein preferentially occurs in a lipid bilayer such as the plasma membrane of the target cell. The polymerized form of the protein acts as an ion-permeable channel in the target cell plasma membrane. If a sufficient number of these channels are present, the target cell will be unable to exclude ions and water, leading to osmotic swelling and lysis. This method of cell killing is analogous to that produced by the membrane attack complex of complement, and the CTL pore-forming protein is structurally homologous to the ninth component of complement, the principal constituent of the membrane attack complex (see Chapter 13). Purified pore-forming protein can be used experimentally to lyse cells. The additional components of the granule, i.e., the serine esterases, the cell toxins, and the proteoglycans, may also injure cells, but the mechanisms by which they do so are less well understood.

The second mechanism of lysis involves the secretion of a cell toxin. This protein toxin, which may or may not be the same as that found in the granule, is secreted independently of, and on occasion in the absence of, granule exocytosis. The CTL–derived toxin may be LT or a structurally related molecule. The toxin kills cells by activating target cell enzymes that cleave DNA in the target cell nucleus. Once the nuclear DNA is fragmented, target cell nuclei also undergo fragmentation, a process called **apoptosis.** Killing of target cells by secreted toxin does not cause osmotic swelling. Conversely, killing of target cells by pore-forming protein does not cause DNA fragmentation or apoptosis. The two methods of killing are thus complementary.

As noted above, CTLs themselves are not killed during the lytic process. However, CTLs can be killed by other CTLs and by high concentrations of the pore-forming proteins or the CTL–derived cell toxin. This raises the question of why CTLs are not injured during target cell lysis. The answer is probably quantitative: *CTLs are relatively resistant to CTL–mediated lysis.* They may express higher levels of membrane proteins that disassemble the pore-forming complex. Moreover, only a portion of the granules undergo exocytosis and a limited quantity of toxin is secreted during the period of contact with the target. CTLs thus preferentially survive.

Much of our understanding of CTL development and function is based on studies of these cells in the experimental setting of allograft rejection. Indeed, CTLs are readily isolated from rejecting allografts and adoptive transfer of mature CTLs can cause allograft rejection (see Chapter 16). Although other experimental systems for their *in vivo* study are less well developed, *it is believed that the physiologic function of CTLs is the eradication of viral infection.* CTLs inhibit viral replication in two ways:

1. *CTLs act to destroy infected host cells that are the source of replicating virus particles.* An important additional action of the CTL secreted cell toxin may be to activate cellular enzymes that degrade viral genomes.

2. *CTLs produce IFN–γ.* Although IFN–γ is primarily an immunoregulatory molecule, it does, as its name implies, have anti-viral activity.

NATURAL KILLER CELLS

Natural killer cells are a subset of lymphocytes found in blood and lymphoid tissues, especially spleen. NK cells are derived from the bone marrow and appear as large lymphocytes with numerous cytoplasmic granules and are sometimes called **large granular lymphocytes** (LGLs). NK cells are best thought of as phylogenetically primitive CTLs that lack the specific T cell receptor (TCR) for antigen recognition. NK cells possess the ability to kill certain tumor cells or normal cells infected by virus. Killing by NK cells is not specific for particular viral antigenic determinants and is not restricted by MHC molecules. Such killing is "natural," in that it is not induced by specific antigen and is thus part of natural rather than specific immunity. Although the target specificity of NK cells is broader than that of CTLs, it is nevertheless not random. NK cells can lyse normal cells infected by some viruses, but not others, and will not lyse uninfected cells. NK activity can cause lysis of certain tumor cell lines, particularly of hematopoietic origin, but not of others. The existence of NK specificity is most clearly demonstrated by the phenomenon of "cold target inhibition"; i.e., one NK target cell type can inhibit lysis of a different NK target type by competing for effector cells, whereas cells that are not NK targets do not compete (Fig. 12–9).

By surface phenotype and lineage, NK cells are neither T nor B cells. NK cells do not undergo thymic

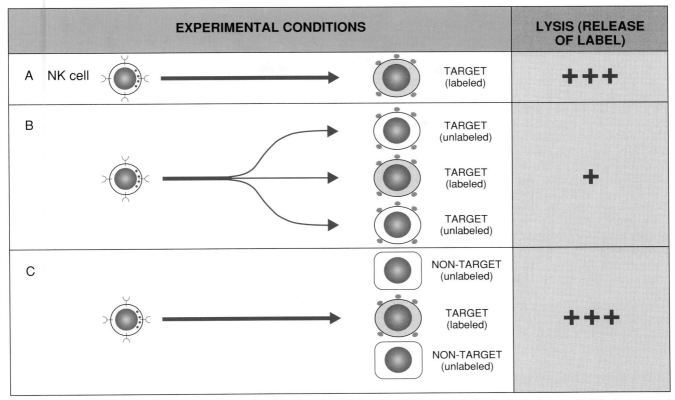

EXPERIMENTAL CONDITIONS	LYSIS (RELEASE OF LABEL)

A NK cell → TARGET (labeled) — **+++**

B → TARGET (unlabeled), TARGET (labeled), TARGET (unlabeled) — **+**

C → NON-TARGET (unlabeled), TARGET (labeled), NON-TARGET (unlabeled) — **+++**

FIGURE 12–9. Demonstration of natural killer (NK) cell specificity by cold target inhibition. NK cells can cause lysis of suitable target cells (A). An excess of unlabeled target cells inhibits NK cell–mediated lysis of labeled targets (B) whereas cells that are not NK targets do not function as competitive inhibitors (C). By this approach, it has been shown that NK cells recognize a variety of virus-infected cells and hematopoietic tumors (all of which serve as cold target inhibitors for one another), but MHC molecules are not involved in this recognition. (In contrast, cold target inhibition of virus-specific CD8+ cytolytic T lymphocyte (CTL) killing requires that the cold target express the same viral antigen and class I MHC molecules as the labeled target.)

maturation and may be increased in animals that lack a thymus. Moreover, NK cells do not undergo Ig or TCR gene rearrangements and do not express CD3 molecules. However, NK cells do express the CD2 molecule and a low-affinity receptor for the Fc portion of IgG, called FcRIII or CD16 (see Chapter 3). NK cells can be induced to proliferate and secrete cytokines by cross-linking either CD2 or CD16. In this regard, it is worth noting that despite lacking CD3, NK cells do express homodimers of the CD3ζ chain, which associate with CD3$\gamma\delta\epsilon$ in MHC–restricted T cells. In NK cells, the ζ chain or a homodimeric protein called γ, which is structurally homologous to ζ, is associated with CD16. Both ζ and γ homodimers are thought to be involved in signal transduction initiated by IgG binding to CD16.

NK cells express the p70 subunit of the IL–2 receptor, but not the p55 subunit, and can be induced to proliferate by high concentrations of IL–2. In addition, NK cells may share with CTLs certain other surface markers. For example, in mice, both CTLs and NK cells express a surface ganglioside called asialo GM–1. Although markers such as asialo GM–1 (and its human equivalent, HNK–1) are useful for identifying NK cells, their relationship to NK function is unclear.

The molecular structure recognized by NK cells

on the surface of susceptible target cells is not yet defined. Unlike CTLs, NK cells do not appear to require prior contact with target antigens to develop cytolytic capacities. They share with CTLs a responsiveness to cytokines, although NK cells do not need antigen contact to acquire cytokine responsiveness. NK cells can be activated to increase their ability to lyse target cells by treatment with type I IFN, IFN–γ, TNF, or IL–2. NK cells can acquire additional specificities by coating target cells with IgG molecules that can be recognized by the NK cell Fc receptor, CD16. This form of cytolysis is called **antibody-dependent cell-mediated cytotoxicity** (ADCC), and NK cells are its principal mediator (see Chapter 3).

Killing of targets by NK cells involves similar mechanisms as killing by CTLs, namely granule exocytosis and secretion of a cell toxin. NK granules, like CTL granules, contain pore-forming protein, cytotoxins, serine esterases, and proteoglycans. It is not known whether the secreted toxin produced by NK cells is the same as or different from that secreted by CTLs. NK cells synthesize TNF but not LT. Under some circumstances, NK cells also appear to secrete IFN–γ; in mice lacking functional T cells, NK cell–derived IFN–γ can activate macrophages to kill infectious organisms such as *L. monocytogenes*.

The role of NK cells in normal immunity is not

clearly established. Since these cells were originally detected, in part, by their ability to kill virally infected cells, it has been hypothesized that they serve to lyse infected cells until antigen-specific CTLs can differentiate from pre-CTLs. Because NK cells can lyse certain tumor cells, it has also been proposed that NK cells serve to kill malignant clones *in vivo*. However, neither viral infection–associated nor tumor-associated inflammatory infiltrates show significant numbers of NK cells. The one setting in which large numbers of NK cells appear to predominate in the histologic pattern of the lesion is in graft-versus-host disease (GVHD) in recipients of bone marrow transplants. We will discuss GVHD in greater detail in Chapter 16; suffice it to say here that NK cells infiltrate into epithelium such as skin and can be found adjacent to necrotic epithelial cells, the hallmark of GVHD. The mechanism by which NK cells lyse normal epithelial cells is not fully known. It has been observed that when NK cells are treated with sufficient concentration of IL–2 to stimulate their p70 receptor, they differentiate into LAK cells. LAK cells demonstrate enhanced cytolytic capacity and demonstrate a very broad target specificity, killing a wide variety of tumor cells (see Chapter 17) and normal cell types, including epithelial cells. Thus, in GVHD, transplanted CD4$^+$ T cells may recognize and respond to the alloantigens of the host. These T cells produce IL–2, which may stimulate the differentiation of NK cells into LAK cells. This is another example of how, in specific cell-mediated immunity, T cells augment the functions and focus the actions of the effector cells of natural immunity.

Summary

Cell-mediated immunity consists of immune responses that are initiated by antigen recognition by specific T lymphocytes and in which T lymphocytes participate in the effector stage as well. There are several forms of cell-mediated immune reactions, which are generally initiated by activation of CD4$^+$ T cells in response to specific antigen. Activated CD4$^+$ T cells secrete cytokines which, in turn, activate various effector cell populations. In delayed type hypersensitivity reactions, CD4$^+$ T cells secrete tumor necrosis factor, which causes endothelial cells to recruit inflammatory leukocytes, and gamma interferon, which activates macrophages to kill microorganisms, initiate acute inflammatory responses and produce tissue remodeling.

Cytolytic T lymphocytes, which usually bear CD8, are important effector cells in settings of virus infection and allograft rejection. CTLs differentiate from pre-CTLs in response to two signals: (1) a target cell bearing endogenously synthesized peptide antigens presented in association with self class I MHC molecules or a target expressing specific foreign class I MHC molecules, and (2) a combination of several CD4$^+$ T cell–derived cytokines. Upon differentiation, CTLs acquire the ability to kill target cells expressing the appropriate MHC–associated antigen. CTL–mediated killing involves two complementary mechanisms: (1) granule exocytosis of a membrane pore-forming protein that causes osmotic lysis of target cells, and (2) secretion of a cell toxin that activates DNA degrading enzymes in target cells.

Natural killer cells are a population of large granular lymphocytes that normally serve to kill target cells bearing an undefined, MHC–independent target molecule or cells coated with specific IgG molecules. NK cell–mediated killing uses the same mechanisms employed in CTL–mediated killing. NK cells are activated by cytokines produced by CD4$^+$ T cells. In response to high levels of IL–2, NK cells differentiate into lymphokine-activated killer cells that kill target cells in relatively indiscriminate fashion. By recruiting and activating NK cells, CD4$^+$ T cells can cause lysis of normal cell types in response to antigen stimulation, characteristic of the reaction found in acute graft-versus-host disease.

Selected Readings

Adams, D. O., and T. A. Hamilton. The cell biology of macrophage activation. Annual Review of Immunology 2:283–318, 1984.

Cerottini, J. C., and H. R. MacDonald (organizers). 17th Forum in Immunology: Molecular mechanism of T-cell–mediated cytotoxicity. Annales de L'Institut Pasteur Immunology 138:287–342, 1987.

Cohen, S. Physiologic and pathologic manifestations of lymphokine action. Human Pathology 17:112–121, 1986.

Herberman, R. B., C. W. Reynolds, and J. Ortaldo. Mechanisms of cytotoxicity by natural killer (NK) cells. Annual Review of Immunology 4:651–680, 1986.

Kupfer, A., and S. J. Singer. Cell biology of cytotoxic and helper T-cell functions. Annual Review of Immunology 7:309–337, 1989.

Mosmann, T. R., and R. L. Coffman. Heterogeneity of cytokine secretion patterns and functions of helper T cells. Advances in Immunology 46:111–147, 1989.

Nabholz, M., and H. R. MacDonald. Cytolytic T lymphocytes. Annual Review of Immunology 1:273–306, 1983.

Osborn, L. Leukocyte adhesion to endothelium in inflammation. Cell 62:3–6, 1990.

Pober, J. S., and R. S. Cotran. Cytokines and endothelial cell biology. Physiological Reviews 70:427–451, 1990.

Trinchieri, G. Biology of natural killer cells. Advances in Immunology 47:187–376, 1989.

Young, J. D., C. C. Liu, P. M. Persechini, and Z. A. Cohn. Perforin-dependent and -independent pathways of cytotoxicity mediated by lymphocytes. Immunological Reviews 103:161–202, 1988.

CHAPTER THIRTEEN

THE

COMPLEMENT

SYSTEM

Soon after the discovery of humoral immunity, Charles Bordet demonstrated that if fresh serum containing an anti-bacterial antibody was added to the bacteria at physiologic temperature (37° C), the bacteria were lysed. If, however, the serum was heated to 56° C or more, it lost its lytic capacity. This was not because of decay of antibody activity, because antibodies are heat-stable and even heated serum was capable of agglutinating the bacteria. Bordet concluded that the serum must contain another heat-labile component that assists or "complements" the lytic function of antibodies. He called this heat-labile substance **complement.** We now know that *complement is not a single protein but a system of functionally linked proteins that interact with one another in a highly regulated manner to provide many of the effector functions of humoral immunity and inflammation.*

The principal biologic functions of the complement system are as follows:

1. Certain activated complement components mediate **cytolysis** by polymerizing on cell surfaces to form pores in the membranes of these cells. In this way, foreign organisms that activate complement can be killed by osmotic lysis.

2. **Opsonization** of foreign organisms or particles occurs by the binding of complement proteins to their surfaces. These complement proteins are called **opsonins.** Phagocytic leukocytes express specific receptors for these opsonins. In this way, opsonins promote phagocytosis of particles or organisms.

3. **Activation of inflammation** occurs in response to the generation of certain proteolytic fragments of complement proteins. Some complement fragments are **chemotactic,** promoting the migration of inflammatory cells into sites of foreign antigen exposure. Other complement fragments act as **anaphylatoxins;** they stimulate leukocytes, including mast cells and granulocytes, to release chemical mediators of inflammation that act primarily on blood vessels.

4. **Immune complexes** that could damage tissues are rendered innocuous by *solubilization, limitation in size, and phagocytic clearance* from the circulation as a result of binding complement proteins.

These functions will be discussed in detail later in the chapter. The complement system has a number of important properties that enable it to function efficiently in host defense against foreign invaders without injuring normal tissues:

1. The soluble serum complement components include multiple proteolytic enzymes, which become sequentially activated only when they themselves are proteolytically cleaved by other previously activated complement system enzymes. Proteins that acquire proteolytic enzymatic activity by the action of other proteases are called zymogens. The process of sequential zymogen activation, i.e., an enzymatic cascade, is also characteristic of the coagulation and kinin systems. *The proteolytic cascades allow for tremendous amplification, since each individual enzyme molecule activated at one step can generate multiple activated enzyme molecules, or active fragments, at the next step.*

2. Although the proteins of the complement system are present in the blood, they are inactive and cannot be activated spontaneously in the circulation. Activation of the complement system normally occurs only at certain localized sites. First, immunoglobulin (Ig) molecules that have bound specific antigens can activate complement, and for this reason *complement serves as a major effector mechanism for specific humoral immunity.* The sequence of complement activation initiated by antibody-antigen complexes is called the **classical pathway.** Second, some complement components are directly activated by binding to the surfaces of infectious organisms. In this way *complement activation also participates in natural immunity.* In the absence of antibody, microbial surfaces often directly initiate the **alternative pathway** of complement activation. The name "alternative" comes from the fact that this pathway was discovered after the classical pathway. Despite its name, the alternative pathway is as important as the classical pathway in host defense against infectious organisms. As we shall see later, these two pathways differ in their initiation but share many late stages and effector functions.

3. The complement system is highly regulated by several soluble and cell membrane–associated proteins that inhibit complement activation at multiple steps. These regulatory mechanisms have two main functions. First, they limit or stop complement activation in response to physiologic stimuli. Second, they prevent abnormal or constitutive complement activation in the absence of microbes and antibodies.

The various biologic functions of the complement system are mediated by (1) complexes of complement components bound to the surfaces or immune complexes where complement is activated, or by (2) soluble fragments of complement proteins that diffuse from the sites where they were generated and bind to specific receptors on other nearby cells.

This chapter describes the biochemistry, function, and regulation of the complement system. The relationship of complement to other components of the immune system will be emphasized.

THE COMPLEMENT CASCADES

Before we describe the individual proteins of the complement system, it is useful to present an overview of complement activation (Fig. 13–1). The central component of the complement system is a protein called **C3,** which is critical for the effector functions of this system. The biologically active forms of C3 are its proteolytic cleavage products. The classical and alternative pathways include distinct protein components that are activated in different ways to generate enzymes called **C3 convertases,** which cleave C3 to produce C3a and C3b. (By convention, lower case letter suffixes denote proteolytic products of each complement protein, "a" referring to the smaller fragment

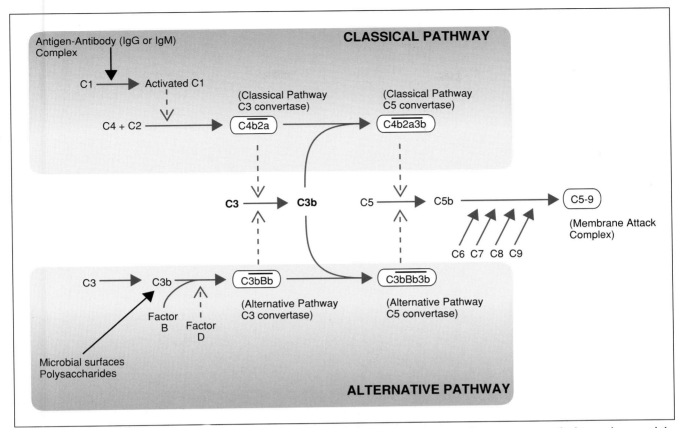

FIGURE 13–1. Overview of complement activation pathways. *The classical pathway is initiated by C1 binding to antigen-antibody complexes, and the alternative pathway is initiated by C3b binding to various activating surfaces, such as microbial cell walls. The C3b involved in alternative pathway initiation may be generated in several ways, including spontaneously, by the classical pathway, or by the alternative pathway itself (see text). Both pathways converge and lead to the formation of the membrane attack complex. In this and subsequent figures, bars over the letter designations of complement components indicate enzymatically active forms and dashed lines indicate proteolytic activities of various components.*

and "b" to the larger one.) In the early steps of the *classical pathway*, antibody molecules that are complexed with specific antigen sequentially bind and proteolytically activate three complement proteins, called C1, C4, and C2, leading to the formation of a $\overline{C4b2a}$ complex, which functions as the **classical pathway C3 convertase.** In the *alternative pathway*, C3b generated spontaneously at low levels, or by the classical pathway, binds to a protein fragment called Bb generated by proteolytic cleavage of a protein called Factor B. The $\overline{C3bBb}$ complex is the **alternative pathway C3 convertase,** functioning, like the classical pathway C3 convertase, to further break down C3 to generate more C3b. The next step in both pathways is the binding of C3b to the C3 convertase enzymes, changing them to **C5 convertases,** which catalyze the proteolytic cleavage of the C5 protein. Although the C5 convertases of the two pathways are molecularly distinct, they catalyze identical reactions and act on identical substrates. Once C5 is cleaved, both pathways share the same terminal steps. These terminal events do not involve proteolysis, but rather the sequential binding of several soluble complement proteins, called C6, C7, C8, and C9, to the activating surface. This leads to the formation of a lipid soluble pore

structure called the **membrane attack complex (MAC),** which causes osmotic lysis of cells.

Different effector functions are mediated by different proteins produced during complement activation. Cytolysis is mediated by the MAC. Opsonization is largely due to a fragment of C3 called C3b, specific receptors for which are expressed on many leukocytes and other cells. Inflammation, consisting of the recruitment and activation of leukocytes, is mediated by cleavage products of C3, C4, and C5, called C3a, C4a, and C5a, respectively. Immune complexes are solubilized by binding of the classical pathway proteins to the Fc regions of antibody molecules. Each of these functions will be discussed in more detail later.

In the following discussion, we describe the various proteins that make up the complement system; these proteins are listed in Table 13–1.

The Classical Pathway

The classical pathway (Fig. 13–2) is the major effector mechanism for antibody-mediated immune responses because it is activated principally by the binding of the first classical pathway component, C1, to the

TABLE 13–1. Protein Components of the Complement Cascades

Component	Molecular Size (kD)	Serum Concentration (μg/ml)	Subunit Chains; Molecular Size Each (kD)	Activation Products	Comments on Function
Classical Pathway					
C1 (C1qr₂s₂)	900				Initiates classical pathway
C1q	410	75	6 of A;24 6 of B;23 6 of C;22		Binds to Fc portion of Ig
C1r	85	50	1	C1̄r	C1̄r is a serine protease; cleaves C1̄s
C1s	85	50	1	C1̄s	C1̄s is a serine protease; cleaves C4 and C2
C4	210	200–500	1 of α;90 1 of β;78 1 of γ;33	C4a C4b	C4a is an anaphylatoxin; C4b covalently binds to activating surfaces where it is part of C3 convertase
C2	110	20	1	C2̄a C2b	C2̄a is a serine protease, part of C3 and C5 convertases
C3 (Also part of alternative pathway)	195	550–1200	1 of α;110 1 of β; 85	C3a C3b	C3a is an anaphylatoxin; C3b covalently binds to activating surfaces, where it is part of C3 and C5 convertases and also acts as opsonin
Alternative Pathway					
Factor B	93	200	1	Ba B̄b̄	B̄b̄ is a serine protease, part of C3 and C5 convertases
Factor D	25	1–2	1	D̄	Protease which circulates in active state; cleaves Factor B
Properdin	220	25	4; 56		Stabilizes alternative pathway C3 convertase
Terminal Lytic Components					
C5	190	70	1 of α;115 1 of β;75	C5a C5b	C5a is an anaphylatoxin C5b initiates MAC assembly
C6	128	60	1		Component of MAC
C7	121	60	1		Component of MAC
C8	155	60	1 of α;64 1 of β;64 1 of γ;22		Component of MAC
C9	79	60	1		Component of MAC; polymerizes to form membrane pores

Abbreviations: kD, kilodalton; MAC, membrane attack complex; Ig, immunoglobulin.

Fc portions of antigen-complexed antibody molecules. There are stringent requirements for antibody-mediated C1 activation that ensure that the classical pathway is activated only under certain conditions:

1. Activation of C1 occurs at significant levels only when it binds to the C_H3 domains of IgM or C_H2 domains of IgG molecules (see Chapter 3). Furthermore, only certain subclasses of IgG are effective C1 activators (human IgG1, IgG2, and IgG3, but not IgG4).

2. A single C1 molecule must bind simultaneously to several (at least two) Fc portions of Ig, each Fc portion having a single C1 binding site. Because secreted IgM is a pentamer containing five Fc regions, even a single IgM molecule can bind C1 and trigger the classical pathway. In contrast, since IgG is a monomer, multiple IgG molecules must be aggregated, bringing multiple Fc regions sufficiently close together, before

C1 can bind. Such aggregation typically occurs if the IgG antibody binds to a multideterminant antigen, such as a bacterial cell surface. Because of these structural differences in the Ig isotypes, IgM is a much more efficient complement binding (also called **complement-fixing**) antibody than IgG.

3. Only antigen-antibody complexes and not free or soluble antibodies activate complement. For IgG this is because of the requirement for aggregation mentioned above. Soluble IgM does not bind C1, even though it is pentameric, apparently because the Fc regions are inaccessible to C1 in solution. Binding of the IgM to an antigen or a cell surface induces a conformational change that exposes the Fc regions, allowing C1 to bind.

Experimental evidence indicates that the classical pathway may also be activated in the absence of Ig,

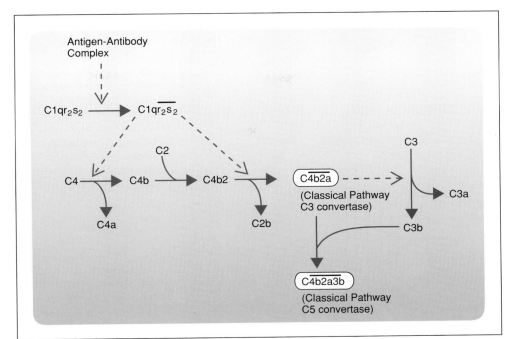

FIGURE 13–2. Classical pathway of complement activation. Antigen-antibody complexes that activate the classical pathway may be soluble or fixed on the surface of cells or trapped in interstitial spaces. The C5 convertase formed by the classical pathway proteolytically cleaves C5 to begin the formation of the membrane attack complex.

on the surfaces of certain infectious organisms such as retroviruses and *Mycoplasma,* and by polyanionic molecules such as DNA, heparin, and chondroitin sulfate. The mechanisms of activation in these cases and the significance of antibody-independent activation of the classical pathway *in vivo* are not known.

C1 is itself a large, multimeric molecular complex, approximately 750 kD, composed of one C1q subunit associated, in a calcium-dependent manner, with two C1r and two C1s molecules. C1q is the subunit that actually binds to Ig molecules, and C1r and C1s are serine esterase zymogens required for the progression of the proteolytic cascade. C1q is a 400 kD protein complex composed of three different kinds of polypeptide chains that combine to form heterotrimeric rod-like structures with a collagen-like triple helix at the amino terminal end and a globular head at the carboxy terminus. Six of these rod-like structures (containing 18 separate polypeptides) combine to form one symmetric molecular complex with a central core composed of the triple helices at one end and a radial array of the globular heads at the other end (Fig. 13–3). C1r and C1s are both single-chain 85 kD proteins which combine, in a calcium dependent manner, to form a flexible linear tetramer composed of two molecules of each type, in the sequence C1s-C1r-C1r-C1s. One tetramer is associated with each C1q molecule. *Binding of two or more of the globular heads of C1q to IgM or IgG molecules leads to the enzymatic activation of the associated C1r.* As a result, the C1r molecules either cleave each other or themselves, generating a 57 kD chain and a 28 kD chain. The 28 kD chain, C1r̄, has **serine esterase** activity, which in turn cleaves the C1s molecules, also into 57 and 28 kD chains. (By convention, enzymatically active subunits of complement fragments are notated by a bar over the subunit name.) Again, the smaller frag-

ment, C1s̄, has serine esterase activity and acts on the next two components of the classical pathway, C4 and C2.

C4 is the second distinct soluble serum protein to be activated in the classical pathway. It is a 210 kD molecule composed of three polypeptide chains, called α, β, and γ. C4 is an unusual protein, in that it contains an internal thioester bond in the α chain, between a cysteine residue and a nearby glutamate residue. This feature is also found in the C3 molecule (Fig. 13–4), discussed below. C1s̄ cleaves the α chain of C4, yielding an 8.6 kD fragment called C4a, and a large remaining molecule, called C4b. (C4a diffuses from the cell surface and has biologic effects discussed later in the chapter.) One C1s̄ molecule can generate multiple C4b molecules. As a result of this proteolytic step, the thioester bond in the α chain of the C4b fragment is susceptible to nucleophilic attack by amine and hydroxyl groups and thus becomes highly unstable. This chemically reactive form of the molecule is called **metastable C4b.** Most of the C4b thioester bonds rapidly react with water molecules, generating a short-lived inactive intermediate, iC4b. However, some C4b thioester bonds undergo transesterification to form covalent amide or ester bonds with cell surface proteins or carbohydrates, respectively. *As a result, the C4b molecule becomes covalently attached to nearby cell surfaces, ensuring that complement activation occurs stably and efficiently at cell surfaces to which antibodies are bound.* C4b may also form covalent bonds with the Ig molecule itself.

C2 is the third soluble serum component of the classical pathway. It is a 110 kD single-chain polypeptide that binds to cell surface bound C4b molecules in the presence of Mg++. Once complexed with C4b, C2 is cleaved by a nearby C1s̄ molecule to generate a 35 kD C2b molecule, which may diffuse off the cell surface,

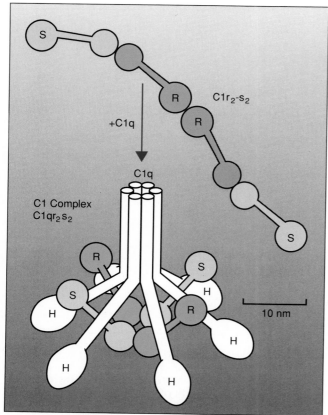

FIGURE 13–3. Structure of C1q,r,s. *C1r and C1s form a tetramer composed of two C1r and two C1s molecules. The larger balls at the ends of C1r and C1s, designated by the letters R and S, are the catalytic domains of these proteins. C1q consists of six identical subunits, arranged to form a central core and symmetrically projecting radial arms. The globular heads at the end of each arm, designated H, are the contact regions for immunoglobulin. One C1r₂s₂ tetramer wraps around the radial arms of the C1q complex in a manner that juxtaposes the catalytic domains of C1r and C1s. (Modified with permission from Arlaud, G. J., M. G. Colomb, and J. Gagnon. A functional model of the human C1 complex. Immunology Today 8:107–109, 1987.)*

and a 75 kD C2a fragment, which remains physically associated with C4a on the cell surface. *The resulting C4b2a complex is the* **classical pathway C3 convertase,** *having the ability to bind to and proteolytically cleave C3.* Binding to C3 is mediated by the C4b component, and proteolysis is catalyzed by the C2b component.

C3 is the fourth soluble serum component of the classical pathway (and also a component of the alternative pathway). The serum concentration of C3, approximately 0.55 to 1.2 mg/ml, is higher than that of any other member of the complement system. C3 is a 195 kD disulfide-linked heterodimeric glycoprotein composed of α and β polypeptide chains. C3 contains the same type of internal thioester bond as the C4 molecule (Fig. 13–4). C3 convertase removes a 9 kD fragment, C3a, from the α chain of C3, leaving a molecule called **metastable C3b** with the thioester bond exposed to potential reactants. (C3a has several biologic activities initiated by binding to C3a receptors

on other cells; these are discussed later in the chapter.)

As with C4b, most of the metastable C3b thioester bonds react with water, yielding inactive C3b by-products, which no longer participate in the complement cascade. Up to 10 per cent of C3b molecules, however, do form covalent bonds with cell surfaces or with the Ig to which the C4b2a is bound. This results in the formation of a new complex, $\overline{\text{C4b2a3b}}$, which functions as the **classical pathway C5 convertase.** As the name implies, this complex catalyzes the enzymatic cleavage of C5, which begins the formation of the MAC, described below.

The Alternative Pathway

The alternative pathway (Fig. 13–5) is activated in the absence of antibody and generates both soluble and membrane-bound forms of C3 convertase, which catalyze the proteolysis of C3. Because stable alternative pathway C3 convertase is formed on microbial cell surfaces but not on the surfaces of autologous cells or cells of the same species, the alternative pathway has a primitive capacity for discriminating between one's own cells and foreign microbes. The alternative pathway includes five proteins — Factors B, D, H, and I and properdin — which are distinct from the proteins of the classical pathway. A sixth alternative pathway protein is the same C3 that is part of the classical pathway.

C3 itself plays a critical role in both the initiation and the progression of the alternative pathway because this pathway is triggered by one of two altered forms of C3. The first is C3b, which is usually generated by the classical pathway. The second is called $C3(H_2O)$, which is produced when the internal thioester bonds of circulating C3 undergo slow spontaneous hydrolysis (Fig. 13–5). C3b or $C3(H_2O)$ binds to the alternative pathway protein, **Factor B,** a single-chain 93 kD protein that is homologous to C2 of the classical pathway. After it is complexed with C3b or $C3(H_2O)$, Factor B becomes susceptible to proteolysis by another alternative pathway protein, **Factor D.** Factor D is a 25 kD serine protease which circulates at very low concentrations in the serum, probably in its enzymatically active form. Factor D proteolytically cleaves bound Factor B, releasing a 33 kD fragment (Ba) and leaving a 63 kD fragment, $\overline{\text{Bb}}$, attached to C3b or $C3(H_2O)$. The resulting complex, $\overline{\text{C3bBb}}$ or $\overline{C3(H_2O)Bb}$ is the **alternative pathway C3 convertase,** with the $\overline{\text{Bb}}$ fragment functioning as a serine protease capable of cleaving C3. This convertase may be in the fluid phase, if formed with $C3(H_2O)$, or particle-bound if formed with particle-bound C3b. Even the $\overline{\text{C3bBb}}$ complex is unstable, however, and it rapidly decays unless another alternative pathway member, **properdin,** binds to the complex. Properdin is a 220 kD protein consisting of four identical, noncovalently linked subunits. This molecule binds to and stabilizes $\overline{\text{C3bBb}}$. In addition, a conformationally altered "active" form of properdin can bind C3b and

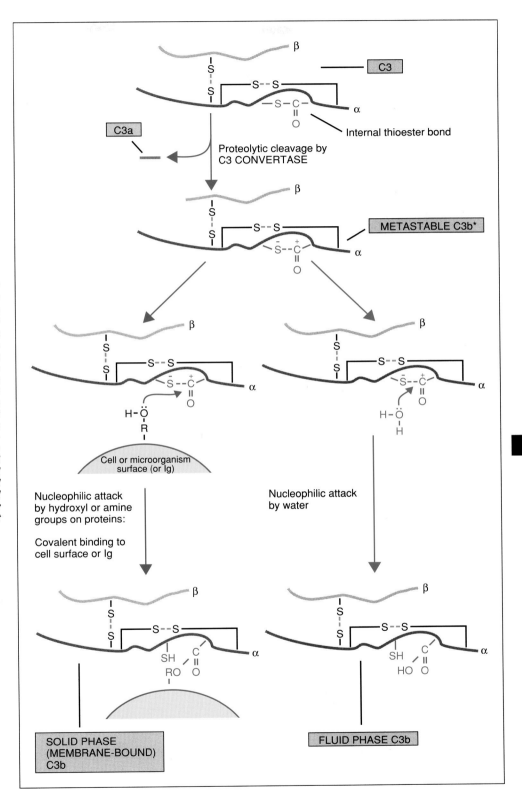

FIGURE 13 – 4. Internal thioester bond of C3. *A schematic view of the internal thioester bond in the C3 molecule and its role in forming covalent bonds with other molecules is shown. Proteolytic cleavage of the β chain converts the C3 molecule into a metastable form (C3b*) in which the internal thioester bond is susceptible to nucleophilic attack by oxygen (or nitrogen) atoms. The result is the formation of covalent bonds with proteins on cell surfaces (solid phase C3b) or with a hydroxyl group donated by water molecules (fluid phase C3b). The C4 molecule has a similar internal thioester bond that is involved in covalent bonding of C4b to cell surfaces in the classical pathway of complement activation (not shown).*

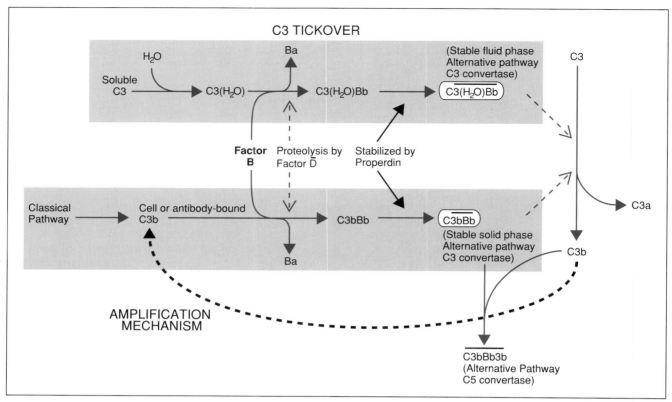

FIGURE 13–5. Alternative pathway of complement activation. *Soluble C3 in serum undergoes a slow spontaneous hydrolysis of its internal thioester bond, generating C3(H_2O) which binds Factor B and forms a fluid phase alternative pathway C3 convertase. The resulting continuous, low-level production of C3b by fluid phase C3 convertase is called C3 tickover. C3b can also be produced by the classical pathway. The C3b formed by either way can then participate in the formation of alternative pathway C3 convertase, which generates C3b from C3. The alternative pathway has a built-in amplification mechanism because the C3b generated by the alternative pathway C3 convertase is also a component of the convertase. The C3 convertase formed by the alternative pathway proteolytically cleaves C5, just as the classical pathway C5 convertase does, to begin the formation of the membrane attack complex.*

enhance its association with Factor B. It should be noted that the formation of the classical and alternative pathway C3 convertases involves homologous proteins and the events are fundamentally similar. For example, Factor B is structurally homologous to C2 and Factor B binding to C3b or C3(H_2O) is analogous to C2 binding to C4b.

The normal function of the alternative pathway is dependent on two important features of the activation and regulation of its components:

1. C3b is continuously generated by alternative pathway C3 convertase, initiated by spontaneous hydrolysis of the internal thioester bond of C3. This is called **C3 tickover** and probably goes on at a low level all the time, even in the circulation. However, it has no deleterious effects because the C3b generated by the C3 tickover mechanism is usually hydrolyzed to an inactive form within a fraction of a second. As a result, significant complement activation does not occur in the fluid phase, i.e., in the circulation. Rare C3b molecules do form covalent bonds with particle surfaces in a random manner. It is at this stage of the alternative pathway that the rudimentary capacity for self/nonself discrimination is apparent. If the C3b is deposited on autologous cell surfaces, it is rapidly inactivated by the action of regulatory proteins, described below, thus stopping the cascade. In contrast, C3b binding to the surfaces of many microbes (which lack the regulatory proteins) leads to the binding of Factor B and, as described above, to the formation of stable enzymatically active particle-bound alternative pathway C3 convertase or $\overline{\text{C3bBb}}$.

2. Alternative pathway activation is an important amplification mechanism for the complement system. The stabilized $\overline{\text{C3bBb}}$ enzyme complex generates many more C3b molecules, and these, in turn, are deposited on the same surface, forming more C3 convertase. *Thus, C3b is both a component of the C3 convertase enzyme complex as well as a product generated by the action of C3 convertase. This situation allows for a positive feedback amplification of the alternative pathway* (Fig. 13–5). In fact, because C3b generated by the classical pathway can trigger the alternative pathway, the alternative pathway C3 convertase is also an amplification mechanism for complement activation initiated by the classical pathway.

Some of the C3b molecules generated by the alternative pathway C3 convertase are deposited on the surface in close proximity and bind to the C3 convertase to form a new complex, $\overline{\text{C3bBb3b}}$. This is the

alternative pathway C5 convertase, analogous to the classical pathway C5 convertase, C4b2b3b, and its function is to proteolytically cleave C5. After this step, the classical and alternative pathways converge and the same terminal sequence of events occurs.

The Membrane Attack Complex

The C5 convertases, generated by either the classical or the alternative pathway, initiate the activation of the terminal components of the complement system, culminating in the formation of the cytocidal membrane attack complex (Fig. 13–6). This process begins with the cleavage of C5 by either of the C5 convertases. This is the last enzymatic step in the complement cascade; subsequent steps involve binding and polymerization of intact proteins. **C5** is a 190 kD disulfide–linked heterodimer with homology to C3 and C4, but without an internal thioester bond. C5 binds to the C3b molecule within either classical or alternative pathway C5 convertases. C5 is then cleaved into an 11 kD C5a fragment that is released and a two-chain 180 kD C5b fragment that remains bound to the cell surface. (C5a has potent biologic effects on several cells; this will be discussed later in the chapter.) C5b transiently maintains a conformation capable of binding the next protein in the cascade, **C6,** a 128 kD single-chain protein. The stable C5b,6 complex remains loosely associated with the cell surface until it binds **C7,** a 121 kD single-chain protein. One C7 molecule binds to each C5b,6 complex. The resulting C5b,6,7 complex is highly lipophilic, and it inserts into the hydrophobic lipid bilayer of plasma membranes, where it becomes a high-affinity integral membrane receptor for one **C8** molecule. The C8 protein is a 155 kD trimer composed of three distinct chains, including a 64 kD α chain that is disulfide linked to a 22 kD γ chain and a noncovalently linked 64 kD β chain. The γ chain inserts into the lipid bilayer of the membrane, and the C5b,6,7,8 complex (C5-8) becomes stably attached to the cell surface. This complex has a limited ability to initiate lysis of the cell to which it is bound.

Full lytic activity of the complement system is conferred by binding of **C9,** the final component of the complement cascades, to the C5-8 complex. C9 is a 79 kD monomeric serum protein that polymerizes at the site of the C5-8 complex to form the MAC. Recent evidence suggests that the MAC is composed of 12 to 15 C9 molecules associated with one C5-8 complex. This "poly-C9" forms pores in plasma membranes with a characteristic electron microscopic appearance. The pores have an internal diameter of about 110 Å, a 115 Å stalk embedded in the lipid bilayer, and a 100 Å long projection above the membrane surface. Viewed *en face,* they appear as doughnuts (Fig. 13–7). This structure is similar to the membrane pores formed by the pore-forming protein, called perforin or cytolysin, found in cytolytic T lymphocytes (CTLs) and natural killer (NK) cells (see Chapter 12).

The pores formed by the MAC permit the passive exchange of small soluble molecules, ions, and water, but they are too small to allow large molecules, such as proteins, to escape from the cytoplasm. This situation results in influx of water and ions into the cells,

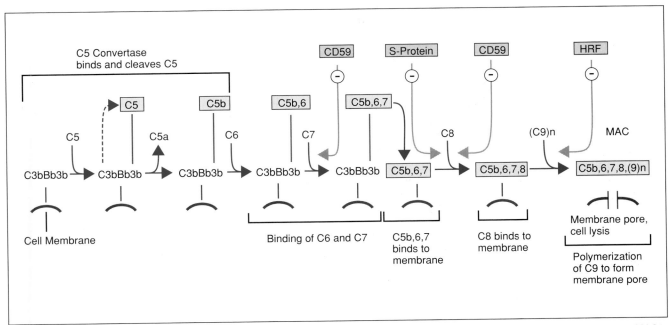

FIGURE 13–6. Formation and regulation of the membrane attack complex (MAC). A schematic view of the cell surface events leading to formation of the MAC is shown. Cell-associated C5 convertase cleaves C5, generating C5b, which becomes bound to the convertase. C6 and C7 bind sequentially, and the C5b,6,7 complex becomes directly inserted into the lipid bilayer of the plasma membrane, followed by a more stable insertion of C8. Up to 15 C9 molecules may then polymerize around the complex to form lytic pores in the membrane. The sites of actions of the regulatory proteins, including S-protein (vitronectin), CD59, and homologous restriction factor (HRF), are indicated.

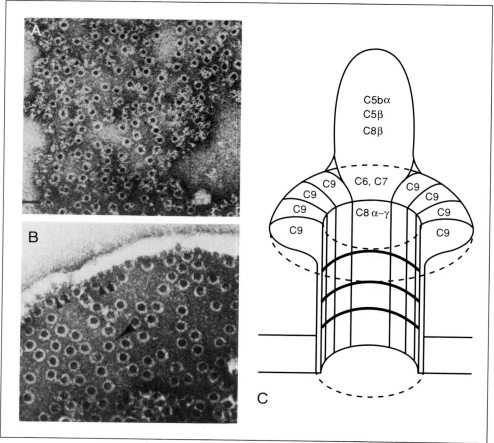

FIGURE 13–7. Structure of the membrane attack complex (MAC) in cell membranes.

A. *Complement lesions in erythrocyte membranes are shown in this electron micrograph. The lesions consist of holes approximately 100 Å in diameter and are formed by polyC9 tubular complexes.*

B. *For comparison, membrane lesions induced on a target cell by a cloned cytolytic T lymphocyte (CTL) line are shown in this electron micrograph. The lesions have a morphology similar to that of complement-mediated lesions, except for a larger internal diameter (160 Å). In fact, CTL and natural killer (NK)–induced membrane lesions are formed by tubular complexes of a polymerized protein (perforin), which is homologous to C9 (see Chapter 12).*

C. *A model of the subunit arrangement in the MAC is shown. The transmembrane region consists of 10 to 15 C9 molecules arranged as a tubule, in addition to single molecules of C6, C7, and C8 α and β chains. The C5bα, C5bβ, and C8β chains form an appendage that projects above the transmembrane pore.*

(Reproduced from Podack, E. R. Molecular mechanisms of cytolysis by complement and cytolytic lymphocytes. Journal of Cellular Biochemistry 30:133–170. 1986. Copyright Alan R. Liss, Inc., 1986.)

leading to osmotic lysis. It is also apparent that some degree of lysis can occur without full poly-C9 polymerization and pore formation. In part, this may be due to the reorientation of the normal lipid arrangement in the membrane as a consequence of the insertion of the hydrophobic portions of the C5-9 complex, creating local areas of leakiness. Furthermore, the insertion of the terminal complement components into a cell membrane may lead to cell death independent of osmotic lysis, by allowing a lethal amount of calcium to passively diffuse into the cell.

REGULATION OF THE COMPLEMENT CASCADES

Uncontrolled activation of complement can lead to formation of the MAC on self tissues and excessive generation of inflammatory mediators. This does not normally happen because both the classical and alternative complement cascades are tightly regulated by several fluid-phase and membrane proteins that interact in specific ways with the various components of the complement system. Furthermore, activation of complement cascades does not occur spontaneously in the blood because the classical pathway is triggered by antigen-antibody complexes, particularly when formed on cell surfaces, and the alternative pathway C3b convertase is unstable unless it is bound to cell surfaces with particular biochemical characteristics. Because of these regulatory mechanisms, a delicate balance of activation and inhibition of the complement cascades is achieved which prevents damage to autologous cells and tissues but promotes the effective destruction of foreign organisms. The pathologic consequences of unregulated complement activation are apparent in various disease states in

TABLE 13–2. Soluble and Membrane Proteins That Regulate Complement Activation

Protein	Molecular Size (kD)/Molecular Characteristics	Serum Concentration (μg/ml) or Cellular Distribution	Specifically Interacts With	Function
Soluble Serum Proteins				
C1 inhibitor (C1 INH)	104 Serpin	200	C$\overline{1r}$, C$\overline{1s}$	Serine protease inhibitor covalently binds to C$\overline{1r}$ and C$\overline{1s}$ and blocks their ability to participate in classical pathway Binds to inactive C1 and prevents spontaneous activation Also inhibits kallikrein, plasmin, and factors XIa and XIIa of coagulation system
C4bp	550 8 SCRs	250	C4b	Accelerates decay of classical pathway C3 convertase (C$\overline{4b2a}$) Acts as cofactor for Factor I–mediated cleavage of C4b
Factor H	150 20 SCRs	480	C3b	Accelerates decay of alternative pathway C3 convertase (C3bBb) Acts as cofactor for Factor I–mediated cleavage of C3b
Factor I	88	35	C4b, C3b	Proteolytically cleaves and inactivates C4b and C3b, using C4bp, factor H, CR1 or MCP as cofactors
Anaphylatoxin inactivator	310 Carboxypeptidase N	35	C3a, C4a, C5a	Proteolytically removes terminal arginine residues and inactivates the anaphylatoxins
S-protein	83 (Vitronectin)	505	C5b-7	Binds to C5b-7 complex and prevents membrane insertion of MAC
SP-40,40	80 Heterodimer	50	C5b-9	Modulates MAC formation
Integral Membrane Proteins				
Complement receptor type 1 (CR1) (CD35)	190–280 34 SCRs	Most blood cells, mast cells	C3b, C4b, iC3b	Accelerates dissociation of classical and alternative pathway C3 convertases Acts as cofactor for Factor I–mediated cleavage of C3b and C4b (Binds immune complexes and promotes their dissolution and phagocytosis)
Membrane cofactor protein (MCP) (CD46)	45–70 4 SCRs; Phosphatidylinositol linkage	Most blood cells (except erythrocytes), epithelial cells, endothelial cells, fibroblasts	C3b, C4b	Acts as cofactor for Factor I–mediated cleavage of C3b and C4b
Decay accelerating factor (DAF)	70 4 SCRs; Phosphatidylinositol linkage	Most blood cells	C4b2b C3bBb	Accelerates dissociation of classical and alternative pathway C3 convertases
Homologous restriction factor (HRF)	65 Phosphatidylinositol linkage	Erythrocytes, lymphocytes, monocytes, neutrophils, platelets	C8 C9	Inhibits lysis of bystander cells (reactive lysis) Blocks C9 binding to C8, preventing MAC insertion into lipid bilayer of autologous cells and lysis; action restricted to C9, C8 of same species
CD59 (membrane inhibitor of reactive lysis [MIRL])	18 Phosphatidylinositol linkage	Erythrocytes, lymphocytes, monocytes, neutrophils, platelets	C7 C8	Inhibits lysis of bystander cells (reactive lysis) Blocks C7, C8 binding to C5b,6, preventing MAC formation and lysis; action restricted to C7, C8 of same species

Abbreviations: SCR, short consensus repeat; MAC, membrane attack complex.

which the regulatory proteins are deficient. The major identified regulatory elements of the complement system, including individual regulatory proteins that work at various points in the cascades, are described next. The regulatory proteins are listed in Table 13–2.

Regulation of the Classical Pathway

Activation of the classical pathway is regulated mainly at two stages:

1. The proteolytic activity of C1 is inhibited by **C1 inhibitor (C1 INH),** a 104 kD, heavily glycosylated serum protein. This molecule is a member of the serine protease inhibitor (serpin) superfamily of proteins, which includes several serine protease inhibitors, such as α-1-antitrypsin, antithrombin II, and α-1-antichymotrypsin. C1 INH regulates the classical complement cascade by forming a stable complex with the activated forms of either C1r or C1s, thereby blocking the ability of these two serine proteases to cleave their normal substrates. As with other serpins, C1 INH accomplishes its task by presenting a "bait" sequence that mimics the normal substrates of C1s and C1r. C1 INH is proteolytically cleaved by C1s or C1r, and this cleavage exposes an active site in the inhibitor, which forms a covalent ester bond with the proteases. C1 INH is the only known inhibitor of C1r and C1s. C1 INH also prevents spontaneous activation of C1, which can occur at a low but significant rate in the absence of antibody. Most of the C1 in blood is bound to C1 INH (present at seven times the molar concentration of C1), and this prevents the conformational changes that cause spontaneous activation. The binding of C1 to an antigen-antibody complex apparently releases C1 from the inhibitory effects of C1 INH.

2. The formation of the classical pathway C3 convertase is inhibited by several proteins.

C4 binding protein (C4bp), an abundant 550 kD soluble serum glycoprotein, and the **type 1 complement receptor (CR1),** an integral membrane protein that is described more thoroughly later, are structurally different but regulate the classical pathway in the same two ways. First, they bind to C4b and competitively inhibit the binding of C2a, thus preventing the assembly of and accelerating the dissociation of the classical pathway C3 convertase, $\overline{C4b2a}$. Second, C4bp and CR1 act as cofactors that promote the proteolysis of C4b by another protein called **Factor I.** Factor I is a 90 kD disulfide-linked heterodimeric serum protein with serine esterase activity. It cleaves C4b to generate two fragments, C4c, which is released into the fluid phase, and a smaller C4d fragment, which remains bound to the original surface. C4d is not able to contribute to C3 convertase activity. In addition to C4bp and CR1, another protein called **membrane cofactor protein** (MCP) also acts as a cofactor for Factor I–mediated cleavage of C4b. MCP is a 45–70 kD integral membrane glycoprotein expressed on leukocytes, lymphocytes, epithelial cells, and fibroblasts. Unlike C4bp and CR1, MCP does not promote dissociation of C4b2a.

The formation of the classical pathway C3 convertase is also inhibited by **decay accelerating factor** (DAF). DAF is a 70 kD phosphatidylinositol-linked or transmembrane glycoprotein found on all peripheral blood cells, endothelium, and various mucosal epithelial cells. Like C4bp, CR1 and MCP, DAF binds to C4b, in competition with C2, thereby inhibiting classical pathway C3 convertase formation and promoting dissociation of C3 convertase after it is formed. Unlike C4bp, CR1 and MCP, DAF does not act as a cofactor for Factor I–mediated cleavage of C4b.

Regulation of the Alternative Pathway

The alternative pathway is also regulated at multiple steps and by several circulating and membrane proteins, some of which function as regulators of the classical pathway as well:

1. Association of the components of the alternative pathway C3 convertase is inhibited, and dissociation is favored, by several different proteins. One of these is a soluble, 150 kD single-chain serum protein called **Factor H.** Factor H competes with Factor B and Bb for binding to C3b. In addition, the two membrane proteins, CR1 and DAF, bind to C3b and competitively inhibit the binding of Factor B, thus preventing the assembly of the alternative pathway C3 convertase. CR1 and DAF also promote the dissociation of Bb from previously formed C3 convertase (Fig. 13–8). These alternative pathway regulatory activities of CR1 and DAF are similar to their role in blocking classical pathway C3 convertase formation, discussed previously.

2. The formation of the alternative pathway C3 convertase, $\overline{C3bBb}$ is inhibited by Factor I–mediated proteolysis of C3b (Fig. 13–9). Factor I cleavage of C3b is promoted by at least three different cofactors, including Factor H, CR1 and MCP. Factor I first cleaves C3b, releasing a 3 kD fragment and leaving an inactive C3b (iC3b) attached to the activating surface. iC3b cannot participate in C3 convertase formation. It is further cleaved by Factor I to yield a 41 kD fragment, C3dg, which remains bound to the activating surface, and a soluble C3c fragment. C3dg is susceptible to proteolysis by any one of several enzymes, including plasmin and trypsin, yielding a 33 kD surface bound C3d molecule and a soluble 8 kD C3g fragment.

In addition to acting directly as cofactors, MCP and CR1 also increase the affinity of surface bound C3b for Factor H relative to Factor B, further reducing the formation of the $\overline{C3bBb}$ complex.

Different cells express different amounts of the regulatory proteins, MCP and CR1, thus controlling the site at which C3b and the alternative pathway C3 convertase are formed. This is particularly important because, as we mentioned earlier, the C3 tickover mechanism is capable of continuously generating C3b, with the potential to form more and more alternative pathway C3 convertase. Most normal cells express high levels of MCP and/or CR1, which protect these cells from complement mediated injury. In contrast, many foreign particles and infectious organisms lack MCP and CR1, so that C3b deposited on these surfaces is not inactivated and binds Factor B with higher affinity than Factor H. This promotes the formation of the $\overline{C3bBb}$ complex, leading to effective complement activation on these foreign surfaces. In addition, this relative preference for Factor B binding to microbial or heterologous cell surfaces may be a function of other biochemical characteristics. For example, high sialic acid content favors Factor H bind-

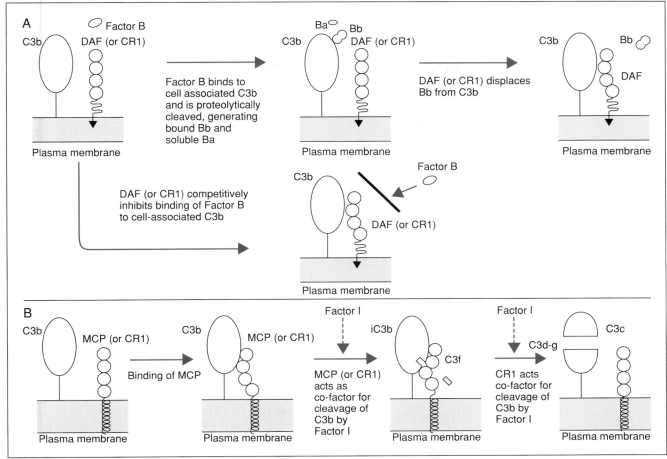

FIGURE 13–8. Membrane protein regulators of the alternative pathway of complement activation.

A. *Decay accelerating factor (DAF) and complement receptor type 1 (CR1) interfere with the formation of the alternative pathway C3 convertase (C3bBb) either by blocking association of Factor B with C3b prior to proteolytic generation of Bb or by promoting dissociation of Bb from C3b. Soluble Factor H has the same effect. Similarly, in the classical pathway, DAF, CR1, and soluble C4 binding protein (C4bp) interfere with the formation of C3 convertase (C4b2b) by blocking interactions of C4 with C2 (not shown).*

B. *Membrane cofactor protein (MCP) and CR1 act as cofactors in the proteolytic inactivation of C3b by Factor I. MCP, CR1, and soluble C4bp also act as cofactors in the Factor I–mediated inactivation of C4b in the classical pathway (not shown).*

(Modified from Hourcade, D., M. Holers, and J. P. Atkinson. The regulators of complement activation (RCA) gene cluster. Advances in Immunology 45:381–416, 1989.)

ing over Factor B, and conversely, cell surfaces with reduced sialic acid content bind Factor B with greater affinity. Many bacteria contain low amounts of surface sialic acid compared to mammalian cells, and this is another reason why complement activation occurs preferentially on bacterial cell surfaces.

Regulation of Membrane Attack Complex Formation

Even after the classical or alternative pathway C3 convertase is formed, excessive complement mediated cell lysis is prevented by a number of proteins that act at the level of the MAC.

1. The formation of the MAC is inhibited by two membrane proteins called **homologous restriction factor (HRF)** and **CD59.** Both of these proteins may be expressed as either phosphatidylinositol-linked forms or as transmembrane forms. HRF (also called C8-binding protein) is a 65 kD protein found on many different cell types which interferes with C9 binding to C8. CD59 (also called **membrane inhibitor of reactive lysis,** or MIRL) is an 18 to 20 kD glycoprotein that inhibits MAC formation probably by blocking C7 and C8 binding to C5b-6. Both HRF and CD59 show the property of homologous restriction; i.e., they efficiently inhibit MAC mediated lysis only when the terminal complement components are from the same species as the cells on which HRF and CD59 are expressed. CD59 and HRF are probably the most important factors protecting normal bystander cells from being lysed when complement is activated on nearby immune complexes or bacteria. Homologous restriction is of no physiological significance, but experimentally, immunologists can easily overcome HRF and CD59 by using heterologous sources of complement proteins to lyse antibody-coated target cells.

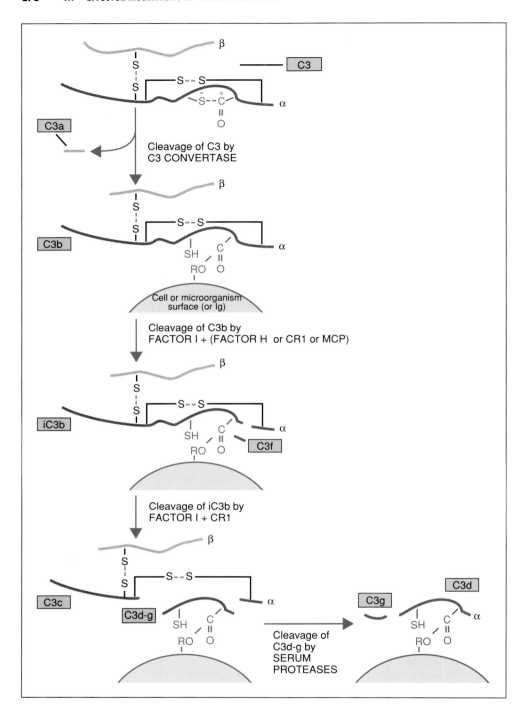

FIGURE 13-9. Sequential proteolytic cleavage of C3. Each proteolytic step generates a soluble fragment and a membrane-bound fragment. Inactive C3b (iC3b), generated by the first Factor I-mediated cleavage, can no longer participate in the formation of C3 convertase. Many of the soluble fragments released in this sequence have biologic activities related to inflammation (see text). Factor I also proteolytically cleaves C4b generated by the classical pathway.

2. The insertion of the terminal complement components into lipid membranes is inhibited by **S protein,** also called **vitronectin,** an 83 kD serum protein related to laminin and fibronectin. It functions by binding to the C5b,6,7 complex and preventing the complex from inserting into lipid membranes. In this way, S protein can diminish the potentially indiscriminate lysis of autologous cell surfaces by insertion of soluble C5bC6C7 complexes released from other activating cell surfaces.

3. The ability of the MAC to lyse cells may be modulated by a circulating protein called **SP-40,40.** SP-40,40 is a heterodimer that has been isolated from soluble C5-9 complexes. It may be a normal component of the MAC whose principal effect is to control the ability of the MAC to lyse cells. The mechanism of action of SP-40,40 is not known.

Receptors for Fragments of the C3 Component of Complement

Many of the biologic activities of the complement system are mediated by the binding of complement fragments to specific integral membrane protein receptors expressed on various cell types. These complement receptors can be divided into three functional categories:

1. Receptors for fragments of C3 that are covalently bound to activating surfaces.
2. Receptors for the soluble C3a and C5a fragments (anaphylatoxins), which mediate the inflammatory effects of complement activation.
3. Receptors that regulate the complement cascades by binding to specific complement proteins and inhibiting their functions.

Receptors for surface bound C3 fragments are the most thoroughly characterized and will be considered in detail in this section of the chapter (Table 13–3). The molecular nature of the anaphylatoxin receptors is not well defined and will be considered briefly in the discussion of the biological activities of complement fragments later in the chapter. The regulatory membrane proteins have been described above.

TABLE 13–3. Receptors for Complement Fragments

Receptor	Molecular Weight (kD) Molecular Features	Ligand	Cell Distribution	Biologic Function
Complement Receptor Type 1 (CR1)	190–280 (Polymorphism) Up to 34 SCRs form entire extracellular region	C3b, C4b, iC3b	Erythrocyte	Clearance of circulating immune complexes; Accelerates dissociation of classical and alternative pathway C3 convertases; Acts as cofactor for Factor I–mediated cleavage of C3b and C4b
			Neutrophils, monocytes, macrophages	Enhances Fc receptor–mediated phagocytosis; Mediates Fc receptor–independent phagocytosis
			Eosinophils	?
			B lymphocytes	?
			T lymphocytes	?
			Glomerular epithelial cells	?Solubilization of trapped immune complexes
			Follicular dendritic cells	?Binding of immune complexes
Complement Receptor Type 2 (CR2)	145 15 SCRs form entire extracellular region	iC3b, C3dg, C3d, C3b (weak) EBV	B lymphocytes	?B cell activation; Mode of EBV infection
			Nasopharyngeal epithelial cells	Mode of EBV infection
			Follicular dendritic cells	?Binding of immune complexes, memory B cell activation
Complement Receptor Type 3 (CR3, CD11bCD18, Mac1)	α:165 β:95 Integrin, common β chain with CR4, LFA–1	iC3b (Cation-dependent)	Monocytes/macrophages, neutrophils, natural killer cells	Cellular adhesion protein required for surface adhesion, chemotaxis, phagocytosis
			Splenic dendritic cells	?
Complement Receptor Type 4 (CR4, CD11cCD18, p150,95)	α:150 β:95 Integrin, common β chain with CR3, LFA–1	iC3b	Neutrophils, monocytes, platelets	Enhances Fc receptor–mediated phagocytosis; Mediates Fc receptor–independent phagocytosis
C3a/C4a Receptor	?	C3a, C4a	Mast cells, basophils	Degranulation releasing histamine and other mediators of inflammation
			Smooth muscle cells	Contraction (?histamine-independent)
			Lymphocytes	?
C5a Receptor	?45	C5a, C5a-des arg	Mast cells, basophils	Degranulation releasing histamine and other mediators
			Endothelial cells	Increases vascular permeability
			Neutrophils, monocytes/macrophages	Promotes chemotaxis

Abbreviations: SCR, short consensus repeat; LFA, leukocyte function–associated antigen; EBV, Epstein-Barr virus.

Complement Receptor Type 1 (CR1, C3b Receptor, CD35). This is a single-chain integral membrane glycoprotein that serves as a high-affinity C3b and C4b receptor. It is present on many cell types, including erythrocytes, neutrophils, macrophages, eosinophils, T and B lymphocytes, and follicular dendritic cells. There are at least four polymorphic forms of CR1 varying in molecular weight from 190 to 280 kD. An interesting feature of CR1 that is shared by several other complement proteins is the presence of multiple, tandemly arranged repeated structures called **short consensus repeats** (SCRs) (Fig. 13–10). Each SCR is 65 to 70 amino acids long, with 11 to 14 conserved amino acid residues, including four highly conserved cysteine residues that form two intrachain disulfide-bonded loops. The most common form of CR1 has 32 tandem SCRs, 28 of which are arranged into four groups, each with seven SCRs. The C3b/C4b binding site of CR1 is located within the second SCR of each group. This repeating structural organization of CR1 ensures that ligand binding sites will be present at some distance from the surface of the CR1–expressing cell, where they may be most effective at binding C3b- or C4b-coated cells and particles. Other complement system molecules that contain SCRs include C4bp, CR2, DAF, and MCP.

CR1 performs at least three important functions. First, CR1 is a regulator of complement activation by virtue of its ability to inhibit C3 convertase activity, discussed previously. Second, CR1 functions as an opsonin receptor that enhances the ability of phagocytic leukocytes to ingest C3b- or C4b-coated particles and microorganisms. Third, CR1 is important for the clearance of immune complexes from the circulation. These functions are described in detail later in the chapter. Recently, a genetically engineered, soluble form of CR1, lacking transmembrane and cytoplasmic domains, has been produced. This soluble CR1 markedly inhibits both alternative and classical pathway activation and limits tissue injury in an *in vivo* model of acute inflammation.

Complement Receptor Type 2 (CR2, C3d Receptor, CD21). This is a 145 kD, single-chain integral membrane glycoprotein present on B lymphocytes, follicular dendritic cells, and epithelial cells. CR2 specifically binds C3dg and C3d, the Factor I generated cleavage products of surface or immune complex bound C3b. The physiologic consequences of this binding are not well understood. CR2 on follicular dendritic cells may serve to trap antigen-antibody complexes in germinal centers, leading to the activation of memory B lymphocytes. *In vitro,* antibody binding to CR2 can enhance or inhibit B cell activation in response to other stimuli, depending on the experimental system. Furthermore, the cytoplasmic tail of CR2 is phosphorylated after surface Ig cross-linking. However, the role of CR2 in physiologic humoral immune responses *in vivo* is not clear. Evidence for such a role comes from studies of geneti-

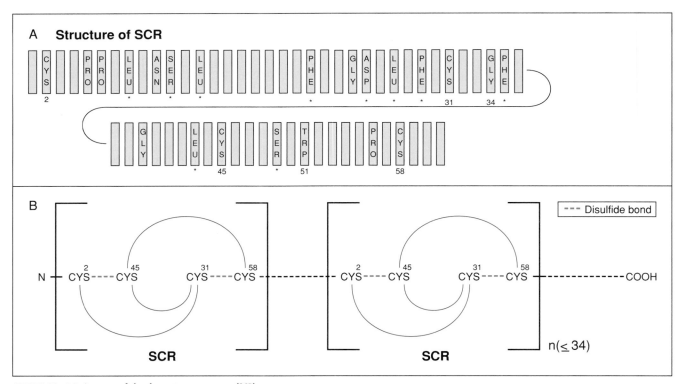

FIGURE 13–10. Structure of the short consensus repeat (SCR).
A. *Amino acid sequences in SCRs which are conserved in at least 44 per cent of SCRs in different molecules are shown in three-letter code. Numbered residues are conserved in 95 to 100 per cent of SCRs, and include four cysteines that form intrachain disulfide bonds. In the residues indicated by asterisks, one or two other amino acids may be used.*
B. *Schematic representation of SCRs with overlapping intrachain disulfide bonds.*
(Modified with permission from Hourcade, D., M. Holers, and J. P. Atkinson. The regulation of complement activation (RCA) gene cluster. Advances in Immunology 45:381–416, 1989.)

cally C3 deficient animals, which often do not show normal secondary antibody responses with IgM to IgG class switching.

CR2 is the cell surface receptor for the **Epstein-Barr virus** (EBV). Ironically, more may be known about the role of CR2 in EBV–related pathology than about the role of this complement receptor in normal physiology. EBV is a human herpes virus that infects most people by adulthood and remains latent within B cells or pharyngeal epithelial cells for the duration of life. Infection may be subclinical or may cause infectious mononucleosis. In addition, EBV is linked to several human malignancies, including African Burkitt's lymphoma (a malignant B cell tumor), B cell lymphomas associated with therapeutic drug-induced or human immunodeficiency virus (HIV)–induced immunodeficiency, and nasopharyngeal carcinoma (a malignant tumor of nasopharyngeal epithelium) (see Chapter 17, Box 17–2). These tumors are derived from the only normal cells known to express CR2. EBV is a potent polyclonal B cell activator, and *in vitro* the virus can transform normal blood B lymphocytes into immortalized lymphoblastoid cell lines. These effects of the virus depend on CR2 expression on the B cells.

COMPLEMENT RECEPTOR TYPE 3 (CR3, iC3b RECEPTOR, Mac-1, CD11bCD18). This is a specific receptor for the iC3b fragment generated by Factor I–mediated cleavage of C3b. This receptor is expressed on many different bone marrow–derived cells, including neutrophils, mononuclear phagocytes, mast cells, and NK cells. CR3 is a member of the integrin family of cell surface receptors (see Chapter 7, Box 7–4). It consists of a 165 kD α chain (CD11b) noncovalently linked to a 95 kD β chain (CD18), which is identical to the β chains of two closely related integrin molecules, lymphocyte function–associated antigen–1 (LFA–1) and p150, 95 (see below).

CR3 is thought to be important for phagocytosis of iC3b-coated microorganisms or particles. Furthermore, CR3 has a specific carbohydrate-binding capacity (i.e., a lectin activity) that may be responsible for complement-independent binding of certain microorganisms to CR3 expressing phagocytic cells. In addition, CR3 on neutrophils and monocytes promotes the attachment of these cells to endothelium, even without complement activation. This may be important for the accumulation of inflammatory cells at sites of tissue injury.

COMPLEMENT RECEPTOR TYPE 4 (CR4, p150,95, CD11cCD18). This is another integrin, with a 150 kD α chain and the same β chain as CR3. It has a similar cellular distribution as CR3 and can bind iC3b as well as C3dg. The function of this receptor may be similar to that of CR3.

BIOLOGIC FUNCTIONS OF COMPLEMENT PROTEINS

The functions of the complement system fall into two broad categories: (1) cell lysis by the MAC and (2) biologic effects of proteolytic fragments of complement. We have previously described how complement activation on cell surfaces leads to the insertion of the MAC into lipid bilayers, causing osmotic lysis of the cell. The many other effects of complement in immunity and inflammation are mediated by the proteolytic fragments generated during complement activation. These biologically active fragments may remain bound to the same cell surfaces where complement has been activated, or they may be released into the fluid phase (e.g., blood or extracellular fluid). In either case, they mediate their effects by binding to specific receptors expressed on a variety of other cell types, including phagocytic leukocytes and endothelium. In this section of the chapter, we will discuss each of these functional roles of the complement system, with reference to the particular fragments and receptors that are involved (Table 13–4).

Complement-Mediated Cytolysis

Complement-mediated lysis of foreign organisms is an important defense mechanism against microbial

TABLE 13–4. Biologic Functions of Complement

Function	Complement Components	Mechanisms
Lysis of cells	C5–C9	MAC formation kills microorganisms
Opsonization/phagocytosis	C3b,iC3b	C3b or iC3b on the surface of microorganisms bind to CR1 (and CR3, CR4) on neutrophils and macrophages, promoting phagocytosis
Inflammation Vascular responses	C5a > C3a ≫ C4a	C5a, C3a, and C4a stimulate mast cell histamine release and smooth muscle contraction
Polymorphonuclear leukocyte activation	C5a	C5a is a chemoattractant for neutrophils and activates neutrophil oxidative metabolism
Immune complex removal	Classical pathway, C3b	Complement activation on Ig molecules inhibits immune complex formation; C3b on immune complexes binds to CR1 on erythrocytes and the immune complexes are cleared from the circulation as the erythrocytes traverse the liver and spleen

Abbreviations: MAC, membrane attack complex; Ig, immunoglobulin.

infection. Specific humoral responses to microbes generate antibodies that bind to the organisms; these antibodies locally activate complement on the surfaces of the microbes and lead to their lysis by the formation of the MAC. Some microorganisms may activate the alternative pathway, in the absence of antibody, also leading to lysis. This mechanism may be important for preventing bacteremia by *Neisseria* bacteria. Acquired resistance to complement-mediated lysis is a mechanism by which some microbes evade host immunity (see Chapter 15). In certain pathologic conditions, the complement system may cause lysis of host cells, leading to tissue injury and disease. For example, some autoimmune diseases are characterized by the production of autoantibodies specific for self proteins expressed on cell surfaces. These autoantibodies may fix complement, and subsequent MAC formation may lead to osmotic lysis of these normal cells (see Chapter 18).

Opsonization and Promotion of Phagocytosis of Microbes

As discussed previously, activation of both classical and alternative pathways leads to the generation of C3b and iC3b covalently bound to cell surfaces. Both C3b and iC3b act as opsonins by virtue of the fact that they specifically bind to receptors on neutrophils and macrophages. C3b and, to a lesser extent, iC3b bind to CR1, and iC3b (but not C3b) binds to CR3 and CR4. Thus, complement activation on the surface of a microbial cell promotes the adherence of the microbe to a phagocytic cell that is competent at phagocytosing and killing the microbe. *C3b- and iC3b-dependent phagocytosis of microorganisms is probably the major defense mechanism against systemic bacterial and fungal infections.*

Complement receptors and Fcγ receptors cooperate to mediate binding and phagocytosis of opsonized particles. For example, if an unactivated neutrophil or monocyte encounters a particle coated with IgG, the particle is phagocytosed relatively slowly via the Fcγ receptors. If the same particle bears iC3b, so that it simultaneously binds to CR3 on the leukocyte, Fcγ receptor-mediated phagocytosis is also greatly enhanced. Similarly, binding of opsonized particles to Fcγ receptors augments CR1- and CR3-mediated phagocytosis. Such observations suggest that Fcγ and complement receptors on leukocytes function not only to bind opsonized particles but also to transduce signals that stimulate the phagocytic capacities of the leukocytes.

Anaphylatoxins and Inflammatory Responses

C3a, C4a, and C5a are called **anaphylatoxins** because they induce the release of soluble inflammatory mediators, which cause rapid increases in vascular permeability characteristic of anaphylaxis (see Chapter 14). As described earlier, C3a is a 9 kD peptide fragment derived from proteolytic cleavage of the C3 α chain by either classical or alternative pathway C3 convertase. C4a is the 8.7 kD peptide released from the α chain of C4 by C2b mediated cleavage in the classical pathway. C5a is the 11 kD peptide released from the α chain of C5 by the action of either classical or alternative pathway C5 convertase. C3a and C4a receptors are expressed on mast cells, basophils, smooth muscle cells, and lymphocytes. C5a receptors are expressed on mast cells, basophils, neutrophils, monocytes/macrophages, and endothelium (see Table 13-3). Ligand binding and functional response data indicate that these receptors are specific, saturable receptors with signal-transducing properties.

The major effects of anaphylatoxin binding to mast cells and basophils are granule exocytosis and release of vasoactive mediators, such as histamine. Histamine increases vascular permeability and stimulates the contraction of visceral smooth muscles. The anaphylatoxins also bind to smooth muscle and stimulate its contraction. C5a is the most potent mediator of these effects, C3a is 20-fold less potent, and C4a is 2500-fold less potent. C5a has important additional effects on neutrophils and endothelial cells not shared by C3a or C4a. C5a is a **chemoattractant** for neutrophils that stimulates directed migration of these cells up a concentration gradient. In addition, C5a stimulates neutrophil oxidative metabolism, granule discharge, and adhesiveness. C5a also may have direct effects on vascular endothelium, causing increased vascular permeability independent of histamine release from mast cells.

The combination of these effects is to promote the accumulation of the cellular and serum protein components required for an effective acute inflammatory response to infections and foreign particles. The specificity of the response for foreign and not self tissues is imparted either by specific antibody activating the complement cascade at the appropriate location, i.e., where the foreign antigen is, or by the capacity of the alternative pathway to be activated on the surface of foreign organisms.

Solubilization and Phagocytic Clearance of Immune Complexes

Small numbers of immune complexes are constantly being formed in the circulation and may increase dramatically when an individual mounts a vigorous humoral immune response to an abundant circulating antigen. These immune complexes are potentially harmful because they may deposit in vessel walls, activate complement, and lead to inflammatory reactions which damage surrounding tissues. Formation of large, potentially harmful, immune complexes requires not only the multivalent binding of Ig Fab regions to antigens but also noncovalent interactions of Fc regions of juxtaposed Ig molecules (see Chapter 3). Complement binding to Ig can sterically block these Fc-Fc interactions, thereby inhibiting new formation of, or destabilizing already formed, immune complexes.

In addition to interfering with immune complex formation, the complement system can promote the clearance of immune complexes from the circulation by the mononuclear phagocyte system. This function is largely mediated by CR1 on the surface of erythrocytes, which, because of their number, account for the great majority of cell-associated CR1 molecules in the circulation. Circulating antigen-antibody complexes activate complement, and the C3b that is generated forms covalent bonds with the antibody. Such complexes may be adsorbed by CR1 expressing erythrocytes because of the high affinity of CR1 for C3b. *In vivo* primate studies have demonstrated that phagocytic cells in the liver (Kupffer cells) and spleen are responsible for removing the immune complexes along with CR1 molecules from the erythrocyte membranes as the erythrocytes traverse the sinusoids of these organs.

COMPLEMENT GENES AND BIOSYNTHESIS

Gene Families Represented by Complement Proteins

The complement system proteins can be categorized as members of various gene families on the basis of sequence homologies. Members of the same gene family often have similar functional characteristics that are dependent on their shared protein structures. Assignment of proteins to one or another gene family (usually based on the amino acid sequences predicted from the nucleotide sequences of the cloned genes) is often useful for studying the structural basis of function. Furthermore, the homologies among genes encoding various complement proteins suggest that members of each gene family may have arisen by duplication of an ancestral gene, followed by the structural diversification that imparts specialized functions to the individual proteins.

The most well-defined complement gene family includes a group of proteins that bind C3b and C4b; these include C4bp, Factor H, CR1, CR2, DAF, MCP, C2, and Factor B. Four of these proteins (C4bp, Factor H, CR1, and MCP) act as cofactors for Factor I catalyzed cleavage of C3b or C4b. The common genetic and structural feature of this family of proteins is the presence of SCRs, described in our discussion of CR1 (see Fig. 13–10). SCRs constitute a significant part of the structure of all these proteins. For example, the amino acid sequence of Factor H is composed entirely of 20 SCRs, and one form of CR1 has 34 SCRs making up the entire extracellular domain. The C3b/C4b binding regions of these molecules are formed, at least in part,

by the SCRs. The presence of SCRs in other complement proteins, including Factor B, C2, C1r, and C1s, reflect exon duplication and fusion with otherwise unrelated genes during evolution. Several non-complement proteins also contain SCRs, including the interleukin-2 receptor, endothelial-leukocyte adhesion molecule–1 (ELAM–1), the lymphocyte homing receptor recognized by the monoclonal antibody MEL–14, and coagulation factor XIII. The significance of SCRs in these molecules is not well understood.

Several complement system proteins are members of other gene families, sharing functions with other family members as well as the amino acid sequences that are critical for those functions. The five serine esterases of the complement system, including Factor I, Factor B, C1r, C1s, and C2, all have sequence homologies with one another and with non-complement serine esterases such as trypsin and chymotrypsin. The serine protease inhibitor, C1 INH, is a member of the serpin family, which includes other protease inhibitors such as α_1-antitrypsin and antithrombin II. C3 and C4 are members of a small family of proteins that also includes α_2-macroglobulin, characterized by the presence of internal thioester bonds. This feature allows the proteins to form covalent bonds with cell surfaces or Ig molecules. CR3 and CR4 are integrins sharing the same β-chain as LFA–1. The membrane pore-forming C9 is homologous to the pore-forming protein (cytolysin or perforin), found in CTLs and NK cells.

Chromosomal Linkage of Complement Genes

At least three groups of complement proteins can be defined by close chromosomal linkage of their respective members. The members of each of these groups probably arose by duplication from a common ancestral gene. CR1, CR2, C4bp, and DAF are highly homologous SCR-containing proteins that are closely linked on a 950 kB DNA segment found on the long arm of chromosome 1. This cluster of genes has been named the **regulation of complement activation (RCA) cluster.** Similarly, the genes encoding the MAC components C6, C7, C8, and C9 are also linked in another region on chromosome 1.

The close proximity of the genes encoding C2, Factor B, and C4 within the major histocompatibility complex (MHC) in man, mouse, and other species is the most thoroughly analyzed example of complement gene linkage. In man, these complement protein genes are present between the class II HLA–DR and class I HLA–B loci on chromosome 6 (Fig. 13–11; see also Chapter 5). MHC-linked complement genes are sometimes called class III genes. Interestingly, as is characteristic of the peptide-binding class I and class II MHC molecules, the class III complement genes are polymorphic. For example, there are over 35 alleles identified for the two closely linked loci that encode the C4 protein. Certain alleles of the C2, Factor B, and

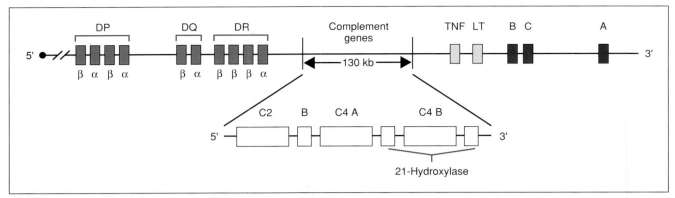

FIGURE 13–11. Complement genes in the human major histocompatibility complex (MHC). *The genes encoding C2, Factor B, and C4 are located between the DR locus and the class I MHC genes, 5' to genes encoding the cytokines tumor necrosis factor (TNF) and lymphotoxin (LT). Two genes encode functionally indistinguishable C4 proteins (C4A and C4B). Both the C2 and C4 genes are polymorphic.*

C4 genes are in linkage disequilibrium, so that they are often inherited *en bloc.* The association of C2 and C4 deficiencies with autoimmune disease (discussed below) may reflect linkage disequilibrium of complement haplotypes containing defective alleles with certain class II "immune response genes" that favor autoimmune responses to self antigens.

Biosynthesis of Complement Proteins

Both hepatocytes and mononuclear phagocytes can synthesize most of the complement proteins present in the serum. The liver probably makes quantitatively more complement proteins, but mononuclear phagocyte synthesis may be significant at sites of inflammation. Interestingly, γ-interferon induces the synthesis of a number of alternative pathway proteins in macrophages. The C1 proteins can also be synthesized by various types of epithelial cells other than hepatocytes. The regulation of synthesis of the various complement proteins is complicated, and incompletely characterized. Many complement proteins are "acute phase reactants" that are synthesized in response to circulating cytokines such as interleukin-1, interleukin-6, and tumor necrosis factor (see Chapter 11, Box 11–2). The C1 and C8 proteins are unusual, in that they are complexes of polypeptide products of more than one gene. The individual chains of each protein are secreted independently, and the mature proteins assemble extracellularly.

HUMAN DISEASES RELATED TO THE COMPLEMENT SYSTEM

The complement system is related to human disease in two general ways. First, deficiencies in any one of the protein components, usually due to abnormalities in gene structure, can lead to abnormal patterns of complement activation. If regulatory components are absent, too much complement activation may occur at the wrong time or wrong site. The absence of an integral component of the classical, alternative, or terminal pathways can result in too little complement activation and a lack of complement-mediated biologic functions. In either case, pathologic consequences may be severe. Second, an intact, normally functioning complement system may be activated in response to abnormal stimuli, such as a persistent microorganism or autoimmune humoral responses to self antigens. In these infectious or autoimmune diseases, the inflammatory or lytic effects of complement may contribute significantly to the pathology of the disease.

Complement Deficiencies

Deficiencies in many of the complement proteins have been described (Table 13–5), and these deficiencies are usually attributable to inherited or spontaneously mutated genes. Alternatively, acquired deficiencies in certain components can arise in individuals with normal complement genes. Deficiencies can be categorized on the basis of the functional type of protein that is lacking. Thus, there are deficiencies of the components of the classical, alternative, and terminal pathways and deficiencies in either soluble or membrane regulatory proteins. Beyond the significance to the affected individuals, an understanding of these diseases provides insights into the normal physiologic roles of the deficient proteins.

1. Genetic deficiencies in *classical and alternative pathway components,* including C1q, C1r, C1s, C4, C2, C3, properdin, and Factor D have all been described; C2 deficiency is the most commonly identified human complement deficiency. C3 deficiency is associated with frequent serious pyogenic bacterial infections that may be fatal. The frequency of pyogenic infections in these patients suggests the importance of C3 for opsonization, enhanced phagocytosis, and destruction of these organisms. Deficiencies in the early components of the classical pathway are associated with immune complex and/or autoimmune diseases,

TABLE 13-5. Complement Deficiencies and Abnormalities

Protein	Resulting Complement Activation Abnormalities	Associated Diseases and Pathology
Classical Pathway		
C1q	Defective classical pathway activation	Systemic lupus erythematosus Glomerulonephritis
C1r	Defective classical pathway activation	Systemic lupus erythematosus Glomerulonephritis Pyogenic infections
C1s	Defective classical pathway activation	Systemic lupus erythematosus Glomerulonephritis Pyogenic infections
C4	Defective classical pathway activation	Systemic lupus erythematosus Glomerulonephritis Pyogenic infections
C2	Defective classical pathway activation	Systemic lupus erythematosus Vasculitis Glomerulonephritis Pyogenic infections
C3	Defective classical/alternative pathway activation	Pyogenic infections Glomerulonephritis
Alternative Pathway		
Properdin	Defective alternative pathway activation	Pyogenic infections
Factor D	Defective alternative pathway activation	Pyogenic infections
Terminal Components		
C5	Defective MAC formation	Disseminated *Neisseria* infections
C6	Defective MAC formation	Disseminated *Neisseria* infections
C7	Defective MAC formation	Disseminated *Neisseria* infections Glomerulonephritis Systemic lupus erythematosus
C8	Defective MAC formation	Disseminated *Neisseria* infections Systemic lupus erythematosus
C9	Defective MAC formation	Disseminated *Neisseria* infections

Abbreviations: MAC, membrane attack complex.

such as glomerulonephritis and systemic lupus erythematosus (SLE) (Chapter 18, Box 18–1). More than 50 per cent of patients with C2 and C4 deficiencies have SLE. This association has been attributed to the requirement of the classical pathway for the clearance and solubilization of circulating immune complexes. Other explanations for the association include genetic linkage of defective complement alleles in the MHC with certain pathogenic immune response genes (see Chapter 18). Somewhat surprisingly, C2 and C4 deficiencies are often not associated with increased infections. This suggests that the alternative pathway may be adequate for the elimination of most bacteria and that a key function of the classical pathway is to remove circulating immune complexes.

2. Deficiencies in members of the *terminal complement components,* including C5, C6, C7, C8, and C9

have also been described. These patients cannot generate the MAC and would therefore be expected to be inefficient in lysing foreign organisms. Interestingly, the only consistent clinical problem in these patients is a propensity for disseminated infections by the intracellular *Neisseria* bacteria, including *N. meningitidis* and *N. gonorrhoeae,* suggesting that MAC formation is particularly important for defense against these organisms. However, the number of patients identified with terminal complement deficiencies is too small to make any firm conclusions on the role of MAC formation in killing one type of organism versus another.

3. Deficiencies in *soluble and membrane-bound complement regulatory proteins* are associated with abnormal complement activation and a variety of related clinical abnormalities (Table 13–6). The absence of

TABLE 13–6. Abnormalities and Deficiencies of Regulatory Complement Proteins

Protein	Resulting Complement Activation Abnormalities	Associated Diseases/Pathology	Disease/Syndrome Name
Regulatory Proteins			
C1 inhibitor	Deregulated classical pathway activation, consumption of C3	Acute, intermittent attacks of skin and mucosal edema	Hereditary angioneurotic edema
		Acute, intermittent attacks of skin and mucosal edema	Acquired angioneurotic edema
		Systemic lupus erythematosus	
		B cell lymphoproliferative diseases	
Factor I	Deregulated classical pathway activation, consumption of C3	Pyogenic infections	
		Vasculitis	
		Glomerulonephritis	
Factor H	Deregulated classical pathway activation, consumption of C3	Pyogenic infections	
		Vasculitis	
		Glomerulonephritis	
		Partial lipodystrophy	
DAF	Deregulated C3 convertase activity	Complement-mediated intravascular hemolysis	Paroxysmal nocturnal hemoglobinuria
HRF	Increased susceptibility of red cells to MAC–mediated lysis	Complement-mediated intravascular hemolysis	Paroxysmal nocturnal hemoglobinuria
CD59 (MIRL)	Increased susceptibility of red cells to MAC–mediated lysis	Complement-mediated intravascular hemolysis	Paroxysmal nocturnal hemoglobinuria
Complement Receptors			
CR1	Deregulated C3 convertase activity	Systemic lupus erythematosus	
CR3		Pyogenic infections	Leukocyte adhesion deficiency

Abbreviations: LFA–1, leukocyte-associated function antigen; MIRL, membrane inhibitor of reactive lysis; DAF, decay accelerating factor; HRF, homologous restriction factor; MAC, membrane attack complex.

classical, alternative, and terminal pathway regulatory proteins have each been described.

a. **Hereditary angioneurotic edema (HANE)** is an *autosomal dominant deficiency in C1 INH.* Clinical manifestations of the disease include intermittent, acute accumulation of edema fluid in skin and mucosa, lasting from 24 to 72 hours. The skin of the face and extremities and the laryngeal and intestinal mucosa are most frequently involved. Serious symptoms resulting from edema in these locations include abdominal pain, nausea and vomiting, diarrhea, and potentially life-threatening airway obstruction. Attacks have been associated with antecedent emotional stress and trauma; the physiologic basis for the association is not understood. The deficiency in C1 INH in HANE patients may be caused either by an absolute reduction in C1 INH protein due to inheritance of a nonfunctional gene or by synthesis of a normal amount of a dysfunctional protein due to mutations in the coding sequences of the gene. Although there is usually one normal allele of the C1 INH gene in these patients, the plasma levels of the C1 INH protein are sufficiently reduced (20 to 30 per cent of normal) so that activation of C1 by immune complexes is not properly controlled. It is clear that during attacks there are elevated plasma levels of activated C1 and decreased levels of the substrates of activated C1, namely C2 and C4. The mediators of edema formation

in HANE patients have not yet been identified. The anaphylatoxins (C3a, C4a, and C5a) that are generated during complement activation are likely participants, and less well characterized proteolytic fragments of C2 may also be involved. The probable role of other mediators in this disease is suspected from the fact that C1 INH is a major regulator of other plasma serine proteases besides C1, including kallikrein and coagulation factor XII. Activated kallikrein and factor XII can both promote increased formation of bradykinin, which can cause edema. Furthermore, C1 INH deficiency can lead to increased plasmin generation, which in turn can proteolytically generate a fragment from C2 with kinin activity.

b. Deficiencies of the *soluble alternative pathway regulators* (Factor I and Factor H) are extremely rare, precluding meaningful analysis of the clinical consequences of the absence of these proteins. Nonetheless, these patients have provided insights into the role of Factor I–mediated cleavage of C3b. Plasma C3 is completely consumed in these patients as a result of unregulated formation of fluid-phase C3 convertase (by the tickover mechanism). This is similar to the effects of an autoantibody called **C3 nephritic factor** (C3NeF), which is specific for alternative pathway C3 convertase (C3bBb). This antibody stabilizes C3bBb and protects the complex from Factor H–mediated dissociation, therefore causing unregulated consumption of C3. Patients with this antibody often have glomerulonephritis, possibly caused by inadequate clearing of circulating immune complexes.

c. Deficiencies in *integral membrane protein regulators of complement activation* include the absence of DAF, HRF, and CD59. All of these proteins are normally bound to the plasma membrane of erythrocytes by phosphatidylinositol linkages. **Paroxysmal nocturnal hemoglobinuria** (PNH) is a disease in which erythrocytes, as well as other cells, lack the ability to express phosphatidylinositol-linked membrane proteins, including DAF, HRF, and CD59. PNH is characterized by recurrent bouts of intravascular hemolysis, at least partially attributable to complement activation on the surface of erythrocytes. This is predictable, since DAF normally functions to inhibit C3 convertase formation on autologous cell surfaces, and HRF and CD59 normally serve to inhibit MAC formation on autologous cell membranes. Erythrocytes are particularly sensitive because other cells express both phosphatidylinositol-linked and transmembrane forms of HRF and CD59.

4. Deficiencies in *complement receptors* include the absence of CR3 and CR4, both resulting from rare mutations in the β chain (CD18) gene common to the CD11CD18 family of integrin molecules. The congenital disease caused by this gene defect is called **leukocyte adhesion deficiency** (see Chapter 19). This disorder is characterized by recurrent pyogenic infections, probably due to a combination of impaired iC3b dependent phagocytosis of bacteria and inadequate adherence of neutrophils to endothelium at tissue sites of infection.

Pathologic Effects of a Normal Complement System

Even when it is properly regulated and appropriately activated, the complement system can cause significant tissue damage. In fact, much of the pathology associated with bacterial infections is attributable to the biologic effects of complement activation. These pathologic effects include the bystander destruction of normal host cells when acute inflammatory responses to infectious organisms take place. For example, a bacterial infection can stimulate a humoral immune response and antibody bound to bacterial antigens can activate complement. Direct activation of the alternative pathway on bacterial surfaces may also occur, in the absence of antibody. The generation of C3a and C5a stimulates the accumulation of neutrophils at the site of infection. The neutrophils adhere to and phagocytose the infecting organisms. In addition, neutrophils release free radicals and proteases that destroy microbes and may damage normal cells in the vicinity as well. Histamine released from mast cells in response to C5a may amplify the inflammatory response by increasing vascular permeability.

Perhaps the clearest example of complement-mediated pathology occurs in immune complex diseases. Systemic vasculitis and immune complex glomerulonephritis may result from deposition of antigen-antibody complexes in the walls of vessels and kidney glomeruli (see Chapter 18). Complement activated by the Ig in these deposited immune complexes initiates the acute inflammatory responses which destroy the vessel walls or glomeruli leading to thrombosis, ischemic damage to tissues, and scarring.

SUMMARY

The complement system includes serum and membrane proteins that interact in a highly regulated manner to produce biologically active protein products. The system includes two convergent proteolytic pathways, composed of several different zymogens. The classical pathway is initiated by antigen-antibody complexes, and the alternative pathway is usually activated directly by the surfaces of infectious organisms. The two pathways converge, both utilizing the C3 protein to form enzymes that initiate the common terminal pathway leading to formation of a cytolytic protein complex called the membrane attack complex. These pathways are regulated by various soluble and membrane-bound proteins, which inhibit different steps in the cascades. The biologic functions of the complement system include cytolysis, opsonization of organisms and immune complexes for phagocytosis, production of inflammation, and solubilization and clearance of immune complexes. Cytolysis is mediated by MAC formation on cell surfaces. Opsonization is largely mediated by proteolytic fragments of C3, as is immune complex clearance. Inflammation is promoted by proteolytic fragments of complement proteins called anaphylatoxins (C3a, C4a, C5a). Specific membrane receptors for complement fragments are required for the opsonin and anaphylatoxin effects. The complement proteins are members of several different gene families, reflecting the common usage of duplicated exons and genes encoding functionally significant domains during the evolution of the system. Many genetic deficiencies in one or more complement components have been described, with associated infections and autoimmune diseases.

SELECTED READINGS

Ahearn, J. M., and D. T. Fearon. Structure and function of the complement receptors, CR1 (CD35) and CR2 (CD21). Advances in Immunology 46:183–219, 1989.

Campbell, R. D., M. C. Carroll, and R. R. Porter. The molecular genetics of components of complement. Advances in Immunology 38:203–244, 1986.

Colten, H. R. Molecular basis of complement deficiency syndromes. Laboratory Investigation 52:468–473, 1985.

Hourcade D., M. Holers, and J. P. Atkinson. The regulators of complement activation (RCA) gene cluster. Advances in Immunology 45:381–416, 1989.

Lubin, D. M., and J. P. Atkinson. Decay-accelerating factor: biochemistry, molecular biology, and function. Annual Review of Immunology 7:35–58, 1989.

Muller-Eberhard, H. J. The membrane attack complex. Annual Review of Immunology 4:503–528, 1986.

Muller-Eberhard, H. J. Molecular organization and function of the complement system. Annual Review of Biochemistry 57:321–347, 1988.

Perlmutter, D. H., and H. R. Colten. Regulation of complement biosynthesis. Annual Review of Immunology 4:231–251, 1986.

Reid, K. B. M., and A. J. Day. Structure-function relationships of the complement components. Immunology Today 10:177–180, 1989.

Schumaker, V. N., P. Zavodszky, and P. H. Poon. Activation of the first component of complement. Annual Review of Immunology 5:21–42, 1987.

Weisman, H. F., T. Bartow, M. K. Leppo, H. C. Marsh, Jr., G. R. Carson, M. F. Concino, M. P. Boyle, K. H. Roux, M. L. Weisfeldt, and D. T. Fearon. Soluble human complement receptor type 1: *In vivo* inhibitor of complement suppressing post-ischemic myocardial inflammation and necrosis. Science 249:146–151, 1990.

CHAPTER FOURTEEN

IMMUNOGLOBULIN E AND MAST CELL/ BASOPHIL-MEDIATED IMMUNE REACTIONS

One of the most powerful effector mechanisms of the immune system is the reaction produced by IgE-dependent stimulation of tissue mast cells and their circulating counterparts, the basophils. When antigen binds to IgE molecules preattached to the surface of these cells, there is a rapid release of a variety of mediators that collectively cause increased vascular permeability, vasodilation, bronchial and visceral smooth muscle contraction, and local inflammation. This reaction is called **immediate hypersensitivity** because it begins rapidly, within minutes of antigen challenge. In its most extreme systemic form, called **anaphylaxis,** mast cell–derived or basophil-derived mediators can restrict airways to the point of asphyxiation and produce cardiovascular collapse leading to death. (The term anaphylaxis was coined to indicate that antibodies, especially IgE antibodies, could confer the opposite of protection [prophylaxis] on an unfortunate individual.) Individuals prone to develop strong immediate hypersensitivity responses are called **atopic** and are said to suffer from **allergies.** Atopy meant "unusual," but we now realize that allergy is in fact quite common. Indeed, allergy is the most common disorder of immunity, affecting 20 per

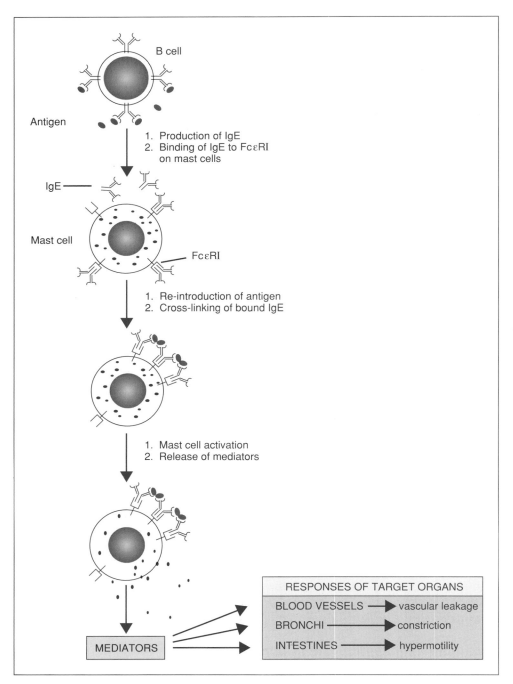

FIGURE 14–1. Sequence of events in immediate hypersensitivity. The initial contact with an antigen leads to specific IgE synthesis by B cells. Secreted IgE binds to mast cells or basophils through high-affinity Fcε receptors (FcεRI). Upon subsequent exposure to antigen, an immediate hypersensitivity reaction is triggered by cross-linking the IgE molecules.

B cell

Antigen

1. Production of IgE
2. Binding of IgE to FcεRI on mast cells

IgE

Mast cell

FcεRI

1. Re-introduction of antigen
2. Cross-linking of bound IgE

1. Mast cell activation
2. Release of mediators

MEDIATORS

RESPONSES OF TARGET ORGANS		
BLOOD VESSELS	→	vascular leakage
BRONCHI	→	constriction
INTESTINES	→	hypermotility

cent of all individuals in the United States. In different individuals, atopy may take different forms such as hay fever, asthma, chronic eczema (skin irritation), or food allergies. All of these conditions are forms of immediate hypersensitivity induced by mast cell or basophil activation.

Mast cell and basophil activation is most characteristically initiated when specific antigen triggers the response by binding to and cross-linking preattached surface IgE molecules. Thus, *the typical sequence of events in immediate hypersensitivity* is as follows: (1) production of IgE by B cells in response to the first exposure to an antigen, (2) binding of the IgE to specific Fc receptors on the surfaces of mast cells and basophils, and (3) interaction of re-introduced antigen with the bound IgE, leading to (4) activation of the cells and release of mediators, some of which are stored in the cytoplasmic granules of the mast cells and basophils (Fig. 14–1). The clinical and pathologic manifestations of immediate hypersensitivity are due to the actions of the released mediators.

This chapter focuses on IgE-mediated reactions. We begin by describing experimental models of immediate hypersensitivity. We then turn to the biology of IgE and to the Fc receptors that bind IgE on the surface of mast cells or basophils. Next, we discuss the biology of mast cells and related cell types, including a description of how these cells are activated in response to antigen. We then describe the structure of the mediators produced by activated mast cells and the biologic effects of these mediators. Finally, we conclude with a more detailed description of different allergic diseases, integrating features of mast cell biology, mast cell mediators, and the responses of various target tissues to explain specific clinical syndromes associated with IgE and mast cell activation.

EXPERIMENTAL MODELS OF IMMEDIATE HYPERSENSITIVITY

The classic example of immediate hypersensitivity in man is the "triple response" or "wheal and flare reaction" (Fig. 14–2). When a sensitized individual is challenged by intradermal injection of an appropriate antigen, the injection site becomes red from locally dilated blood vessels engorged with red blood cells. In the second phase, the site rapidly swells as a result of leakage of plasma from the venules. This soft swelling is called a **wheal** and can involve an area of skin as large as several centimeters in diameter. In the third phase, blood vessels at the margins of the wheal dilate and become engorged with red blood cells, producing a characteristic red rim called a **flare.** The full wheal and flare reaction can appear within 5 to 10 minutes after administration of antigen and usually subsides in less than an hour. By electron microscopy, the venules in the area of the wheal show slight separation of the endothelial cells, which accounts for the escape of macromolecules and fluid, but not cells, from the vascular lumen.

The first clue to the mechanism of this reaction also came from histologic examination. Mast cells in the area of the wheal and flare show evidence of release of pre-formed mediators, i.e., their cytoplasmic granules have been discharged. A causal association of IgE and mast cells with immediate hypersensitivity has been deduced from three kinds of experiments:

1. Immediate hypersensitivity reactions can be elicited in nonresponsive individuals if the local skin site is first injected with IgE from a responsive individual. *Thus, IgE is responsible for specific recognition of antigen and can be used to adoptively transfer immediate hypersensitivity.* Such adoptive transfer experiments were first performed with serum from immunized individuals in the 1920s. Some 40 years later, it was shown that the serum protein responsible for transferring this reaction was a class of antibody, which was named IgE. This serum factor was originally called "reagin," and for this reason IgE molecules are still sometimes called "reaginic antibodies."

2. *Immediate hypersensitivity reactions can be mimicked by injecting anti-IgE antibody instead of antigen.* Anti-IgE elicits a reaction both in atopic individuals who have high levels of antigen-specific IgE antibodies and in non-atopic individuals who have low but measurable levels of IgE. Anti-IgE antibodies act as an analog of antigen and directly activate mast cells and basophils which have bound IgE on their surface. This use of anti-IgE to activate mast cells is similar to the use of anti-IgM or anti-IgD antibodies as analogs of antigen to activate B cells (see Chapter 9), except that in the case of mast cells or basophils, secretory IgE, made by B cells, is attached to the cell surface by high-affinity Fc receptors rather than being synthesized as membrane IgE.

3. *Immediate hypersensitivity reactions can also be mimicked by injection of other agents that directly cause mast cell activation, such as C5a, and can be inhibited by agents that prevent mast cell activation.*

Although these classic experiments in immediate hypersensitivity were originally performed in man, immunologists often use animal models to permit greater ease of experimental manipulation. The guinea pig consistently mounts strong immediate hypersensitivity reactions and has proved to be the most useful animal model.

After many, but not all, elicited immediate hypersensitivity reactions, a second **late phase reaction** begins between 2 and 4 hours after the original challenge with antigen. At this time, the wheal and flare of the immediate hypersensitivity reaction have subsided. This late phase reaction consists of accumulation of inflammatory leukocytes, including neutrophils, eosinophils and basophils. In some respects, the late phase reaction resembles a delayed type hypersensitivity (DTH) reaction (see Chapter 12) involving sequential accumulation of polymorphonuclear leukocytes and then mononuclear cells. The inflammation is maximal by about 24 hours and then gradually subsides. Late phase reactions in atopic individuals are rich in eosinophils. Atopic individuals

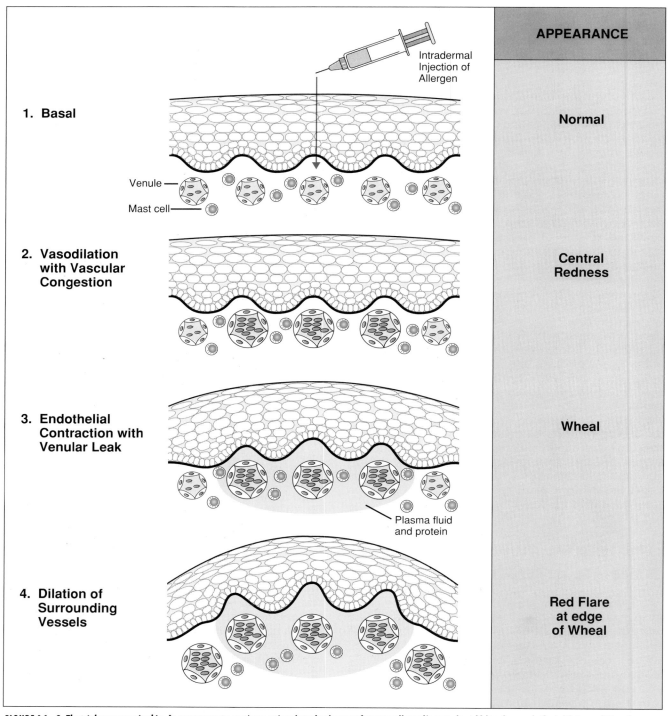

FIGURE 14–2. The triple response in skin. *In response to antigen-stimulated release of mast cell mediators, local blood vessels first dilate and then become leaky to fluid and macromolecules, producing redness and local swelling (a wheal). Subsequent dilation of vessels on the edge of the swelling produces the appearance of a red rim (the flare).*

have elevated numbers of eosinophils in their peripheral blood, and the composition of the infiltrate may simply reflect the blood count. The late phase reaction is part of immediate hypersensitivity, since, like the wheal and flare reaction, it can be adoptively transferred with IgE and can be mimicked with anti-IgE antibodies or mast cell activating agents.

A fundamental unanswered question about immediate hypersensitivity is: What physiologic function is served by this reaction? In fact, the principal consequences of IgE and mast cell–mediated reactions are pathologic and sometimes even fatal. Nevertheless, this effector mechanism of specific immunity has been conserved through evolution. It is noteworthy that many parasites elicit strong IgE responses. Based on this, it has been speculated that the primary role of

IgE-dependent mast cell activation is the expulsion of antigenic parasites by mobilizing peristalsis of the gut and constriction of the airways. The outpouring of mucus which accompanies this reaction is also thought to contribute to the clearance function. However, it is not completely established that such a reaction is protective. Recently, a mutant mouse strain has been developed that, because of a single gene mutation, has only 1 per cent of the normal number of mast cells. These mice fail to resist infection by certain tick larvae. Immunity can be provided to mast cell–deficient mice by adoptive transfer of specific IgE and mast cells together, but not by either component alone. The ticks are eradicated by inflammatory cells and not because of the wheal and flare reaction. These observations suggest that the IgE and mast cell–mediated late phase inflammatory reaction may serve a host defensive function.

BIOLOGY OF IgE

As we have noted, IgE antibody provides recognition of antigen for immediate hypersensitivity reactions. IgE is the isotype of immunoglobulin that contains the ϵ heavy chain (see Chapter 3). It circulates as a bivalent antibody and is normally present in plasma at a concentration of less than 1 μg/ml. In pathologic conditions, such as severe atopy, this level can rise to over 1000 μg/ml. The IgE heavy chain V regions and IgE light chains are derived as products of the same genes as other Ig molecules. The heavy chain C regions are encoded by the ϵ gene located in the Ig heavy chain gene cluster. Thus, IgE is produced as a result of heavy chain isotype switching (see Chapter 4).

Regulation of IgE Synthesis

There is a critical difference between atopic and normal individuals: The former produce high levels of IgE in response to particular antigens, whereas the latter generally synthesize other Ig isotypes, such as IgM and IgG, and only small amounts of IgE. Four interacting factors contribute to regulation of IgE synthesis: (1) heredity, (2) the natural history of antigen exposure, (3) the nature of the antigen, and (4) helper T cells and their cytokines.

HEREDITY

Abnormally high levels of IgE synthesis and associated atopy often run in families. Although the full inheritance pattern is probably multigenic, family studies have shown that there is clear autosomal transmission of atopy. However, the target organ of atopic disease is variable. Thus, hay fever, asthma, eczema, and food allergies can be present to various degrees in different members of the same kindred. All of these individuals, however, will show higher than average plasma IgE levels. In addition to this general proclivity to synthesize IgE, the ability to make specific IgE antibodies to certain antigens, e.g., ragweed pollen, is also inherited and may be linked to particular class II major histocompatibility complex (MHC) alleles. This may be an example of an "immune response gene" (Ir gene) effect (see Chapter 6). In the case of a complex antigen such as ragweed pollen, different class II alleles may serve to present different peptides to specific T cells.

NATURAL HISTORY OF ANTIGEN EXPOSURE

The natural history of antigen exposure is an important determinant of the level of specific IgE antibodies. In general, repeated exposure to a particular antigen is necessary to develop an atopic reaction to that antigen. Individuals with allergic rhinitis or asthma often benefit from a geographic change of residence with a change in indigenous plant pollens, although local antigens in the new residence may trigger an eventual return of the symptoms. Food allergies are often worse in early childhood, perhaps because the mucosal barrier of the gastrointestinal tract is not as mature. Clinically, this has two consequences. First, if an individual does not encounter an antigenic food until later in life, an atopic reaction is less likely to develop. Second, many individuals often "outgrow" a particular allergy. The most dramatic examples of the influence of the natural history of exposure to antigen are seen in cases of insect, e.g., bee, stings. The protein toxins in the insect venoms are usually not of concern on the first encounter because the atopic individual has no pre-existing specific IgE antibodies. However, a large IgE response may occur after a single encounter with antigen and a second sting by an insect of the same species may induce fatal anaphylaxis!

NATURE OF THE ANTIGEN

Antigens that elicit strong immediate hypersensitivity reactions are called **allergens** and are proteins or chemicals bound to proteins. It is not known why some antigens cause strong allergic responses whereas other antigens, which may be encountered by the same route of administration, are simply not allergenic and instead result in non-IgE humoral or cell-mediated immune responses. The property of being allergenic may reside in the antigen itself, perhaps in epitopes seen by certain T cells. Some drugs, such as penicillin, characteristically elicit strong IgE responses. It is thought that these drugs bind to self proteins, forming hapten-carrier conjugates that function as "neoantigens."

Some protein antigens are naturally encountered with adjuvant substances that favor IgE synthesis. For example, an antigen and an adjuvant may be present in the same parasite. The nature of the adjuvant may determine the type of antigen presenting cell (APC) that is activated or recruited and is likely to present the antigen to T cells. A particular type of APC may provide costimulators that favor the activation of helper T cells that are especially potent at stimulating IgE synthesis.

HELPER T CELLS AND CYTOKINES

Isotype switching to IgE is dependent upon helper T cells; i.e., T cell–independent antigens do not elicit IgE. Interleukin-4 (IL–4) secreted by activated helper T lymphocytes is responsible for isotype switching of B cells to IgE synthesis. Studies of mouse T cell clones have shown that only a subset of CD4[+] T cells produce IL–4. In other species, IL–4 may not be produced by a distinct subset of CD4[+] cells. Atopic individuals may contain larger numbers of allergen-specific IL–4-producing T cells than non-atopic persons. Moreover, in atopic individuals, the allergen-specific T cells may secrete more IL–4 per cell than in normal persons. Both factors probably contribute to the increased IgE production associated with atopy. T cells that produce large quantities of interferon (IFN–γ) can inhibit isotype switching to IgE because IFN–γ antagonizes the actions of IL–4.

It has recently been observed that murine mast cells also produce IL–4 in response to cross-linking of IgE bound to Fc receptors. Thus, the introduction of allergens and subsequent IgE-mediated mast cell activation may trigger a positive feedback loop that results in more IL–4 secretion and the synthesis of more IgE.

In addition to these well-characterized cytokines, there are reports of other putative T cell–derived regulatory molecules that are differentially expressed between atopic and non-atopic individuals. Some activities, more common in atopic individuals, are proposed to enhance IgE synthesis, whereas others, more common in non-atopics, serve as inhibitors. These cytokine activities can be separated from IL–4 and IFN–γ biochemically, but until their structure is elucidated and purified molecules are available, it is not possible to fully evaluate their biologic significance.

Fc Receptors for IgE

IgE, like all other antibody molecules, is exclusively made by B cells, yet IgE functions as an antigen receptor on the surface of mast cells and basophils. On these cells, IgE is bound by Fc receptors specific for ϵ heavy chains, called FcϵR. Two classes of FcϵR have been identified on different cell types. Mast cells and basophils express high-affinity receptors, called FcϵRI. The dissociation constant (K_d) of these receptors for IgE is between 1×10^{-8} M and 1×10^{-9} M. The serum concentration of IgE, although quite low compared with other Ig isotypes in normal individuals (i.e., no more than 50 μg/ml or approximately 2.5×10^{-7} M), is still sufficiently high to bind to the FcϵRI receptors. B cells, macrophages, and possibly eosinophils express various forms of a second lower-affinity receptor, called FcϵRII, which may not be occupied unless IgE levels rise.

Each FcϵRI molecule contains four separate polypeptides, one α, one β, and two identical γ chains (Fig. 14–3). As deduced from transfection experiments, all

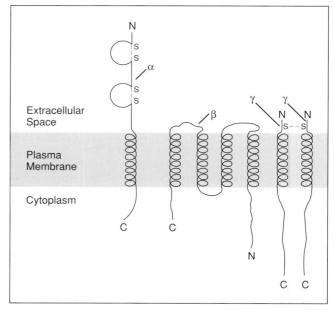

FIGURE 14–3. The polypeptide chain structure of the high-affinity IgE Fc receptor (FcϵRI). IgE binds to the Ig-like domains of the α chain. The β chain and the γ chains are thought to mediate signal transduction.

three subunits must be present to have cell surface expression. The α chain mediates binding of IgE. The predicted amino acid sequence of the α chain of the rat FcϵRI contains 222 amino acid residues, yielding a predicted size of 25 kilodaltons (kD). The 180 amino terminal residues form two extracellular 90 amino acid residue repetitive sequences that are members of the Ig gene superfamily. The IgE binding site is highly homologous to the IgG binding sites of the FcRII and FcRIII receptors described in Chapter 3. Each FcϵRI α chain has an approximately 20 amino acid residue hydrophobic sequence that is believed to cross the cell membrane once and approximately 20 carboxy terminal amino acids that are believed to form a cytoplasmic domain. The β chain of the rat FcϵRI is a 243 amino acid residue hydrophobic polypeptide whose predicted structure crosses the membrane four times. The two identical γ chain polypeptides are only 62 amino acid residues long and are highly homologous to the ζ chains of the CD3 complex (see Chapter 7). From its predicted structure, only five amino terminal amino acid residues of the γ chain are extracellular. Each γ chain crosses the membrane once, and the remaining residues are believed to be intracellular.

Although the details of FcϵRI polypeptide association are not yet known, it is proposed that the β chain serves to link the α chain to γ homodimers and that γ homodimers mediate coupling of FcϵRI to an intracellular signaling pathway. This is the same function ascribed to the CD3 ζ homodimer in T lymphocytes. In natural killer (NK) cells, FcRIII (CD16) may be associated with either a CD3 ζ or an FcϵRI γ chain, further emphasizing the potential similarities between these molecules. It is of further note that between the α, β, and γ chains, the complex has seven transmembrane helices, a motif shared by several membrane receptors known to interact with guanosine triphosphate (GTP)–binding (G) proteins, such as the β-adrenergic receptor and rhodopsin.

Less is known about the structure and function of FcεRII. The affinity of this receptor appears to vary considerably among different cell types. In addition, several monoclonal antibodies appear to distinguish FcεRII expressed on eosinophil cell lines from those on B cells. Recent molecular cloning studies of the IgE binding chain of FcεRII suggest that two polypeptides may be generated by alternative splicing of messenger RNA (mRNA) from the same gene. One product is B cell–specific and is expressed constitutively (FcεRIIa); the other product (FcεRIIb, also called CD23) is induced on B cells, monocytes, and perhaps eosinophils by IL–4. FcεRII may also exist in soluble form, where it has been postulated to interact with IgE and regulate IgE synthesis.

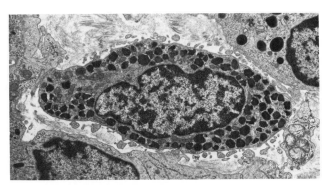

FIGURE 14–4. *Electron micrograph of a human mast cell. Note the characteristic numerous cytoplasmic granules, known to contain histamine, heparin, and various enzymes. (Courtesy of Dr. Noel Weidner, Department of Pathology, Brigham and Women's Hospital, Boston.)*

BIOLOGY OF MAST CELLS AND RELATED CELL TYPES
Mast Cells and Basophils

All mast cells are derived from progenitors present in the bone marrow. Normally, mast cells are not found in the circulation. Progenitors are believed to migrate to the peripheral tissues as immature cells and undergo differentiation *in situ*. Mature mast cells are found throughout the body, predominantly located near blood vessels, near nerves, or beneath epithelia. By light microscopy, human mast cells may be round, oval, or even spindle-shaped. The nuclei are typically round. The cytoplasm contains populations of membrane-bound granules and often lipid bodies (Fig. 14–4). The granules contain acidic proteoglycans, which bind basic dyes. Some of these dyes assume a different color when bound by the granules than they do when staining nuclear DNA, so that the granules are sometimes called "metachromatic."

A recent advance in the understanding of mast cell biology is the appreciation that in rodents mature mast cells may assume one of two phenotypes (Table 14–1). Mast cells found in the mucosa of the gastrointestinal tract have chondroitin sulfate as their major granule proteoglycan. Such "mucosal" mast cells contain little histamine. The second phenotype has

been found in the lung and in the serosa of body cavities. These "connective tissue" mast cells contain heparin as their major granule proteoglycan and produce large quantities of histamine. Mast cells may also be cultured from rodent bone marrow in the presence of IL–3 and IL–4. Such cultured mast cells resemble mucosal mast cells based on granule content of chondroitin sulfate and low histamine. Moreover, the presence of mucosal mast cells *in vivo* appears to depend upon T cells, the presumed source of IL–3 and IL–4, since they are absent in athymic mice. Bone marrow–derived mucosal mast cells can be changed to a connective tissue mast cell phenotype by co-culture with fibroblasts. Recent repopulation experiments in mast cell–deficient mice further suggest that the mucosal and connective tissue phenotypes are not fixed and that bidirectional changes may be possible in suitable microenvironments. However, it is likely that in normal development there is a maturational sequence of bone marrow precursor to mucosal type mast cell to connective tissue mast cell. The key point is that *the precise nature of the mast cell and the mediators it can produce vary with its anatomic location.*

In humans, the factors that regulate mast cell growth and development are less well defined. There appears to be a similar pattern of T cell–independent connective tissue mast cells and T cell–dependent mucosal mast cells. However, human mast cells cannot yet be cultivated from bone marrow and the cytokines that cause phenotypic change are not well defined. In addition, human mast cell phenotypes are not as clearly differentiated as those of the mouse.

TABLE 14–1. Mast Cell Heterogeneity

	Connective Tissue	Mucosal	Bone Marrow–Derived
T cell dependence	No	Yes	Yes
Histamine content	High	Low	Low
Major proteoglycan	Heparin	Chondroitin sulfate	Chondroitin sulfate
Major arachidonate metabolite	PGD_2	$LTC_4 > PGD_2$	$LTC_4 = PGD_2$

In rodents, mast cells isolated from connective tissue or gastrointestinal mucosa, or cultured from bone marrow in the presence of IL–3, differ in several properties, the most important of which are listed here.

Abbreviations: PGD_2, prostaglandin D_2; LT, leukotrienes.

Major differences between types of human mast cells reside in the composition of serine proteases found in the granule (trypsin-like or chymotrypsin-like in substrate specificity) and in the ultrastructural morphology of the granules. Nevertheless, it does appear that in humans as well as in mice the pattern of mediators produced by mast cells may vary with anatomic location.

Basophils share a number of similarities with mast cells. Like mast cells, basophils are derived from bone marrow progenitors and contain granules that bind basic dyes. Basophils are capable of synthesizing many of the same mediators as mast cells. Most significantly, both basophils and mast cells express the same high-affinity Fcε receptor (FcεRI) and can be triggered by antigen binding to IgE. Therefore, basophils, like mast cells, may mediate immediate hypersensitivity reactions to antigen. Despite these similarities, basophils appear to be a distinct cell type from the mast cell. Basophils mature in the bone marrow and circulate in their differentiated form. Like other granulocytes, basophils enter tissues only when they are recruited into inflammatory sites. Thus, basophils are best thought of as an inflammatory granulocyte, with structural and functional similarities to mast cells but derived from a different cell lineage.

Eosinophils

The inflammatory infiltrates of late phase reactions are typically rich in eosinophils. Eosinophils are bone marrow–derived granulocytes whose granules contain basic proteins that bind acidic dyes such as eosin. Indeed, the two major proteins of the eosinophil granule are called major basic protein and major cationic protein. Major basic protein is toxic for helminths, and eosinophils are the principal effector cells of antibody-dependent cell-mediated cytotoxicity (ADCC) against helminthic infections.

The increased presence of eosinophils in the blood of atopic individuals suggests that eosinophil production in the bone marrow may be under the control of the same T cells that regulate IgE synthesis. Interleukin-5 (IL–5) has been shown to be an eosinophil activating factor, converting resting eosinophils to a larger "hypodense" state that is more potent at mediating ADCC. IL–5 also appears to act as the factor that augments eosinophil production, and this is supported by the ability of anti–IL–5 antibody to inhibit the eosinophilia that occurs in mice infected with helminthic parasites. In mice, the Th2 T cell clones that produce IL–4, the IgE switching factor, also synthesize IL–5, suggesting that this subset of helper T cells regulates multiple components of the allergic response. Activated mast cells may also synthesize IL–5, more closely linking eosinophils to atopy.

As mentioned earlier, it is not currently known whether eosinophils are selectively recruited into inflammatory reactions of the late phase or whether their presence is simply reflective of increased numbers in the blood. Eosinophils, like neutrophils, bind to endothelial cells expressing endothelial leukocyte adhesion molecule–1 (ELAM–1) (see Chapter 12). Mast cell–derived cytokines, including tumor necrosis factor (TNF), can cause endothelial cells to express ELAM–1, and the recruitment of eosinophils into late phase reactions can be explained on this basis.

Activation of Mast Cells and Basophils

The event that initiates immediate hypersensitivity is the binding of antigen to IgE on the mast cell or basophil surface. Mast cells and basophils are activated by cross-linking of FcεRI molecules, which is thought to occur by binding of multivalent antigens to the attached IgE molecules (Fig. 14–5). Experimentally, antigen binding can be mimicked by polyvalent anti-IgE or by anti-FcεRI antibodies. In fact, such antibodies can activate mast cells from atopic as well as non-atopic individuals, whereas allergens activate mast cells only in atopic persons. The reason for this is that in an individual allergic to a particular antigen, a significant proportion of the IgE bound to mast cells is specific for that antigen. Administration of the antigen will cross-link sufficient IgE molecules to trigger mast cell activation. In contrast, in non-atopic individuals, the mast cell–associated IgE is specific for many different antigens (all of which may have induced low levels of IgE production). Therefore, no single antigen will cross-link enough of the IgE molecules to cause mast cell activation. Anti-IgE antibodies, on the other hand, can cross-link these IgE molecules and lead to comparable triggering of mast cells from both atopic and non-atopic individuals.

Activation of mast cells (and basophils) results in three types of biologic responses:

1. Mast cells undergo regulated secretion in which the *pre-formed contents of their granules are released by exocytosis.*
2. Mast cells enzymatically synthesize *lipid mediators* derived from precursors stored in cell membranes and, in some cases, in the lipid bodies.
3. Mast cells initiate transcription, translation, and *secretion of cytokines.* Basophils also undergo degranulation and synthesize lipid mediators; it is not yet known whether basophils synthesize cytokines.

The mechanisms of granule exocytosis are partly understood, largely from studies of rat mast cell and basophil leukemia cell lines. The cross-linking of FcεRI results in activation of a G protein that, in turn, activates a membrane-bound phospholipase C to catalyze phosphatidyl inositol bisphosphate breakdown to inositol triphosphate (IP_3) and diacylglycerol (DAG). IP_3 causes elevation of cytoplasmic calcium, and DAG activates protein kinase C. These events are similar to the processes described in Chapter 7 for T cell activation induced by cross-linking the TCR:CD3 complex. In the basophil, the activated protein kinase

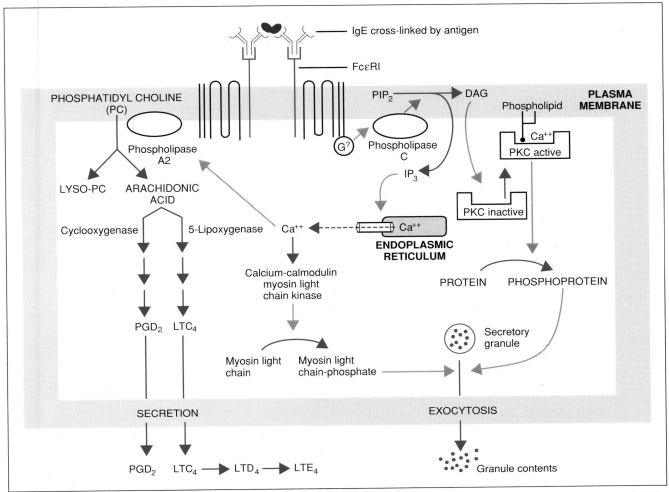

FIGURE 14-5. Biochemical events of mast cell activation. *Cross-linking of bound IgE by antigen is thought to activate a guanosine triphosphate (GTP)–binding (G) protein that in turn causes activation of a phosphatidyl inositol bisphosphate (PIP$_2$)–specific phospholipase C. This enzyme catalyzes release of inositol triphosphate (IP$_3$) and diacyl glycerol (DAG) from membrane PIP$_2$. IP$_3$ causes release of intracellular calcium (Ca^{2+}) from the endoplasmic reticulum. Ca^{2+} in the cytoplasm directly activates certain enzymes, such as phospholipase A$_2$, and, in complex with calmodulin, activates other enzymes such as myosin light chain kinase. Ca^{2+} and DAG combine with membrane phospholipids to activate protein kinase C (PKC). These intracellular events are similar to those that occur in T and B cells in response to cross-linking their antigen receptors (see Fig. 7–11). In mast cells, the result of activation is the generation of lipid mediators, such as prostaglandin D$_2$ (PGD$_2$) or leukotriene C$_4$, and the exocytosis of secretory granules.*

C phosphorylates myosin light chains. This event is thought to lead to disassembly of actin-myosin complexes beneath the plasma membrane, thus allowing fusion of the granules with the plasma membrane and resulting in exocytosis of the granule contents. The role of elevated calcium is less clear, but calcium binding to calmodulin leads to activation of myosin light chain kinase, which phosphorylates myosin light chain at distinct amino acid residues from protein kinase C.

Several other biochemical events of uncertain significance also occur. Cross-linking of FcϵRI activates the enzyme adenylate cyclase through a different G protein. This, in turn, elevates cyclic adenosine monophosphate (cAMP) levels that activate protein kinase A. Protein kinase A inhibits degranulation, suggesting that this pathway is a negative feedback loop. Two other enzyme activities are also activated.

Shortly after receptor cross-linking, membrane methyl transferases convert phosphatidyl ethanolamine to phosphatidyl choline. In addition, serine proteases of unknown substrate specificities are activated. The relationship of the activation of these enzymes to degranulation is not known. It is also not known how FcϵRI cross-linking is coupled to the activation of phospholipase A2, the enzyme that catalyzes the rate-limiting step in synthesis of lipid mediators (see below), although this enzyme may be regulated by cytoplasmic calcium.

Mast cells may be activated by mechanisms other than cross-linking FcϵRI. For example, mast cells or basophils may respond to interleukin-8 (IL-8) or other mononuclear phagocyte–derived cytokines produced as part of natural immunity (see Chapter 11), to as yet undefined T cell–derived cytokines produced as part of cell-mediated immunity (Chapter 12), and to complement-derived anaphylatoxins, such as C5a, produced during humoral immune responses (see Chapter 13). Mast cells may also be recruited into inflammatory reactions and activated by neutrophil granule contents or by neurotransmitters such as nor-epinephrine and substance P. These latter agents are potentially important as links between the nervous system and the immune system. The nervous system is known to affect the expression of immediate hypersensitivity reactions. The "flare," produced at the edge of the wheal in elicited immediate hypersensitivity reactions, is in part mediated by the nervous system, as shown by the observation that the flare is markedly diminished in skin sites lacking innervation.

MAST CELL–DERIVED AND BASOPHIL-DERIVED MEDIATORS

This section of the chapter describes the various mediators of immediate hypersensitivity released by mast cells or basophils upon activation. It should be remembered that mast cells are heterogeneous and that not all mast cells will release the same mediators or the same combinations of mediators. Nevertheless, the same general classes of mediators appear to be made by most mast cells as well as by basophils. These may be divided into **preformed mediators,** which include biogenic amines and granule macro-molecules, and **newly synthesized mediators,** which include lipid-derived mediators and cytokines.

Biogenic Amines

The granules of mast cells contain non-lipid, low molecular weight vasoactive mediators. In humans, the prototypic mediator of this class is **histamine,** but in certain rodents serotonin may be of equal or greater import. Because these substances have in common the structural features of an amine group and share common functional effects on blood vessels, they have been collectively called "biogenic" or "vasoactive" amines. Histamine acts by binding to target cell receptors, and different cell types express distinct classes of receptors (e.g., H1, H2, H3) that can be distinguished by pharmacologic inhibitors. Upon binding to cellular receptors, histamine initiates intracellular events, such as phosphatidyl inositol breakdown to IP_3 and DAG, which cause different changes in different cell types. In vascular endothelial cells, binding of histamine leads to endothelial cell retraction and paracellular leakage of plasma into the tissues. Histamine also causes endothelial cells to synthesize vascular smooth muscle cell relaxants, such as prostacyclin and nitric oxide, which cause vasodilatation. These actions of histamine produce the wheal and flare response of immediate hypersensitivity. Moreover, histamine receptor antagonists (commonly called antihistamines) can inhibit the wheal

and flare response to intradermal allergen or anti-IgE antibody.

Histamine also causes constriction of intestinal and bronchial smooth muscle. Thus, histamine may contribute to the increased peristalsis or bronchospasm associated with food allergies or asthma, respectively. However, in these instances, especially in asthma, antihistamines are not effective at blocking the reaction. Moreover, bronchoconstriction in asthma is more prolonged than the effects of histamine, which is rapidly removed from the extracellular milieu by amine specific transport systems. Thus, other mast cell–derived mediators are clearly important in some forms of immediate hypersensitivity.

Granule Proteins and Proteoglycans

In addition to vasoactive amines, mast cell granules contain several enzymes, such as serine proteases and aryl sulfatase, as well as proteoglycans such as heparin or chondroitin sulfate. The enzymes may alter the local tissue environment when released upon mast cell degranulation. One function of the negatively charged proteoglycans may be to bind and store the positively charged biogenic amines. However, it is not clear how important these substances are in immediate hypersensitivity reactions.

Lipid Mediators

Three classes of lipid mediators are synthesized by activated mast cells (Fig. 14–6). In general, these reactions are all initiated by the actions of phospholipase A_2, which releases substrates from precursor phospholipids stored in membranes or in the lipid bodies. The substrates are then converted by enzyme cascades into the ultimate mediators.

1. The first mast cell lipid mediator to be described was **prostaglandin D_2** (PGD_2). Released PGD_2 binds to receptors on smooth muscle cells and acts as a vasodilator and as a bronchoconstrictor. Moreover, PGD_2 is released from lung mast cells during asthmatic bronchoconstriction. PGD_2 is synthesized from arachidonic acid derived from phospholipid by the sequential actions of enzymes. Like other prostaglandins, PGD_2 synthesis depends upon the enzyme cyclooxygenase, and PGD_2 synthesis can be prevented by inhibitors of cyclooxygenase such as aspirin or nonsteroidal anti-inflammatory agents. Surprisingly, doses of these drugs that completely prevent PGD_2 synthesis paradoxically exacerbate asthmatic bronchoconstriction. Thus, PGD_2 is unlikely to be a key mediator of this form of immediate hypersensitivity.

2. The second class of mast cell arachidonic acid–derived mediators are the **leukotrienes.** Mast cells convert arachidonic acid, by the action of 5-lipoxygenase and other enzymes, into three main

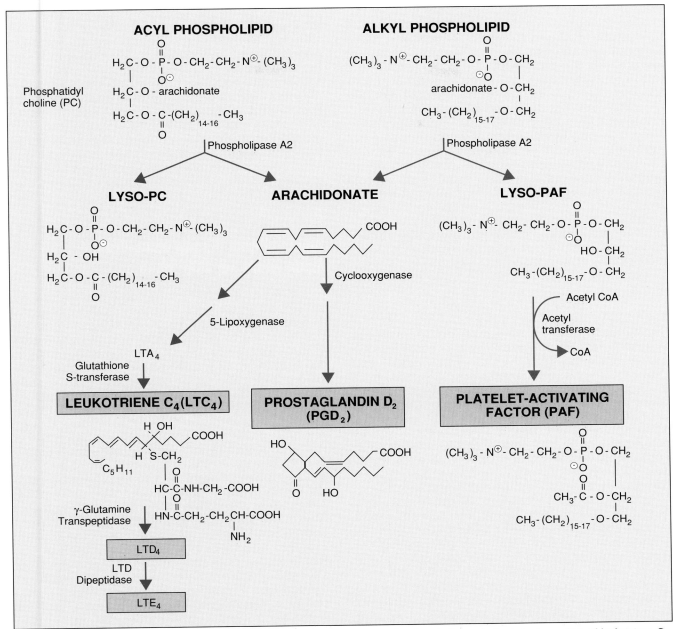

FIGURE 14-6. Biosynthesis of lipid mediators. *Breakdown of membrane phospholipids by phospholipase A₂ leads to generation of leukotriene C₄, prostaglandin D₂, and platelet-activating factor (PAF).*

leukotrienes (LT), LTC$_4$, LTD$_4$, and LTE$_4$. (Lesser amounts of LTB$_4$ may be made as well, but this leukotriene is more characteristically a product of blood phagocytes.) Mast cell–derived leukotrienes bind to specific receptors on smooth muscle cells, different from the receptors for PGD$_2$, and cause prolonged bronchoconstriction. When injected into skin, these leukotrienes produced a characteristic long-lived wheal and flare reaction. Collectively, LTC$_4$, LTD$_4$, and LTE$_4$ constitute what was once called "slow-reacting substance of anaphylaxis" (SRS–A) and are now thought to be major mediators of asthmatic bronchoconstriction. Pharmacologic inhibitors of 5-lipoxy-

genase also block anaphylactic reactions in experimental systems; as yet, there are no drugs approved for human use with this mechanism of action. The probable reason why aspirin exacerbates asthma is that PGD$_2$ and leukotriene synthesis are the two major competitive fates for arachidonic acid in mast cells, and inhibition of cyclooxygenase shunts arachidonic acid into the 5-lipoxygenase pathway, leading to increased leukotriene production.

3. The third lipid mediator produced by basophils and probably mast cells is called **platelet-activating factor** (PAF) for its original bioassay as an inducer of rabbit platelet aggregation. PAF is synthe-

sized by acylation of lysoglyceryl ether phosphoryl-choline, which is derived from a membrane phospholipid by phospholipase A_2 release of a fatty acid. (If the fatty acid is arachidonic acid, then phospholipase A_2 can generate the precursors of all three lipid mediators in one reaction.) PAF has direct bronchoconstricting actions. It also causes retraction of endothelial cells and can relax vascular smooth muscle. However, PAF is very hydrophobic and is rapidly destroyed by enzymes in plasma. It is uncertain whether mast cell–released or basophil-released PAF can reach its target cells. Nevertheless, pharmacologic inhibitors of PAF receptors do ameliorate some aspects of immediate hypersensitivity in rabbit lung. PAF may be of particular importance in late phase reactions, where it can activate inflammatory leukocytes. In this situation, the major source of PAF may be the surface of vascular endothelial cells (stimulated by histamine) rather than mast cells or basophils.

Cytokines

Within the last few years, it has been appreciated that cultured mast cells are significant sources of cytokines, including TNF, IL–1, IL–4, IL–5, IL–6, and various colony-stimulating factors (CSFs) such as IL–3 and granulocyte-monocyte colony-stimulating factor (GM–CSF). Many of these cytokines, especially IL–3, IL–4, and IL–5, were once thought to be exclusively produced by T cells. The relative contributions of mast cells versus T cells to the production of these molecules *in vivo* is not yet clear. Nevertheless, it now appears likely that cytokines, released upon IgE-mediated mast cell activation, are predominantly responsible for the late phase reaction. TNF in particular may account for sequential polymorphonuclear and mononuclear cell infiltrates by the same mechanisms described in Chapter 12 for DTH reactions. Indeed, the same sequential pattern of endothelial cell changes can be noted in the post-capillary venules in both reactions. A principal distinction between the late phase reaction of immediate hypersensitivity and the inflammatory phase of DTH is the cellular source of the cytokines as revealed by adoptive transfer: The late phase reaction is transferred by IgE and is mediated by mast cells, whereas DTH is transferred by T cells, which directly secrete the relevant cytokines.

CLINICAL ALLERGY IN HUMANS

Now that we have described the cells and mediators of immediate hypersensitivity, we can return to consideration of various allergic diseases. As we noted earlier, atopic individuals are characterized by markedly elevated levels of serum IgE. In addition, these individuals have slightly greater numbers of mast cells, more high-affinity $Fc\epsilon$ receptors on each mast cell, and a larger proportion of these receptors are occupied by IgE compared with non-atopic individuals.

Atopic individuals characteristically present with one or more manifestations of atopic disease. The most common forms of atopic disease are allergic rhinitis (hay fever), bronchial asthma, atopic dermatitis (eczema), and food allergies. The clinical and pathologic features of allergic reactions vary with the anatomic site because of several factors: (1) the point of contact with and the nature of the allergen, (2) the concentrations of mast cells in various target organs, (3) the local mast cell phenotype, and (4) the sensitiv-of target organs to mast cell-derived mediators. Furthermore, only certain kinds of antigens, including plant pollens, dust mites, and some drugs and foods, typically produce immediate hypersensitivity reactions.

Immediate Hypersensitivity Reactions in the Skin

When an allergen is introduced into the skin of a sensitized, atopic individual, the reaction that ensues is mediated largely by histamine. Histamine binds to venular endothelial cells, which express numerous histamine receptors. Most immediately, the endothelial cells synthesize and release prostacyclin, nitric oxide, and PAF. These mediators cause vascular smooth muscle cell relaxation, and the injection site becomes red from local accumulation of red blood cells. The endothelial cells also retract, allowing plasma to extravasate. The initial redness (erythema) is then replaced by soft swelling, the wheal. Finally, the blood vessels on the edge of the wheal dilate in a reaction augmented by the nervous system, producing the flare. Antihistamines can block this response almost completely. Skin mast cells appear to produce little in the way of long-acting mediators, such as leukotrienes, and the wheal and flare response typically subsides after about 15 to 20 minutes. Clinically, this reaction can occur after contact of the skin with an allergen, or after an allergen enters the circulation via the intestinal tract or by injection. The cutaneous reaction to systemic allergens, called urticaria, may persist for several hours, probably because antigen exposure is sustained.

In many atopic patients, a late phase reaction begins after about 2 to 4 hours. Tumor necrosis factor and other cytokines, probably derived from mast cells, act on the venular endothelial cells to promote inflammation, involving the production of vasodilators, adhesion molecules, IL–8, and related chemokinetic factors that facilitate leukocyte diapedesis (see Chapter 12). As may be expected for a cytokine-mediated response, the late phase inflammatory reaction is not inhibited by antihistamines. It can be blocked by pretreatment with corticosteroids which inhibit cytokine synthesis. The clinical manifestation of the late phase reaction in the skin is chronic eczema. Eczema is often treated with topical corticosteroids.

Contact sensitivity to chemicals is an immune-mediated dermatitis that resembles chronic eczema clinically. However, contact sensitivity is caused by a

T cell–mediated delayed type hypersensitivity reaction rather than IgE-dependent immediate hypersensitivity. Histologically, eosinophils are more numerous in eczema than in contact sensitivity.

Immediate Hypersensitivity Reactions in the Lung

Immediate hypersensitivity (asthmatic) reactions in the lung resemble skin reactions in some ways, but differ in others. In the lung, mast cell mediators act not only on the blood vessels but also on bronchial smooth muscle (Fig. 14–7). Bronchial asthma is characterized by paroxysms of bronchial constriction and increased production of thick mucus which leads to bronchial obstruction and exacerbates respiratory difficulties. Bronchitis and infections are frequent complications. Most cases of asthma are due to immediate hypersensitivity, and the bronchial mucosa contains increased numbers of mast cells and eosinophils. However, less frequently asthma may not be associated with atopy.

Antihistamines, as we have noted earlier, do not block the bronchial immediate response to allergen, and lung mast cells are thought to exert their effects predominantly by release of leukotrienes. Antihistamines can make asthma appear worse because these drugs often, as a side effect, cause production of thicker, more viscous mucus that can plug airways, exacerbating the breathing difficulties. As there are no drugs available that specifically block leukotriene synthesis or receptor binding, asthma is often treated by using drugs that directly relax bronchial smooth muscle, countering the target cell actions of leukotrienes. Epinephrine is the prototypic drug, and it is often administered to disrupt acute asthmatic attacks. Epinephrine acts by elevating cAMP levels in bronchial smooth muscle cells, and therapy for asthma often includes epinephrine combined with drugs such as theophylline, which block the degradation of cAMP by phosphodiesterase. Inhalant analogs of epinephrine combined with oral theophylline are often used to prevent relapse as epinephrine actions wear off. Although the major target of phosphodiesterase inhibitors is thought to be the smooth muscle cell, these drugs also raise cAMP in mast cells, inhibiting their activation. In severe asthma, corticosteroids are needed to disrupt the late phase reaction. Chronic asthma sufferers may require maintenance therapy with corticosteroids. Asthmatic attacks can be pre-

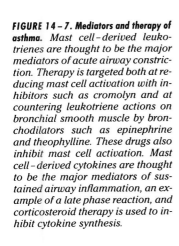

FIGURE 14–7. Mediators and therapy of asthma. *Mast cell–derived leukotrienes are thought to be the major mediators of acute airway constriction. Therapy is targeted both at reducing mast cell activation with inhibitors such as cromolyn and at countering leukotriene actions on bronchial smooth muscle by bronchodilators such as epinephrine and theophylline. These drugs also inhibit mast cell activation. Mast cell–derived cytokines are thought to be the major mediators of sustained airway inflammation, an example of a late phase reaction, and corticosteroid therapy is used to inhibit cytokine synthesis.*

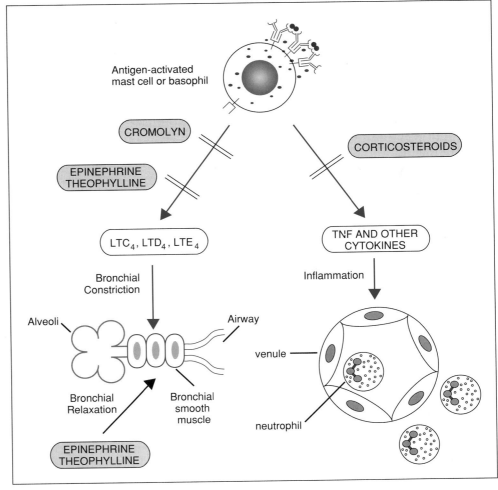

vented by inhalation of sodium cromolyn, a drug whose important action may be to render mast cells less susceptible to activation.

Systemic Immediate Hypersensitivity

In systemic immediate hypersensitivity, such as **anaphylactic shock,** vasodilatation and vascular exudation of plasma occur in vascular beds throughout the body. This usually implies the systemic presence of antigen, either by injection, insect sting, or absorption across an epithelial surface, such as the gut. The decrease in vascular tone and leakage of plasma lead to a fall in blood pressure, or shock, that may be fatal. The most important mast cell mediators of anaphylactic shock are not fully known. However, antihistamines are beneficial in anaphylaxis, suggesting a role for histamine in this reaction. In some animal models, PAF receptor antagonists also offer some protection. It is also possible that TNF is an important mediator of anaphylactic shock, much as it is in septic shock (see Chapter 11). The mainstay of treatment is systemic epinephrine, which can be life-saving, reversing the bronchoconstrictive and vasodilatory effects of the various mast cell mediators. Epinephrine also improves cardiac output, further aiding survival from threatened circulatory collapse.

Immunotherapy for Allergy

In addition to therapy aimed at the consequences of immediate hypersensitivity, clinical immunologists often try to limit the onset of allergic reactions by treatments aimed at reducing the quantity of IgE present in the individual. Despite the fact that the regulation of IgE synthesis is not fully understood, several empirical protocols have been developed to diminish specific IgE synthesis. In one approach, called **desensitization,** small but increasing quantities of antigen are administered subcutaneously over a period of hours or more gradually over weeks or months. As a result of this treatment, specific IgE levels decrease. IgG titers often rise, perhaps further inhibiting IgE production by neutralizing the antigen and by antibody feedback (see Chapter 10). However, the beneficial effects of desensitization may occur in a matter of hours, much earlier than changes in Ig levels. Although the precise mechanism is unknown, this approach has been very successful in preventing acute anaphylactic responses to protein antigens (e.g., insect venoms) or vital drugs (e.g., penicillin). It is more variable in its effectiveness for chronic atopic conditions such as hay fever.

Summary

Binding of antigen to IgE attached to mast cells or basophils leads to immediate hypersensitivity, an ef-

fector reaction mediated by mast cell or basophil released products. Immediate hypersensitivity is characterized by rapid vascular leakage of plasma, vasodilatation, bronchoconstriction, and, at later times, inflammation. In extreme cases (anaphylaxis) death may result from asphyxiation and circulatory collapse. Individuals prone to immediate hypersensitivity reactions are called atopic and have more IgE, more mast cells, and more IgE receptors per mast cell than do non-atopic individuals. IgE synthesis is regulated by heredity, exposure to antigen, and T cell products. Mast cells are derived from bone marrow and mature in the tissues. In mice, mast cells can be classified as connective tissue type, maturing under the influence of fibroblast-derived factors, and mucosal type, responding to T cell–derived cytokines such as IL–3 and IL–4. Human mast cells may also consist of distinct subsets, but these are not as well defined. Basophils are granulocytes that accumulate at inflammatory sites. They are functionally similar to mast cells but appear to be a distinct cell lineage. Eosinophils, recruited into inflammatory reactions by mast cells, are also important components of allergic reactions.

Upon binding of antigen to IgE on the surface of mast cells or basophils, the Fcε high-affinity receptor becomes cross-linked and activates intracellular second messengers. Activated mast cells and basophils produce three important classes of mediators: biogenic amines, such as histamine; lipid mediators, such as prostaglandin D_2, leukotrienes C_4, D_4, and E_4 and platelet-activating factor; and cytokines. Biogenic amines and lipid mediators produce the rapid components of immediate hypersensitivity, such as vascular leakage, vasodilatation, and bronchoconstriction. Cytokines probably mediate the late phase reaction.

Various organs show distinct forms of immediate hypersensitivity involving different mediators and target cell types. Drug therapy is aimed at inhibiting mast cell mediator production and at blocking the effects of mediators on target organs. The goal of immunotherapy is to prevent or reduce immediate hypersensitivity reactions to specific antigens.

Selected Readings

Feuerstein, G., and J. M. Hallenbeck. Prostaglandins, leukotrienes and platelet activating factor in shock. Annual Review of Pharmacology and Toxicology 27:301–313, 1987.

Gleich, G. J., and D. A. Loegring. The immunobiology of eosinophils. Annual Review of Immunology 2:429–459, 1984.

Harper, J. F. Stimulus-secretion coupling: second messenger-regulated exocytosis. Advances in Second Messenger and Phosphoprotein Research 22:193–318, 1988.

Ishizaka, K. Regulation of immunoglobulin E biosynthesis. Advances in Immunology 47:1–44, 1989.

Ishizaka, K., T. Ishizaka, and M. M. Hornbrook. Physicochemical properties of human reaginic antibody. IV. Presence of a unique immunoglobulin as a carrier of reaginic activity. Journal of Immunology 97:75–85, 1966.

Metzger, H., J.-P. Kinet, H. Blank, L. Miller, and C. Ra. The receptor with high affinity for IgE. *In* D. Chadwick, D. Evered, and J. Whelan (eds.). IgE, Mast Cells, and the Allergic Response. Ciba Foundation Symposium 147, 1989, pp. 93–101.

Plaut, M., J. H. Pierce, C. J. Watson, J. Hanley-Hyde, R. P. Nordan, and W. E. Paul. Mast cell lines produce lymphokines in response to cross-linkage of Fcε-RI or to calcium ionophores. Nature 339:64–67, 1989.

Romagnani, S. Regulation and deregulation of human IgE synthesis. Immunology Today 11:316–321, 1990.

Schwartz, L. B., and K. F. Austen. Structure and function of the chemical mediators of mast cells. Progress in Allergy 34:271–321, 1984.

Stevens, R. L., and K. F. Austen. Recent advances in the cellular and molecular biology of mast cells. Immunology Today 10:381–386, 1989.

Wershil, B. K., Y. A. Mekori, and S. J. Galli. The contribution of mast cells to immunological responses with IgE and/or T cell-mediated components. In S. J. Galli and K. F. Austen (eds.). Mast Cell and Basophil Differentiation and Function in Health and Disease. New York, Raven Press, 1989, pp. 229–246.

IMMUNITY

IN DEFENSE

AND

DISEASE

In this final section, we apply our knowledge of the fundamental mechanisms of specific immunity to understanding immunologic defenses against potential pathogens and tumors, and the principles of diseases that are caused by abnormalities in immune responses. We begin with a discussion of the role of specific immunity in combating microbial infections in Chapter 15. Chapter 16 is devoted to tissue transplantation, an increasingly promising therapy for a variety of diseases, in which the major limitation is immunologic rejection. Chapter 17 describes immune responses to tumors as well as the mechanisms by which cancer cells evade elimination by the immune system. Chapter 18 deals with diseases caused by excessive and abnormal immune responses, with an emphasis on autoimmunity and its clinical and pathologic consequences. In Chapter 19 we discuss the cellular and molecular bases of congenital and acquired immunodeficiencies, including the acquired immunodeficiency syndrome (AIDS), and the pathologic complications of deficient immunity.

CHAPTER FIFTEEN

IMMUNITY TO

MICROBES

The principal physiologic function of the immune system is to protect the host against pathogenic microbes. Resistance to infections formed the basis for the original identification of acquired immunity. As our understanding of specific immune responses has increased, we are better able to explain the mechanisms of anti-microbial immunity. Throughout this book we have mentioned examples of specific immune responses to particular microbes, largely to illustrate the physiologic relevance of various aspects of lymphocyte function. In this chapter, we discuss in more detail the main features of immunity to different types of pathogenic microorganisms.

The evolution of an infectious disease in an individual involves a sequence of interactions between the microbe and the host. These include entry of the microbe, invasion and colonization of host tissues, evasion from host immunity, and tissue injury or functional impairment. Some microbes produce disease by liberating toxins, even without extensive colonization of host tissues. Many features of microorganisms determine their virulence, and many diverse mechanisms contribute to the pathogenesis of infectious diseases. These are largely beyond the scope of this book and will not be discussed in detail. Rather, our discussion will focus on the host immune response to pathogenic microorganisms. There are several important general features of immunity to microbes:

1. *Defense against microbes is mediated by both natural and acquired immunity.* Microbial infections provide clear demonstrations of the role of specific immunity in enhancing the protective mechanisms of natural immunity and in directing these mechanisms to sites where they are needed.

2. *Different types of microbes stimulate distinct lymphocyte responses and effector mechanisms.* Because microbes differ greatly in patterns of host invasion and colonization and in their immunogenicity, their elimination requires diverse effector systems. Studies in humans and experimental models have led to reports of virtually every type of immune response to infections by different classes of microorganisms. Our subsequent discussions will attempt to highlight the principal mechanisms of specific immunity against different bacteria, viruses and parasites.

3. *The survival and pathogenicity of microbes in a host are critically influenced by their ability to evade or resist protective immunity.* Microorganisms have developed a variety of strategies for surviving in the face of powerful immunologic defenses.

4. *Tissue injury and disease consequent to infections may be caused by the host response to the microbe and its products rather than by the microbe itself.* Immunity, like many other homeostatic mechanisms, is necessary for host survival but also has the potential of causing injury to the host.

This chapter considers four types of pathogenic microorganisms: (1) extracellular bacteria, (2) intracellular bacteria, (3) viruses, and (4) parasites. In each group, selected examples will be used to highlight key points. As we shall see, these four groups of microbes illustrate the diversity of antimicrobial immunity and the physiologic significance of many of the responses and effector functions of lymphocytes discussed in earlier chapters.

IMMUNITY TO EXTRACELLULAR BACTERIA

Extracellular bacteria are capable of replicating outside host cells, e.g., in the circulation, in extracellular connective tissues, and in various tissue spaces such as the airways and intestinal lumens. These bacteria include gram-positive pus-forming, or pyogenic, cocci *(Staphylococcus, Streptococcus),* gram-negative cocci (meningococcus and gonococcus, two species of *Neisseria*), many gram-negative bacilli (including enteric organisms such as *Escherichia coli*) and some gram-positive bacilli (particularly anaerobes such as the *Clostridium* species).

Extracellular bacteria cause disease by two principal mechanisms. First, they induce inflammation, which results in tissue destruction at the site of infection. Pyogenic cocci are responsible for a large number of suppurative infections in humans. Second, many of these bacteria produce **toxins,** which have diverse pathologic effects. Such toxins may be **endotoxins,** which are components of bacterial cell walls, or **exotoxins,** which are actively secreted by the bacteria. The endotoxin of gram-negative bacteria, also called **lipopolysaccharide** (LPS), has been mentioned in earlier chapters as a potent stimulator of cytokine production, an adjuvant, and a polyclonal activator of B cells. Many exotoxins are primarily cytotoxic, and they kill cells by poorly defined mechanisms. There are also many other examples of exotoxins whose mode of action is known in precise detail. For instance, diphtheria toxin inhibits protein synthesis, by enzymatically modifying and thereby blocking the function of elongation factor–2, which is necessary for the synthesis of all polypeptides. Cholera toxin synthesis stimulates cyclic adenosine monophosphate (cAMP) production in intestinal epithelial cells, leading to active chloride secretion, water loss, and intractable diarrhea. Tetanus toxin is a neurotoxin that binds to motor end plates at neuromuscular junctions and causes persistent muscle contraction, which can be fatal if it affects the muscles involved in breathing. Clostridial toxins cause extensive tissue necrosis and lead to gas gangrene. *Immune responses against extracellular bacteria are aimed at eliminating the bacteria and at neutralizing the effects of their toxins.*

Natural Immunity to Extracellular Bacteria

Because extracellular microbes are rapidly killed by the microbicidal mechanisms of phagocytes, a principal mechanism of natural immunity to these microbes is phagocytosis by neutrophils, monocytes, and tissue macrophages. The resistance of bacteria to phagocytosis and digestion within macrophages is an important determinant of virulence. Activation of the complement system, in the absence of antibody, also plays an important role in the elimination of these bacteria. Gram-positive bacteria contain a peptidoglycan in their cell walls that activates the alternative pathway of complement by promoting the formation of the alternative pathway C3 convertase (see Chapter 13). LPS in the cell walls of gram-negative bacteria was one of the first agents shown to activate the alternative complement pathway, in the absence of antibody. LPS may provide a site for C3b deposition where the bound C3b is protected from inactivation by factors H and I. It may also directly bind C1q and activate the classical pathway of complement, without a requirement for antibody. One result of complement activation is the generation of C3b, which opsonizes bacteria and enhances phagocytosis. In addition, the membrane attack complex (MAC) lyses bacteria, and complement by-products participate in inflammatory responses by recruiting and activating leukocytes.

Endotoxins, such as LPS, stimulate the production of cytokines by macrophages and by other cells, e.g. vascular endothelium. These cytokines include tumor necrosis factor (TNF), interleukin-1 (IL–1), interleukin-6 (IL–6), and low molecular weight inflammatory cytokines, which are members of the interleukin-8 (IL–8) family. The structure and functional effects of these cytokines have been discussed in Chapter 11. The principal physiologic functions of macrophage-derived cytokines are to stimulate nonspecific inflammation and to enhance the activation of specific lymphocytes by bacterial antigens. Thus, cytokines induce the adhesion of neutrophils and monocytes to vascular endothelium at sites of infection, which is followed by migration, local accumulation, and activation of the inflammatory cells. These inflammatory cells serve to eliminate the bacteria; injury to adjacent normal tissues is a pathologic side effect of these defense mechanisms. Cytokines also induce fever and stimulate the synthesis of acute phase proteins, two responses whose physiologic roles are not well understood (see Chapter 11, Box 11–2). Many of the same cytokines function as costimulators of T and B lymphocytes, providing amplification mechanisms for specific immunity.

Large amounts of cytokines or their uncontrolled production can be harmful and are responsible for some of the clinicopathologic manifestations of infections by extracellular bacteria. The most severe cytokine-induced pathologic consequence of infection by gram-negative bacteria is progressive disseminated intravascular coagulation (DIC) and vascular collapse, also called "septic shock" or "endotoxin shock." As discussed in Chapter 11, TNF is the principal mediator of endotoxin shock.

Specific Immune Responses to Extracellular Bacteria

Humoral immunity is the principal protective specific immune response against extracellular bacteria.

Some of the most immunogenic components of the cell walls and capsules of these microbes are polysaccharides, which are prototypical thymus-independent antigens. Such antigens directly stimulate B cells, giving rise to strong specific IgM responses. In addition, other immunoglobulin (Ig) isotypes may be produced, probably as a result of the production of cytokines that promote heavy chain isotype switching (see Chapter 9). The best documented example of heavy chain class switching induced by a T cell–independent antigen is the humoral immune response to pneumococcal capsular polysaccharides in humans, which is dominated by IgG2 antibodies.

The principal T cell response to extracellular bacteria consists of CD4+ T cells responding to protein antigens in association with class II major histocompatibility complex (MHC) molecules. As discussed in Chapter 6, extracellular microbes and soluble antigens are phagocytosed by antigen presenting cells (APCs), the antigens are processed, and fragments of the processed proteins preferentially associate with class II MHC molecules. It is not known whether macrophages, B cells, or other cell types are the most important APCs for such bacterial protein antigens *in vivo.* CD4+ T cells function as helper cells to stimulate antibody production and to activate the phagocytic and microbicidal functions of macrophages.

Recently, it has been observed that some bacterial toxins stimulate large numbers of CD4+ T cells. Any one of these toxins can stimulate all the T cells in an individual that express a particular set or family of V_β T cell receptor genes. Such toxins have been called **super-antigens** (Box 15–1). Their importance lies in their ability to activate many T cells, resulting in large amounts of cytokine production and clinicopathologic abnormalities that may be similar in some respects to endotoxin shock.

Both IgM and IgG antibodies against bacterial surface antigens and toxins stimulate three types of **effector mechanisms:**

1. *IgG antibodies opsonize bacteria and enhance phagocytosis* by binding to Fcγ receptors on monocytes, macrophages, and neutrophils (see Chapter 3). Both IgM and IgG antibodies activate complement, generating C3b and iC3b, which bind to specific type 1 and type 3 complement receptors, respectively, and further promote phagocytosis. Individuals deficient in C3 are extremely susceptible to pyogenic infections.

2. *Both IgG and IgM antibodies neutralize bacterial toxins,* prevent their binding to target cells, and promote their clearance by phagocytosis. Passive immunization against tetanus toxin by injection of antibody is a potentially life-saving treatment in acute tetanus infections. IgA antibody present in various secretions, e.g., in the gastrointestinal and respiratory tracts, is important for neutralizing the toxins of bacteria in these organs and for preventing colonization of extraluminal tissues.

3. *Both IgM and IgG antibodies activate the complement system,* leading to the production of the microbicidal MAC and the liberation of by-products that

BOX 15-1. BACTERIAL 'SUPER-ANTIGENS'

Staphylococcal enterotoxins (SEs) are exotoxins produced by the gram-positive bacterium *Staphylococcus aureus,* and consist of five serologically distinct groups of proteins: SEA, SEB, SEC, SED, and SEE. These toxins are the most common cause of food poisoning in humans. A related toxin, TSST, causes a disease called the **toxic shock syndrome** (TSS), which is associated with tampon use. Pyrogenic exotoxins of streptococci, and exotoxins produced by mycoplasma may be structurally and functionally related to these enterotoxins.

The immune response to staphylococcal enterotoxins and related proteins has a number of features that make these bacterial products quite unique in terms of biologic and pathologic effects:

1. *Staphylococcal enterotoxins are among the most potent naturally occurring T cell mitogens known.* They are capable of stimulating the proliferation of normal T lymphocytes at concentrations of 10^{-9} M or less. The observed mitogenic effect of staphylococcal protein A preparations is actually due to contaminating enterotoxins. As many as one in five normal T cells in mouse lymphoid tissue or human peripheral blood may respond to a particular enterotoxin.

2. *The T cells that respond to each enterotoxin express a V_β gene from a particular V_β family in the antigen receptors.* Responsiveness is apparently not related to other components of the T cell receptor (TCR), i.e., V_α, J, or D segments. Different enterotoxins stimulate T cells expressing V_β genes from different families (see table). Because T cells expressing only certain TCRs recognize and respond to each enterotoxin, these proteins are called antigens and not polyclonal mitogens. However, since the frequency of enterotoxin-responsive T cells is much higher than the frequency of cells specific for conventional protein antigens, the enterotoxins have been named "super-antigens."

3. *Responses to staphylococcal enterotoxins require antigen-presenting cells that express class II MHC molecules.* Depletion of class II–bearing cells or addition of anti–class II antibody inhibits the T cell proliferative response to these toxins.

4. *Staphylococcal enterotoxins directly bind to class II MHC molecules on accessory cells.* This complex is then recognized by T cells expressing antigen receptors with a particular V_β. It is likely that enterotoxins do not need to be processed, like other protein antigens, before they bind to MHC molecules, and they do not associate with MHC molecules in the peptide-binding cleft. The same enterotoxin binds to class II molecules of different alleles, indicating that the polymorphism of the MHC does not influence presentation of these antigens.

The remarkably high frequency of staphylococcal enterotoxin-responding CD4+ T cells has several functional implications. Acutely, exposure to high concentrations of enterotoxins leads to systemic reactions like fever, DIC, and cardiovascular shock. These abnormalities are probably mediated by cytokines, such as TNF, produced directly by the T cells or by macrophages that are activated by the T cells. This is the likely pathogenesis of the toxic shock syndrome, which is characterized by shock, skin exfoliation, conjunctivitis, and severe gastrointestinal upset, and can progress to renal and pulmonary failure and death. More prolonged administration of enterotoxins to mice results in wasting, thymic atrophy, and profound immunodeficiency, also probably secondary to chronic high levels of cytokine, e.g., TNF, production.

Staphylococcal enterotoxins are proving to be useful tools for analyzing T lymphocyte development. Administration of SEB to neonatal mice leads to intrathymic deletion of all T cells expressing $V_\beta 3$ and $V_\beta 8$ TCR genes. This mimics the postulated self antigen–induced clonal deletion of self-reactive T cells during thymic maturation.

The concept of super-antigens may extend beyond bacterial products. Mice express polymorphic genes called *Mls* (for "minor lymphocyte stimulating" antigen) that are not linked to the MHC complex and are detected by the ability to stimulate strong mixed-lymphocyte reactions. Thus, T cells from mice expressing one *Mls* allele proliferate in response to stimulator cells expressing a different *Mls* allele, even if the two strains are identical at all MHC loci. The *Mls* gene product functions as a super-antigen, because any allelic difference stimulates virtually all T cells expressing a V_β gene from a particular V_β family. As expected, in mice expressing one *Mls* allele, all T cells whose antigen receptors contain V_β reactive with that allele are deleted during thymic development.

V_β Expression in Responding T Cells		
Enterotoxin	Mice	Humans
SEB	$V_\beta 3, 7, 8.1 - 8.3, 17$	$V_\beta 3, 12, 14, 15, 17, 20$
SEC 2	$V_\beta 3, 8.2, 10, 17$	$V_\beta 12, 13.1, 13.2, 14, 15, 17, 20$
SEE	$V_\beta 11, 15, 17$	$V_\beta 5.1, 6.1 - 6.3, 8, 18$
TSST	$V_\beta 3, 15, 17$	$V_\beta 2$

Abbreviations: SE, staphylococcal enterotoxin, TSST, toxic shock syndrome toxin.

are mediators of acute inflammation. It is likely, however, that the lytic function of the MAC is important for the elimination of only some microbes. As we mentioned in Chapter 13, deficiencies of the late components of complement, C5 to C9, which are involved in the formation of the complex, are associated with increased susceptibility to *Neisseria* but not other bacterial infections.

As mentioned earlier, acute inflammation and endotoxin shock are two of the injurious consequences

of defense against extracellular bacteria. A late complication of the humoral immune response to bacterial infections may be the generation of disease-producing antibodies. The best-defined examples are two sequelae of streptococcal infections of the throat or skin, which are manifested weeks or even months after the infections are controlled. In **rheumatic fever,** pharyngeal infection with some serologic types of β-hemolytic streptococci leads to the production of antibodies against a bacterial cell wall protein (M protein). Some of these antibodies cross-react with myocardial sarcolemmal proteins and myosin, leading to antibody deposition in the heart and subsequent inflammation (carditis). In **post-streptococcal glomerulonephritis,** infection of the skin or throat with other serotypes of β-hemolytic streptococci leads to the formation of immune complexes of bacterial antigen and specific antibody. The complexes deposit in kidney glomeruli and produce nephritis. It is worth noting that thorough antibiotic therapy is recommended for "sore throats" caused by β-hemolytic streptococci, not because of the severity of the pharyngitis but to prevent the later development of rheumatic fever.

Other bacterial infections may lead to different sequelae. The polyclonal lymphocyte activation induced by bacterial endotoxins and super-antigens may also contribute to the development of autoimmunity. Such bacterial infections may lead to the stimulation of many lymphocytes, among which are self-reactive clones that are normally anergic to stimulation by self antigens. This concept, and other possible links between infections and autoimmune diseases, are discussed more fully in Chapter 18.

Evasion of Immune Mechanisms by Extracellular Bacteria

The virulence of extracellular bacteria has been linked to a number of mechanisms that favor tissue invasion and colonization. These include adhesive properties of bacterial surface proteins, anti-phagocytic mechanisms, and inhibition of complement or inactivation of complement products. For instance, the capsules of many gram-positive and gram-negative bacteria contain one or more sialic acid residues that inhibit complement activation by the alternative pathway. Encapsulated bacteria also resist phagocytosis and, therefore, are much more virulent than homologous strains lacking a capsule.

One mechanism utilized by bacteria to evade specific immunity is *genetic variation of surface antigens.* Surface antigens of many bacteria, such as gonococci and *E. coli,* are contained in the pili, which are the structures primarily involved in bacterial adhesion to host cells. The major antigen of the pili is a protein of approximately 35 kilodaltons (kD) called pilin. The pilin genes of gonococci consist of one or two expression loci. In addition, there are ten to 20 silent loci, each containing six coding sequences, called "minicassettes." Antigenic variation results from a high rate of conversion between silent and expression loci. A gene conversion event replaces the minicassette on the expression locus with a duplicate of one of the minicassettes from one of the silent loci (Fig. 15-1). From ten silent loci, each with six minicassettes, it is possible to create 10^6 combinations whose protein products are antigenically distinct. This mechanism helps the bacteria to escape specific antibody attack, although its principal significance for the bacteria may be to select for pili that are more adherent for host cells so that the bacteria are more virulent.

IMMUNITY TO INTRACELLULAR BACTERIA

A number of bacteria, and all viruses, survive and replicate within host cells. Among the bacteria, some of the most pathogenic are ones that are resistant to degradation in macrophages and are therefore capable of surviving within phagocytes. Two of the best known examples are mycobacteria and *Listeria monocytogenes.* Since these microbes are able to find a niche where they are inaccessible to circulating antibodies, their elimination requires immune mechanisms that are very different from the mechanisms of defense against extracellular bacteria. Many fungi are also capable of surviving within host cells, and defense against them is mediated by mechanisms similar to those against intracellular bacteria.

Natural Immunity to Intracellular Bacteria

The principal mechanism of natural immunity against intracellular microbes is phagocytosis. However, pathogenic intracellular bacteria are relatively resistant to degradation within mononuclear phagocytes. It is, therefore, not surprising that usually *natural immunity is quite ineffective in controlling colonization by and spread of these microorganisms.* Resistance to phagocytosis is also the reason why such bacteria tend to cause chronic infections that may last for years, often recur or recrudesce after apparent cures, and are difficult to eradicate.

Specific Immune Responses to Intracellular Bacteria

The major protective immune response against intracellular bacteria is cell-mediated immunity. Cell-mediated immunity was first identified by George Mackaness in the 1950s as protection against the intracellular bacterium *L. monocytogenes.* This form of immunity could be adoptively transferred to naive animals with lymphoid cells but not with serum from infected or immunized animals. We now know that the specificity of cell-mediated immunity is due to T lymphocytes, but the effector function of bacterial elimination is mediated by macrophages that are activated by T cell–derived cytokines, particularly γ-interferon (IFN-γ) (Fig. 15-2). The immune response to such bacteria is analogous to delayed type hypersensitivity (DTH) reactions to soluble protein antigens (see Chapter 12).

PILIN GENES	PHENOTYPE

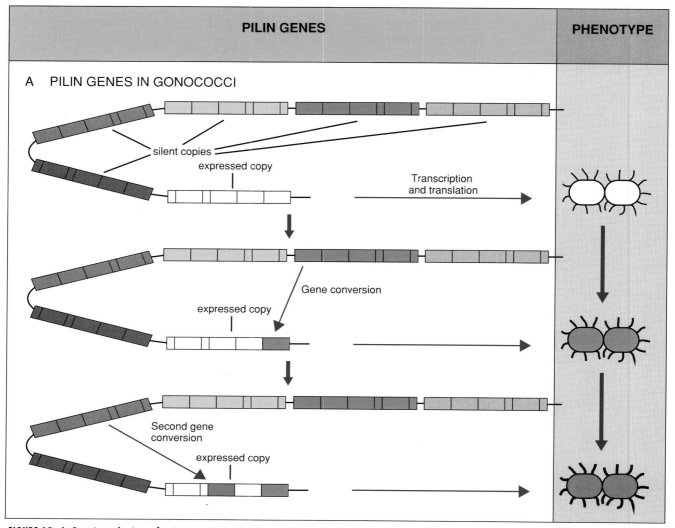

FIGURE 15–1. Genetic mechanisms of antigenic variation in microorganisms.
A. *In gonococci, a segment of the expressed pilin gene may be replaced by nucleotides from a DNA segment ("minicassette") in a silent pilin gene by a process of gene conversion, generating a new pilin gene and expressed protein. (Sizes of DNA segments are not to scale, and only five silent copies of the pilin gene are shown.)*

The protein antigens of intracellular bacteria stimulate strong T cell responses. Many such microbes contain cell wall constituents that activate macrophages directly and therefore function as adjuvants. An example of such an adjuvant is muramyl dipeptide, present in the cell walls of mycobacteria. Adoptive transfer experiments have shown that both CD4+ and CD8+ T cells contribute to protective immunity against intracellular bacteria. These T cell subsets may recognize and respond to different types of antigens. For instance, in mycobacterial infections, antigens such as the purified protein derivative (PPD) stimulate CD4+ T cells and these cells mediate DTH reactions to skin challenge with PPD in previously infected persons. CD8+ T cells may recognize bacterial antigens that are produced in infected cells. The relative contribution of CD4+ and CD8+ T cells to immunity against different intracellular bacteria is not known. However, the principal function of both T cell subsets in cell-mediated immunity is the production

of cytokines, particularly IFN-γ.

The consequence of IFN-γ production by specific T cells is the activation of macrophages, including ones that are infected. IFN-γ stimulates phagocytic and degradative functions of macrophages, leading to enhanced bacterial killing. As a result of macrophage activation, the number of viable bacteria may be drastically reduced and often completely eradicated. However, intracellular microbes have evolved to resist phagocytes and often persist for long periods, even in individuals with effective cell-mediated immunity. Persistent organisms provide chronic antigenic stimulation. This may lead to local collections of activated macrophages, called **granulomas** (Chapter 12, Fig. 12–6), surrounding the microbes and preventing their spread. The histologic hallmark of many mycobacterial and fungal infections is granulomatous inflammation. This type of inflammation is associated with tissue necrosis and extensive fibrosis, leading to severe functional impairment. *Thus, the host immune*

VARIABLE SURFACE GLYCOPROTEIN (VSG) GENES	PHENOTYPE

B   VSG GENES IN TRYPANOSOMES

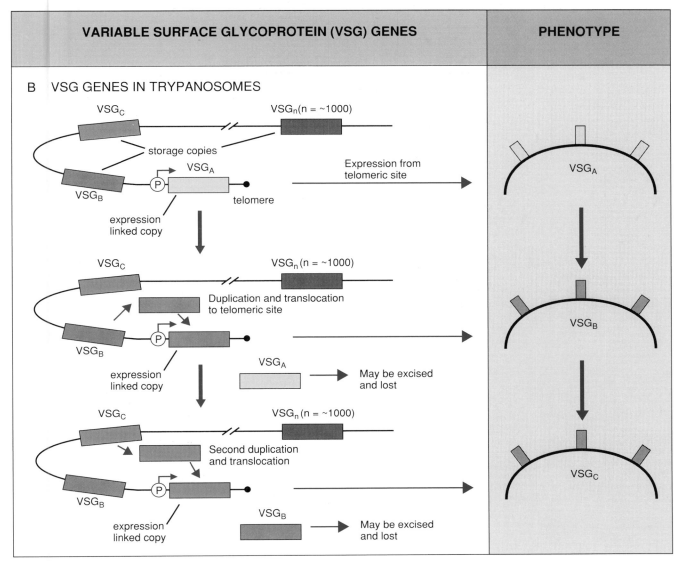

FIGURE 15 – 1. *Continued*

B. *In trypanosomes, the expressed variable surface glycoprotein (VSG) is encoded by a gene located close to the telomere. Another VSG gene may be duplicated and translocated to this telomeric expression site, generating a new VSG. The fate of the previously expressed VSG gene is not known, but it may be excised and lost (as shown).* (P), *promoter.*

response is the principal cause of tissue injury and disease in infections by some intracellular bacteria. This is most clearly illustrated in mycobacterial infections. Mycobacteria do not produce any known toxins or enzymes that directly injure infected tissues. The first exposure to *Mycobacterium tuberculosis* induces a local cellular inflammation, and the bacteria initially proliferate within phagocytes. They may then die or lie dormant. At the same time, the infected individual develops specific T cell immunity. After immunity has developed, severe granulomatous reactions can occur at sites of bacterial persistence or upon subsequent exposures to the bacteria. Thus, both protective immunity and the hypersensitivity reaction that produces tissue injury are manifestations of the same type of specific immune response.

Differences among individuals in the patterns of im- *mune responses to intracellular microbes are important determinants of disease progression and clinical outcome.* An example of this is leprosy, caused by *Mycobacterium leprae*. There are two polar forms of the disease, although many patients fall in less clear intermediate groups. In lepromatous leprosy, patients have high specific antibody titers but weak cell-mediated responses to *M. leprae* antigens. Mycobacteria proliferate within macrophages, presumably because of poor cell-mediated immunity. The bacterial growth and macrophage activation result in destructive lesions of skin and underlying bones. In contrast, patients with tuberculoid leprosy have strong cell-mediated immunity but low antibody levels. This pattern of immunity is reflected in granulomas that form around nerves, giving rise to sensory peripheral nerve defects and secondary traumatic skin lesions. Such

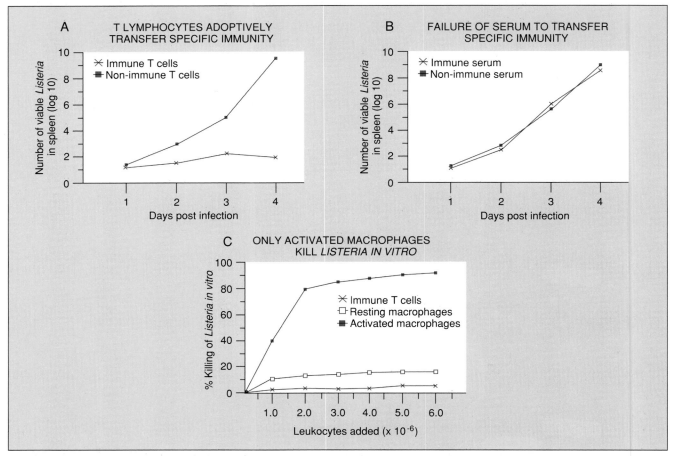

FIGURE 15 – 2. Cell-mediated immunity to Listeria monocytogenes. *Immunity to* L. monocytogenes *is measured by inhibition of bacterial growth in the spleens of animals inoculated with a known dose of viable bacteria. Such immunity can be transferred to normal mice by T lymphocytes* (A) *but not by serum* (B) *from syngeneic mice previously immunized with killed* Listeria monocytogenes. *However, the actual killing of bacteria in* vitro *is mediated by activated macrophages and not by T cells, even from immune animals* (C).

differences suggest that in different individuals *M. leprae* stimulates the production of cytokines that either selectively help B cells or activate macrophages. This may be due to varying levels of T cell activation, or differential expansion of distinct T cell subsets that may be analogous to the Th1 and Th2 clones described in mice (mentioned in Chapters 9 and 10). In fact, T cells from patients with lepromatous leprosy produce less IL – 2 and IFN – γ in response to *M. leprae* than cells from tuberculoid leprosy patients. Furthermore, intradermal injection of IFN – γ has a beneficial effect on the skin lesions of lepromatous leprosy.

Several recent studies have shown that mycobacteria activate T cells bearing the $\gamma\delta$ form of the T cell receptor (TCR). Mice infected with *M. tuberculosis* show increased numbers of $\gamma\delta^+$ cells in draining lymph nodes. If peripheral blood lymphocytes are stimulated by *M. tuberculosis*–infected macrophages, $\gamma\delta$-expressing T cells are preferentially expanded. Furthermore, molecular cloning of mycobacterial antigens has shown that some of the immunodominant antigens are homologous to **heat shock proteins,** which are also known to activate $\gamma\delta$ T cells. Heat shock proteins are evolutionarily conserved molecules

found in many prokaryotes and eukaryotes. They are induced upon exposure to different types of stress, including heat, contact with free radicals, and deprivation of oxygen, nutrients, or essential ions. Intracellular bacteria are exposed to anoxia and free radicals within phagocytes and to fever associated with infection. All these stimuli could lead to the production of heat shock proteins by the bacteria and, perhaps, by infected host cells as well. It has been postulated that the reaction of $\gamma\delta$-bearing T cells to heat shock proteins is an example of a primitive and rather nonspecific mechanism of defense against some microbes and their protein products. However, at present we do not know the significance of this rare T cell subset in immunity to mycobacteria and other intracellular microbes.

Evasion of Immune Mechanisms by Intracellular Bacteria

An important mechanism for survival of intracellular bacteria is their ability to resist elimination by phago-

cytes. Mycobacteria do this by inhibiting phagolysosome fusion, perhaps by interfering with lysosome movement. The phenolic glycolipid of *M. leprae* functions as a scavenger of reactive oxygen species. Virulent strains of *L. monocytogenes* produce a protein called hemolysin, which promotes intracellular bacterial survival, probably by forming pores in the phagosome membrane, thereby releasing bacteria into the cytoplasm and preventing their degradation in phagolysosomes. (Hemolysin may also block antigen processing by macrophages and reduce the specific T cell response.) *Legionella pneumophila* is an intracellular bacterium that is the causative organism of Legionnaire's disease. Mutants of these bacteria that lose their ability to inhibit phagolysosome fusion also lose their virulence.

IMMUNITY TO VIRUSES

Viruses are obligatory intracellular microorganisms that replicate within cells, often using the nucleic acid and protein synthetic machineries of the host. Many viruses enter host cells by binding to physiologically important, normal cell surface molecules. Three well-known examples are (1) human immunodeficiency virus–1 (HIV–1), which binds to the CD4 molecule on human T cells; (2) Epstein-Barr virus (EBV), which binds to the type 2 complement receptor on human B cells; and (3) rhinovirus, the agent of the common cold, which binds to intercellular adhesion molecule (ICAM–1) expressed on a variety of cell types, including airway epithelium.

After entering cells, viruses can cause tissue injury and disease by any of several mechanisms. Viral replication interferes with normal cellular protein synthesis and function, leading to injury to and ultimately death of the infected cell. This is one type of **cytopathic effect of viruses,** and the infection is said to be "lytic" because the infected cell is lysed. Noncytopathic viruses may cause latent infections, during which they reside in host cells and produce proteins that are foreign to the host and stimulate specific immunity. As a result, infected cells are recognized and killed by viral antigen-specific cytolytic T lymphocytes (CTLs). Released viral proteins may also stimulate DTH reactions. *In these situations, cell injury is a direct consequence of physiologic immune responses to the virus.* Relatively little is known about the pathogenic mechanisms in many other viral infections, e.g., slow virus–induced demyelination and hepatitis virus–induced liver injury. Human immunodeficiency virus is discussed in Chapter 19.

Protective immunity against viruses operates at two stages: in the *initial phase of infection*, before a virus has invaded host cells, and *after invasion into cells*, when the virus is inaccessible to antibodies and phagocytes. Furthermore, because different viruses can infect a wide variety of cell types, anti-viral immunity must be capable of acting on diverse populations of infected cells.

Natural Immunity to Viruses

There are two principal mechanisms of natural immunity against viruses:

1. *Viral infection directly stimulates the production of type I IFN by infected cells.* Type I IFN functions to inhibit viral replication. The characteristics of the cytokine-induced "anti-viral state" have been described in Chapter 11.

2. *Natural killer (NK) cells lyse a wide variety of virally infected cells.* NK cells may be one of the principal mechanisms of immunity against viruses early in the course of infection, before specific immune responses have developed (see Chapter 12). Type I IFN can enhance the ability of NK cells to lyse infected target cells.

In addition, complement activation and phagocytosis serve to eliminate viruses from extracellular sites and from the circulation.

Specific Immune Responses to Viruses

Immunity against viral infections is mediated by a combination of humoral and cellular immune mechanisms. *Specific antibodies are important in defense against viruses early in the course of infection.* Neutralizing anti-viral antibodies bind to envelope or capsid proteins and prevent viral attachment and entry into host cells. Opsonizing antibodies may enhance phagocytic clearance of viral particles. Somewhat perversely, however, opsonizing antibodies may actually enhance the invasion of Fc receptor–bearing cells by viruses; this has been postulated to be a mechanism for HIV–1 infection of mononuclear phagocytes. Secretory immunoglobulins of the IgA isotype may be important for neutralizing viruses that enter via the respiratory or intestinal tract. Induction of secretory immunity is one of the bases for oral immunization against poliomyelitis. Complement activation may also participate in antibody-mediated viral immunity, mainly by promoting phagocytosis and possibly by direct lysis of viruses with lipid envelopes.

The success of prophylactic vaccination with attenuated or killed viruses is largely related to the ability of these vaccines to stimulate specific antibody responses. The importance of humoral immunity is suggested by the observation that resistance to a particular virus, induced either by infection or vaccination, is often specific for the serologic type of the virus and seems to correlate with antibody specificity. An example of this is influenza virus, in which exposure to one serologic type does not confer resistance to other serotypes of the virus. However, several points about the role of humoral immunity in protection against viruses should be emphasized. First, antibodies are of protective value only in the early phase of viral infection, before the microorganism has gained a foothold in its sequestered location inside host cells.

Second, it has generally proved difficult to transfer anti-viral immunity to naive animals with purified antibodies. Third, the neutralizing capacity of an antibody *in vitro* usually shows little or no correlation with its protective capacity *in vivo*. Taken together, these observations suggest that antibodies are an important component of immunity to viruses but may not be sufficient for eliminating many viral infections.

The principal mechanism of specific immunity against established viral infections is CTLs. The best-defined virus-specific CTLs are CD8[+] cells that recognize endogenously synthesized viral antigens in association with class I MHC molecules on virtually any cell type. A smaller but detectable proportion of virus-specific CTLs in humans and mice consists of CD4[+] CTLs that recognize viral antigens presented in association with class II MHC molecules. CD4[+] CTLs can be effective only against infected cells that express class II molecules, whereas CD8[+] CTLs have a much broader range of cellular reactivity. The full differentiation of CD8[+] CTLs requires cytokines produced by CD4[+] helper cells, which recognize endogenously synthesized or shed viral antigens in association with class II molecules. As discussed in Chapter 12, the anti-viral effects of CTLs are due to lysis of infected cells, stimulation of intracellular enzymes that degrade viral genomes, and secretion of cytokines with interferon activity.

The importance of CTLs in the outcome of viral infections has been demonstrated in many experimental systems. Mice can be protected against influenza virus by adoptive transfer of virus-specific, class I–restricted CTLs and by cloned lines of such T cells. Interestingly, a large proportion of influenza-specific CTLs are not serotype-specific because they recognize peptides derived from internal proteins (like matrix protein and nucleoprotein) rather than the envelope proteins (hemagglutinin, neuraminidase) that determine serotype. Nevertheless, as mentioned above, actively acquired immunity to influenza virus is serotype-specific. These findings support the view that both antibodies and CTLs cooperate to protect the host against viruses — the former act to block viral binding and entry into host cells, and the latter inhibit viral replication in infected cells.

In some infections with non-cytopathic viruses, CTLs may be responsible for tissue injury. The best example is lymphocytic choriomeningitis virus (LCMV), which induces inflammation of the spinal cord meninges in mice. LCMV infects meningeal cells but does not injure them. It stimulates the development of specific CTLs that lyse meningeal cells during a physiologic attempt to eradicate the viral infection. T cell–deficient mice infected with LCMV become chronic carriers of the virus but pathologic lesions do not develop, whereas in normal mice meningitis develops. On face value, this observation appears to contradict the usual situation, in which immunodeficient individuals are more susceptible to infectious diseases than normal individuals. Hepatitis B virus infection in humans shows some similarities to murine LCMV, in that immunodeficient persons who become infected do not develop the disease, but become carriers who can transmit the infection to otherwise healthy persons. The livers of patients with acute hepatitis contain large numbers of CD8[+] T cells, but the antigenic specificity and MHC restriction of these cells have not been defined.

Viral infections, and immune responses to them, may be involved in producing disease in two other ways. First, a consequence of persistent infection with some viruses, such as hepatitis B, is the formation of circulating immune complexes composed of viral antigens and specific antibodies. These complexes deposit in blood vessels and lead to widespread, destructive vasculitis (see Chapter 18). Second, some viruses are known to contain amino-acid sequences that are also present in some self antigens. It has been postulated that because of this "molecular mimicry" anti-viral immunity can lead to immune responses against self antigens.

Evasion of Immune Mechanisms by Viruses

The intracellular persistence of viruses is the most obvious mechanism by which they can be hidden from immune effector cells and molecules. Viruses have evolved other mechanisms for evading host immunity:

1. *Many viruses are capable of great antigenic variation,* and large numbers of serologically distinct strains of these viruses have been identified. The influenza pandemics that occurred in 1918, 1957, and 1968 were all due to different strains of the virus, and subtler variants arise more frequently. As a result, the virus becomes insusceptible to immunity generated in the population by previous infections. There are so many existing serotypes of rhinovirus that specific immunization against the common cold may not be a feasible preventive strategy. In these situations, prophylactic vaccination may have to be directed against invariant viral proteins, such as surface molecules that mediate virus binding and entry into host cells.

2. *Viruses suppress immune responses by various mechanisms.* Some viruses may infect the cells of the immune system, impairing their function and resulting in inhibition of specific immunity. The most obvious example of this is, of course, HIV–1–induced acquired immunodeficiency syndrome (AIDS). Immune suppression has been described in infections with retroviruses, Epstein-Barr virus (EBV), and numerous others, but the mechanisms are not well defined. One intriguing possibility has been suggested by the recent observation that an EBV gene is homologous to a mammalian gene that encodes a cytokine called "cytokine synthesis inhibitory factor" or "CSIF." CSIF inhibits the production of other cytokines, including IL–2 and IFN–γ. Thus, pathogenic viruses may contain or may have acquired genes whose products inhibit antiviral immune responses.

IMMUNITY TO PARASITES

In infectious disease terminology, "parasitic infection" refers to infection with animal parasites, such as protozoa, helminths, and ectoparasites (e.g., ticks and mites). Such parasites currently account for greater morbidity and mortality than any other class of infectious organisms, particularly in developing countries. It is estimated that about 30 per cent of the world's population suffers from parasitic infestations. Malaria alone affects almost 300 million people worldwide, with about 1 million deaths annually. The magnitude of this public health problem is the principal reason for the great interest in immunity to parasites and for the development of immunoparasitology as a distinct branch of immunology.

Most parasites go through a complex life cycle, part of which is in humans (or other vertebrates) and part is in intermediate hosts such as flies, ticks, and snails. Humans are infected usually by bites from infected intermediate hosts or by sharing a particular habitat with an intermediate host. For instance, malaria and trypanosomiasis are transmitted by insect bites and schistosomiasis is transmitted by exposure to water in which infected snails reside.

A fundamental feature of most parasitic infections is their chronicity. There are many reasons for this, including weak natural immunity and the ability of parasites to evade or resist elimination by specific immune responses. Furthermore, many anti-parasite antibiotics are toxic and/or relatively ineffective. Individuals living in endemic areas require repeated chemotherapy because of continued exposure, and this is often not possible because of expense and logistical problems. Because of these reasons, attempts to develop prophylactic vaccines for parasites have long been considered an area of great priority for developing countries. The persistence of parasites in human hosts also leads to immunologic reactions that are chronic and may result in pathologic tissue injury as well as abnormalities in immune regulation. Therefore, some of the clinicopathologic consequences of parasitic infestations are due to the host response and not the infection itself.

Natural Immunity to Parasites

Protozoan and helminthic parasites that enter the blood stream or tissues are often able to survive and replicate because they are well adapted to resisting natural host defenses. The invertebrate stages of many parasites, which are recovered from the non-human intermediate hosts, activate the alternative pathway of complement and are lysed by the MAC. However, parasites recovered from the vertebrate, e.g., human, host are usually resistant to lysis by complement. This may be due to many reasons, including loss of surface molecules that bind complement or the acquisition of host regulatory proteins such as decay accelerating factor (DAF). Macrophages can phagocytose protozoa, but many pathogenic organisms are resistant to phagocytic killing and may even replicate within macrophages. The tegument of helminthic parasites makes them resistant to the cytocidal mechanisms of both neutrophils and macrophages.

Specific Immune Responses to Parasites

Different protozoa and helminths vary greatly in their structural and biochemical properties. It is, therefore, not surprising that different parasites elicit quite distinct specific immune responses, which are also different from the responses to bacteria and viruses. Although virtually every type of response to parasites has been reported, the major patterns of specific immunity to protozoa and helminths are the following:

1. *Production of specific IgE antibody and eosinophilia are frequently observed in helminthic infections.* Helminths such as *Nippostrongylus*, filaria, and schistosomes induce higher levels of IgE than any other infectious organisms. These responses are attributed to the propensity of helminths to stimulate specific CD4+ helper T cells that secrete IL-4 and IL-5. Such helper T cells resemble the Th2 clones identified in mice that were mentioned in Chapter 9. The chronic antigenic stimulation caused by parasites may be especially effective at inducing the differentiation of T cells to functionally distinct subsets such as Th1 and Th2 cells. In mice infected with *Nippostrongylus brasiliensis* or *Schistosoma mansoni*, the elevation in serum IgE is blocked by injection of a neutralizing antibody specific for IL-4 and eosinophilia is inhibited by anti-IL-5 antibody. *In vitro* experiments suggest that IgE antibody-dependent cytotoxicity mediated by eosinophils may be particularly effective at resisting helminthic infections, because the major basic protein of eosinophil granules may be more toxic for helminths than the proteolytic enzymes and reactive oxygen species produced by neutrophils and macrophages. Thus, IgE antibody binds to helminths, eosinophils attach to these opsonized organisms by Fc receptors specific for IgE, the eosinophils are activated and secrete their granule contents, and the major basic protein lyses the parasites. Other antibodies and effector cells may also participate in host defense. Activated macrophages directly kill schistosome larvae through the action of nitrogen oxides and TNF. In rats, immunity to schistosomiasis can be passively transferred with IgG2 antibodies from infected animals. Such antibodies may activate the complement system or may opsonize parasites for phagocytosis or killing by activated macrophages and neutrophils.

2. *Some parasites and their products induce granulomatous responses with concomitant fibrosis. S. mansoni* eggs deposited in the liver stimulate CD4+ T cells, which in turn activate macrophages as in DTH reactions. This results in the formation of granulomas around the eggs. The granulomas serve to contain the

schistosome eggs, but severe fibrosis associated with this chronic cell-mediated immune response leads to disruption of venous blood flow in the liver, portal hypertension, and cirrhosis. In lymphatic filariasis, the parasites lodge in lymphatic vessels, leading to chronic cell-mediated immune reactions without granulomatous inflammation and ultimately to fibrosis. This results in lymphatic obstruction and severe, chronic lymphedema.

3. *CD4$^+$ helper T cells and cytokines may be involved in the resolution and exacerbation of some parasitic infections.* Perhaps the best documented example of this is *Leishmania major* infection in mice. Resistance to the infection is associated with the production of IFN-γ and TNF by CD4$^+$ T cells, whereas exacerbation of lesions is associated with high levels of IL-4. Inbred strains of mice that are susceptible to fatal leishmaniasis produce more IL-4 in response to the infection than resistant strains, and the injection of anti-IL-4 antibody induces resistance in the susceptible strains. In contrast, resistant strains produce higher amounts of IFN-γ and TNF and antibodies against these cytokines make the mice susceptible to the infection. IFN-γ and TNF presumably activate macrophages and enhance intracellular killing of leishmania. High levels of IL-4 may inhibit activation of macrophages by TNF and IFN-γ, and may block the production of cytokines, such as TNF, by the macrophages. In other parasitic infections, TNF may actually contribute to the pathology and clinical symptoms. For instance, fatal cerebral malaria in mice can be prevented by anti-TNF antibody and TNF production is associated with the cachexia seen in African trypanosomiasis. Such observations indicate that different parasites may stimulate unique patterns of specific T cell activation and cytokine production. Attempts to alter the outcome of these infections in experimental animals with cytokines or cytokine antagonists are going on in many laboratories at present.

4. *Protozoa that replicate inside cells may stimulate specific CTLs.* The CTL response to malaria is an important defense against the spread of this intracellular protozoon (Box 15-2). The poor efficacy of vaccination with malarial antigens is attributed to the inability of such immunizations to stimulate CTLs.

Chronic and persistent parasitic infestations are often associated with the formation of complexes of parasite antigens and specific antibodies. The complexes can deposit in blood vessels and kidney glomeruli, producing vasculitis and nephritis, respectively (see Chapter 18). Immune complex disease has been described in schistosomiasis and malaria. Malaria infections and African trypanosomiasis are also

---

BOX 15-2.   IMMUNITY TO MALARIA

Malaria is an example of a parasitic disease that illustrates many fundamental concepts of anti-parasite immunity. The life cycle of the protozoan malaria parasite (*Plasmodium*) is well known. Infection is initiated by the bite of an infected mosquito, resulting in the inoculation of hundreds of sporozoites. Most of the sporozoites are cleared from the circulation by phagocytes in the liver and spleen. Some enter liver cells, where they develop by schizogony for about a week. Thousands of merozoites are then released. They invade red blood cells, and this stage is responsible for the clinical manifestations of all forms of malaria. Sexual stage gametocytes develop in red blood cells, are taken up by mosquitoes during a blood meal, and fertilize and develop in the mosquito. Immature sporozoites develop in 2 to 3 weeks and travel to the salivary glands, where they mature. The clinical features of malaria caused by the four common species of *Plasmodium* are fever spikes, anemia, and, in severe cases, ischemic damage to the brain and kidneys caused by hemolysis and capillary obstruction by parasitized red blood cells. Cytokines, such as TNF, may mediate the vascular lesions of cerebral malaria.

Immunity to malaria is stage-specific; i.e., immunization with sporozoites protects against sporozoite challenge but not against the blood stage of infection. Numerous immune mechanisms may participate in host defense against malarial infections. Mature sporozoites have a 44 kD coat protein called the circumsporozoite (CS) protein that has been a major focus of investigations of protective immunity. The CS protein is the immunodominant B cell antigen of sporozoites and the principal target of neutralizing antibodies. Most of these antibodies are specific for a central region of the CS protein that is composed of multiple repeats whose precise structure varies in different species. In *Plasmodium falciparum*, the central core of the CS protein contains about 40 tandem repeats of the sequence Asn-Ala-Asn-Pro (NANP). Antibodies against the CS protein or against (NANP)n offer partial protection of mice against challenge with small numbers (up to 500) of sporozoites. This is at least tenfold less than the protection induced by immunization with irradiated sporozoites. Based on these observations, it has been postulated that antibodies alone are insufficient and T cells also play an important role in specific anti-malarial immunity.

Recent experiments have shown that in mice resistance to sporozoite challenge can be adoptively transferred to naive animals with T cells from immunized donors. Furthermore, if mice vaccinated with irradiated sporozoites are depleted of CD8$^+$ cells by the injection of anti-CD8 antibody, they lose their acquired resistance. Depletion of CD4$^+$ T cells does not have the same effect. These results suggest that CD8$^+$ CTLs may be the principal mechanism of protective immunity against the extra-erythrocytic, e.g., sporozoite, stages of the parasite. The protective effect of CD8$^+$ T cells appears to be TNF- and IFN-γ-dependent, so that cytokine production rather than cytolysis may be the critical effector function of these cells. Both TNF and IFN-γ inhibit replication of parasites within hepatocytes, but the mechanism is unknown. It also appears that the major T cell epitopes of the CS protein of *P. falciparum* lie outside the (NANP)n regions. Furthermore, the T cell epitopes correspond to the most variable residues of the CS protein. This suggests that variation or polymorphism of the antigens of the surface coat may have arisen as a result of selection pressures imposed by specific T cell responses. Immunity against blood-stage forms is mediated primarily by CD4$^+$ T cells.

associated with the production of autoantibodies reactive with many self tissues. The myocarditis and neuropathy seen in Chagas' disease, which is caused by *Trypanosoma cruzi*, are probably autoimmune reactions because few or no parasites are present even in active lesions. Autoantibody production may also be secondary to polyclonal lymphocyte stimulation by the parasites (see Chapter 18). In contrast, in many cases of malaria and African trypanosomiasis, there is a severe and generalized suppression of the immune system. This may be secondary to the production of immunosuppressive cytokines by activated macrophages and/or T cells.

Evasion of Immune Mechanisms by Parasites

The ability of parasites to survive in vertebrate hosts reflects evolutionary adaptations that permit these organisms to evade or resist immune effector mechanisms. Different parasites have developed remarkably effective ways of resisting specific immunity. The most important of these fall into two categories: (1) parasites can reduce or alter their own antigenicity, or (2) they can actively inhibit host immune responses.

1. *Anatomic sequestration is commonly observed with protozoa.* Some (e.g., malaria parasites, *Toxoplasma*) survive and replicate inside cells, and others (like *Entamoeba* and *Trichinella*) develop cysts that are resistant to immune effectors. Some helminthic parasites reside in intestinal lumens and are sheltered from cell-mediated immune effector mechanisms. It is likely, however, that anatomic concealment is a temporary and only partially effective mechanism for evading immune responses.

2. *Antigen masking is an intriguing phenomenon in which a parasite, during its residence within a host, acquires on its surface a coat of host proteins.* The larvae of *S. mansoni* enter the skin and travel to the lungs and then into the circulation. By the time they enter the lungs, these larvae are coated with ABO blood group glycolipids and MHC molecules derived from the host. It is likely that many other host molecules attach to the surface of the schistosome larvae. It has been postulated that as a result of this coat of self proteins, parasite antigens are masked and the organism is seen as self by the host immune system. Although this is an interesting hypothesis, the significance of antigen masking is not clear because schistosome larvae do elicit specific immunity in vertebrate hosts.

3. *Parasites become resistant to immune effector mechanisms during their residence in vertebrate hosts.* Lung stage schistosome larvae develop a tegument that is resistant to damage by antibodies and complement or by CTLs directed against surface-bound antigens. This resistance is presumably due to a biochemical change in the surface coat. The structural complexity of the larval tegument has made it difficult to define the molecular alterations that are associated with acquired resistance. Infective forms of *T. cruzi* synthesize membrane glycoproteins similar to decay accelerating factor that inhibit complement activation. *Leishmania major* promastigotes induce rapid breakdown or release of the membrane attack complex thus reducing complement-mediated lysis. Parasites also evade macrophage killing by various mechanisms. *Toxoplasma gondii* inhibits phagolysosome fusion, and *T. cruzi* lyses the membranes of phagosomes and enters the cytoplasm before fusion with lysosomes can occur. Finally, some parasites express ectoenzymes that cleave bound antibody molecules and thus become resistant to antibody-dependent effector mechanisms.

4. *Parasites have developed effective mechanisms for varying their surface antigens during their life cycle in vertebrate hosts.* Two forms of antigenic variation are well defined.

a. The first is a stage-specific change in antigen expression, such that the mature tissue stages of parasites produce different antigens from the infective stages. For example, the infective sporozoite stage of malaria parasites is antigenically distinct from the merozoites that reside in the host and are responsible for chronic infection. By the time the immune system has responded to the infection, the parasite expresses new antigens and is no longer a target for immune elimination.

b. The most remarkable antigenic variation in parasites is the continuous variation of major surface antigens seen in African trypanosomes such as *Trypanosoma brucei* and *Trypanosoma rhodesiense*. Infected individuals show waves of blood parasitemia, and each wave consists of one antigenically unique parasite. The same phenomenon can be reproduced in experimental animals infected with a single clone of a trypanosome (Fig. 15–3). Thus, by the time the host produces antibodies against the parasite, an antigenically different organism has replicated. Over a hundred such recrudescent waves of parasitemia can occur in an infection. The major surface antigen of African trypanosomes is a glycoprotein dimer of approximately 50 kD, called the **variable surface glycoprotein** (VSG), which is attached to the surface by a phosphatidyl-inositol linkage. Trypanosomes contain more than 1000 different VSG genes, which vary markedly in their sequences except for the most C-terminal 50 amino acids (which are responsible for the surface linkage). Any one VSG gene is expressed in a particular clone at a particular stage of infection. Expression of a new gene may involve duplication and transposition of that gene to a more telomeric chromosomal site at which active transcription ensues (Fig. 15–1). This mechanism is different from the gene conversion events that lead to variation of antigens in the pili of gonococci. However, gene conversion and activation of previously silent VSG genes are additional mechanisms that may contribute to antigenic variation. Continuous antigenic variation in trypanosomes is neither induced by nor dependent on the specific antibody response and is probably due to a programmed variation in the expression of VSG genes. The molecular

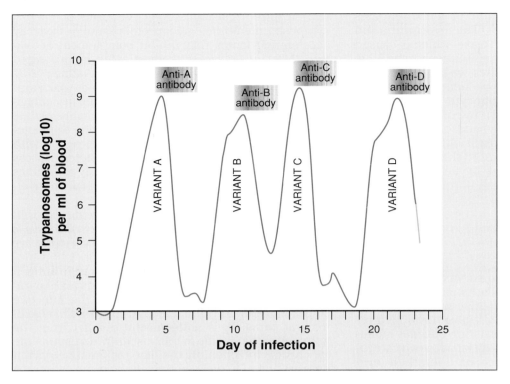

FIGURE 15–3. Parasitemia following trypanosome infections. In a mouse infected experimentally with a single clone of Trypanosoma rhodesiense, the blood parasite counts show cyclical waves. Each wave is due to a new antigenic variant of the parasite (labeled A, B, C, and D) that expresses a new VSG, and each decline is a result of a specific antibody response to the variant. The durations of peak antibody production as shown are approximate. Similar waves of parasitemia are seen in natural infections in humans. (Courtesy of Dr. John Mansfield, University of Wisconsin, Madison.)

mechanisms that regulate this phenomenon are the focus of active investigation in many laboratories.

One consequence of antigenic variation in parasites is that it is difficult to effectively vaccinate individuals against these infections. In fact, prophylactic immunization against one parasite antigen may itself stimulate additional antigenic variation, as has been seen in experimental malarial infections.

5. *Parasites shed their antigenic coats, either spontaneously or after the binding of specific antibodies.* Examples of active membrane turnover and loss of surface antigens have been described with *Entamoeba histolytica*, schistosome larvae, and trypanosomes. Shedding of antigens and bound antibodies renders the parasites relatively resistant to immune effector mechanisms.

6. *Parasites alter host immune responses by multiple mechanisms.* Specific anergy to parasite antigens has been described in severe schistosomiasis involving the liver and spleen and in filarial infections. The mechanisms of immunologic unresponsiveness in these patients are not well understood. In lymphatic filariasis, infection of lymph nodes with subsequent architectural disruption may contribute to deficient immunity. More nonspecific and generalized immunosuppression, e.g., in systemic leishmaniasis, has been mentioned earlier. It has been variously attributed to abnormalities in cytokine production, deficient T cell activation, immunosuppressive macrophages, and "suppressor cells." Better structural definition of parasite antigens and analysis of specific lymphocyte responses are now being done by many research groups.

The worldwide implications of parasitic infestations for health and economic development are well appreciated. Attempts to develop effective vaccines against these infections have been actively pursued for many years (Box 15–3). Although the progress has been slower than one would have hoped, elucidation of the fundamental mechanisms of immune responses to and immune evasion by parasites holds great promise for the future.

SUMMARY

The interaction of the immune system with infectious organisms is a dynamic interplay of host mechanisms aimed at eliminating infections and microbial strategies designed to permit survival in the face of powerful effector mechanisms. Different types of infectious agents stimulate distinct patterns of immune responses and have evolved unique mechanisms for evading specific immunity.

The principal protective immune response against extracellular bacteria consists of specific antibodies, which opsonize the bacteria for phagocytosis and activate the complement system. Toxins produced by such bacteria are also neutralized and eliminated by specific antibodies. Some bacterial toxins are powerful inducers of cytokine production, and cytokines account for much of the systemic pathology associated with severe, disseminated infections with these microbes.

Intracellular bacteria are capable of surviving and replicating within host cells, including phago-

BOX 15 - 3. STRATEGIES FOR VACCINE DEVELOPMENT

The birth of immunology as a science may be dated from Edward Jenner's successful vaccination against smallpox, which was reported in 1798. The importance of prophylactic immunization against infectious diseases is best illustrated by the fact that worldwide programs of vaccination have led to the complete or near complete eradication of many of these diseases in developed countries. Smallpox and polio are perhaps the two most impressive examples. The development of effective vaccines against viruses, bacteria, and parasites remains an important goal of immunologists worldwide.

The aim of all vaccination is to induce specific immunity that prevents microbial invasion, eliminates microbes that enter hosts, and neutralizes microbial toxins. Since effective vaccination as a public health measure requires long-lasting immunity, the ability of vaccines to stimulate memory T and B lymphocytes is an important consideration in vaccine design. The success of active immunization in eradicating infectious disease is dependent on numerous factors. For instance, infections that are limited to human hosts and are caused by poorly infectious agents whose antigens are relatively invariant are more likely to be controlled by vaccination. On the other hand, antigenic variation, the existence of animal or environmental reservoirs of infection, and high infectivity of microbes make it less likely that vaccination alone will eradicate a particular infectious disease.

Many types of infectious agents and their products have been used as vaccines.

ATTENUATED AND INACTIVATED BACTERIAL AND VIRAL VACCINES.
Live, attenuated bacteria were first shown by Louis Pasteur to confer specific immunity. Among the attenuated bacterial vaccines in use today are *Mycobacterium tuberculosis* bacille Calmette-Guérin (BCG), avirulent mutants of *Salmonella typhi*, inactivated *Vibrio cholerae*, and inactivated *Bordetella pertussis*. Many of these vaccines induce limited protection and are effective for relatively short periods. Live, attenuated viral vaccines are generally much more effective. The most frequently used approach for producing such vaccines is to derive attenuated viruses from long-term cell culture. More recently, temperature-sensitive and deletion mutants are being generated with the same goal in mind. Polio, measles, and yellow fever are three examples of effective attenuated viral vaccines. Inactivated viruses are also used as vaccines, e.g., in influenza, rabies, and Japanese encephalitis. Viral vaccines often induce long-lasting specific immunity, so that immunization of children is sufficient for life-long protection.

PURIFIED ANTIGEN (SUBUNIT) VACCINES.
One effective use of purified antigens as vaccines is for the prevention of diseases caused by bacterial toxins. Toxins can be rendered harmless without loss of immunogenicity and such "toxoids" induce strong antibody responses. Diphtheria and tetanus are two infections that have been largely controlled because of immunization of children with toxoid preparations. Vaccines composed of bacterial polysaccharide antigens are used against pneumococcus and *Haemophilus influenza*. They are effective in high-risk individuals, but they induce short-lived protection because polysaccharide antigens are inefficient at stimulating the development of memory cells. Subunit vaccines composed of purified peptides have been used for hepatitis B and influenza viruses and are in clinical trials for *Bordetella pertussis* and cholera.

SYNTHETIC ANTIGEN VACCINES.
Early approaches for developing synthetic antigens as vaccines relied on the synthesis of linear and branched polymers of three to ten amino acids based on the known sequences of microbial antigens. Such peptides are weakly immunogenic by themselves and need to be coupled to large proteins to induce antibody responses. This is much like generating antibody responses to hapten-carrier conjugates (see Chapter 9).

Two advances have revolutionized the development of synthetic peptide vaccines. First, it is now possible to deduce the protein sequences of microbial antigens from nucleotide sequence data and to prepare large quantities of proteins by recombinant DNA technology. Second, by testing overlapping peptides and by mutational analysis, it is possible to identify epitopes or even individual residues that are recognized by B or T cells or that bind to MHC molecules for presentation to MHC-restricted T lymphocytes. Empirical trial of peptides containing single or multiple amino acid substitutions has led to the construction of antigens with enhanced binding to MHC molecules or enhanced capacity to activate T cells. To date, such studies have been done largely in inbred mice.

Because T cell antigen recognition is influenced by the polymorphism of MHC molecules, it is likely that in outbred human populations it will be much more difficult to "custom design" peptides with enhanced immunogenicity. Nevertheless, there is great potential in this approach for creating at will vaccines that are of high potency. Using recombinant DNA technology, synthetic peptide vaccines have been produced that correspond to immunogenic epitopes of hepatitis B virus, herpes simplex virus, and foot-and-mouth disease virus (a major pathogen for livestock). The same method is being explored in many other infectious diseases.

LIVE VIRAL VECTORS.
Perhaps the most exciting new approach to vaccine development is to introduce genes encoding microbial antigens into a nonpathogenic virus and infect individuals with this virus. Thus, the virus serves as a source of the antigen in the inoculated individual. This technique has been used most commonly with vaccinia virus vectors. The gene encoding the desired antigen is inserted by a process of homologous recombination into the vaccinia virus genome at the site of the nonessential viral thymidine kinase gene. Thymidine kinase-negative recombinant viruses are selected in culture medium containing bromodeoxyuridine (which kills all cells that produce thymidine kinase). At least 25,000 base pairs (bp) of foreign DNA can be inserted into the viral genome, and the upper limit of the size of the foreign gene may be much greater. With this method, recombinant vaccinia viruses producing hepatitis B surface antigen, herpes simplex virus proteins, influenza virus hemagglutinin and neuraminidase, malaria circumsporozoite protein, and many other microbial antigens have been generated. Inoculation of recombinant viruses into many species of animals induces both humoral and cell-mediated immunity against the antigen produced by the foreign gene (and, of course, against vaccinia virus antigens as well). Attempts are under way to improve the construction and efficiency of expression of viral vectors, to reduce the pathogenicity of the vaccinia virus, to enhance the immunogenicity of the expressed antigen, and to incorporate adjuvants or use delivery systems to maximize vaccine potency. Such live recombinant viruses have not been used in human trials to date because of safety concerns, but their enormous potential is undisputed.

Finally, protective immunity can also be conferred by **passive immunization**, e.g., by transfer of specific antibodies. In the clinical situation this is most commonly used for diseases caused by toxins, such as tetanus. Antibodies against snake venoms can be life-saving treatments for poisonous snake bites. Passive immunity is short-lived, because the host does not respond to the immunization and protection lasts only as long as the injected antibody persists. Moreover, passive immunization does not induce specific memory, so that the immunized individual is not protected against subsequent exposures to the toxin or microbe.

cytes, because they have developed mechanisms for resisting lysosomal degradation. Immunity against these microbes is principally cell-mediated and consists of CD4+ T cells activating macrophages (as in delayed type hypersensitivity) as well as CD8+ cytolytic T lymphocytes. The characteristic pathologic response to infection by intracellular bacteria is granulomatous inflammation.

Viruses are obligatory intracellular microbes. Natural immunity against viruses is mediated by type I interferons and NK cells. Specific antibodies protect against viruses early in the course of infection. However, the major defense mechanism against established infections consists of specific CTLs. CTLs effectively lyse infected cells and may contribute to tissue injury even when the infectious virus is not cytopathic by itself.

Animal parasites, such as protozoa and helminths, give rise to chronic and persistent infections, because natural immunity against them is weak and because parasites have evolved multiple mechanisms for evading and resisting specific immunity. The structural and antigenic diversity of pathogenic parasites is reflected in the heterogeneity of the specific immune responses they elicit. Different parasites induce specific IgE antibodies and eosinophilia, granulomatous inflammation, cytokine production, and specific CTLs. Parasites evade the immune system by masking and shedding their surface antigens and by varying their antigens during residence in vertebrate hosts. In addition, various parasites cause specific and generalized suppression of lymphocyte activation. The chronicity of parasitic infestations often leads to secondary immunopathologic consequences, including the formation of immune complexes and the development of autoimmunity.

Selected Readings

Askonas, B. A., A. J. McMichael, and R. G. Webster. The immune response to influenza viruses and the problem of protection against infection. In A. S. Beare (ed.). Basic and Applied Influenza Research. Boca Raton, Fla, CRC Press, 1982, p. 159.

Cross, G. A. M. Cellular and genetic aspects of antigenic variation in trypanosomes. Annual Review of Immunology 8:83–110, 1990.

Gaylord, H., and P. J. Brennan. Leprosy and the leprosy bacillus: recent developments in the characterization of antigens and immunology of the disease. Annual Review of Microbiology 41:645–675, 1987.

Good, M. F., J. A. Berzofsky, and L. H. Miller. The T cell response to the malaria circumsporozoite protein: an immunological approach to vaccine development. Annual Review of Immunology 6:663–688, 1988.

Joiner, K. A. Complement evasion by bacteria and parasites. Annual Review of Microbiology 42:201–230, 1988.

Kaufman, S. H. E. CD8+ T lymphocytes in intracellular microbial infections. Immunology Today 9:168–173, 1988.

Liew, F. Y. Functional heterogeneity of CD4+ T cells in leishmaniasis. Immunology Today 10:40–45, 1989.

Mahmoud, A. A. F. Parasitic protozoa and helminths: biological and immunological challenges. Science 246:1015–1022, 1989.

Morrison, D. C., and J. L. Ryan. Endotoxins and disease mechanisms. Annual Review of Medicine 38:417–432, 1987.

Scott, P., E. Pearce, A. W. Cheever, R. L. Coffman, and A. Sher. Role of cytokines and CD4+ T-cell subsets in the regulation of parasite immunity and disease. Immunological Reviews 112:161–182, 1989.

Sher, A. Vaccination against parasites: special problems imposed by the adaptation of parasitic organisms to the host immune response. In P. T. Englund and A. Sher (eds.). The Biology of Parasitism: A Molecular and Immunologic Approach. New York, Alan R. Liss, 1988.

Young, R. A. Stress proteins and immunology. Annual Review of Immunology 8:401–420, 1990.

CHAPTER SIXTEEN

IMMUNITY

TO TISSUE

TRANSPLANTS

Transplantation is the process of taking cells, tissues, or organs, called a **graft,** from one individual and placing them into a (usually) different individual. The individual who provides the graft is referred to as the **donor,** and the individual who receives the graft is referred to as either the **recipient** or the **host.** If the graft is placed into its normal anatomic location, the procedure is called *orthotopic transplantation;* if the graft is placed in a different site, the procedure is called *heterotopic transplantation.* Transfusion is transplantation of circulating blood cells and/or plasma from one individual to another.

Although attempts at transplantation date back to ancient times, the impetus behind modern transplantation was World War II and the Battle of Britain. Royal Air Force pilots were often severely burned when their planes crashed. The mortality associated with burns corresponds to the size of the area of skin that has been injured, and survival can be improved if burned skin is replaced. For this reason, British doctors turned to skin transplantation from other human donors as a mode of therapy. However, attempts to replace damaged skin with skin from unrelated donors were uniformly unsuccessful. Over a matter of several days, the transplanted skin would undergo necrosis and fall off. This problem led many investigators, including Peter Medawar, to study skin transplantation in animal models. These experiments established that the failure of skin grafting was caused by an inflammatory reaction that was called **rejection.** More importantly, several features indicated that *rejection is a form of specific immunity.* The key experimental results may be summarized as follows (Table 16–1):

1. A skin graft transplanted between genetically unrelated individuals, e.g., from a strain A mouse to a strain B mouse, is rejected by a naive host in 7 to 10 days. This process is called **first set rejection.** A subsequent skin graft transplanted from the same donor to the same recipient is rejected more rapidly, i.e., in only 2 or 3 days. This accelerated response, called **second set rejection,** is an example of memory, one of the cardinal features of acquired immunity.

2. Second set rejection ensues if the first and second skin grafts are derived from the same donor or from genetically identical donors, e.g., strain A mice. However, if the second graft is derived from an indi-

vidual unrelated to the donor of the first graft, e.g., strain C, there is no second set rejection; the new graft elicits only a first set rejection. Thus, the phenomenon of second set rejection shows specificity, another cardinal feature of acquired immunity.

3. The ability to mount second set rejection against a graft from strain A mice can be adoptively transferred to a naive strain B recipient by immunocompetent lymphocytes taken from a strain B animal previously exposed to a graft from strain A mice. This experiment demonstrated that second set rejection is mediated by sensitized lymphocytes and provided the definitive evidence that rejection is a form of acquired immunity.

Transplant immunologists have developed a vocabulary to describe the kinds of cells and tissues encountered in the transplant setting. A graft transplanted from one individual to the same individual is called either an **autologous graft** (shortened to **autograft**) or an **isograft.** A graft transplanted between two genetically identical or syngeneic individuals is called a **syngeneic graft** (or **syngraft.**) A graft transplanted between two genetically different individuals of the same species is called an **allogeneic graft** (or **allograft**). A graft transplanted between individuals of different species is called a **xenogeneic graft** (or **xenograft**). The molecules that are recognized as foreign on allografts are called **alloantigens,** and those on xenografts are called **xenoantigens.** The lymphocytes or antibodies that react with alloantigens or xenoantigens are described as being **alloreactive** or **xenoreactive,** respectively.

The remainder of this chapter focuses on allogeneic transplantation because it is far more commonly practiced and better understood than xenogeneic transplantation. We will consider both the basic immunology and some aspects of the clinical practice of transplantation. Transplantation of organs such as kidney, heart, and liver is currently in widespread use, and the practice is growing. In addition, the transplantation of many other organs is now being attempted. The immunology of transplantation is important for two reasons. First, the immunologic rejection response, along with problems of organ procurement, are the two major barriers to transplantation today. Second, although the encounter with alloantigens appears to be an unlikely happenstance in the

TABLE 16–1. First Set and Second Set Allograft Rejection

| Animal | Skin Graft Donor | Recipient | | Rejection |
		Strain	*Prior Treatment*	
1	Strain A	Strain B	None	Slow (first set)
2	Strain A	Strain B	Sensitized by previous graft from strain A donor	Rapid (second set); demonstration of immunologic memory
3	Strain A	Strain B	Injected with lymphocytes from animal No. 1	Rapid (second set); demonstration of role of lymphocytes in graft rejection
4	Strain C	Strain B	Sensitized by previous graft from strain A donor	Slow (first set); demonstration of immunologic specificity

normal life of an organism, the immune response to allogeneic molecules is very strong and has therefore been a useful model for elucidating the mechanisms of lymphocyte activation.

TRANSPLANTATION IMMUNOLOGY

The immune response to alloantigens can be either cell-mediated or humoral. In general, cell-mediated immune reactions are more important for rejection of transplanted organs, but antibodies may contribute. Most studies of the immune responses to tissue transplants have focused on T cell responses to allogeneic molecules. There are three major questions addressed by these studies:

1. What antigens in grafts stimulate alloreactivity?
2. What types of lymphocytes respond to foreign transplants?
3. Why do individuals react against tissues that they do not encounter normally?

Molecular Basis of Allogeneic Recognition

In Chapter 5, we presented evidence that recognition of transplanted cells as self or foreign is determined by inheritance of co-dominant genes. This conclusion was based on the results of experimental transplantation between inbred strains of mice.

1. Cells or organs transplanted between individuals of the same inbred strain of mice are never rejected.
2. Cells or organs transplanted between individuals of different inbred strains of mice are almost always rejected.
3. The offspring of a mating between two different inbred strains will never reject grafts from either parent. In other words, an (A × B)F1 animal will not reject grafts from an A or B strain animal.
4. A graft derived from the offspring of a mating between two different inbred strains will almost always be rejected by either parent. In other words, a graft from an (A × B)F1 animal will be rejected by either an A or a B strain animal.

These genetic experiments led to the hypothesis that certain polymorphic gene products, co-dominantly expressed on a graft, are recognized by the immune system to identify a graft as self or foreign. Co-dominant expression means that an (A × B)F1 animal expresses both A strain and B strain alleles. This is why an (A × B)F1 animal is tolerant to both A and B strain grafts and why both A and B strain animals will recognize an (A × B)F1 graft as foreign. As described in Chapter 5, George Snell and colleagues were able to identify about 40 polymorphic genes that served as the molecular targets of rejection in mice. Specifically, they found that polymorphic molecules encoded by

genes in histocompatibility locus 2 (H-2), now known as the mouse major histocompatibility complex, were responsible for almost all the strong (rapid) rejection reactions. *As many as 2 per cent of a host's T cells are capable of recognizing and responding to a single foreign MHC molecule.* This high frequency of T cells reactive with allogeneic MHC molecules is the reason why allograft rejection is a strong response *in vivo*.

An important question in transplantation is the molecular structure of the determinants on allogeneic MHC molecules that are recognized by alloreactive T cells. We now know that mature T cells express receptors that are specific for foreign peptides bound to the peptide-binding cleft of self class I or class II MHC molecules. Any given T cell receptor (TCR) simultaneously recognizes amino acid residues of the bound foreign peptide and residues of self MHC molecules. Foreign MHC molecules differ from self MHC molecules by variations (polymorphisms) in amino acid sequence, and, as we noted in Chapter 5, these polymorphic residues are confined to the top, sides, and floor of the peptide-binding cleft. The determinants of foreign MHC molecules recognized by specific alloreactive T cells are formed largely by these polymorphic residues. It is believed that the three-dimensional surface of the determinant recognized on the foreign MHC molecules resembles self MHC plus a bound foreign peptide. Thus, *recognition of foreign MHC molecules is a cross-reaction of a normal T cell receptor which was selected to recognize self MHC plus foreign peptide.* Three kinds of experiments support this conclusion:

1. A T cell clone or hybridoma that contains one set of functionally rearranged T cell receptor genes specific for self MHC plus a foreign peptide may also recognize one or more foreign MHC molecules in the absence of the specific foreign peptide.
2. Monoclonal antibodies reactive with idiotypic determinants on the TCR molecule of such a T cell clone or hybridoma may inhibit recognition of both self MHC–associated foreign peptide and foreign MHC molecules.
3. Transfection of rearranged α and β T cell receptor genes into a recipient T cell confers specificity both for self MHC plus foreign peptide and for foreign MHC molecules.

Because in these *in vitro* systems exogenously added foreign peptides were not necessary for allorecognition, the results initially seemed to support the conclusion that bound peptide does not contribute to the determinant formed by a foreign MHC molecule. However, MHC molecules expressed on cell surfaces may always contain bound peptides. Even in artificial systems, such as lipid bilayers containing purified foreign MHC molecules, peptides could be provided by the culture medium or by the responding T cell or could remain associated with the MHC molecules through purification. Moreover, some alloreactive T cell clones have now been shown to be specific for foreign MHC plus bound peptide. The peptides recognized in association with foreign MHC molecules may be self peptides because thymic education does not produce tolerance to self proteins plus foreign MHC. The importance of the contribution of bound peptide to recognition by most alloreactive T cells is not yet known.

It is surprising that many more mature T cells recognize particular foreign MHC molecules than recognize any specific foreign peptide. This raises the question of why alloreactive cells are so common. Two explanations have been offered to account for widespread cross-reactivity.

1. *Foreign MHC molecules differ from self MHC molecules at multiple different amino acid residues, each of which individually or in combination may produce a determinant recognized by a different cross-reactive T cell clone.* Thus, each foreign MHC molecule is recognized by multiple clones of T cells whose receptors are specific for different foreign peptides in association with self MHC molecules. In this model, widespread cross-reactivity is caused entirely by multiple variations in the sequence of the foreign MHC molecule. For example, foreign MHC molecule X will be recognized by T cell 1, specific for self MHC molecule Y plus peptide A and by T cell 2, specific for self MHC molecule Y plus peptide B.

2. *Different bound self peptides, in combination with one foreign MHC molecule, may produce determinants recognized by different cross-reactive T cell clones.* The result, once again, is that many T cell clones recognize and respond to each foreign MHC molecule, but in this model, widespread cross-reactivity is caused by many different self peptides combining with a lesser degree of variation in the sequence of the foreign MHC molecule. For example, foreign MHC molecule X plus self peptide A will be recognized by T cell 1, specific for self MHC molecule Y plus foreign peptide B and foreign MHC molecule X plus self peptide C will be recognized by T cell 2 specific for self MHC molecule Y plus foreign peptide D.

These two models of alloantigen recognition are not mutually exclusive. It seems likely that associated self peptides will be more important (model 2) in those cases in which the self and foreign MHC molecules are structurally similar, and less important (model 1) when the self and foreign MHC molecules are structurally dissimilar to each other.

Polymorphic alloantigens other than MHC molecules generally produce weak or slower (gradual) rejection reactions and are called minor histocompatibility antigens. Most minor histocompatibility antigens are proteins that are processed and presented to host T cells in association with either self MHC or graft MHC molecules. In contrast, foreign MHC molecules can be recognized directly by host T cells without any requirement for processing or association with self MHC molecules.

Cellular Basis of Allogeneic Recognition

Vigorous rejection reactions of allografts generally result from recognition of the transplanted tissues by both CD4+ and CD8+ T cells. The **mixed leukocyte reaction** (MLR) has been a useful model for understanding the cellular basis of alloantigen recognition by different T cell subpopulations.

THE MIXED LEUKOCYTE REACTION

As we have discussed above, MHC genes were initially identified for their role in graft rejection, which is often a T cell–mediated process. The MLR is an *in vitro* model of T cell recognition of foreign MHC gene products and is used as a predictive test of cell-mediated graft rejection.

The MLR is induced by culturing mononuclear leukocytes (which include T cells, B cells, mononuclear phagocytes, and dendritic cells), from one individual or inbred strain with mononuclear leukocytes derived from another individual or strain. In humans, these cells are typically isolated from peripheral blood; in the mouse or rat, mononuclear leukocytes are usually purified from spleen or lymph nodes. If there are differences in the alleles of the MHC genes between the two individuals, a large proportion of the mononuclear cells will proliferate over a period of 4 to 7 days. This proliferative response, usually measured by incorporation of ^{3}H-thymidine into DNA during cell replication, is called the **allogeneic MLR** (Fig. 16–1). In the experiment described above, the cells from each donor react and proliferate against the other, resulting in a "two-way MLR." To simplify the analysis, one of the two mononuclear leukocyte populations can be rendered incapable of proliferation, either by gamma irradiation or by treatment with mitomycin C, an antimitotic drug, prior to culture. In this "one-way MLR," the treated cells serve exclusively as **stimulators** and the untreated cells, still capable of proliferation, serve as the **responders.**

Two populations of alloreactive T cells are stimulated during an allogeneic MLR, and each responding T cell subset recognizes a different MHC gene product. One type of T cell expresses the CD8 but not the CD4 molecule, usually functions as a cytolytic T lymphocyte (CTL), and is indistinguishable from self class I MHC–restricted CTLs specific for foreign protein antigens. The CTLs generated during an allogeneic MLR lyse target cells derived from the same individual or strain as the original stimulator cell population. The molecules on stimulator and target cells that are recognized by CD8+ CTL are the class I MHC molecules, namely, HLA–A, B, or C in humans or H-2K, D, or L in mice. Several lines of evidence have indicated that foreign class I MHC gene products are the actual molecular targets recognized by the CD8+ CTLs generated in the MLR:

1. If there are no differences in class I MHC alleles between the stimulator and responder cell populations in the MLR, CD8+ CTLs are not generated.

2. The CTLs generated against one stimulator cell population will lyse third-party target cells only if these targets share a class I MHC allele with the original stimulators.

3. Antibodies directed against class I MHC allelic

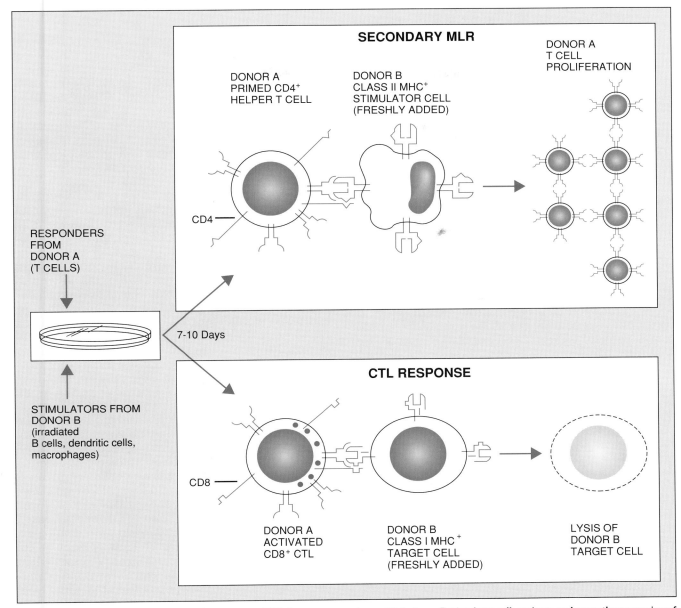

FIGURE 16 – 1. Responder T cells in the mixed leukocyte reaction (MLR). *In a one-way primary MLR, donor B stimulator cells activate and cause the expansion of two types of donor A responder T cells: CD4+ helper T cells, which can be detected in a secondary MLR by rapid proliferation to antigen-presenting cells (APCs) bearing donor B class II molecules; and CD8+ cytolytic T lymphocytes (CTLs), which can be detected in a specific killing assay using target cells bearing donor B class I molecules.*

gene products on the stimulator cells protect target cells against lysis.

4. Transfection and expression of an allelic class I MHC gene can render a cell susceptible to lysis by a CTL population specific for that allele.

The full differentiation of CTLs in the MLR requires stimulation by class I MHC molecules as well as help that is optimally provided by CD4+ T cells present in the same culture (see Chapter 12).

Within the CD8+ CTL population derived from an MLR, each individual CTL is specific for only one particular class I MHC gene product. However, the bulk population contains CTLs directed against all class I

MHC allelic differences between the original stimulator and responder populations. Furthermore, in an outbred individual, all the class I MHC alleles inherited from both parents are co-dominantly expressed on every class I–expressing cell, so that an individual target cell can be lysed by several different CTLs, each with a different class I MHC specificity.

The second type of T cell that is generated during the MLR was initially called a primed responder cell, because when such T cells are recultured with stimulator cells from the same donor individual (or strain) used in the original MLR, a secondary MLR ensues that is stronger and more rapid; i.e., peak proliferation occurs by 2 or 3 days. It is now appreciated that primed responder cells are interleukin-2 (IL–2)–producing T cells that play a role in the development of CD8+ CTLs. Such T cells express the CD4 but not the CD8 surface molecule and are indistinguishable from IL–2–producing CD4+ helper T cells specific for foreign protein antigens. Alloreactive CD4+ helper T cells are specific for allogeneic class II MHC molecules, i.e., HLA–DR, DP, and DQ in humans and I-A and I-E in mice. The class II MHC molecules have been established as the molecules seen by the CD4+ helper cells by the same kinds of evidence that established class I MHC molecules as the targets of CD8+ CTL.

1. Alloreactive CD4+ T cells are stimulated only if there are differences in class II MHC alleles between the original stimulator and responder cells in the primary MLR.

2. Alloreactive CD4+ T cells respond to third-party stimulator cells only if they share class II MHC alleles with the original stimulator population.

3. Antibodies directed against class II MHC gene products prevent development of the secondary MLR.

4. Transfection of appropriate allelic class II MHC genes can convert a cell from a non-stimulator to a stimulator of a CD4+ T cell population specific for that MHC allele.

Alloreactive CD4+ T cells, like self MHC–restricted antigen-specific helper cells, can be stimulated only by cells that express class II MHC molecules and provide costimulatory signals. The most efficient stimulators are dendritic cells, B lymphocytes, and mononuclear phagocytes. In humans, vascular endothelial cells are also able to stimulate proliferative responses of alloreactive CD4+ T cells. Each individual CD4+ helper T cell is specific for one particular class II gene product. However, the bulk population contains helper cells reactive with all class II allelic differences between the original stimulator and helper cell population. Furthermore, since there is no allelic exclusion of class II genes on individual cells and all the parental alleles are co-dominantly expressed, one stimulator cell can activate several different helper T cells, each with a different class II MHC specificity.

It should be emphasized that the functional subdivision of CD4+ and CD8+ alloreactive T cells into helper cells and CTLs is not absolute. CD4+ class II specific CTLs can be detected in the MLR, particularly in humans. Moreover, at least some CD8+ T cells produce IL–2, γ-interferon (IFN–γ), tumor necrosis factor (TNF), and lymphotoxin (LT), which is similar to the cytokine profile of many CD4+ cells. As discussed in Chapters 6 and 7, the same exceptions have been found for self MHC–restricted T cells specific for foreign protein antigens.

A more specific analysis of the role of class I and class II molecules in allogeneic immune responses has been performed by considering the one-way MLR when only isolated class I or class II differences exist between the stimulator and responder cell populations (Table 16–2). In the extreme case, this has been done by using cells from mouse strains that differ only by a small mutation in a single class I or class II gene product. Proliferation is strongest when stimulators and responders differ by a class II gene product and can directly stimulate CD4+ T cells. Fewer CTLs arise in this instance, and many of these are CD4+ class II-specific CTLs. When only class I differences exist between stimulator and responder cells, the proliferative response is small. Nevertheless, there is a proliferative response and CD8+ CTLs specific for the class I difference do arise. In this situation, proliferation and the development of CTLs may be mediated by cytokines produced by the CD8+ T cells themselves responding to the foreign class I molecules. Alternatively, if class II MHC+ accessory cells are present, they may take up, process, and present foreign class I molecules in the form of peptides associated with self class II molecules. In this setting, the foreign class I molecules behave like other foreign protein antigens that are recognized by CD4+ T cells present in the responder population. This process is far less efficient than direct recognition of foreign class II molecules. Therefore, stimulator cell populations that differ from

TABLE 16–2. Induction of Mixed Leukocyte Reaction by Class I and Class II Major Histocompatibility Complex (MHC) Mismatches

MHC Differences Between Stimulator and Responder Cells			Induction of	
Class I	Class II	Proliferation	Primed Helper (Cytokine-Producing) Cells	CTLs
Yes	Yes	++++	++++ (CD4+, class II-specific)	++++ (CD8+, class I-specific)
Yes	No	+	+ (CD8+, class I-specific)	+++ (CD8+, class I-specific)
No	Yes	+++	+++ (CD4+, class II-specific)	+ (CD4+, class II-specific)

In a one-way MLR between stimulator and responder cells that differ at class I or class II MHC loci or both, the major types of cytokine-producing helper (proliferating) cells and CTL are different.

Abbreviations: CTL, cytolytic T lymphocyte.

the responders at both the class I and class II MHC loci induce many more allospecific CTLs than stimulators that differ at only class I loci.

Two additional points about the MLR should be noted:

1. *The MLR is the only* in vitro, *antigen-specific response of T cells that can be readily observed without prior immunization* in vivo. This is because T cells reactive with allogeneic MHC molecules are much more numerous in an unstimulated population than are the T cells specific for any single foreign protein antigen. In addition, an allogeneic stimulator cell may express a large number of foreign MHC molecules that are capable of stimulating alloreactive T cells. In contrast, on an antigen presenting cell (APC) that is normally presenting a foreign peptide antigen, a minor fraction of the MHC molecules may be complexed with the specific peptide. As a result, many more alloreactive than foreign antigen-specific, self MHC–restricted T cells are stimulated by such APCs.

2. Although the MLR is initiated by allogeneic stimulation, the majority of helper T cells and CTLs that proliferate in the primary MLR are actually not specific for the allogeneic MHC gene products on the stimulator cells. Rather, they are driven to proliferate by growth factors, such as IL–2, produced by a small number of specifically stimulated alloreactive cells. However, the specifically stimulated alloreactive cells preferentially increase in number, compared with any other T cell, and thus become the only cells sufficiently numerous to be detectable as CTLs or primed helper cells after the primary MLR.

STIMULATION OF ALLOREACTIVE T CELLS *IN VIVO*

In the case of allografts that differ from hosts at both class I and class II loci, both CD8+ and CD4+ T cells are activated by recognition of alloantigens of the grafts. CD8+ cells recognize foreign class I MHC molecules, which are expressed by all the cells in the graft. The differentiation of these CTLs is largely dependent upon CD4+ T cells being stimulated by allogeneic class II molecules present on APCs in the allograft. Therefore, one can predict that tissue allografts that stimulate strong rejection contain class II–bearing APCs.

The importance of APCs in stimulating an alloantigenic immune response *in vivo* has most clearly been demonstrated by experiments in rodents. If class II–bearing cells (which include APCs) are removed from a graft prior to transplantation, such grafts are usually rejected slowly or may even be accepted despite class I MHC differences. (Experimentally, class II bearing cells may be eliminated from such grafts by several treatments, including prolonged culture; treatment with anti-class II antibody plus complement; or, in some cases, extensive perfusion of graft blood vessels to "wash out" the APCs.) When rat kidney allografts are purged of class II–bearing cells by perfusion, infusion of dendritic cells derived from the organ donor concomitant with transplantation restores allorecognition and leads to rapid rejection. These observations have led to several conclusions, collectively described as the **passenger leukocyte hypothesis.**

BOX 16–1. IMMUNITY TO AN ALLOGENEIC FETUS

The mammalian fetus, except in those instances in which the mother and father are syngeneic, will express paternally-inherited antigens that are allogeneic to the mother. Nevertheless, fetuses are not normally rejected by the mother. An understanding of how the fetus escapes the maternal immune system may be relevant for transplantation.

Three experimental observations indicate that the anatomic location of the fetus is a critical factor in the absence of rejection:

1. Wholly allogeneic fetal blastocysts that lack any maternal genes can successfully develop in a pregnant or pseudopregnant mother. Thus, neither specific maternal nor paternal genes are necessary for survival of the fetus.
2. Hyperimmunization of the mother with cells bearing paternal antigens does not compromise placental and fetal growth.
3. Pregnant mothers are able to recognize and reject allografts syngeneic to the fetus placed at extrauterine sites without compromising fetal survival.

The failure to reject the fetus has focused attention upon the region of physical contact between the mother and fetus. The fetal tissues of the placenta that most intimately contact the mother may be classified as *vascular trophoblast,* which is exposed to maternal blood for purposes of mediating nutrient exchange, and *implantation site trophoblast,* which diffusely infiltrates the uterine lining (decidua) for purposes of anchoring the placenta to the mother.

One simple explanation for fetal survival is that trophoblast cells fail to express paternal MHC molecules. So far, class II molecules have not been detected on trophoblast. In mice, cells of the implantation trophoblast, but not vascular trophoblast, do express paternal class I molecules. In humans, the situation may be more complex, in that trophoblast cells may express only a non-polymorphic class I–like molecule. However, even if these cells do express classical MHC molecules, they may lack costimulator functions and fail to act as APCs.

A second explanation for lack of rejection is that the uterine decidua may be an immunologically privileged site that is not accessible to functional T cells. In support of this idea is the observation that mouse decidua is highly susceptible to infection by *Listeria monocytogenes* and cannot support a delayed type hypersensitivity response. The basis of immunologic privilege is clearly not a simple anatomic barrier because maternal blood is in extensive contact with trophoblast. Rather, the barrier is likely to be functional inhibition. Cultured decidual cells directly inhibit macrophage and T cell functions, perhaps by producing inhibitory cytokines such as transforming growth factor–β (see Chapter 11). Some of these inhibitory decidual cells may be resident suppressor T cells, although the evidence for this proposal is not convincing.

1. In order to stimulate a rejection reaction, host CD4[+] helper T cells are activated by foreign cells that express allogeneic class II molecules and provide costimulators. The CD4[+] T cells then stimulate the growth and differentiation of alloreactive CD8[+] CTLs.

2. The cells that provide such costimulatory functions are traditional APCs and are usually present as "passenger leukocytes" carried along with the graft.

3. Elimination of passenger leukocytes serves to reduce the incidence and severity of rejection, by reducing the activation of helper T cells.

Although the role of passenger leukocytes is well documented in rodents, attempts to remove such cells have not been useful in human transplantation. The probable explanation is that human, but not rodent, endothelial cells provide costimulator functions, activate alloreactive CD4[+] helper T cells, and are sufficient to initiate rejection even in the absence of passenger leukocytes.

In contrast to T cell alloreactivity, much less is known about the mechanisms that lead to the production of alloantibodies against foreign MHC molecules. Presumably, B cells specific for alloantigens are stimulated by mechanisms similar to those involved in stimulation of B cells reactive with other foreign proteins.

Before we conclude this section of the chapter, we should point out that many of the issues that arise in discussing alloreactivity and graft rejection are also relevant to maternal-fetal interactions. The fetus expresses paternal MHC molecules and is, therefore, semiallogeneic to the mother. Nevertheless, the fetus is not rejected by the maternal immune system. Many possible mechanisms have been proposed to account for this, and it is not yet clear which of these mechanisms are the most significant (Box 16–1, p. 323).

Effector Mechanisms in Allograft Rejection

So far we have described the molecular basis of allogeneic recognition and the cells involved in the recognition of and responses to allografts. We now turn to a consideration of the effector mechanisms used by the immune system to reject allografts. In different experimental models, alloreactive CD4[+] or CD8[+] T cells or specific alloantibodies are all capable of mediating allograft rejection upon adoptive transfer. Furthermore, graft rejection can be inhibited by anti-CD4 or anti-CD8 antibodies. It is now clear that these different immune effectors cause graft rejection by different mechanisms.

1. Alloreactive CD4[+] T cells can recruit and activate macrophages, initiating graft injury by a delayed type hypersensitivity (DTH) response (see Chapter 12).

2. Alloreactive CD8[+] T cells directly lyse graft endothelial and parenchymal cells.

3. Alloantibodies activate the complement system and injure graft blood vessels.

For historical reasons, graft rejection is usually classified on the basis of histopathology rather than on immune effector mechanisms. Based upon the experience of renal transplantation, the histopathologic pattern is called hyperacute, acute, or chronic.

The names of the various forms of rejection imply a temporal sequence of events, but this is not strictly true. Although hyperacute rejection is always a very rapid process immediately following transplantation, acute and chronic rejection can occur at almost any time after transplantation. Indeed, acute and chronic rejection often co-exist in the same graft. Histology, rather than the length of time following transplantation, is the major criterion for classifying rejection reactions. However, in the current era of renal transplantation, in many centers biopsies are performed less frequently than in the past and diagnosis is often made on the basis of clinical features and post-transplantation time without histologic confirmation.

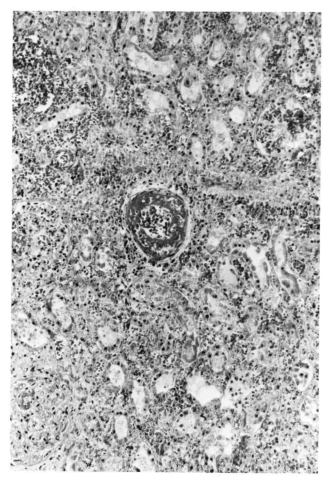

FIGURE 16 – 2. Hyperacute rejection in the kidney. Preformed antibodies reactive with vascular endothelium of a kidney allograft activate complement and trigger rapid intravascular thrombosis and necrosis of the vessel wall, often preceding the development of an inflammatory reaction. (Courtesy of Dr. Helmut Rennke, Department of Pathology, Brigham and Women's Hospital, Boston.)

HYPERACUTE REJECTION

Hyperacute rejection is characterized by rapid thrombotic occlusion of the graft vasculature that begins within minutes after host blood vessels are anastomosed to graft vessels (Fig. 16–2, p. 324). Thrombosis occurs prior to the development of inflammation. *Hyperacute rejection is mediated by pre-existing antibodies that bind to endothelium and activate complement.* The endothelial cells are stimulated to secrete high molecular weight forms of von Willebrand factor that mediate platelet adhesion and aggregation. Complement activation also leads to endothelial cell injury, initiation of coagulation, and exposure of subendothelial basement membrane proteins that activate platelets. These processes contribute to thrombosis and vascular occlusion, and the organ suffers irreversible ischemic damage.

In the early days of transplantation, hyperacute rejection was often mediated by pre-existing IgM antibodies which were present at high titer prior to any exposure to alloantigens. Such "natural antibodies" are believed to arise in response to carbohydrate antigens expressed by the bacteria that normally colonize the bowel. The best known examples of such antibodies are those directed against the ABO blood group antigens expressed on red blood cells (Box 16–2). ABO antigens are also expressed on vascular endothelial cells. Today, hyperacute rejection by anti-ABO antibodies is not a clinical problem because all graft donors and recipients are selected so that they have the same ABO type. However, less well characterized natural antibodies have become the major barrier to xenotransplantation across species, limiting the use of animal organs for human transplantation.

In the more recent clinical experience, hyperacute rejection of allografts is infrequent. When it does occur, it is usually mediated by antibodies directed against protein alloantigens such as foreign MHC molecules or against an incompletely described alloantigen system expressed on endothelial cells and blood monocytes but not lymphocytes, called E-M antigens. Such antibodies generally arise as a result of prior exposure to alloantigens through blood transfusion, prior transplantation, or multiple pregnancies. These alloantibodies are often of the IgG isotype. By testing recipients for the presence of such antibodies reactive with the cells of potential donors, hyperacute rejection has been virtually eliminated from clinical transplantation.

ACUTE REJECTION

ACUTE HUMORAL REJECTION.
Acute humoral rejection is characterized by necrosis of individual cells of the graft blood vessels. The histologic pattern is one of vasculitis (Fig. 16–3) rather than the bland thrombotic occlusion seen in hyperacute rejection. *Acute humoral rejection is often mediated by IgG antibodies against endothelial cell alloantigens (either MHC molecules or E-M antigens) and involves activation of com-*

BOX 16–2. ABO BLOOD GROUP ANTIGENS

The first alloantigen system to be defined was a family of red blood cell surface antigens called ABO. Differences in the ABO system between donors and recipients limit blood transfusions by causing antibody and complement-dependent lysis of the foreign red blood cells. IgM antibodies to these red blood cell antigens pre-exist in a naive host prior to transfusion, and it has been speculated that they arise as responses to cross-reactive microbial antigens. The red blood cell antigen responsible for these transfusion reactions is expressed as a cell surface glycosphingolipid. All normal individuals synthesize a common core glycan, called the O antigen, that is attached to a sphingolipid. A single genetic locus encodes three common alleles of a glycosyl transferase enzyme. The O allele gene product is devoid of enzymatic activity, whereas the A allele gene product transfers a terminal N-acetyl galactosamine moiety and the B allele gene product transfers a terminal galactose moiety. Individuals who are homozygous O cannot attach terminal sugars to the O antigen and express only the O antigen. In contrast, individuals who possess an A allele (AA homozygotes, AO heterozygotes or AB heterozygotes), form the A antigen by adding terminal N-acetyl galactosamine to some of their O antigens. Similarly, individuals who express a B allele (BB homozygotes, BO heterozygotes, or AB heterozygotes) form the B antigen by adding terminal galactose to some of their O antigens. AB heterozygotes form both A and B antigens from some of their O antigens. Because all individuals express the O antigen, all individuals are tolerant to the O antigen. Individuals with A or B glycosyl transferase alleles are also tolerant to A or B antigens, respectively. However, OO and AO individuals form anti-B IgM antibodies, whereas OO and BO individuals form anti-A IgM antibodies. If a patient receives a transfusion of red blood cells from a donor who expresses a form of the antigen not expressed on self red blood cells, massive red cell lysis will result. It follows that AB individuals can tolerate transfusions from all potential donors and are therefore called **universal recipients;** similarly, OO individuals can tolerate transfusions only from OO donors but can provide blood to all recipients and are therefore called **universal donors.** The terminology has been simplified so that OO individuals are said to be blood type O; AA and AO individuals are blood type A; BB and BO individuals are blood type B; and AB individuals are blood type AB.

The same glycosphingolipid that carries the ABO determinants can also be modified by other glycosyl transferases to generate minor blood group differences which elicit milder transfusion reactions. In general, differences in minor blood groups lead to red cell lysis only after repeated transfusions produce a secondary antibody response. Almost all individuals possess a fucosyl transferase that adds a fucose moiety to a side branch of the ABO glycosphingolipid. Upon fucosylation, the O antigen is technically called the H antigen and the whole antigenic system is often called ABH rather than ABO. Addition of fucose moieties at other side branch positions can be catalyzed by different fucosyl transferases and results in epitopes of the Lewis antigen system.

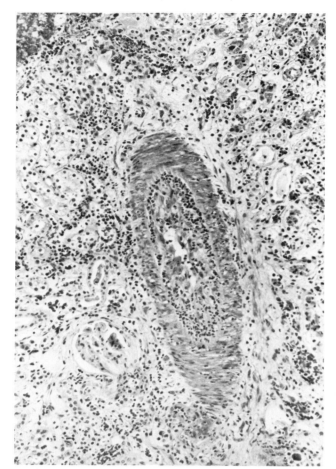

FIGURE 16 – 3. Acute vascular rejection in the kidney. *Antibodies reactive with graft endothelial cells arise in a transplant recipient and cause a destructive inflammatory reaction in the vessel wall. T lymphocytes reactive with graft alloantigens may also participate in vascular injury. (Courtesy of Dr. Helmut Rennke, Department of Pathology, Brigham and Women's Hospital, Boston.)*

undergoing acute cellular rejection are markedly enriched for CD8+ CTLs specific for graft alloantigens. Second, cloned lines of alloreactive CD8+ CTLs can be used to adoptively transfer acute cellular graft rejection. And third, most vascular and parenchymal cells express class I MHC molecules and are susceptible to lysis by CD8+ CTLs but are usually resistant to killing by activated macrophages and NK cells.

The identification of both antibody and CTLs as important effector mechanisms in acute graft rejection suggests that this process is similar to normal anti-viral immune responses (see Chapter 15). The basis of this similarity probably arises from the fact that the foreign class I MHC molecules present in the graft are recognized as if they were self MHC molecules associated with endogenously synthesized, e.g., viral, peptides.

CHRONIC REJECTION

Chronic rejection is characterized by fibrosis with loss of normal organ structures (Fig. 16 – 5). The

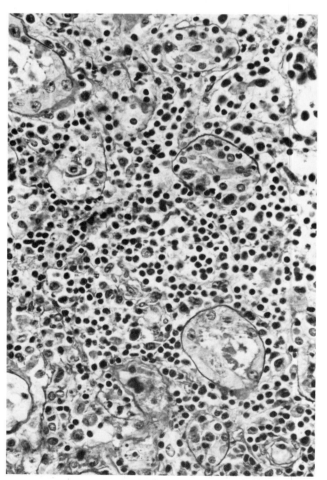

FIGURE 16 – 4. Acute cellular rejection in the kidney. *T lymphocytes reactive with alloantigens in a kidney graft mediate necrosis of tubular epithelial cells as well as of interstitial cells and microvascular endothelial cells. (Courtesy of Dr. Helmut Rennke, Department of Pathology, Brigham and Women's Hospital, Boston.)*

plement. Because lymphocytes may also be involved, an alternative and more accurate name for this process is **acute vascular rejection.** Lymphocytes may contribute by responding to alloantigens present on vascular endothelial cells, leading to direct lysis of these cells, or they may produce cytokines that activate inflammatory cells, causing endothelial necrosis.

ACUTE CELLULAR REJECTION. This type of rejection is characterized by necrosis of parenchymal cells and is usually accompanied by lymphocyte and macrophage infiltrates (Fig. 16 – 4). These infiltrating leukocytes are responsible for the lysis of the graft parenchymal cells. *Several different effector mechanisms may be involved in acute cellular rejection including CTL-mediated lysis, activated macrophage-mediated lysis (as in delayed type hypersensitivity [DTH]), and natural killer (NK) cell-mediated lysis (see Chapter 12). Several lines of evidence suggest that recognition and lysis of foreign cells by alloreactive CD8+ CTLs is probably the most important mechanism in acute cellular rejection.* First, the cellular infiltrates that are present in grafts pathogenesis of chronic rejection is less well understood than that of acute rejection. The fibrosis of chronic rejection may represent wound healing following the cellular necrosis of acute rejection. However, in many instances, chronic rejection develops without evidence that acute rejection ever occurred. Two other possible explanations of the fibrosis are that chronic rejection represents a form of chronic DTH in which activated macrophages secrete mesenchymal cell growth factors such as platelet-derived growth factor (see Chapter 12) or, alternatively, that chronic rejection is a response to chronic ischemia caused by injury to blood vessels. Vascular injury could result from repeated bouts of antibody-mediated acute humoral rejection, or it may result from cell-mediated injury of microvascular endothelial cells. The stimulus for fibrosis as a result of ischemia is not precisely known.

A variant form of chronic rejection, characterized by proliferation of intimal smooth muscle cells in the walls of muscular arteries, has been described in renal

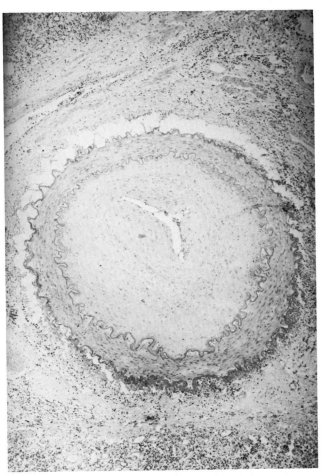

FIGURE 16–6. *Transplant associated accelerated arteriosclerosis in the kidney. In this variant of chronic rejection, the vascular lumen is replaced by accumulation of smooth muscle cells and connective tissue in the vessel intima.*

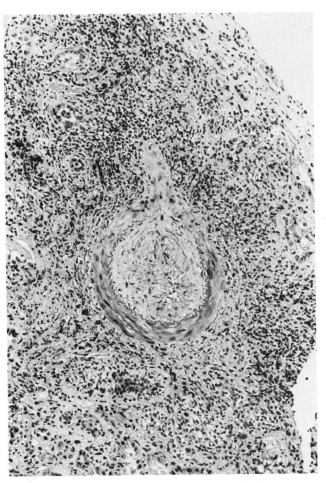

FIGURE 16–5. *Chronic rejection in the kidney. The normal cells of the renal interstitium and tubules are replaced by fibrous tissue. As described in the text, this reaction may represent healing of acute rejection, chronic delayed type hypersensitivity to graft alloantigens, or chronic ischemia. (Courtesy of Dr. Helmut Rennke, Department of Pathology, Brigham and Women's Hospital, Boston.)*

and cardiac transplants (Fig. 16–6). This accelerated arteriosclerosis is the major cause of late graft loss as the involved vessels become completely occluded. In many cases, there is no histologic evidence of prior arterial injury. The smooth muscle cell proliferation in the vascular intima may represent a specialized form of chronic DTH, in which lymphocytes activated by alloantigens in the graft vessel wall induce macrophages to secrete smooth muscle cell growth factors. This is similar to the proposed model of chronic rejection as a form of chronic DTH, except that in the vessel wall smooth muscle cells rather than fibroblasts proliferate and produce collagen.

Prevention and Treatment of Allograft Rejection

If the recipient of an allograft has a fully functional immune system, transplantation almost invariably results in some form of rejection. Two approaches have been used in clinical practice and in experimental models to avoid or delay rejection:

1. *The graft may be made less immunogenic.*

a. In rodents, as discussed above, this may be accomplished by elimination of passenger leukocytes from grafts, an approach that has not worked in humans and other primates.

b. In human transplantation, the major strategy to reduce graft immunogenicity has been to minimize alloantigenic differences between the donor and recipient by selection. For example, to avoid hyperacute rejection, the ABO blood group antigens of the donor and recipient are always compatible. In addition, MHC molecule allelic differences are also considered at both class I and class II loci. For kidney transplantation, all potential donors and recipients are "tissue-typed" to determine the identity of the HLA molecules that are expressed (Box 16–3). Good matches, involving identity at three or four alleles out of four HLA–A,B loci, are favored. Matching is possible because donor kidneys can be stored in organ banks prior to transplantation until a well-matched recipient can be identified and because, with dialysis, patients needing a kidney allograft can be clinically treated until a well-matched organ is available. In the case of heart and liver transplantation, organ preservation is more difficult and potential recipients are

often in critical condition. For these reasons, HLA typing is simply not considered in pairing of potential donors and recipients.

2. *The donor's immune system may be suppressed.* Immunosuppression is the major approach to prevention and management of transplant rejection. Several methods of immunosuppression are commonly used.

a. *Levels of preformed antibodies, such as those that mediate hyperacute rejection, can be reduced by plasmapheresis.* (Plasmapheresis is the removal of blood plasma *ex vivo* and return of washed cells to the body.) Plasmapheresis can also be employed to treat acute humoral rejection, but this has proved to be less successful.

b. *Tolerance to allografts may be induced prior to transplantation by exposure to alloantigens through blood transfusion.* Such transfusions may induce T or B cell tolerance, i.e., may inactivate alloreactive T or B cells, or may stimulate other cells that inhibit alloreactivity.

c. *T cells may be inhibited or lysed by various immunosuppressive treatments. Immunosuppressive drugs are the principal treatment regimen for graft rejection.* Commonly used immunosuppressive therapies include corticosteroids, metabolic toxins, such as azathioprine and cyclophosphamide; irradiation of lymphoid organs; specific immunosuppressive drugs, the prototype of which is cyclosporin A (also known

---

BOX 16–3. TISSUE TYPING

Tissue typing, also called HLA typing, is the determination of the particular MHC alleles expressed by an individual. The classic approach to tissue or HLA typing is testing whether sera collected from certain donors mediate complement-dependent lysis of an individual's lymphocytes. The sera used for this purpose are obtained from donors who have been inadvertently immunized with foreign cells bearing MHC molecules by transfusion, transplantation, or multiple pregnancies. Such sera characteristically have a low specific antibody titer and react with multiple foreign MHC molecules encoded by several loci. To determine whether an individual expresses HLA–A2, for example, lymphocytes would be tested with a panel of sera, each of which can recognize HLA–A2 bearing cells but may differ in the other specificities they recognize. Only if all of the appropriate sera react and cause lysis is the individual "typed" as HLA–A2 positive. Naturally, well-characterized human sera are in short supply. Therefore the assays have been honed to a microscale, where 1 μl of serum plus 1 μl of complement can be tested against 50 target cells in 3 μl of solution in the bottom of a tiny well, kept from evaporating by an overlaid oil drop! In general, tissue typing is still performed this way using standardized sera that have been tested and characterized by many different laboratories. It is hoped that conventional typing sera will be replaced by monoclonal antibodies reactive with specific HLA molecules. Unfortunately, these reagents are not yet available for most specificities.

The HLA types defined by serologic methods are not necessarily single alleles. Some common HLA types contain several different closely related alleles that may be "split" as new reagents become available that can distinguish among them. Typing

with antibodies for class II alleles is especially imprecise. Alloreactive T cells often recognize some but not all of the cells that are said to share a DR specificity. The information from secondary MLRs can thus be useful at splitting class II types. Interestingly, some of the T cell responses that are used to split DR types are actually directed against DQ molecules present in linkage disequilibrium with a subset of the DR molecules within a type.

Recently, two new approaches have been introduced that should permit more precise typing of the class II loci, replacing both serology and secondary MLRs. The first approach takes advantage of the fact that serologically similar MHC allelic products may be biochemically quite different and can be separated by an analytical technique such as two-dimensional gel electrophoresis combining isoelectric focusing and sodium dodecyl sulfate–polyacrylamide gel electrophoresis (SDS-PAGE) (see Box 3–3, Chapter 3). The position of a "spot" on a two-dimensional gel can thus be used to split a serologic type. The second method is even more precise. The polymorphic residues of class II MHC molecules are largely located within exon 2 of both the α and β chains (i.e., within the α1 and β1 polypeptide regions; see Chapter 5). This entire region of the gene can be amplified by **polymerase chain reaction (PCR)** methods using primers that bind to conserved sequences within the 5' and 3' ends of these exons. The amplified segment of DNA can then be readily sequenced. Thus the actual predicted amino acid sequence can be directly determined for the HLA–DR, DQ, and DP alleles of any cell, providing precise molecular tissue typing. Indeed, it is exactly for this purpose that the method of polymerase chain reaction was initially developed by Henry Erlich and colleagues.

as cyclosporine); and antibodies reactive with T cell surface molecules.

Corticosteroids have two proposed mechanisms of action. First, they may cause selective lysis of T cells. Corticosteroids are known to cause lysis of immature cortical thymocytes as well as certain T cell lines by activating endogenous nucleases that cleave DNA. However, corticosteroids do not lyse mature medullary thymocytes or mature T cells isolated from blood or peripheral lymphoid organs. A second and more likely proposed mechanism is that corticosteroids act by blocking cytokine gene transcription in and cytokine secretion from mononuclear phagocytes. Inhibition of IL–1, IL–6 and tumor necrosis factor (TNF) synthesis by corticosteroids has been demonstrated both *in vitro* and *in vivo*. Lack of IL–1 and TNF will limit the development of inflammatory reactions. Moreover, IL–1, TNF, and IL–6 may be important costimulators of T cell activation and their relative deficiency may impair specific immunity.

The metabolic toxins in clinical use, namely azathioprine and cyclophosphamide, inhibit the growth of lymphocytes (and other leukocytes) from hematopoietic precursors and may cause preferential lysis of T cells. Irradiation was similarly used as an immunosuppressive agent because T cells are radiosensitive.

The most important immunosuppressive agent in current clinical use is cyclosporin A. Cyclosporin A is a cyclic peptide that is found as a natural metabolite in a species of fungus. The major action of cyclosporin A on T cells is to inhibit transcription of certain genes, most notably the IL–2 gene. Cyclosporin A binds with high affinity to a ubiquitous small molecular size (approximately 12 kilodaltons [kD]) cellular protein called cyclophilin. Cyclophilin has recently been found to have an enzymatic activity that is to catalyze *cis-trans* isomerizations around proline imide bonds in proteins; this peptidyl-prolyl isomerase, or "rotamase," activity serves to catalyze the correct folding of proteins. Cyclosporin A binds to the active site of cyclophilin and blocks catalytic activity. Cyclophilin is not a DNA–binding protein, and it is not known whether or how cyclophilin participates in gene transcription. It is speculated that cyclophilin normally functions to catalyze the proper folding of a positively activating transcription factor and that cyclosporin A blocks this activity. At least two separate DNA–binding proteins that interact with the 5' regulatory sequences of the IL–2 gene are inhibited in cyclosporin A–treated T cells.

Regardless of its precise mechanism of action, the consequence of cyclosporin A treatment is a profound inhibition of cell-mediated immunity. In the absence of adequate IL–2 and other cytokines, T cells fail to mount an effective immune response. IL–2 is essential for T cell growth and contributes to CTL differentiation. Other T cell genes inhibited by cyclosporin A include *c-myc* and IFN–γ; the failure of these genes to be expressed may also contribute to lack of T cell growth and effector cell activation, respectively.

The introduction of cyclosporin A into clinical practice opened the modern era of transplantation. Prior to the use of cyclosporin A, the majority of transplanted hearts and livers were rejected. Nevertheless, cyclosporin A is not a panacea for transplantation. Drug levels needed for optimal immunosuppression cause kidney damage. For this reason, there is much excitement about a newly characterized fungal metabolite called FK506. FK506 is structurally unrelated to cyclosporin A, but it also binds to a rotamase that catalyzes isomerization about proline imide bonds. The FK506 binding protein, however, is different from cyclophilin. Strikingly, FK506 shares with cyclosporin A the ability to selectively inhibit the transcription of cytokine and certain other genes in T cells. FK506 is active at lower concentrations than cyclosporin A and it may be less toxic. It should be noted, however, that cyclosporin A was also thought to be nontoxic when it was introduced. Nevertheless, FK506, either alone or in combination with cyclosporin A, may expand the scope of clinical transplantation.

Antibodies reactive with T cell surface structures are important agents for treating acute rejection episodes. In the 1960s, commonly used agents for this purpose were polyclonal horse antisera reactive with human lymphocytes or thymocytes. Since the 1980s, mouse monoclonal antibodies to specific T cell surface markers have been more commonly used. The most widely used antibody is OKT3, the first anti-CD3 antibody. It may seem surprising that one would use a potential polyclonal activator such as anti-CD3 to reduce T cell reactivity. *In vivo*, however, OKT3 acts either as a lytic antibody, activating the complement system to eliminate T cells, or opsonizes T cells for phagocytosis. Those T cells that escape probably do so by capping and endocytosing ("modulating") CD3 off their surface, but these may be rendered transiently nonfunctional. Newer antibodies are being tested for immunosuppressive effects without causing T cell elimination. For example, antibodies to the p55 subunit of the IL–2 receptor are in clinical trial because these antibodies can prevent T cell activation by blocking IL–2 binding to activated T cells. The major limitation on the use of mouse monoclonal antibodies is that human recipients rapidly develop anti-mouse Ig antibodies that eliminate the injected mouse Ig. For this reason, attempts are being made to produce human monoclonal antibodies or human-mouse chimeric antibodies that may be less immunogenic.

In addition to these accepted methods of immunosuppression, newer experimental approaches are also in development. One is the use of soluble allogeneic MHC molecules or fragments of MHC molecules to tolerize recipients against specific donor alloantigens. Such peptides are thought to bind competitively to the antigen receptors of alloreactive T cells. A second approach, which has been effective in animal models, is the use of protein toxins, such as diphtheria toxin or ricin A chain, targeted to activated T cells. Targeting can be achieved by conjugating protein toxins to anti-T cell antibodies or by generating fusion proteins. For example, an IL–2-diphtheria toxin hybrid protein blocks the rejection of allografts in rats by binding to and killing T cells bearing IL – 2 receptors. The targeted toxin approach has a theoretical advantage over more conventional monoclonal antibody therapy, in that toxins may mediate more effective elimination of targeted cells, providing more sustained immunosuppression. In addition, a single dose of such toxins may be effective, so that neutralizing host antibodies do not develop. It remains to be seen if toxins, even when targeted, can be used without serious side effects.

Interestingly, in experimental models, if acute allograft rejection is prevented, the graft continues to survive and function even after immunosuppressive therapy is curtailed. It has been postulated that the reason for this is that the recipient becomes tolerant to graft alloantigens or that "suppressor cells" specific for the alloantigens are induced. The relevance of this to human transplantation is uncertain because in humans maintenance immunosuppressive therapy has to be continued permanently.

CLINICAL ORGAN TRANSPLANTATION

We now turn our attention to some of the important clinical issues that have arisen in the practice of solid organ transplantation. Kidney transplants have been successfully performed for the longest period (since the 1950s), and the renal allograft experience has formed the basis of considering transplantation of other organs. For this reason, our discussion will focus on the kidney, but will refer to other organs for comparison when appropriate.

Selection of donor and recipient matches in renal transplantation is based on blood group (ABO) matching, absence of pre-formed antibodies against donor cells in the blood of the recipient (called cross-matching), and human leukocyte antigen (HLA) typing. Analysis of the results of graft survival as a function of HLA type has led to four conclusions:

1. The larger the number of HLA – A and B alleles that are matched between donor and recipient (e.g., three or four of four loci), the better is graft survival, especially in the first year following transplantation. (HLA – C is not routinely matched and is believed to be less important as a target of T cell recognition.)

2. Matches at HLA – DR alleles are important, independent of the number of HLA – A,B matches. Because HLA – DR and DQ are in strong linkage disequilibrium, matching at the DR locus often also matches at the DQ locus. DP typing is not in common use and its importance is unknown.

3. Matching is more predictive of outcome in Europe, where populations are more inbred, than in the United States, where extensive outbreeding has probably diminished linkage disequilibrium among HLA loci.

4. The recipient HLA – DR types influence graft survival independent of the degree of matching. This effect of HLA – DR type of the recipient has been interpreted as an "immune response" gene effect, presumably because host HLA – DR molecules were involved in selecting the mature T cell repertoire. Thus, in recipients who express particular DR alleles, the T cell repertoire may not contain cells specific for some alloantigens, so that grafts bearing these antigens would fail to induce immune responses and would be accepted.

In renal transplantation, immunosuppression with corticosteroids, azathioprine, and anti – T cell antibodies was sufficient to allow survival of unrelated cadaveric donor grafts of 50 to 60 per cent at 1 year and survival of living related donor grafts of 90 per cent at one year. Since cyclosporin A has been introduced, survival of unrelated cadaveric donor grafts has approached about 80 per cent.

In the early years of renal transplantation, rejection was often assessed by biopsy. In the 1970s, biopsy was used less commonly in many transplant centers and rejection severity was usually assessed by following renal function, e.g., as measured by plasma creatinine levels. However, cyclosporin A, which is now universally used in kidney transplantation, is itself a cause of renal injury and can elevate plasma creatinine levels. Thus, a common clinical dilemma is to distinguish declining renal function caused by rejection from that caused by cyclosporin A toxicity. This is usually done by histopathologic examination of biopsy specimens of the transplanted kidney. A useful distinction may be made by examining kidney cells collected by needle biopsy or fine needle aspiration biopsy with an immunocytochemical stain for class II MHC molecule expression. If renal tubular cells express HLA – DR molecules, one may infer that IFN – γ is being produced locally by activated T cells and that renal failure is likely due to rejection. If, on the other hand, HLA – DR is not expressed by tubular cells, the kidney is apparently failing in the absence of local T cell cytokine production and the likely cause is cyclosporin A toxicity. (The functional role or consequence of class II MHC molecule expression on renal tubular cells is unknown.)

Monitoring the rejection of other transplanted organs is somewhat different. Liver allograft rejection can often be measured by assessing liver functions; cyclosporin A is not as toxic to the liver, and failure of bile excretion is a good measure of rejection. Needle biopsies may be used if the clinical pattern is confusing, and expression of HLA – DR molecules by biliary epithelial cells may be indicative of rejection. In the case of heart allografts, functional impairment usually indicates that the rejection process is already quite severe and potentially irreversible. For this reason, cardiac allograft biopsies are performed on regular schedules to assess rejection regardless of cardiac function. (Such biopsy specimens are obtained through a catheter passed into the right ventricle via the venous circulation. Biopsies of the intraventricular septum may be taken with little risk to the patient, since even punctures of the septum will likely scar without sequelae.) Studies are currently in progress to learn whether these histologic and functional tests may be supplemented or replaced by serologic assays of T cell activation, such as the presence of shed p55 subunit of the IL–2 receptor in the blood.

Acute rejection, when present, is often managed by rapidly intensifying immunosuppressive therapy. This may involve a large "pulse" of corticosteroids or administration of an antibody such as OKT3. Cyclosporin A doses can also be increased. Although acute rejection can cause loss of a graft, most rejection episodes can be reversed by such therapeutic intervention. In modern transplantation, chronic rejection has become the more common cause of allograft failure, especially in cardiac transplantation. Chronic rejection is more insidious than acute rejection, and it is much less reversible. It seems likely that prevention rather than treatment will be the best approach to this problem, but successful intervention will probably require a better understanding of pathogenesis.

Graft survival is dependent upon adequate immunosuppression. This has introduced a clinical dilemma because transplant patients often manifest two other clinical problems caused by immunosuppressive therapy. First, they are particularly susceptible to infections, especially by viruses. Infection by cytomegalovirus, a herpes family virus, is particularly common and may be fatal in the immunosuppressed patient. Second, transplant patients have an increased proclivity to development of certain tumors (see Chapter 17). The three malignancies commonly seen in these patients are B cell lymphomas, squamous cell carcinoma of the skin, and Kaposi's sarcoma. The B cell lymphomas are thought to be sequelae of unchecked infection by Epstein-Barr virus (EBV), another herpes family virus. EBV is a polyclonal activator of B cells, and such polyclonal proliferations appear to predispose to development of monoclonally derived malignant cells (see Chapter 17, Box 17–2). The squamous cell carcinomas of the skin are associated with human papilloma virus and probably also represent virally induced malignancies. Kaposi's sarcoma is now well known for its prevalence in patients with the acquired immunodeficiency syndrome (AIDS) (see Chapter 19) and may be yet another example of a virally induced or provoked malignancy.

In patients receiving immunosuppression for transplantation, clinical problems related to viral infection and virally induced or virally potentiated malignancies are not coincidental. The major thrust of transplant-related immunosuppression is to reduce CTL function, the key effector mechanism of acute cellular rejection. It should thus be no surprise that defense against viruses, the physiologic function of CTLs, is preferentially undermined.

BONE MARROW TRANSPLANTATION

Bone marrow transplantation is really the transplantation of pluripotent hematopoietic stem cells (see Chapter 2). Upon transplantation, these cells then repopulate the recipient's bone marrow with their differentiating progeny. Clinically, allogeneic bone marrow transplantation may be used to remedy acquired defects in the hematopoietic system or in the immune system, since both types of cells develop from a common stem cell. It has also been proposed as a means of correcting inherited enzyme deficiencies, by providing a self-renewing source of enzyme-producing cells. In addition, allogeneic bone marrow transplantation may be used as part of the treatment of bone marrow malignancies, i.e., leukemias. In this case, the chemotherapeutic agents needed to destroy leukemia cells also destroy normal marrow elements and bone marrow transplantation is used to "rescue" the patient from the side effects of chemotherapy. For other malignancies, when the marrow is not involved by tumor or when it can be purged of tumor cells, the patient's own bone marrow may be harvested and reinfused after chemotherapy. This procedure, called autologous bone marrow transplantation, lacks the immunologic problems associated with allogeneic bone marrow transplantation and will not be discussed further.

There are several unique problems associated with allogeneic bone marrow transplantation that lead us to consider it separately from solid organ transplantation:

1. The transplanted stem cells must "home" to establish themselves in the appropriate environment; surgeons cannot "place" the stem cells in a particular location in the bone marrow. Moreover, experimental and clinical experience suggests that there are only a limited number of "niches" within marrow cavities and if these are occupied at the time of transplantation, the graft cells cannot establish themselves. The recipient often must be "prepared" with intense radiation and chemotherapy prior to transplantation to deplete his or her own marrow cells and vacate these sites.

2. Allogeneic stem cells are readily rejected by even a minimally immunocompetent host. The mechanisms of rejection are not completely known, but it has been suggested that in addition to specific immune mechanisms, hematopoietic stem cells may also be rejected by NK cells. The recipient's immune system must be nearly ablated to permit successful bone marrow transplantation. Again, this is accomplished by intense "preparation" of the recipient with radiation and chemotherapy.

3. Graft cells may mount a rejection response against the host. This response, called the **graft-versus-host reaction,** can injure the host and cause graft-versus-host disease (GVHD) (see below). The graft-versus-host reaction arises only in the setting of extreme injury to the host immune system, a consequence of the preparation necessary to avoid stem cell rejection.

4. Recipients of allogeneic bone marrow transplants often show prolonged and profound immunodeficiencies. In human bone marrow transplantation, this is a major cause of morbidity and mortality.

Graft-versus-Host Disease

Graft-versus-host disease is the principal limitation on the use of bone marrow transplantation. As in solid organ transplantation, GVHD may be classified on the basis of histologic patterns into acute and chronic categories.

Acute GVHD involves epithelial cell necrosis in three principal target organs, skin, liver, and the gastrointestinal tract (Fig. 16–7). In the liver, the biliary epithelial cells but not the hepatocytes are involved. Clinically, acute GVHD is characterized by skin rash, jaundice, and diarrhea. When the epithelial necrosis is extensive, the skin or lining of the gut may simply slough off. In this circumstance, acute GVHD may be fatal.

Chronic GVHD is characterized by fibrosis and atrophy of one or more of the same organs, without evidence of acute cell necrosis (Fig. 16–7). On occasion, necrosis and fibrosis can be present at the same time, leading to a diagnosis of acute and chronic GVHD. When severe, chronic GVHD leads to complete dysfunction of the affected organ and may also be fatal.

In animal models, acute GVHD is initiated by ma-ture T cells present in the bone marrow inoculum. Elimination of mature donor T cells from the graft can prevent development of GVHD. Efforts to eliminate T cells from human marrow inoculum have reduced the incidence of GVHD, but also appear to reduce the efficiency of engraftment; mature T cells, perhaps through production of IL–3 and other colony-stimulating factors (CSFs), significantly improve stem cell repopulation. Since failure to engraft is even more lethal than GVHD, it is not yet clear whether the removal of T cells will be clinically beneficial. An alternative approach in current clinical trial is to combine removal of T cells with supplemental IL–3 and/or granulocyte-macrophage colony-stimulating factor (GM–CSF) to promote engraftment.

Although GVHD is initiated by T cell recognition of host alloantigens, the effector cells that produce epithelial cell necrosis are less well defined. Histologically, NK cells are often attached to the dying epithelial cells, suggesting that NK cells are the effector cells of acute GVHD. This has raised the issue of how NK cells lyse normal epithelial cells, since they do not recognize alloantigens and cannot lyse epithelial cells *in vitro*. It has been proposed that the NK cells are activated by locally produced IL–2 to differentiate into lymphokine-activated killer (LAK) cells. As we

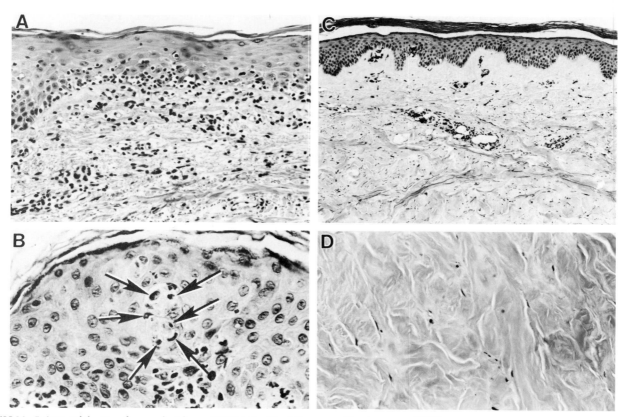

FIGURE 16–7. Acute and chronic graft-versus-host disease (GVHD) in the skin. *At low magnification, acute GVHD appears as a sparse lymphocytic infiltrate at the dermal-epidermal junction (A); at higher magnification (B), lymphocytes can be identified in the epidermis adjacent to injured epithelial cells (arrows). In contrast, chronic GVHD (C) shows fibrosis of the dermis and epidermal thinning. At higher magnification (D), dermal appendages can be seen to be trapped in the dense fibrosis. (Courtesy of Dr. George Murphy, Departments of Dermatology and Pathology, University of Pennsylvania, Philadelphia.)*

discussed in Chapter 12, LAK cells can lyse normal cell types, including epithelium, and are not restricted by MHC molecules.

The relationship of chronic GVHD to acute GVHD is unknown and raises issues similar to those of relating chronic allograft rejection to acute allograft rejection. For example, chronic GVHD may represent the fibrosis of wound healing secondary to epithelial cell necrosis. However, chronic GVHD can arise without evidence of prior acute GVHD. An alternative explanation is that chronic GVHD may represent a response to ischemia caused by vascular injury.

Both acute and chronic GVHD are commonly treated with intense immunosuppression. It is not clear that either condition responds very well. A possible explanation is that conventional immunosuppression is targeted against T lymphocytes, especially CTLs. This works well in allogeneic rejection of solid organs, but is less efficacious for NK cell–mediated or LAK cell–mediated responses. Much effort has focused on prevention of GVHD. HLA typing is very important for preventing GVHD. Indeed, most human bone marrow transplants are performed between siblings who are completely identical at all HLA loci and clinical GVHD is due to differences at minor histocompatibility loci. Transplantation between parent and child may be performed when necessary, but only with stringent elimination of mature T cells.

Immunodeficiency Following Bone Marrow Transplantation

As noted above, bone marrow transplantation is often accompanied by clinical immunodeficiency. Several factors may contribute to defective immune responses in recipients:

1. Bone marrow transplant recipients may be unable to regenerate a completely new T cell repertoire. The transplanted bone marrow may not contain a sufficient number and variety of self-renewing lymphoid progenitors, and the thymus gland of the recipient may have undergone irreversible changes during or after involution in early childhood.

2. The ablation of the specific immune system in preparation for bone marrow transplantation unmasks a "natural suppression" system that prevents adequate regeneration of a specific immune system. Some immunologists have referred to specific populations of "natural suppressor" cells, observed after whole body irradiation. Such natural suppressor cells may be identical or related in lineage to NK cells.

3. The allogeneic host environment may overwhelm the developing immune system with alloantigenic stimuli that prevent development of a normal repertoire. An alternative statement of this explanation is that the graft-versus-host reaction pre-empts normal immunity. Many immunologists regard immunodeficiency as part of GVHD. However, immunodeficiency may well exist in bone marrow transplant recipients who lack clinically overt or histologically detectable GVHD.

The consequence of immunodeficiency is that bone marrow transplant recipients are very susceptible to viral infections, especially with cytomegalovirus. They are also susceptible to EBV–provoked B cell lymphomas. However, there has not been an increased incidence of other malignancies, namely squamous cell carcinoma of the skin and Kaposi's sarcoma, noted in solid organ transplant recipients. The basis for this difference is unclear.

SUMMARY

Transplantation of tissues from one individual to a genetically nonidentical recipient leads to a specific immune response, called rejection, that can destroy the graft. The major molecular targets in transplant rejection are non–self allelic forms of class I and class II MHC molecules.

The reaction to foreign class I and class II molecules can be analyzed in vitro in the MLR. In general, foreign class I molecules stimulate alloreactive CD8+ CTLs whereas foreign class II molecules stimulate alloreactive CD4+ helper T lymphocytes, although the largest reactions occur when there are differences at both class I and class II loci.

In vivo, rejection is mediated by antibodies and by CTLs. Help, provided by CD4+ T cells, is often necessary to initiate the rejection reaction. Alloreactive CD4+ T cells may be stimulated by foreign class II MHC–positive APCs in the graft.

Several patterns of rejection can occur in solid organ transplants. Pre-existing antibodies, often IgM directed against ABO antigens on endothelial cells, can cause hyperacute rejection characterized by thrombosis of graft vessels. Antibodies produced in response to the graft cause blood vessel cell necrosis, called acute humoral or vascular rejection. Infiltrating alloreactive CTLs cause parenchymal cell necrosis, called acute cellular rejection. Chronic rejection, characterized by fibrosis, may represent healing of acute rejection or may represent a chronic delayed type hypersensitivity reaction. A variant of chronic rejection in the walls of muscular arteries can produce accelerated arteriosclerosis and ischemic injury of the graft.

Rejection may be minimized by reducing the immunogenicity of the graft, often by limiting the number of differences between donor and recipient MHC alleles. Rejection is both prevented and treated by immunosuppression. The most commonly used immunosuppressive drugs are agents that reduce T cell function and number. Such agents include corticosteroids; cytotoxic drugs with specificity for T cells, such as azathioprine; immunosuppressive drugs, such as cyclosporin A; and antibodies directed against T cell surface molecules.

Patients receiving solid organ transplants may

experience complications related to their therapy. These include viral infections, especially with cytomegalovirus, and virus-related malignancies, such as B cell lymphoma, squamous cell carcinoma of the skin, and Kaposi's sarcoma.

Bone marrow transplant recipients are very susceptible to graft rejection and require intense preparatory immunosuppression. In addition, two unique problems not seen with solid organ transplants may develop. First, lymphocytes in the bone marrow graft may respond to alloantigens of the host, producing GVHD. Acute GVHD is characterized by epithelial cell necrosis in the skin, liver, and gut, causing a rash, jaundice, and diarrhea, respectively. When severe, acute GVHD may be fatal. Chronic GVHD is characterized by fibrosis and atrophy of one or more of these same target organs and may also be fatal. Second, bone marrow transplant recipients often have immunodeficiencies, rendering them susceptible to infections.

SELECTED READINGS

Auchincloss, H., Jr., T. Mayer, R. M. Ghobrial, and H. J. Winn. T cell subsets, b^m mutants, and the mechanism of allogeneic skin graft rejection. Immunologic Research 8:149–164, 1989.

Borel, J. F. Pharmacology of cyclosporine (Sandimmune). IV. Pharmacological properties *in vivo*. Pharmacological Reviews 41:259–371, 1989.

Busch, G. J., E. S. Reynolds, E. G. Galvanek, W. E. Braun, and G. J. Dammin. Human renal allografts: the role of vascular injury in early graft failure. Medicine 50:29–83, 1971.

Clift R., and R. Storb. Histoincompatible bone marrow transplants in humans. Annual Review of Immunology 5:43–64, 1987.

Faustman, D., V. Hauptfeld, P. Lacy, and J. Davie. Prolongation of murine islet allograft survival by pretreatment of islets with antibody directed to Ia determinants. Proceedings of the National Academy of Sciences USA 78:5156–5159, 1981.

Ferrara, J. L. M., and S. J. Burakoff. The pathophysiology of acute graft-vs.-host disease in a murine bone marrow transplant model. *In* Burakoff, S. J., H. J. Deeg, J. L. M. Ferrara, and K. Atkinson (eds.). Graft-vs.-Host Disease: Immunology, Pathophysiology and Treatment. New York, Marcel Dekker, Inc., 1990, pp. 9–30.

Kahan, B. D. Cyclosporine. New England Journal of Medicine 321:1725–1738, 1989.

Krensky, A. M., A. Weiss, G. Crabtree, M. M. Davis, and P. Parham. T-lymphocyte–antigen interactions in transplant rejection. New England Journal of Medicine 322:510–517, 1990.

Lafferty, K. J., S. J. Prawse, R. J. Simeonovic, and H. S. Warren. Immunobiology of transplantation. Annual Review of Immunology 1:143–173, 1983.

Lechler, R. I., G. Lombardi, J. R. Batchelor, N. Reinsmoen, and F. H. Bach. The molecular basis of alloreactivity. Immunology Today 11:83–88, 1990.

Mason, D. W., and P. J. Morris. Effector mechanisms in allograft rejection. Annual Review of Immunology 4:119–145, 1986.

CHAPTER SEVENTEEN

IMMUNITY

TO

TUMORS

Malignant tumors, or cancers, grow in an uncontrolled manner, invade normal tissues, and often metastasize and grow at sites distant from the tissue of origin. In general, cancers are derived from one or only a few normal cells that have undergone a poorly understood process called malignant transformation. Cancers can arise from almost any tissue in the body. Those derived from epithelial cells, called carcinomas, are the most common kinds of cancers. Sarcomas are malignant tumors of mesenchymal tissues, arising from cells such as fibroblasts, muscle cells, and fat cells. Solid malignant tumors of lymphoid tissues are called lymphomas, and marrow and blood-borne malignant tumors of lymphocytes and other hematopoietic cells are called leukemias.

Hypothetically, a major function of the immune system could be to recognize and destroy spontaneously arising malignantly transformed cells, so-called "mutant clones," before they grow into tumors. This idea, called **immunosurveillance,** was articulated by Macfarlane Burnet and Lewis Thomas in the 1950s and 1960s. In addition, immune responses to malignant cells may be protective even after these cells have grown into tumors. If malignant cells and tumors can stimulate immune responses, it follows that they must express **tumor antigens** that are recognized as foreign by the tumor-bearing host. Furthermore, if the concept of immunosurveillance is valid, immune effector cells, such as B cells, helper T cells, cytolytic T lymphocytes (CTLs), or natural killer (NK) cells must be able to recognize tumor antigens and mediate the killing of tumor cells.

A common histologic observation which suggests that tumors may be immunogenic is the presence of mononuclear cell infiltrates, composed of T cells, NK cells, and macrophages, surrounding many tumors. Although such infiltrates may often result after tissue destruction caused by the tumor, they are more frequently present around certain types of tumors, including testicular seminomas, thymomas, medullary breast carcinoma, and malignant melanomas in the skin, irrespective of the presence of other inflammatory stimuli such as infection or tissue necrosis. In fact, the presence of lymphocytic infiltrates in medullary breast carcinomas and malignant melanomas is associated with a better prognosis compared with histologically similar tumors without infiltrates. Another histopathologic indication that tumors stimulate immune responses is the frequent finding of lymphocytic proliferation (hyperplasia) in lymph node draining sites of tumor growth. Furthermore, there is often evidence of cytokine effects in tumors, such as class II MHC expression on tumor cells and endothelial cells of tumor vessels, suggesting an active immune response at the sites of the tumors.

At one time, the major effector mechanism for tumor immunosurveillance was considered to be the CTL. In fact, when CTLs were first discovered, their only demonstrated function was the artificial role of killing allogeneic cells in a transplant or a mixed leukocyte reaction (MLR), and antitumor activity was the assumed physiologic role for these cells. More re-

cently, we have come to appreciate that CTLs are most important in anti-viral immunity. Furthermore, a critical evaluation of the immunosurveillance hypothesis suggests that it is not generally valid for most forms of cancer. For example, if the immune system is required to prevent the frequent occurrence of cancers, one would expect that many more malignant tumors would develop in individuals with congenital or acquired immunodeficiencies than in immunocompetent individuals. In fact, this is not the case for most common forms of cancers, such as carcinomas of the colon, lung, or breast. There is, however, a strikingly increased incidence of certain forms of cancer in immunosuppressed individuals, and many of these cancers may result from infections with tumor-causing viruses (as discussed later in the chapter). Thus, the concept of immunosurveillance may be most relevant for the limited subset of cancers caused by oncogenic viruses.

The idea that the immune system responds to tumors has served as the stimulus for a branch of immunology called **tumor immunology.** The field of tumor immunology encompasses the study of specific acquired immune responses to tumors, the antigens on tumor cells which induce immune responses, immunologic effector mechanisms that kill tumor cells, and immunologic approaches for detecting, diagnosing and treating cancers. The great progress we have made over the last decade in understanding the physiology of normal immune responses is already being applied to the important practical problems of prevention and treatment of tumors. This chapter discusses these different aspects of tumor immunology, referring to the basic principles of the cognitive and effector arms of the immune response which have already been described in detail in previous chapters.

TUMOR ANTIGENS

The abnormal growth behaviors of malignant tumors are the reflection of complex abnormalities in physiology which result from expression of mutated or viral genes and/or deregulated expression of normal genes. It is a reasonable assumption, therefore, that cancer cells express certain proteins that are either not expressed at all or are present in much lower quantities in normal cells. Such proteins may be the tumor antigens, that are seen as foreign by a tumor host, resulting in specific immune responses to tumor cells. In addition, surface proteins peculiar to tumors may serve as targets for effectors of natural immunity, such as NK cells.

The fact that tumor cells express antigens that can stimulate immune responses in the host has been clearly demonstrated in both experimental animal models and in human cancer patients. Two main approaches have been used to identify tumor antigens. First, antibodies can be produced by immunizing an animal with the tumor cells, and these antibodies can then be used as probes for different molecules expressed on the tumor cell surface. Second, tumor antigens can be operationally defined as molecules that stimulate T cell–mediated rejection of tumor transplants in an animal previously immunized with the tumor. The tumor antigens that are defined by rejection experiments are called **tumor-specific transplantation antigens** (TSTAs); they include tumor cell proteins that have been processed and presented by the tumor cell in association with major histocompatibility complex (MHC) molecules. Some tumor antigens are unique to particular tumors, whereas others are present on many or all cancers of a specific type.

A fundamental, and as yet unanswered, challenge in the field of tumor immunology is to determine the role that immune responses to tumor antigens play in the control of naturally occurring tumors. For example, there is no compelling evidence that the presence of anti-tumor antibodies serves to block tumor growth. It is also clear that immune responses to TSTAs often do not block the outgrowth of artificially induced tumors and may be effective only in the experimental situation of tumor transplantation into a specifically immunized animal. It should be kept in mind, however, that our difficulty in demonstrating the physiologic significance of tumor antigens may be a reflection of our limited (but improving) ability to analyze the complex biology of tumor growth and *in vivo* immune responses.

This portion of the chapter describes several types of tumor antigens that have been studied in some detail, providing various insights into the biology of tumor-host interactions.

Unique Tumor Antigens

Studies in the 1950s of chemical-induced or radiation-induced tumors in inbred strains of mice demonstrated the existence of antigens expressed exclusively by the cells of one individual tumor. Although analogous unique tumor antigens have not been demonstrated in naturally occurring human tumors, this model of tumor antigens is significant because it is the clearest demonstration that the immune system can

specifically prevent the growth of malignant tumors. In a typical study of this sort, a sarcoma is induced in an inbred mouse by painting its skin with the chemical carcinogen, methylcholanthrene (MCA). These MCA–induced sarcomas can be excised from the original host mouse and introduced into other mice or back into the original animal. Upon transplantation of these tumors into other syngeneic mice, the tumors grow and eventually kill the new host. In contrast, reintroduction of the tumor into the original host results in a specific immunologic rejection of the tumor. Adoptive transfer experiments show that rejection is mediated mainly by tumor-specific CTLs. Alternatively, the cells of a tumor from one mouse can be killed by irradiation and used to immunize a second syngeneic mouse. Subsequent introduction of live cells from the original tumor into the immunized mouse results in immunologic rejection of the tumor transplant (Fig. 17–1). These experiments demonstrate that the *rejection of the transplanted tumors displays two cardinal features of specific immune responses, namely specificity and memory.* In addition, they suggest that CTLs are an important effector mechanism for anti-tumor immunity. Since the tumor antigens in this experimental system are defined on the basis of rejection of transplanted tumor cells, they are called TSTAs. A remarkable property of these TSTAs is their enormous diversity, reflected by the specificity of the immune responses to each individual tumor. For example, one MCA–induced sarcoma does not induce protective immunity against another MCA–induced sarcoma, even if both tumors are derived from the same mouse (Table 17–1, experiment 1).

Although TSTAs were described over 30 years ago, attempts to define their molecular nature were for a long time largely unsuccessful. For many years, investigators tried, and failed, to raise monoclonal antibodies specific for these antigens. Recently, however, genes encoding some of these TSTAs have been identified. The strategy used was to artificially mutagenize a tumorigenic (tum$^+$) mouse cell line and isolate non-tumorigenic (tum$^-$) variant cell lines. It was established that the tum$^-$ phenotype was due to the

TABLE 17–1. Transplantation Antigens on Chemically and Virally Induced Tumors

Experiment	Immunization with Killed Tumor Cells from	Challenge with Live Tumor Cells from	Result	Conclusion
	Treatment of Mouse			
1	Chemically induced sarcoma A	Chemically induced sarcoma A	No growth	Immunity to chemically induced tumors is specific for individual tumors.
	Chemically induced sarcoma A	Chemically induced sarcoma B	Growth of chemically induced sarcoma B	
2	MSV–induced sarcoma A	MSV–induced sarcoma A	No growth	Immunity to virus-induced tumors is virus-specific.
	MSV–induced sarcoma A	MSV–induced sarcoma B	No growth of sarcoma B	
	MSV–induced sarcoma A	Chemically induced sarcoma C	Growth of chemically induced sarcoma C	
	MSV–induced sarcoma A	MuLV–induced sarcoma D	Growth of MuLV-induced sarcoma D	

Abbreviations: MSV, murine sarcoma virus; MuLV, murine leukemia virus.

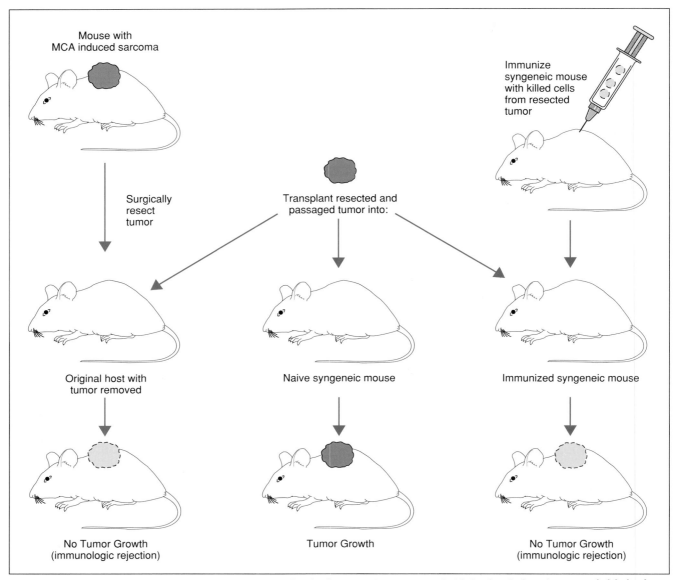

FIGURE 17–1. Tumor-specific transplantation antigens (TSTAs) of chemically induced sarcomas. *A mouse treated with the chemical carcinogen methylcholanthrene (MCA) develops a sarcoma. If this tumor is resected and transplanted into a normal syngeneic mouse, the tumor will grow. In contrast, the original tumor-bearing animal that was cured by surgical resection will reject a subsequent transplant of the same tumor. Injection of killed cells from the same tumor into a syngeneic mouse induces the same type of protective immunity.*

presence of unique TSTAs that were not present on the parent tum$^+$ cells. These TSTAs stimulated a specific CTL-mediated rejection of transplanted tum$^-$ cells. In other words, the tum$^-$ variant expresses TSTAs and is immunogenic whereas the tum$^+$, TSTA–negative parent line is not immunogenic. A cosmid library of genes was derived from the tum$^-$ line, and these genes were then transfected into the tum$^+$ line. By this approach, genes were identified that encoded the TSTAs and that would convert the cells to a nontumorigenic, i.e., immunogenic, phenotype (Fig. 17–2). In this system, the TSTA–encoding genes are highly diverse and apparently represent point mutations of various unrelated normal cellular genes. It is plausible that a similarly diverse group of mutated

genes code for the unique TSTAs in the MCA–sarcoma model described above.

The proteins produced by such tumor-specific genes are endogenously synthesized, processed, and presented to the host immune system, usually in association with class I MHC molecules. The processing and presentation of endogenously synthesized proteins presumably occurs normally in many or all cells. If the proteins are normal self proteins, they do not induce immune responses because of the absence of self reactive T cells. If, however, the proteins are altered or mutated forms of normal proteins, they will be recognized by specific CTLs and will serve as targets for cell lysis and rejection. Thus, *in different tumors, the TSTAs may be altered forms of different cellu-*

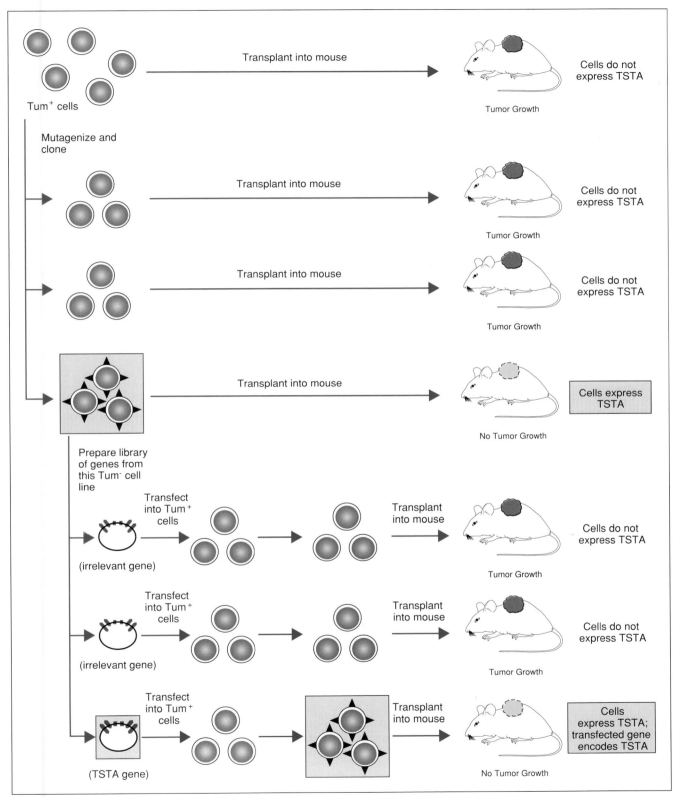

FIGURE 17 – 2. Identification of genes encoding tumor-specific transplantation antigens (TSTAs). *Cells expressing TSTAs and genes encoding TSTAs are shown in shaded boxes. The genes identified by this approach encode a variety of apparently unrelated cellular proteins, with point mutations resulting in one or a few amino acid differences from normal proteins. These mutated proteins induce immune responses that result in tumor transplant rejection.*

lar proteins. The fact that most of these unique TSTAs are only present on the cell surface in the form of peptides bound to MHC molecules is probably why it has been difficult to raise antibodies against them. The relationship (if any) of the mutations to the malignant phenotype of the tumor cells is not known. The mutations may be a result of the high doses of mutagens or carcinogens used to generate the experimental tumors and tumor variants. A similar rate of mutations and the resultant expression of unique tumor antigens may not occur in human tumors, since human tumors are rarely caused by such high doses of mutagens.

Antigens Shared by Different Tumors

Most tumor antigens studied are not unique to individual tumors, but are shared by different tumors. Furthermore, most, if not all, of these diverse groups of antigens may be found on normal cells or benign tumor cells. Such antigens are often called **tumor-associated antigens** (TAAs). There are several classes of these antigens, and many different ones may be expressed on the same tumor. An example of the diversity of TAAs is seen in the phenotype of human melanomas (Box 17–1).

SILENT GENES

Some cellular genes that are not normally expressed in an individual may become transcriptionally active in tumor cells, and therefore their protein products may be recognized by the host as foreign antigens. These genes are called "silent" genes. For example, the non-polymorphic class I MHC–like molecule called the thymic leukemia antigen (Tla) is not normally expressed at any time in some strains of mice, whereas other strains express the antigen on developing thymocytes. T cell leukemias from any strain of mice invariably express Tla molecules, and these antigens can elicit antibody responses in normally Tla–negative mice. Tla however, does not appear to elicit tumor rejection responses, and its role in protective immunity is not known. Human counterparts of tumor-associated silent gene products have not yet been described.

ONCOFETAL ANTIGENS

Oncofetal antigens make up another class of tumor-associated antigens. They are normally ex-

---

BOX 17–1.   MELANOMA ANTIGENS

Malignant melanomas are aggressive, frequently metastatic and fatal tumors derived from either melanocytes or melanocyte related nevus cells. They make up 3 per cent of all skin cancers. Melanomas are among the most thoroughly characterized human tumors with respect to surface antigen expression. This is a reflection of the facts that the primary skin tumors are frequently excised and that melanoma cells can be grown in tissue culture more easily than many other tumor types. Furthermore, melanoma cells express several highly immunogenic surface molecules, including chondroitin sulfate proteoglycan and gangliosides. The fact that melanomas can stimulate immune responses *in vivo* is suggested by the frequent presence of intense lymphocytic infiltrates adjacent to these tumors.

The major strategy for characterizing melanoma antigens is to immunize mice with tumor cells and to produce monoclonal antibodies that recognize melanoma cell surface molecules. Occasionally, monoclonal antibodies that recognize intracellular proteins as well are produced. With the use of this strategy, more than 40 different **melanoma-associated antigens** (MAAs) have been defined. These antigens can be grouped into several categories, including MHC molecules, growth factor receptors, cation binding proteins, high molecular weight extracellular matrix binding molecules, gangliosides, and nevomelanocytic differentiation antigens (see Table). Many of these antigens are expressed on normal cells of various types, but others are expressed only on cells in nevi or on normal or neoplastic cells of neural crest origin. Several of the high molecular weight, substrate interacting surface molecules are considered to be oncofetal antigens, since their expression is usually limited to developing tissues. Although

antibodies to a few MAAs are detected in the serum of melanoma patients, there is no evidence that immune responses to these antigens play any role in protective immunity against the tumors.

Monoclonal antibodies specific for MAAs are used for three major purposes:

First, the biology of tumor progression has been studied by comparing the patterns of antigen expression on cells representing different stages in melanoma development, including melanocytes, nevus cells, *in situ* melanomas, and metastatic lesions. Correlation of the functional properties of these molecules with the growth phenotype of the cells on which they are expressed may help to elucidate mechanisms of tumor progression. For example, expression of melanoma ganglioside 2 (GD2) is restricted to advanced *in situ* and metastatic melanoma cells and GD2 is implicated as a cell adhesion molecule. Interestingly, GD2 is perhaps the most immunogenic MAA defined.

Second, monoclonal antibodies to MAAs are used for immunodiagnostic purposes, by immunohistochemical detection of MAAs on biopsy sections and serodiagnosis of melanoma based on detection of shed MAAs in the blood. Radioactive imaging of metastatic melanoma lesions in patients has been undertaken using radioactively labeled antibodies to melanotransferrin, chondroitin sulfate proteogylcan, and other MAAs.

Third, monoclonal antibodies against MAAs have been tried for immunotherapy. Unconjugated antibodies specific for gangliosides have been administered to melanoma patients, with limited success. Immunotoxins specific for MAAs are being evaluated in animal models. The strategies and limitations of antibody immunotherapy for tumors are discussed in the text.

Continued

Melanoma-Associated Antigens

Category	Example	Biochemical Characteristics	Significant Features
High molecular weight substrate interacting antigens	Chondroitin sulfate proteoglycan	>400 kD; 250 kD polypeptide core	Expressed on membrane spikes; involved in intercellular adhesion, and matrix attachment; highly immunogenic
	Melanoma-associated cellular adhesion molecule	105 and 130 kD	Role in matrix adhesion
	Placental membrane antigen	120 and 94 kD	Role in matrix adhesion
	High molecular weight proteins with ganglioside-like distribution pattern	260 kD	Role in matrix adhesion; highly specific to melanomas
Gangliosides	GD2 9-O-acetylated GD3 GD3 GM2	Gangliosides	Expressed in brain and tumors of neural crest origin only; implicated in cell adhesion; GD2 and GD3 expression characteristic of advanced or metastatic lesions; highly immunogenic
Growth factor receptors	Epidermal growth factor receptor (EGF-R)		Expressed on advanced tumors; EGF is mitogenic for melanoma cells in vitro
	Nerve growth factor receptor (NGF-R) Insulin growth factor receptor Platelet-derived growth factor receptor (PDGF-R) Transforming growth factor β receptor (TGF-β-R)		Expressed on all cultured melanoma cells
Cation transport and binding proteins	Melanotransferrin	97 kD monomeric sialoglycoprotein; related to transferrin	Expressed on all cultured melanoma cells; highly immunogenic
	Calcium-binding S-100	21 kD highly acidic cytoplasmic protein	Member of calcium-binding protein family; expressed by neural crest-derived tumors and normal tissues; widely used for immunohistochemical diagnosis of nonpigmented melanomas.
Class II MHC	HLA-DR		Expressed on many primary tumor explants; no correlation with behavior in vivo
ICAM-1/2	—	90 kD	Ligands for LFA-1
Pigmentation-associated antigen		70-80 kD	Found in melanosomes of pigmented normal and malignant melanocytes
Differentiation antigens	Nevus antigen Gangliosides Galactocerebrosides Myelin-associated glycoprotein Others	Variable	Antigens on melanoma cells which correspond to antigens expressed on normal nevomelanocytes

Abbreviations: HLA, human leukocyte antigen; kD, kilodalton; MHC, major histocompatibility complex; GD, ganglioside; ICAM-1/2, intercellular adhesion molecule-1/2; LFA-1, leukocyte function-associated antigen-I.

pressed on developing (fetal) but not adult tissues. The expression of these proteins on tumor cells is the result of the derepression of genes by unknown mechanisms. As techniques for detecting these antigens have improved in sensitivity, it has become clear that their expression in adults is not strictly limited to tumors. These proteins are found in tissues in various inflammatory conditions, and even in small quantities in normal tissues. Furthermore, oncofetal antigens are not antigenic in the host, since they are expressed as self proteins during development. Not surprisingly, therefore, no evidence exists indicating that an individual mounts an immune response to these antigens on tumor cells. Nonetheless, the study of oncofetal antigens is useful for diagnostic purposes and provides some insights into tumor biology. The two most thoroughly described oncofetal antigens are **alphafetoprotein** (AFP), and **carcinoembryonic antigen** (CEA).

AFP is a 70 kilodalton (kD) α-globulin glycoprotein normally synthesized and secreted in fetal life by the yolk sac and liver. Fetal serum concentrations can be as high as 2 to 3 mg/ml, but in adult life the protein is replaced by albumin and only low levels are present in the serum. Serum levels of AFP can be significantly elevated in patients with hepatocellular carcinoma, germ cell tumors, and occasionally gastric and pancreatic cancers. Elevated serum AFP is a useful indicator of advanced liver or germ cell tumors or of recurrence of these tumors after treatment. Furthermore, the detection of AFP in tissue sections by immunohistochemical techniques can help in the pathologic identification of tumor cells. The diagnostic value of AFP as a tumor marker is limited by the fact that elevated serum levels are also found in non-neoplastic liver diseases such as cirrhosis.

CEA is a highly glycosylated 180 kD integral membrane protein that is a member of the Ig gene superfamily. CEA is also released into the extracellular fluid. Normally, high CEA expression is restricted to the gut, pancreas, and liver during the first two trimesters of gestation and reduced expression is found in normal adult colonic mucosa and lactating breast. CEA expression is greatly increased in colonic carcinomas, resulting in a rise in serum levels. Assays for serum CEA are used to monitor the spread of colon carcinoma or its recurrence after primary treatment. Recent studies have demonstrated that CEA functions as an intercellular adhesion molecule, promoting CEA–expressing cells to bind to one another. Thus, CEA may play a role in the way tumor cells interact with one another and with the tissues into which they are growing.

ANTIGENS ENCODED BY GENOMES OF ONCOGENIC VIRUSES

Viral antigens represent the most immunogenic molecules on malignant tumors and may be the most significant type of tumor antigens for protective tumor immunity. Both RNA and DNA viruses are implicated in the development of tumors in both experimental animals and humans. Virally induced tumors usually contain integrated proviral genomes in their cellular genomes and often express viral genome-encoded proteins. These endogenously synthesized proteins can be processed, and complexes of processed viral peptides with MHC molecules (usually class I) may be expressed on the tumor cell surfaces. Thus, tumor cells expressing viral proteins can stimulate and/or become the targets of specific T cell immune responses. Structurally and biologically distinct antigens are produced by various DNA and RNA tumor viruses.

DNA viruses are probably involved in the development of several different tumors. The papova viruses (including polyoma virus and SV40) and the adenoviruses induce a variety of malignant tumors in neonatal or immunodeficient adult rodents. Several different genes in these viruses cooperate to cause malignant transformation of infected cells. In humans, DNA viruses are associated with the development of several different tumor types. Examples include the association between Epstein-Barr virus (EBV) and B cell lymphomas (Box 17–2), human papilloma virus (HPV) and cervical carcinoma, and hepatitis B virus (HBV) and hepatocellular carcinoma. The viral genes responsible for producing the malignant phenotype in these human tumors are not well defined.

In most cases, DNA virus–induced tumor cells do not produce viral particles, and virally encoded protein antigens that are not components of infectious viral particles may be found in the nucleus, cytoplasm, or plasma membrane of the tumor cells. Specific immunity to DNA virus–encoded nuclear antigens protects against tumor development in animals. For example, SV40-induced tumors in mice express antigens that induce specific protective immunity against subsequent challenge with other SV40-induced tumors, but not against tumors induced by other viruses. Because these antigens are targets for tumor transplant rejection, they are functionally defined as TSTAs, as are the TSTAs of chemically induced tumors described earlier. The viral TSTAs, however, are not unique for each tumor but are shared by all tumors induced by the same type of virus (Table 17–1).

Different effector mechanisms mediate rejection of DNA virus–induced tumors, and different viral antigens serve as the immunologic targets. For example, the T antigen is a virally encoded nuclear protein expressed in SV40 transformed cells. The T antigen is required to produce the malignant phenotype, and it is not part of infectious virus particles. Immunization of experimental animals with this protein induces protective immunity against the development of SV40-induced tumors, and this immunity is mediated by class I MHC–restricted CTLs. Human adenovirus-induced rodent tumors express a virally encoded protein called E1A, which is found largely in the nucleus and is the principal determinant of the transformed phenotype of the infected cells. E1A is not part of infectious adenovirus particles. When class I–restricted CTLs specific for a processed peptide derivative of the E1A protein are adoptively transferred into mice with adenovirus-induced tumors, these CTLs kill the tumors (Fig. 17–3). There is no comparably well characterized DNA virus–encoded tumor antigen that is known to induce protective immunity in human tumors.

Both humoral and cell-mediated immune responses to DNA virus–encoded proteins expressed on tumor cells are clearly demonstrable in animals and humans. A protective role of the immune system in controlling the growth of DNA virus–induced tumors is suggested by the higher frequency of these tumors in immunodeficient individuals. In humans, EBV–associated lymphomas and HPV–associated skin cancers arise much more frequently in immunosuppressed individuals, such as allograft recipients receiving immunosuppressive therapy and acquired immunodeficiency syndrome (AIDS) patients, than in normal individuals. Adenovirus infection induces tumors much more frequently in neonatal or nude (congenitally T cell–deficient) mice, compared with nor-

Epstein-Barr virus is a double-stranded DNA virus of the herpesvirus family. The virus is transmitted by saliva, infects nasopharyngeal epithelial cells and B lymphocytes, and is ubiquitous in human populations worldwide. It infects human B cells by binding specifically to the type 2 complement receptor (CR2), followed by receptor-mediated endocytosis. Two types of cellular infections can occur. In a lytic infection, viral DNA, RNA, and protein synthesis begin, followed by assembly of viral particles and lysis of the host cell. Alternatively, a latent non-lytic infection can occur, in which the viral DNA is incorporated into the host genome indefinitely. Various virally encoded antigens are detectable in infected cells. **Epstein-Barr nuclear antigens** (EBNAs) include at least four different nuclear proteins that are expressed early in lytic infections and may also be expressed by some latently infected cells. EBNAs are the only well-characterized EBV antigens that have been shown to be targets for specific CTLs. Other viral structural protein antigens are expressed within infected cells and on released viral particles during lytic infections, including **viral capsid antigens** (VCAs). Antibodies specific for VCAs are present in acutely infected, recovering, and remotely infected individuals. Epstein-Barr virus has profound effects on B lymphocyte growth characteristics *in vitro*. First, the virus is a potent, T cell–independent polyclonal activator of B cell proliferation. Second, EBV can immortalize normal human B cells so that they will proliferate in culture indefinitely. The resulting long-term B lymphoblastoid cell lines are latently infected with the virus and may express EBNA proteins, but they do not have a malignant phenotype. The molecular basis for these effects of EBV on B cells is presently unknown.

There is a wide spectrum of sequelae to infection by EBV. Most people are infected during childhood, they do not experience any symptoms, and viral replication is apparently controlled by humoral and T cell–mediated immune responses. In previously uninfected young adults, **infectious mononucleosis** typically develops upon EBV infection. This disease is characterized by sore throat, fever, and generalized lymphadenopathy. Large morphologically atypical T cells are abundant in the peripheral blood of infectious mononucleosis patients. These cells are activated CTLs with specificity for EBV–encoded antigens. Previously infected, healthy individuals harbor the virus for the rest of their lives in latently infected B cells and, perhaps, in nasopharyngeal epithelium. It is estimated that one of every million B cells in a previously infected individual is latently infected. EBV infection is also strongly implicated as one of the etiologic factors for the development of certain malignancies, including nasopharyngeal carcinoma in Chinese populations, Burkitt's lymphoma in Equatorial Africa, and histologically variable B cell lymphomas in immunosuppressed patients.

There is compelling evidence that T cell–mediated immunity is required for control of EBV infections and, in particular, for the killing of EBV–infected B cells. First, individuals with deficiencies in T cell–mediated immunity often have uncontrolled, widely disseminated, and perhaps lethal acute EBV infections. Second, EBV–infected B cells isolated from patients with infectious mononucleosis can be propagated *in vitro* indefinitely, but only if the patient's T cells are thoroughly removed or inactivated by drugs such as cyclosporin A. In fact, immortalization of normal peripheral blood B cells by *in vitro* infection with EBV is usually successful only if the donor's T cells are removed or inactivated. Third, CTLs specific for EBV–encoded antigens are present in acutely infected and completely recovered infectious mononucleosis patients. Cloned CTL lines have been established *in vitro* that specifically lyse EBV–infected B cells, and these CTLs most often recog-

nize peptide fragments of EBNA proteins in association with class I MHC molecules. It is possible that EBV–specific T cells are required *in vivo* to limit the polyclonal proliferation of infected B cells as well as to kill potentially immortalized clones of latently infected B cells. A loss of normal T cell–mediated immunity may allow latently infected B cells to progress toward malignant transformation. We discuss this hypothesis below.

The epidemiology and molecular genetics of Burkitt's lymphoma and other EBV–associated lymphomas have been the subject of intense investigation, and they offer fascinating insights into various aspects of viral oncogenesis and tumor immunity. Burkitt's lymphoma refers to a histologic type of malignant B cell tumor composed of monotonous small malignant B cells. The African form of the disease is endemic in regions where both EBV and malaria infection are common. In these regions, the tumor occurs frequently in young children, often beginning in the jaw. Virtually 100 per cent of African Burkitt's lymphoma patients have evidence of prior EBV infection, and their tumors almost all carry the EBV genome and express EBV–encoded antigens. Malarial infections in this population are known to cause T cell immunodeficiencies, and this may be the link between EBV infection and the development of lymphoma. Sporadic Burkitt's lymphoma occurs less frequently in other parts of the world, and although these B cell tumors are histologically similar to the endemic form, only approximately 20 per cent carry the EBV genome. Both endemic and sporadic Burkitt's lymphoma cells have reciprocal chromosomal translocations involving immunoglobulin (Ig) gene loci and the cellular *myc* gene on chromosome 8 (see Box 4–5, Chapter 4).

B cell lymphomas occur at a high frequency in T cell–immunodeficient individuals, including individuals with congenital immunodeficiencies, AIDS patients, and kidney or heart allograft recipients receiving immunosuppressive drugs. Only some of these tumors can be called Burkitt's lymphomas, based on histologic appearance. Regardless of histologic appearance, most of these tumors share with Burkitt's lymphoma one or both of the features described above, namely *myc* translocations to Ig loci and latent infection with EBV.

These observations can be synthesized into a hypothesis about the pathogenesis of EBV–associated B cell tumors. African children with malaria, allograft recipients, congenitally immunodeficient children, and AIDS patients all have deficiencies in normal T cell function. EBV infection proceeds unchecked in these individuals, and EBV–induced polyclonal proliferation of B cells is uncontrolled. This rapid, exuberant proliferation of B cells increases the chances of errors made by recombinases or isotype switching enzymes, resulting in a relatively high frequency of genetic translocations to Ig loci. If the translocation involves the *myc* gene, this gene becomes transcriptionally deregulated. The resulting abnormal expression of *myc* may be causally related to malignant transformation and outgrowth of a neoplastic clone of cells. It is possible that other genetic events are required as well. For example, the integrated EBV genome may contribute to the malignant phenotype in EBV–positive lymphomas. This proposed scheme predicts that early in their course, EBV–associated B cell tumors may be polyclonal, since they arise from a polyclonally stimulated population of normal B cells. Later, one or a few clones may obtain selective growth advantages, perhaps because of deregulation of *myc*. As a result, the polyclonal proliferation evolves into a monoclonal or oligoclonal tumor. In fact, this has been shown to be the case by Southern blot analysis of Ig gene rearrangements in EBV–positive B cell tumors from immunosuppressed patients.

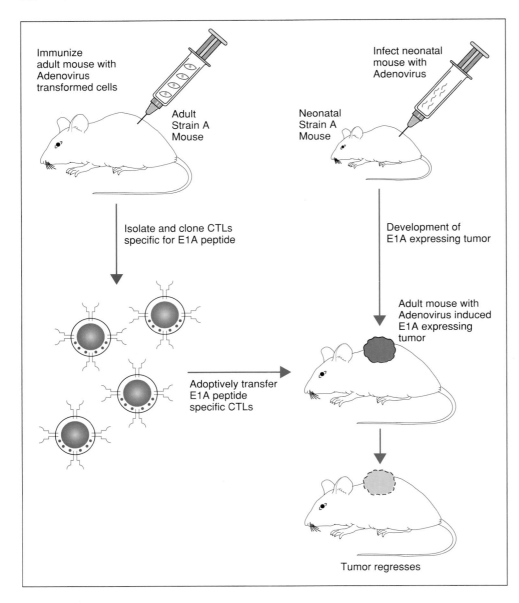

Immunize
adult mouse with
Adenovirus
transformed cells

Adult
Strain A
Mouse

Infect neonatal
mouse with
Adenovirus

Neonatal
Strain A
Mouse

Isolate and clone CTLs
specific for E1A peptide

Development of
E1A expressing tumor

Adult mouse with
Adenovirus induced
E1A expressing
tumor

Adoptively transfer
E1A peptide
specific CTLs

Tumor regresses

FIGURE 17–3. Viral antigen-specific cytolytic T lymphocytes (CTLs) kill virally infected tumors in vivo. *If neonatal mice are infected with adenovirus, they develop malignant tumors as adults and these tumors express the virally encoded E1A protein. The CTL clones isolated from a syngeneic mouse immunized with E1A-expressing cells can kill these E1A-expressing tumors when the CTLs are adoptively transferred to the tumor-bearing animal.*

mal adult mice. *Thus, a competent immune system may play a role in tumor immunosurveillance, not as a specialized anti-tumor function but because of its ability to recognize and kill virally infected cells.*

One of the clearest examples of viral oncogenesis is the development of tumors in animals infected with certain types of retroviruses (RNA tumor viruses). Some of these viruses carry well-defined oncogenes, induce tumors in days to weeks after infection, and are called acute transforming retroviruses. Examples of these acute transforming retroviruses include Rous sarcoma virus (carrying the *src* oncogene), avian myelocytomatosis virus (carrying the *myc* oncogene), and Kirsten murine sarcoma virus (carrying the v-K-*ras* oncogene). Other retroviruses, such as the murine leukemia viruses (MuLVs), cause tumors months after infection and do not carry any well-defined oncogenes. These slow-transforming retroviruses may cause tumors by inserting near, and deregulating

transcription of, cellular genes that are responsible for growth control and differentiation.

The genomes of retroviruses are small, and there is a limited number of potentially immunogenic proteins that they may express in their host tumor cells. These proteins include products of the envelope *(env)* gene; core protein *(gag)* gene; and, in the case of acute transforming retroviruses, the oncogene. Retroviral oncogenes represent slightly altered forms of normal mammalian cellular genes, and therefore the viral oncogene products are usually not highly immunogenic. In contrast, humoral and cell-mediated immune responses to the *env* and *gag* products on tumor cells can be observed experimentally. Furthermore, *env* and *gag* products behave as TSTAs, stimulating CTL–mediated rejection of transplanted tumors. These TSTAs are shared by all tumors induced by the same type of retrovirus.

The only well-established human RNA tumor

virus is human T lymphotropic virus-1 (HTLV-1), which is the etiologic agent for adult T cell leukemia/lymphoma (ATL), an aggressive malignant tumor of CD4+ T cells. Although immune responses specific for HTLV-1 encoded antigens have been demonstrated, it is not clear whether they play any role in protective immunity against development of tumors in virally infected people. Furthermore, ATL patients are often profoundly immunosuppressed, perhaps because of an effect of the virus on CD4+ T cells, which the virus preferentially infects.

TISSUE-SPECIFIC (DIFFERENTIATION) ANTIGENS ON TUMOR CELLS

Tissue-specific, or differentiation, antigens are present on the surfaces of normal cells and are characteristic of a particular tissue type at a particular stage of normal differentiation of that tissue. Tumors that arise from a certain tissue often express the differentiation antigens of that tissue. Since these antigens are part of normal cells, they do not stimulate immune responses against the tumors on which they are expressed. The clinical significance of differentiation antigens on tumors relates to their use as targets for immunotherapy, discussed later, and also as diagnostic markers of the tissue of origin of tumors. The histologic appearance of a tumor may not be characteristic enough to permit a diagnosis of the type of normal tissue from which the tumor arose. Therefore, antibody probes for the expression of tissue-specific antigens may be required. For example, malignant lymphomas arising from the malignant transformation of a developing B cell may often be diagnosed as a B cell lineage tumor by the detection of a surface marker characteristic of normal pre-B cells, called CD10 (previously called common acute lymphocytic leukemia antigen, or CALLA). Tumors arising from more mature B cells are characterized by the presence of surface immunoglobulin. Examples of tissue-specific antigens expressed on tumors are listed in Table 17-2.

THE ROLE OF MHC MOLECULES IN ANTI-TUMOR IMMUNITY

The expression of MHC proteins on tumor cells may be critical for immunologic recognition and destruction of the tumor cells. This is clearly the case if T cells are required for the cognitive and/or effector stages of specific anti-tumor immune responses, since T cells can recognize antigens only in association with MHC molecules. It is possible, therefore, that tumors that stimulate protective immune responses express adequate amounts of MHC molecules whereas other tumors that are not immunogenic fail to express enough or any MHC molecules. However, when the level of MHC expression on a broad range of experimentally induced or human tumor cells is compared with the growth properties of those cells, no clear correlation exists. For example, metastatic tumors, which presumably have evaded immune attack, do not express, on the average, any more or less MHC proteins than non-metastatic tumors. Although extensive analysis of the role of MHC expression on tumor growth *in vivo* has not permitted us to make any broadly applicable conclusions, some experimental models have established the importance of the MHC in the immune response to certain virally induced tumors.

Resistance to induction of neoplasms by tumor viruses often correlates with MHC gene haplotypes in inbred animals. For example, some murine RNA tumor viruses induce tumors only in some inbred strains of mice and not others, suggesting a requirement that certain MHC alleles be expressed in order for an anti-tumor immune response to occur. Such an immune response may be largely specific for a particular viral protein. If the immunodominant peptide from that protein binds only to a particular class I MHC allele, that peptide will be immunogenic only in strains of mice that express the allele. Thus, only certain inbred strains of mice will mount a protective anti-tumor immune response against tumors expressing the viral antigen. This is an example of an immune response (Ir) gene effect linked to class I rather than class II MHC molecules.

A more direct experimental analysis of the effects of MHC expression on tumor growth *in vivo* has been performed using rat cells transformed *in vitro* with viral oncogenes and then transplanted into syngeneic immunocompetent rats. We have described previously that the adenovirus E1A gene product is a tumor antigen that serves as a target for class I-restricted CTLs. Rat cells transformed by the Ad12 strain of adenovirus readily grow into tumors when injected into animals. In contrast, Ad5 strain adenovirus-transformed cells are not tumorigenic. This difference is correlated with the profound suppression of class I MHC expression in cells transformed by

TABLE 17-2. Examples of Tissue-Specific Tumor Antigens Used in Clinicopathologic Analysis of Tumors

Tissue of Origin	Tumor	Antigens
B lymphocytes	B cell leukemias and lymphomas	CD10 (CALLA) Immunoglobulin
T lymphocytes	T cell leukemias and lymphomas	Interleukin-2 receptor (p55 chain) T cell receptor CD45R CD4/CD8
Prostate	Prostatic carcinoma	Prostate-specific antigen Prostatic acid-phosphatase
Neural crest-derived	Melanomas	S-100
Epithelial cells	Carcinomas	Cytokeratins

Abbreviations: CALLA, common acute lymphocytic leukemia antigen.

Ad12, but not Ad5, virus. The suppression of MHC expression is an effect of the adenovirus E1A oncogene, but neither the mechanism of suppression nor the molecular basis of the differences between Ad5 and Ad12 strains is well understood. When class I MHC expression on AD12-transformed cells is increased by γ-interferon (IFN-γ) treatment or by transfection of autonomously transcribed class I MHC genes, these cells acquire the same non-tumorigenic phenotype as their Ad5-transformed counterparts (Fig. 17–4). Thus, class I expression is apparently required for inhibition of tumor growth in this model, consistent with the finding that class I MHC–restricted CTLs mediate killing of adenovirus-induced tumors. However, differences in the *in vivo* growth of Ad5 versus Ad12 transformed cells may be influenced by other factors, besides class I MHC expression, such as resistance to lysis by NK cells.

EFFECTOR MECHANISMS IN ANTI-TUMOR IMMUNITY

Tumor antigens elicit both humoral and cell-mediated immune responses *in vivo,* and many immunologic effector mechanisms are capable of killing tumor cells *in vitro.* The challenge for tumor immunologists is to determine which, if any, of these effector mechanisms are important in protective immune responses

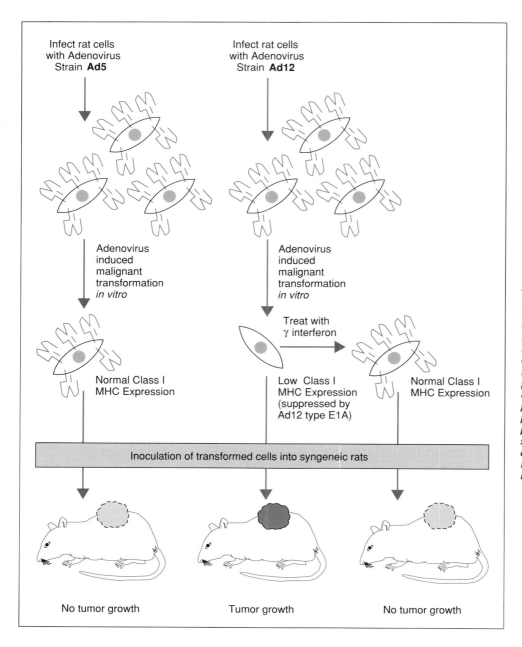

FIGURE 17–4. Relationship between class I MHC expression and tumorigenicity in adenovirus-induced tumors. Rat cells that are malignantly transformed in vitro *by infection with the Ad5 strain of adenovirus express normal levels of class I MHC molecules and are not tumorigenic in syngeneic rats. In contrast, rat cells that are malignantly transformed* in vitro *by infection with the Ad12 strain of adenovirus express low levels of class I MHC molecules and are tumorigenic. Ad12-infected tumors can be induced to express higher levels of class I MHC molecules by γ-interferon, and this treatment renders them non-tumorigenic. An interpretation of this experiment is that class I MHC expression on a virally induced tumor permits the host animal to mount a protective immune response, presumably against a virally encoded antigen presented by the tumor cell in association with class I MHC molecules.*

to spontaneously arising (non-experimental) tumors. In this section of the chapter, we briefly review the evidence for tumor killing by these various effector mechanisms and discuss which are the most likely to be relevant to human tumors.

Antibody Responses

Tumor-bearing hosts mount **antibody responses** specific for tumor antigens. The antigens that stimulate these immune responses are predictably limited to proteins that have not been expressed on normal tissues in a way that would induce tolerance. For example, as mentioned above, antibodies specific for the Tla are easily detected in normally Tla–negative mice bearing thymic leukemias. Patients with EBV–associated lymphomas have serum antibodies against EBV–encoded antigens expressed on the surface of their tumor cells. No evidence exists, however, for a role of such humoral responses in inhibiting tumor development or growth. A great variety of tumor cells can be lysed by antibody-dependent mechanisms *in vitro*. In these experimental situations, the antibodies against tumor surface proteins are often generated in other species and their tumoricidal activity is attributable to complement activation or to antibody-dependent cell-mediated cytotoxicity (ADCC) in which Fc receptor–bearing macrophages or NK cells mediate the killing. Whether or not these antibody-dependent mechanisms of tumor killing play a role *in vivo* remains unknown.

Cytolytic T Lymphocytes

CTLs provide effective anti-tumor immunity *in vivo*, as demonstrated in experimental tumor transplantation studies discussed earlier. In these cases, the effector cells are predominantly class I MHC–restricted CTLs which are fundamentally similar to virus specific or alloreactive CTLs described in Chapters 12 and 16. As discussed previously, the role for CTLs in immunosurveillance of non-virally induced tumors is questionable, since such tumors do not arise frequently in T cell–deficient animals or people or in patients with suppressed T cell immunity caused by therapeutic drugs or human immunodeficiency virus (HIV) infection. On the other hand, peripheral blood lymphocytes from patients with advanced tumors, including carcinomas and melanomas, contain CTLs that lyse explanted tumors from the same patients. Furthermore, mononuclear cells derived from the inflammatory infiltrate in human solid tumors, called tumor-infiltrating lymphocytes (TILs), also include CTLs with the capacity to lyse the tumor from which they were derived. However, the specificity of the anti-tumor CTLs derived from peripheral blood or tumors is not well established, since they often also show reactivity against unrelated tumor cells.

Natural Killer Cells

NK cells may be effector cells of natural and acquired immune responses to tumors. They utilize the same lytic mechanisms as CTLs to kill cells; however, they do not express T cell antigen receptors, and they kill targets in an MHC–unrestricted manner (see Chapter 12). NK cells lyse both virally infected cells and certain tumor cell lines, especially hematopoietic tumors, *in vitro*. In fact, lysis of such lines serves as a bioassay for NK activity. There appears to be a degree of specificity to NK killing, since many virally infected cells or tumor cells and most normal cells are not susceptible to NK lysis *in vitro*. The basis of this specificity is not understood. In addition, NK cells can be targeted to antibody-coated cells because they express low-affinity Fc receptors (CD16) for IgG molecules. The tumoricidal capacity of NK cells is increased by cytokines, including interferons, tumor necrosis factor (TNF), and interleukin-2 (IL–2). Therefore, their role in anti-tumor immunity may depend on the concurrent stimulation of T cells and macrophages which produce these cytokines. There is great interest in the role of IL–2 activated NK cells in tumor killing. These cells, called **lymphokine-activated killer (LAK) cells,** are derived *in vitro* by high-dose IL–2 treatment of peripheral blood cells or TILs from tumor patients. LAK cells exhibit a markedly enhanced and nonspecific capacity to lyse other cells, including tumor cells. The use of LAK cells in adoptive immunotherapy of tumors is discussed later.

A possible role for NK cells in tumor immunity *in vivo* is suggested by a variety of indirect evidence. For example, the incidence of tumors in different strains of inbred mice, or in mice of different ages, correlates inversely with the functional capacity of NK cells in these mice. Interestingly, T cell–deficient nude mice have normal or elevated numbers of NK cells and they do not have a high incidence of spontaneous tumors. Thus, it is possible that NK cells play a role in immunosurveillance against developing tumors, especially those expressing viral antigens. However, there is not a high degree of NK activity in the cellular infiltrates associated with solid human tumors, before *in vitro* expansion with IL–2.

MACROPHAGES

Macrophages are potentially important cellular mediators of anti-tumor immunity. Their role is largely inferred from the demonstration that activated macrophages preferentially lyse tumor cells and not normal cells *in vitro*. The basis for this preferential susceptibility of tumor cells to macrophage mediated lysis is unknown. Like NK cells, macrophages express Fcγ receptors and they can be targeted to tumor cells coated with antibody. There are probably several mechanisms of macrophage killing of tumor target cells, some of which are essentially the same as the mechanisms of macrophage killing of infectious organisms. These include the release of lysosomal enzymes and reactive oxygen metabolites. Other reactive chemical species, such as nitric oxide, may also play a role.

Activated macrophages also secrete the cytokine TNF, which, as its name implies, was first characterized as an agent which can kill tumors but not normal cells. The various actions of TNF have been discussed in Chapter 11. There is convincing evidence that a major component of macrophage-mediated killing of tumors is due to TNF secretion. For example, tumor cells selected *in vitro* for resistance to killing by TNF are often also resistant to killing by macrophages. Killing by both mechanisms is slow (24 to 48 hours), is augmented by protein or RNA synthesis inhibitors, and involves nuclear DNA fragmentation rather than osmotic lysis.

TNF kills tumors by at least two different mechanisms. First, *binding of TNF to high-affinity cell surface receptors is directly toxic to tumor cells.* The toxicity may be a result of the production of free radicals. Normal cells respond to TNF by synthesizing superoxide dismutase, an enzyme that participates in the inactivation of free radicals. In contrast, many tumor cells fail to make superoxide dismutase in response to TNF. Thus, part of the explanation of selective tumor cell killing by TNF may be loss of responses in these cells that serve to protect normal cells. Direct toxic effects of TNF may also involve disruption of cytoskeletal proteins, or interference with gap junction formation. Second, *in vivo, TNF causes tumor necrosis by mobilizing various host responses.* In fact, even tumor cells lacking TNF receptors can be eradicated in mice by treatment with TNF. The key observation is that TNF selectively eradicates vascularized tumors and is much less effective in killing avascular implants. Histologically, the response to TNF, described as hemorrhagic necrosis, looks very much like the localized Shwartzman reaction described in Chapter 11. This resemblance has led to the suggestion that TNF acts selectively on tumor vessels to produce a Shwartzman-like reaction leading to thrombosis of the vessels and ischemic necrosis of tumors. Tumor vessels, unlike normal vessels, may be already "primed" to trigger the Shwartzman response once they encounter TNF. The differences between normal and tumor vessels are a subject of intense study.

MECHANISMS OF EVASION OF THE IMMUNE SYSTEM BY TUMORS

Although many malignant tumors are weakly immunogenic, there are numerous examples of tumor antigens that can stimulate strong immune responses. A major focus of tumor immunology is to understand the ways in which tumor cells evade immune destruction, despite their potential immunogenicity. The process of evasion, often called "tumor escape," may be a result of one or more mechanisms.

1. Some tumors may be poorly immunogenic in a particular host because the host does not express the appropriate MHC molecules necessary for binding and presenting processed derivatives of tumor antigens. This immune response gene effect is hypothesized to be the reason why some strains of mice are resistant to tumor induction by murine leukemia viruses whereas others are not.

2. MHC expression may be down-regulated on tumor cells so that they cannot form immunologically recognizable complexes of processed tumor antigens and MHC molecules. We have previously discussed the correlation of MHC down-regulation and tumorigenicity in adenovirus-induced tumors.

3. A host may be tolerant to some tumor antigens, either because of neonatal exposure to such antigens or because the tumor cell may present its antigens to the immune system in a tolerogenic form, e.g., in high doses or without the proper costimulators (see Chapter 10). Neonatally induced tolerance has been demonstrated for tumors caused by the murine mammary tumor virus. This virus causes breast tumors in adult mice that have acquired the viral infection by neonatal nursing. Although these tumors are not seen as foreign in these mice and do not stimulate an immune response, they are highly immunogenic when transplanted to syngeneic virus-free mice. Another example of neonatally induced tolerance to virally encoded tumor antigens is seen in SV40-transgenic mice. Strains of SV40-transgenic mice that express SV40 genes during early development and have a high incidence of tumors do not mount immune responses against the SV40 T antigen. In contrast, other SV40-transgenic mice that have a low incidence of tumors are immunologically reactive to the SV40 T antigen.

4. The kinetics of tumor growth may allow for the establishment of immunologically resistant tumors before an effective immune response develops. This phenomenon, called "sneaking through," has been experimentally modeled by transplantation studies. Transplantation of small numbers of tumor cells may lead to the establishment of lethal tumors, whereas larger transplants of the same tumor are rejected. One postulated reason for this apparent contradiction is that low doses of tumor antigens are not sufficiently stimulatory to the immune system, and by the time a large number of tumor cells grow in the transplant recipient, mutations in tumor antigen genes may have occurred that reduce the chance of immune recognition.

5. Anti-tumor immunity may result in selection of mutant tumor cells that have lost expression of immunogenic proteins, especially if such proteins are not critical for the malignant phenotype of the tumor. Given the generally high mitotic rate of tumor cells and their genetic instability, such mutations are theoretically likely. Analysis of tumors that are serially transplanted from one animal to another has shown that the loss of antigens recognized by tumor-specific CTL clones correlates with increased growth and metastatic potential.

6. The loss of surface expression of tumor antigens as a result of antibody binding, called **antigenic modulation,** leads to acquired resistance to immune effector mechanisms. Antigenic modulation is due to either endocytosis or shedding of the antigen-antibody complexes. Thus, some non-complement–fixing anti-tumor antibodies may protect tumor cells from other, complement-activating antibodies. Antigenic modulation is perhaps most relevant as a problem complicating attempted passive immunotherapy with anti-tumor antibodies.

7. Antigens shed by tumors, and complexes of antibody with shed tumor antigens, have been postulated in the past to act as blocking factors that interfere with immune responses to tumors. The mechanisms of action of blocking factors remain obscure but could involve functional blockade of NK cell Fc receptors, or induction of "suppressor cells" which specifically down-regulate the function of tumor antigen-specific helper T cells.

8. Tumor cell surface antigens may be hidden from the immune system by glycocalyx molecules, including sialic acid–containing mucopolysaccharides. This is called "antigen masking" and may be a consequence of the fact that tumor cells often express more of these glycocalyx molecules than do normal cells. Similarly, some tumors may shield themselves from the immune system by activating the coagulation system, thereby investing themselves in a "fibrin cocoon."

9. Immunosuppression may be induced by tumor products or by the chemical, physical, or infectious agents that induce malignant transformation of cells. An example of an immunosuppressive tumor product is transforming growth factor–β (TGF–β), which is secreted in large quantities by many tumors. TGF–β inhibits a wide variety of lymphocyte and macrophage functions (see Chapter 11). Immunosuppressive carcinogenic agents include ionizing radiation, chemotherapeutic agents, and certain viruses. These agents can kill or functionally inhibit lymphocytes.

IMMUNOTHERAPY OF TUMORS

The potential for treating cancer patients by immunologic approaches has held great promise for immunologists and cancer biologists over much of this century. Recent advances in our understanding of the immune system have encouraged a variety of new strategies. Next we describe some of the modes of tumor immunotherapy that have been tried in the past or are currently being investigated.

Stimulation of Immune Effectors

The development of virally induced tumors can be blocked by vaccination with viral antigens. This approach is successful in reducing the incidence of feline leukemia virus–induced hematologic malignancies in cats and in preventing the herpesvirus-in-duced lymphoma called Marek's disease in chickens. In humans, it is possible that the ongoing vaccination program against the hepatitis B virus may reduce the incidence of hepatocellular carcinoma, a cancer that is associated with HBV infection of the liver.

Many different approaches have been used for the immunotherapy of already established tumors. Nonspecific immune stimulation of tumor patients with adjuvants, such as the bacille Calmette-Guérin (BCG) mycobacterium injected at the sites of tumor growth, has been tried many times. This treatment serves predominantly to activate macrophages. Oncologists are still assessing the potential of local BCG administration in bladder carcinomas and melanomas. Another experimental approach to nonspecific immune stimulation is the administration of low doses of anti-CD3 antibodies to mice with transplanted fibrosarcomas. This treatment results in polyclonal activation of T cells and, concomitantly, prevention of tumor growth. The dose of anti-CD3 is of critical importance since, as described in Chapter 16, high doses of anti-CD3 antibody are widely used as an immunosuppressant to prevent allograft rejection.

Immunization of tumor-bearing hosts with tumor cells is an experimental approach previously attempted in experimental animals and in humans. Leukemic patients have been immunized with killed leukemic cells from other patients with little success. In attempts to make them more immunogenic, animal tumors have been altered by covalently linking haptens (such as trinitrophenol) to their surface or by infecting the tumor cells with viruses (such as vaccinia virus). These altered cells are then used to immunize tumor-bearing animals. The rationale for this approach is based on the assumption that immune responses to the altered tumor cells will then be effective on the unaltered tumor cells, although the basis for this cross-reaction is not clear. The results suggest that such procedures may enhance active anti-tumor immunity, but their feasibility in the clinical situation is unproven.

Antibody Therapies

There are many variations on the use of *antibodies specific for tumor antigens* in tumor therapy (Table 17–3). The theoretical potential of using tumor-specific antibodies as "magic bullets" remains alluring to many investigators:

1. *Anti-idiotypic antibodies* have been used in the treatment of B cell lymphomas expressing surface Ig with particular idiotypes. The idiotype is a highly specific tumor antigen, since it is expressed only on the neoplastic clone of B cells and on no other cells. (Anti-idiotypic antibodies are raised by immunizing rabbits with a patient's B cell tumor, and depleting the serum of reactivity against all other human immunoglobulins.) This strategy relies on complement fixation or ADCC in order for the lymphoma cells to be killed. The approach is not generally successful, and

TABLE 17-3. Examples of Immunotherapy with Anti-tumor Antibodies

Approach	Examples	Tumors	Current Status
Free antibody	Anti-Ig idiotype	B cell lymphomas	Human trials
	Anti-IL-2R	T cell lymphomas	Human trials
	Anti-ganglioside	Melanoma	Human trials
	Anti-*neu* oncogene product	Sarcoma	*In vivo* animal model
Ig-toxin conjugates	Ricin A-anti-CD5	T cell lymphomas	*In vitro*
	Ricin A-anti-CD22	B cell lymphomas	Human trials
	Ricin A-anti-CD19	B cell lymphomas	*In vitro*
	Ricin A-anti-melanoma	Melanoma	Human trials
Ig-drug conjugates	Chlorambucil-anti-melanoma	Melanoma	Human trials
Ig-radioisotope conjugates	^{211}Bismuth-anti-Thy-1	T cells	*In vitro*
Dual-specificity heteroconjugate Ig	Anti-CD3:Anti-TAA	Sarcoma	*In vitro*
Ig-hormone heteroconjugate	Anti-CD3: Melanocyte-stimulating hormone	Melanoma	*In vitro*

Abbreviations: Ig, immunoglobulin; IL-2R, interleukin-2 receptor; TAA, tumor-associated antigen.

there are many theoretical reasons why it may not work. Since surface Ig expression is not functionally related to the malignant phenotype of the cell, selective outgrowth of non-Ig-expressing tumor cells can occur. Alternatively, the high degree of somatic mutation known to occur in Ig genes could result in the selective outgrowth of tumor cells with altered idiotypes no longer reactive with the anti-idiotypic antibody. Furthermore, since the rabbit antibodies are foreign proteins, the tumor patient may develop antirabbit Ig antibodies and these may interfere with the efficacy of the rabbit-anti-tumor antibodies. Attempts to circumvent these problems by producing human monoclonal antibodies or by injecting cocktails of several different antibodies have also not proven successful.

2. *Antibodies directed against growth factor receptors (IL-2 receptors)* have been used in the experimental therapy of human T lymphocyte malignancies, including HTLV-1 associated leukemias and lymphomas. The rationale of this approach is that IL-2 may serve to stimulate the growth of these tumor cells, and such antibodies may cause modulation or functional blockade of IL-2 receptors (IL-2R). Alternatively, such antibodies could cause complement-mediated lysis of the IL-2R expressing tumor cells. Anti-IL-2R therapy is not tumor specific and may be immunosuppressive because normal T cells would be rendered nonfunctional. There is also no evidence to support an obligatory role of IL-2 as an autocrine or paracrine growth factor for HTLV-1-induced tumors *in vivo*. Although initial trials have met with little success, anti-growth factor receptor antibodies could theoretically be useful for the treatment of other tumors.

3. *Antibodies specific for an oncogene product* might be able to inhibit tumor growth if that oncogene product is essential for the transformed phenotype. Monoclonal antibodies against the *neu* oncogene encoded cell surface protein cause *neu*-transformed cells to revert to a nontransformed phenotype *in vitro*, and the same antibodies can inhibit tumor growth in mice.

4. *Anti-tumor antibodies coupled to toxic molecules, radioisotopes, and drugs* are being used in immunotherapy trials in cancer patients and in experimental animals. Toxins such as ricin or diphtheria toxin are highly potent inhibitors of protein synthesis and are theoretically useful at extremely low doses if they are bound to tumor-specific antibodies to form **immunotoxins.** This approach requires the covalent attachment of the toxin to an antibody molecule without loss of toxicity or antibody specificity. Furthermore, the immunotoxin must be endocytosed and delivered to the appropriate intracellular site of action. Another approach is to covalently attach anti-neoplastic drugs or cytocidal radioisotopes to anti-tumor antibodies. Two practical difficulties must be overcome for this technique to be successful. First, the specificity of the antibody must be such that there is not significant binding to non-tumor cells. As we have discussed, there are few truly tumor-specific antigens to select when designing an antibody-based immunotherapy approach. Second, it may be difficult to ensure that a sufficient amount of antibody reaches the appropriate target, before clearance of the antibody by Fc receptor-bearing phagocytic cells. Such clearance may not only reduce anti-tumor effectiveness, but also may damage phagocytic cells. F(ab')$_2$ conjugated toxins may minimize the latter problem.

5. *Heteroconjugate antibodies* may allow targeting of cytotoxic effector cells onto tumor cells. In this approach, an antibody specific for a tumor antigen is covalently coupled to an antibody directed against a surface protein on cytotoxic effector cells, such as NK cells or CTLs. Such heteroconjugates promote binding of the NK cells or CTLs to appropriate tumor targets. A heteroconjugate consisting of an anti-CD3 antibody coupled to an antibody against a tumor cell surface protein enhances CTL-mediated lysis of the tumor

cell. In this case, the anti-CD3 antibody serves not only to bring the CTL into proximity of the target cell but also to activate the CTL.

6. *Conjugates of antibodies and hormones* can be used to target CTLs to tumor cells expressing hormone receptors. For example, anti-CD3 antibodies coupled to melanocyte-stimulating hormone enhance *in vitro* destruction of hormone-binding human melanoma cells by CTLs. A related (but not strictly immunologic) strategy is to generate fusion proteins with toxic activity and tumor-binding capacity. This is done by engineering and expressing genetic constructs in which bacterial toxin genes are linked to the genes encoding the binding domains of hormones or other ligands that bind to the tumor cells. Fusion proteins combining IL-2 and protein toxins have been used as T cell lytic agents in experimental transplantation (see Chapter 16).

7. *In vitro depletion of bone marrow tumor cells by antibody plus complement-mediated lysis* is used in autologous bone marrow transplants in B cell lymphoma patients. In this protocol, some of the patient's bone marrow is removed and the patient is given lethal doses of irradiation and chemotherapy, which destroy tumor cells. This treatment also destroys the remaining normal marrow cells in the patient. The bone marrow that was removed earlier is then treated with antibodies directed against B lymphocyte-specific antigens, which are expressed on the B cell-derived lymphoma cells. Complement is then added to promote lysis of the lymphoma cells that have bound antibody. The bone marrow, having been purged of lymphoma cells, is reinjected into the patient to reconstitute the hematopoietic system destroyed by irradiation and chemotherapy.

Adoptive Cellular Immunotherapy

Adoptive cellular immunotherapy refers to the transfer of cultured immune cells that have anti-tumor reactivity into a tumor-bearing host. Two variations to this approach are currently in clinical trials:

1. *Lymphokine-activated killer cell therapy* involves the *in vitro* generation of LAK cells by culturing peripheral blood leukocytes removed from tumor patients in high concentrations of IL-2. The LAK cells are then injected back into the cancer patient. As we discussed previously, LAK cells are derived mainly from NK cells. Adoptive therapy with autologous LAK cells, in conjunction with *in vivo* administration of IL-2 or chemotherapeutic drugs, has had impressive results in mice, with regression of solid tumors. Human LAK therapy trials have so far been largely restricted to advanced cases of metastatic tumors, and the efficacy of this approach cannot yet be fully evaluated.

2. *Tumor-infiltrating lymphocyte therapy* involves the generation of LAK cells from mononuclear cells originally derived from the inflammatory infiltrate present in and around solid tumors, obtained from surgical resection specimens. The rationale for this approach is that TILs may be enriched for tumor-specific killer cells. In fact, TILs include activated NK cells and CTLs, both of which appear to kill cells nonspecifically. High doses of IL-2 may impart CTLs with the capacity to kill targets without specific T cell receptor (TCR)-mediated binding. Human trials with TIL therapy are ongoing.

Cytokine Therapy

Cytokines are also used for the treatment of various tumors. This type of experimental therapy has become feasible only recently with the production of highly purified or recombinant cytokines in sufficient quantities. The rationale for using cytokines is based on their ability to enhance one or more components of cellular immune function; the effects of the cytokines are not specific for anti-tumor-directed immune effector cells.

1. IL-2, administered in high doses, is being used alone or in conjunction with adoptive cellular immunotherapy. This treatment is effective in inducing measurable tumor regression in 20 to 40 per cent of patients with melanoma and renal cell carcinoma. Presumably, the IL-2 works by activating NK cells and/or CTLs, i.e., inducing LAK cell differentiation *in vivo*. The treatment can be highly toxic, causing fever, pulmonary edema, and often shock. These toxic effects are probably indirectly mediated by IL-2 acting on other lymphocytes to enhance production of TNF, IFN-γ, and lymphotoxin. Interleukin-4 (IL-4) also can activate CTLs and is currently being tested in clinical trials as an alternative agent with potentially fewer side effects.

2. TNF has been used in preliminary cancer treatment protocols in patients with advanced carcinomas. Although TNF clearly has potent anti-tumor effects *in vitro*, it has many undesirable pathologic effects and can be highly toxic at the doses that are required for tumor killing *in vivo*.

3. Alpha-interferon (IFN-α) is a type I interferon, produced largely by leukocytes (see Chapter 11). It has antiproliferative effects on cells *in vitro*, increases the lytic potential of NK cells, and increases class I MHC expression on various cell types. This cytokine has been used in extensive clinical trials, with promising results. Objective tumor regression responses occur in 10 to 15 per cent of renal cell carcinomas, melanomas, and Kaposi sarcomas; 40 to 50 per cent of various lymphomas; and 80 to 90 per cent of hairy cell leukemias (a B cell lineage tumor). In fact, IFN-α treatment of hairy cell leukemia is now standard practice and is currently the only reliable cytokine therapy for a human cancer.

4. IFN-γ has been used in clinical trials for the treatment of various hematopoietic and solid tumors, with little success. It was hoped that the macrophage and NK cell-activating properties of this cytokine, as

well as its ability to up-regulate MHC molecule expression, would help to enhance anti-tumor immunity. Intraperitoneal administration of IFN-γ for the treatment of ovarian carcinomas is currently being evaluated.

5. Hematopoietic growth factors, including granulocyte-macrophage colony-stimulating factor (GM – CSF) and granulocyte colony-stimulating factor (G-CSF) are used in cancer treatment protocols, although not strictly to enhance immune responses against tumors. Rather, they shorten periods of neutropenia following chemotherapy or after autologous bone marrow transplantation by stimulating the maturation of granulocyte precursors.

An interesting experimental approach to cytokine treatment of tumors is the transfection of tumor cells *in vitro* with cytokine genes followed by transplantation of the cells into tumor-bearing animals. In this way, immunostimulatory cytokines are produced in abundance specifically at the site of tumor growth. This has been accomplished in different animal tumors with IL – 2, IL – 4, and IFN – γ genes. In each case, transfection of the cytokine gene inhibits tumor growth *in vivo* and in each case the inhibition is due to stimulation of a different immune effector mechanism by the secreted cytokine. For example, IL – 4 transfected tumor cells stimulate an intense eosinophilic inflammatory response *in vivo* and do not grow into lethal tumors and IL – 2 transfected colon carcinoma cells stimulate a protective CTL response in mice. The potential of this type of strategy for treatment of human tumors remains hypothetical.

SUMMARY

Malignant tumors express a variety of antigens that may stimulate and serve as targets for anti-tumor immunity. Protective anti-tumor immune responses have been convincingly demonstrated in experimental animal models. It has been more difficult to demonstrate that natural or acquired immune responses to most common human tumors serve to control their development or growth, but this may reflect the limitations of analysis of immune responses in humans. The development of tumors induced by viruses, which express virally encoded antigens, is likely to be inhibited by specific immune responses. Antigens unique to individual tumors, which stimulate specific rejection responses upon transplantation, have been demonstrated only in experimental animal tumors. Other tumor antigens that can stimulate immune responses are shared by different tumors, and these include viral antigens and products of derepressed genes. Tumors may also express tissue differentiation antigens or embryonic antigens to which the host is tolerant; these molecules are useful diagnostic markers. MHC molecule expression may vary from tumor to tumor; in some tumors, MHC expression may be necessary for protective immune responses.

Virtually every immunologic effector mechanism known can destroy tumor cells *in vitro*. One or more of these mechanisms may work on tumor cells *in vivo*, and different mechanisms may be effective on different tumors. Natural killer cells, CTLs and macrophages are probably the major effectors of anti-tumor immunity *in vivo*. Various mechanisms have been proposed to explain how potentially immunogenic tumors escape destruction by the immune system. These mechanisms include MHC – linked genetic unresponsiveness of the host, down-regulation of MHC molecules, induction of tolerance to tumor antigens, loss of expression of immunogenic proteins due to mutations, modulation of tumor antigens by anti-tumor antibodies, antigen masking by extracellular proteins, and immunosuppression of the host. A variety of immunologic approaches for treating cancers, including anti-tumor antibodies, adoptive cellular immunotherapy, and cytokine treatment are currently in clinical trials.

SELECTED READINGS

Burnet, F. M. The concept of immunological surveillance. Progress in Experimental Tumor Research 13:1–27, 1970.

Goodenow, R. S., J. M. Vogel, and R. L. Linsk. Histocompatibility antigens on murine tumors. Science 230:777–783, 1985.

Hanto D. W., G. Frizzera, K. J. Gajl-Peczalska, and R. L. Simmons. Epstein-Barr virus, immunodeficiency, and B cell lymphoproliferation. Transplantation 39:461–472, 1985.

Herlyn, M., and H. Koprowski. Melanoma antigens: immunological and biological characterization and clinical significance. Annual Review of Immunology 6:283–308, 1988.

Klein, G., and E. Klein. Evolution of tumors and the impact of molecular biology. Nature 315:190–195, 1985.

Lurquin C., A. V. Pel, B. Mariame, E. D. Plaen, J. -P. Szikora, C. Janssens, M. J. Reddehase, J. Lejune, and T. Boon. Structure of the gene of Tum⁻ transplantation antigen P91A: the mutated exon encodes a peptide recognized with L^d by cytolytic T cells. Cell 58:293–303, 1989.

Prehn, R. T., and M. J. Main. Immunity to methylcholanthrene-induced sarcomas. Journal of the National Cancer Institute 18:769–778, 1957.

Purtilo, D. T. Defective immune surveillance in viral carcinogenesis. Laboratory Investigation 51:373–385, 1984.

Rosenberg, S. A., and M. T. Lotze. Cancer immunotherapy using interleukin-2 and interleukin-2 activated lymphocytes. Annual Review of Immunology 4:681–709, 1986.

Rosenberg, S. A., P. Spiess, and R. Lafreniere. A new approach to the adoptive immunotherapy of cancer with tumor-infiltrating lymphocytes. Science 233:1318–1321, 1986.

Schreiber, H., P. L. Ward, D. A. Rowley, and H. J. Strauss. Unique tumor-specific antigens. Annual Review of Immunology 6:465–483, 1988.

Tonaka K., T. Yoshioka, C. Bieberich, and G. Jay. The role of the major histocompatibility complex class I antigens in tumor growth and metastasis. Annual Review of Immunology 6:359–380, 1988.

Vitetta, E. S., and J. W. Uhr. Immunotoxins. Annual Review of Immunology, 3:197–212, 1985.

CHAPTER EIGHTEEN

DISEASES CAUSED

BY HUMORAL AND

CELL-MEDIATED

IMMUNE REACTIONS

Specific immunity is a powerful homeostatic mechanism for eliminating pathogenic microbes and other foreign antigenic substances. The effector mechanisms of specific immunity, such as complement, phagocytes, inflammatory cells, and cytokines, are not themselves specific for foreign antigens. Therefore, immune responses and attendant inflammation are often accompanied by local and systemic injury to normal self tissues. Normally, however, such pathologic side effects are controlled and self-limited and they abate as the foreign antigen is eliminated. Furthermore, normal individuals are tolerant of their own antigens and do not develop immune responses against autologous tissues. *Failure to control physiologic immune responses against foreign antigens or to maintain self-tolerance leads to diseases in which the primary pathogenic mechanism is immunologic.* Disorders that result from aberrant, excessive, or uncontrolled immune reactions are also called **hypersensitivity diseases.** This term arises from the clinical definition of immunity as "sensitivity," which is based on the observation that an individual who is immune to an antigen responds to, or is "sensitive to," exposure to that antigen. (As applied to the historical definition of immunity to microbes, such a "sensitive" individual, of course, would usually be resistant to infection by that microbe.) Immunologic diseases that are thought to be due to immune responses against self antigens are called **autoimmune diseases.**

In this chapter we first discuss the mechanisms by which humoral and cell-mediated immune responses lead to diseases, using examples of clinical and experimental disorders to illustrate the current understanding of their etiology and pathogenesis. We then discuss the mechanisms that might lead to autoimmunity and describe some of the approaches that are being used to elucidate these mechanisms.

TYPES OF IMMUNOLOGIC DISEASES

Immunologic diseases comprise a clinically heterogeneous group of disorders. The two principal factors that determine the clinical and pathologic manifestations of such diseases are (1) the type of immune response that leads to tissue injury, and (2) the nature and location of the antigen that initiates or is the target of this response.

The most frequently used *classification of immunologic diseases is based on the principal pathogenic mechanism responsible for cell and tissue injury* (Table 18–1). Immediate hypersensitivity caused by IgE antibodies and mast cells, which is also called type I hypersensitivity, has been described in Chapter 14. Antibodies other than IgE can cause tissue injury by recruiting and activating inflammatory cells and the complement system. These antibodies may be specifically reactive with one's own antigens or with foreign antigens that are deposited in or are antigenically cross-reactive with self antigens. Such disease-producing antibodies may be detectable in two forms. Some can be found bound to their target antigens or in the circulation in a free form, and the diseases they cause are called type II hypersensitivity. Other antibodies may form immune complexes in the circulation, and the complexes subsequently deposit in tissues, particularly in blood vessels, and cause injury. Diseases caused by immune complexes are classified under type III hypersensitivity. Finally, tissue injury may be due to activated T lymphocytes and the principal effector cells of delayed type hypersensitivity (DTH), namely activated macrophages; these are called type IV hypersensitivity disorders.

In our discussion, we will use descriptions that identify the pathogenic mechanisms rather than the less informative numerical designations. This classification is useful because distinct types of pathogenic immune responses show quite different patterns of tissue reactions and may vary in their tissue specificity. As a result, they produce disorders with distinct clinical and pathologic features. However, immunologic diseases in the clinical situation are often complex and are due to various combinations of humoral and cell-mediated immune responses and multiple effector mechanisms. This is not surprising, given that a

TABLE 18–1. Classification of Immunologic Diseases

Type of Hypersensitivity	Pathologic Immune Mechanisms	Mechanisms of Tissue Injury and Disease
Type I: Immediate hypersensitivity	IgE antibody	Mast cells and their mediators (vasoactive amines, arachidonic acid metabolites, cytokines)
Type II: Antibody-mediated	IgM, IgG antibodies against tissue or cell surface antigen	1. Complement activation 2. Recruitment and activation of leukocytes (neutrophils, macrophages) 3. Abnormalities in receptor functions
Type III: Immune complex–mediated	Immune complexes of circulating antigens and IgM or IgG antibodies	1. Complement activation 2. Recruitment and activation of leukocytes
Type IV: T cell–mediated	1. CD4$^+$ T cells (delayed type hypersensitivity) 2. CD8$^+$ CTLs (T cell–mediated cytolysis)	1. Activated macrophages, cytokines 2. Direct target cell lysis, ? cytokines

Abbreviations: Ig, immunoglobulin; CTL, cytolytic T lymphocyte.

single antigen may normally induce both humoral and cell-mediated immunity.

Immunologic diseases can also be subdivided based on the source of the antigens against which the pathogenic immune responses are directed. Such a classification is often impractical in the clinical situation, because in many immunologic disorders the antigen against which the pathologic immune response is generated has not been identified. Nevertheless, it is important to try to classify these diseases by the specificity of the immune response, because specificity may provide valuable insights into the mechanisms by which immunologic diseases are initiated.

1. *Immune responses to foreign antigens may be pathogenic in several situations.* First, some microbes persist for prolonged periods because they resist elimination by immune and inflammatory mechanisms. This leads to persistent antigenic stimulation, resulting in a response of increasing magnitude associated with severe tissue injury. Second, some foreign antigens may share antigenic determinants with self tissues and lead to immune responses that cross-react with self antigens. Third, the foreign antigen may be deposited or "planted" in a particular tissue because of a physicochemical affinity with normal tissue components, so that an immune response directed against the foreign antigen becomes targeted to the tissue in which this antigen is fixed. Fourth, normal immune responses may become defective in their self-regulation, so that they continue unabated even after the initiating foreign antigen is eliminated. Examples of diseases caused by these different kinds of immune responses to foreign antigens are mentioned later in this chapter.

2. *Immune responses against self (autologous) antigens, called* **autoimmunity,** *are usually abnormal.* In normal individuals, potentially self-reactive lymphocytes that encounter self antigens prior to attaining a stage of functional maturity are either deleted or inactivated (see Chapters 8 and 10). Many mechanisms have been implicated in the loss of self-tolerance and the induction of autoimmunity, and these are discussed later in this chapter. Pathologic autoimmunity is a frequent cause of immunologic diseases in humans, estimated to affect 1 to 2 per cent of the United States population.

DISEASES CAUSED BY ANTIBODIES

The first immunologic diseases in which the pathogenic mechanisms were identified were diseases caused by deposition of antibodies in tissues. This was largely because techniques for detecting abnormal circulating autoantibodies and immunoglobulins (Ig) deposited in tissues were developed well before methods for identifying and isolating T cells from lesions or from the blood of patients. Moreover, in experimental models of immunologic diseases, it was possible to cause tissue injury by transferring purified Ig before pure or clonal populations of tissue-reactive

T cells became available. For historic reasons, therefore, many of the general principles of immunologic diseases are based on antibody-mediated disorders.

Antibody-mediated diseases are of two types, which differ in their clinicopathologic manifestations and are due to the deposition of antibodies in distinct forms (Fig. 18–1):

1. *Immunologic diseases may be produced by* **immune complexes** *composed of a soluble antigen and specific antibody; such complexes are formed in the circulation and may deposit in vessel walls virtually anywhere in the body.* This leads to local activation of leukocytes and the complement system, with resultant tissue injury. The antigens that induce the pathogenic humoral immune response can be foreign or self antigens, and the antibodies in the complexes are usually IgM or IgG because these isotypes are most efficient at activating complement and/or inflammatory cells. The pathologic features of such diseases reflect the site(s) of immune complex deposition and are not determined by the cellular source of the antigen. Therefore, immune complex–mediated diseases tend to be systemic, with little or no specificity for a particular antigen located in a particular tissue or organ.

2. *Antibodies against circulating cells or fixed tissue antigens cause diseases that are specific for that cell or tissue.* The lesions are due to the binding of specific antibodies and not to the deposition of immune complexes formed in the circulation. In most cases, such antibodies are autoantibodies, although occasionally they may be produced against a foreign antigen that is immunologically cross-reactive with a component of self tissues. Such antibodies are usually of the IgM or IgG class, and they cause disease by activating the same effector mechanisms as immune complexes. Some immunologic diseases are due to antibodies specific for cellular structures, such as hormone receptors, that are important for normal function. In these situations, diseases may occur because of interference with the normal functions of these structures and not because of antibody-mediated inflammation or complement activation leading to actual tissue injury.

In order to prove that a particular disease is caused by antibodies, one would need to demonstrate that the lesions can be induced in a normal animal by the adoptive transfer of Ig purified from the blood or affected tissues of individuals with the disease. An experiment of nature is occasionally seen in children of mothers suffering from antibody-mediated diseases. These infants may be born with transient expression of the diseases because of transplacental passage of antibodies. However, in the usual clinical situations it is not possible to experimentally transfer diseases with antibodies. Therefore, the *diagnosis* of antibody-mediated disease is usually based on the following criteria: (1) the demonstration of antibodies or immune complexes deposited in tissues, (2) the presence of anti-tissue antibodies or immune complexes in the circulation, and (3) clinicopathologic similarities with experimental diseases that are proved to be antibody-mediated by adoptive transfer.

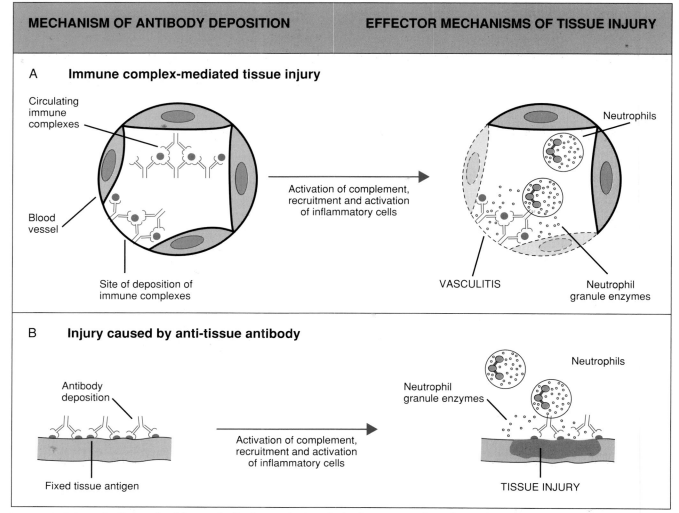

FIGURE 18 – 1. Types of antibody-mediated diseases. *Antibodies may be deposited as immune complexes that are formed in the circulation* (A) *or by binding specifically to tissue antigens* (B). *In both cases, similar effector mechanisms lead to tissue injury at the sites of antibody deposition.*

Mechanisms of Antibody-Mediated Tissue Injury and Functional Abnormalities

In normal immune responses, the protective functions of antibodies are mediated by neutralization of the antigen, activation of the complement system, and recruitment of host inflammatory cells. The same effector mechanisms are responsible for the pathologic consequences of antibody deposition. Which effector systems are involved in mediating the protective functions or pathologic effects of different antibodies is determined largely by the isotype of the Ig and the nature of the target antigen:

1. *Complement-mediated lysis of cells* occurs after IgM and some classes of IgG antibodies bind to their specific antigens (see Chapter 13). Complement activation leads to the generation of the membrane attack complex (MAC), which causes osmotic lysis of cells (Fig. 18–2A).

2. *Recruitment and activation of inflammatory cells,* mostly neutrophils and, to a lesser extent, monocytes, occur at sites of antibody deposition. This is largely in response to the local generation of complement by-products, particularly C5a (Fig. 18–2B). In addition, neutrophils and macrophages express surface receptors specific for the Fc portions of γ heavy chains and can, therefore, bind to and be activated by antigen-complexed IgG antibodies even in the absence of complement activation. Activated neutrophils and macrophages produce hydrolytic enzymes, reactive oxygen species, arachidonic acid metabolites, and cytokines, which can all contribute to cell and tissue injury.

3. *Phagocytosis of antibody-coated cells* (Fig. 18–2C) may lead to selective depletion of those cells.

ANTIBODY BINDING	EFFECTOR MECHANISMS	RESULT

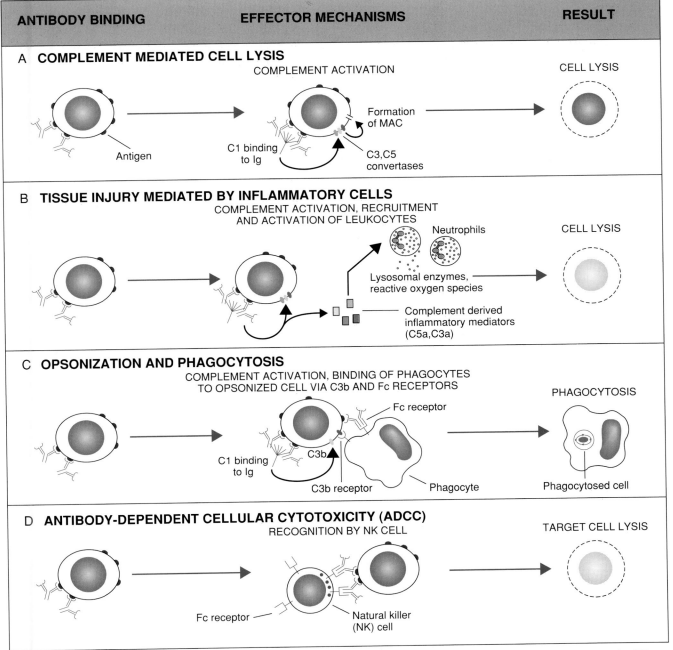

FIGURE 18-2. *Effector mechanisms in antibody-mediated cell injury. Binding of antibodies, such as IgG, to antigens on a cell may cause injury by different effector mechanisms (A–D).*
A. *Activation of complement and formation of the cytocidal membrane attack complex (MAC).*
B. *Recruitment and activation of neutrophils by complement by-products, followed by neutrophil degranulation and release of cytocidal substances.*
C. *Phagocytosis of opsonized cells by macrophages or neutrophils.*
D. *Cytolysis by natural killer (NK) cells and other leukocytes bearing Fcγ receptors.*

For instance, in autoimmune hemolytic anemia, autoantibodies are produced against self erythrocytes. The opsonized erythrocytes are phagocytosed by macrophages in the liver and spleen. This leads to depletion of the erythrocytes and hence gives rise to anemia.

4. *Lysis of antibody-coated cells by natural killer (NK) cells* (Fig. 18–2D) has been postulated as a mechanism for tissue injury in some diseases, such as autoimmune thyroiditis.

5. *Antibodies can cause pathologic effects by binding to functionally important molecules and altering cellular functions.* Examples of such diseases are described later in the chapter.

Immune Complex – Mediated Diseases

The occurrence of diseases due to immune complexes was suspected as early as 1911 by an astute physician named Clemens von Pirquet. At that time, diphtheria infections were being treated with serum from horses immunized with the diphtheria toxin. This is an example of passive immunization against diphtheria toxin by the transfer of serum containing anti-toxin antibodies. Von Pirquet noted that patients injected with the anti-toxin containing horse serum were developing joint inflammation (arthritis), skin rash, and fever. Two clinical features of this reaction suggested that it was not due to an infection or a toxic component of the serum itself. First, these symptoms appeared even after the injection of horse serum not containing the anti-toxin, so that the lesions could not be attributed to the anti-diphtheria antibody. Second, the symptoms appeared at least a week or so after the first injection of the horse serum and more rapidly with each repeated injection. Von Pirquet concluded that this disease was due to a host response to some component of the serum. He suggested that the host made antibodies to horse serum proteins, these antibodies formed complexes with the injected proteins and the disease was due to the antibodies or immune complexes. We now know that his conclusions were entirely accurate. He called this disease "serum disease"; it is now more commonly known as **serum sickness,** and is the prototype for immune complex–mediated disorders.

EXPERIMENTAL MODELS OF SERUM SICKNESS

Much of our current knowledge of immune complex diseases is based on analysis of experimental models of serum sickness, performed in detail by Frank Dixon and his associates in the 1960s using techniques for accurately measuring the levels of antigens and antibodies in the blood and tissues. These investigators showed that if a rabbit is injected intravenously with a single dose (greater than 50 mg/kg of body weight) of a foreign protein antigen, bovine serum albumin (BSA), within a few days the rabbit begins to produce specific anti-BSA antibodies (Fig. 18–3). These antibodies complex with circulating BSA, leading to enhanced phagocytosis and clearance of the antigen by macrophages in the liver and spleen. Immune complexes are initially detected in the circulation and then deposit in tissues, where they activate complement, with a concomitant fall in serum complement levels. Complement activation leads to recruitment and activation of inflammatory cells, predominantly neutrophils, at the sites of immune complex deposition, and the neutrophils cause tissue injury. Since the complexes deposit mainly in arteries, renal glomeruli, and the synovia of joints, the clinical and pathologic manifestations are vasculitis, nephritis, and arthritis. The clinical symptoms are usually short-lived, and the lesions heal unless the antigen is injected again. This type of disease is an example of **acute serum sickness.** It is produced by the administration of a single large dose of a foreign antigen and is characterized by the deposition of large immune complexes. A more chronic disease, called **chronic**

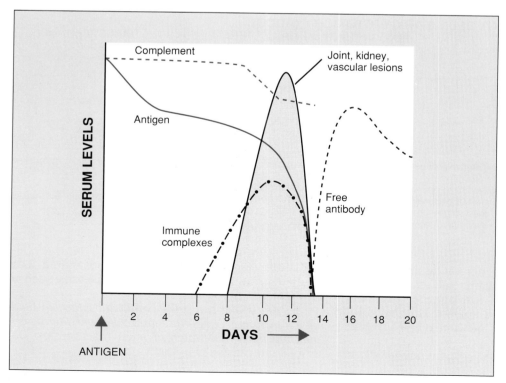

FIGURE 18–3. Sequence of immunologic responses in experimental acute serum sickness. *Injection of bovine serum albumin into a rabbit leads to the production of specific antibody and the formation of immune complexes. These complexes deposit in tissues, activate complement (leading to a fall in serum complement levels), and cause lesions, which resolve as the complexes as well as the remaining antigen are removed. (Adapted with permission from Cochrane, C. G. Immune complex-mediated tissue injury. In Cohen, S., P. A. Ward, and R. T. McCluskey (eds.). Mechanisms of Immunopathology. New York, John Wiley & Sons, Inc., 1979, pp. 29–48.)*

serum sickness, is produced by multiple injections of antigen, which lead to the formation of smaller complexes that deposit most often in kidneys, arteries, and lungs.

A localized form of experimental immune complex–mediated vasculitis is called the **Arthus reaction.** It is induced by injecting an antigen subcutaneously into a previously immunized animal. The animal contains circulating antibodies that bind to the injected antigen, forming immune complexes that deposit in the walls of small arteries at the injection site. This gives rise to a local cutaneous vasculitis with necrosis. As we shall discuss later, various diseases in humans are believed to be the clinical counterparts of acute and chronic serum sickness and the Arthus reaction.

FACTORS THAT INFLUENCE IMMUNE COMPLEX DEPOSITION

From analyses of these experimental models of immune complex–mediated diseases, it is now known that several factors determine the extent of immune complex deposition.

1. The *size of circulating immune complexes* is a major factor, because very small complexes are not deposited and large ones are phagocytosed by mononuclear phagocytes and cleared. Usually, small and intermediate-sized immune complexes are prone to tissue deposition, but this may vary with different combinations of antigens and antibodies.

2. The extent of immune complex deposition in tissues is inversely proportional to the *ability of the host to clear immune complexes from the circulation.* Removal of circulating immune complexes is determined by the functional integrity of the mononuclear phagocyte system and the binding of complement proteins, which function to enhance the clearance of the complexes. Defective phagocytosis may promote the persistence and subsequent tissue deposition of immune complexes. In patients with genetic deficiencies of proteins of the classical complement pathway, such as C2 and C4 (see Chapter 13), immune complex-mediated diseases often develop, because defective production of C3b by antigen-antibody reactions and the absence of complement receptor-mediated phagocytosis lead to persistence of immune complexes in the blood. In this situation, immune complexes that deposit in tissues presumably recruit inflammatory cells by complement-independent mechanisms or by activating the alternative complement pathway.

3. The *physicochemical properties of antigens and antibodies,* including charge, valence, avidity of interaction, and Ig isotype, may influence immune complex formation and deposition. For instance, complexes containing cationic antigens bind avidly to negatively charged components of the basement membranes of kidney glomeruli. Such complexes typically produce severe and long-lasting tissue injury.

4. *Anatomic and hemodynamic factors* are important determinants of the sites of immune complex deposition. Capillaries in renal glomeruli and synovia are vessels in which plasma is ultrafiltered (to form urine and synovial fluid, respectively) by passing through the capillary wall at high hydrostatic pressure, and these are among the most common sites of immune complex deposition.

5. Finally, it is thought that immune complexes bind to inflammatory cells and stimulate *local secretion of cytokines and vasoactive mediators,* which cause increased vascular permeability and enhanced deposition of immune complexes in vessel walls by enlarging interendothelial spaces. This may lead to amplification of tissue injury and disease.

ROLE OF IMMUNE COMPLEXES IN TISSUE INJURY AND DISEASE

It is likely that antigen-antibody complexes are produced during many immune responses but are of pathologic significance only if the quantity, structure, or clearance of the complexes or local functional and anatomic properties is such that abnormally large amounts are deposited in tissues. The *morphologic hallmarks of immune complex–mediated tissue injury are* (1) *necrosis,* which often contains fibrin because of leakage of plasma proteins and is also called *"fibrinoid necrosis,"* and (2) *cellular infiltrates composed predominantly of neutrophils.* Irregularly shaped (granular) deposits of antibody and complement components can be detected in these tissues by immunofluorescence, and if the antigen is known, it is possible to also identify antigen molecules in the deposits.

There is compelling evidence supporting a primary *pathogenic role of immune complexes in many human systemic immunologic diseases* (Table 18–2).

TABLE 18–2. Examples of Human Immune Complex Diseases

Disease	Antigen	Antibody	Clinicopathologic Manifestations
Post-streptococcal glomerulonephritis	Streptococcal cell wall antigens(s)	Anti-streptococcal antibody	Nephritis with glomerular lesions
Systemic lupus erythematosus	DNA, nucleoproteins, others	Autoantibodies (various)	Nephritis, arthritis, vasculitis (disseminated)
Polyarteritis nodosa	Hepatitis B surface antigen (HBs Ag)	Anti-HBs antibody	Arteritis (disseminated)

BOX 18 – 1. SYSTEMIC LUPUS ERYTHEMATOSUS

Systemic lupus erythematosus (SLE) is a chronic, remitting and relapsing, multisystem autoimmune disease that affects predominantly women, with an incidence of 1 in 700 among women between the ages of 20 and 60 (about 1 in 250 among black women) and a female : male ratio of 10 : 1. The principal clinical manifestations are skin rashes, arthritis, and glomerulonephritis, but hemolytic anemia, thrombocytopenia, and central nervous system involvement are also common. Many different autoantibodies are found in patients with SLE. The most frequent are antinuclear, particularly anti-DNA, antibodies, and others include antibodies against ribonucleoproteins, histones, and nucleolar antigens. Immune complexes formed of these autoantibodies and their specific antigens are thought to be responsible for glomerulonephritis, arthritis, and vasculitis involving small arteries throughout the body. Hemolytic anemia and thrombocytopenia are due to autoantibodies against erythrocytes and platelets, respectively. The principal diagnostic test for the disease is the presence of antinuclear antibodies; antibodies against double-stranded native DNA are quite specific for SLE. The presence of so many distinct autoantibodies suggests that SLE is due to polyclonal lymphocyte stimulation and/or abnormalities in lymphocyte regulation rather than antigen-specific activation of an abnormal clone(s) of autoreactive lymphocytes. Genetic factors also contribute to the disease. The relative risk for individuals with HLA-DR2 or DR3 is 2 to 3, and if both haplotypes are present, the relative risk is about 5. (The mechanisms of autoimmunity and the roles of immunologic abnormalities and genetic factors are discussed elsewhere in this chapter.) Deficiency of the complement protein, C4, occurs in about 10 per cent of SLE patients but in only 1 per cent of the normal population.

Animal models of lupus provide valuable experimental systems for analyzing the pathogenesis of this disease. Several inbred mouse strains have been discovered to spontaneously develop autoimmune diseases that resemble human SLE to varying degrees.

The first to be described, and the one most like SLE, is the NZB strain and the (NZB X NZW)F1. Female mice develop kidney lesions and hemolytic anemia and produce anti-DNA autoantibodies spontaneously. Extensive breeding studies have shown that non-MHC genes in the F1 that are inherited from both parental strains contribute to the evolution of the disease. The B cells of (NZB X NZW)F1 mice are hyperresponsive to foreign antigens as well as to polyclonal activators and cytokines, and this may be the primary immunologic abnormality in these mice. The biochemical basis of the B cell hyperresponsiveness is unknown.

A second model of lupus is the MRL congenic strain called MRL-*lpr/lpr,* referring to an MRL mouse into which a gene for "lymphoproliferation" has been bred. The MRL-*lpr/lpr* (also called MRL/*lpr*) strain develops massive lymphadenopathy due to a spontaneous polyclonal proliferation involving mostly phenotypically immature CD4⁻ CD8⁻ T cells. These mice also produce autoantibodies and develop arthritis and kidney lesions. MRL mice are prone to developing autoimmunity, and the *lpr* gene greatly accelerates the disease. Autoantibody production may occur because the proliferating T cells constitutively secrete cytokines that stimulate B cell growth and differentiation. A role for T cells is further supported by the observation that neonatal thymectomy prevents the development of lymphoproliferation and autoimmunity in MRL/*lpr* mice. The cause of lymphoproliferation is unknown, but unidentified genes from the MRL background as well as *lpr* genes are necessary to develop the severe disease. The disease of MRL/*lpr* mice is not sex-related.

A third inbred strain that develops a lupus-like disease is a recombinant called BXSB, in which disease susceptibility is linked to the Y chromosome and only the males are affected. These mice produce anti-DNA antibodies and develop severe nephritis and vasculitis.

Systemic lupus erythematosus (SLE) (Box 18–1) is an autoimmune disease in which numerous autoantibodies are produced. Its many clinical manifestations include glomerulonephritis and arthritis, which are attributed to the deposition of immune complexes composed of self DNA or nucleoprotein antigens and specific antibodies (Fig. 18–4). The glomerular lesions of SLE often resemble the lesions seen in chronic serum sickness. Some cases of a form of systemic vasculitis called **polyarteritis nodosa** occur as a late sequel of hepatitis B virus infection and are due to arterial deposition of immune complexes composed of hepatitis virus surface antigen (HBsAg) and specific antibodies. **Post-streptococcal glomerulonephritis** is a kidney disease that develops 1 to 3 weeks after streptococcal skin and throat infections. It is thought to be due to glomerular deposits of immune complexes composed of streptococcal antigen and anti-streptococcal antibodies. However, post-streptococcal glomerulonephritis differs from typical immune complex–mediated diseases because it involves only the kidneys and there are no systemic manifestations. It is, therefore, possible that this disease may be due to initial binding of streptococcal antigen to glomeruli followed by deposition of the antibody, so that the pathogenic mechanism is not deposition of circulating complexes but free antibody against a "planted" bacterial antigen. Granular deposits of antibody and complement have been demonstrated in injured tissues in many other forms of cutaneous necrotizing vasculitis, arthritis and glomerulonephritis. Some skin diseases associated with vasculitis are morphologically similar to experimental Arthus reactions. Such diseases are postulated to be due to immune complexes, but the nature of the antigens is unknown.

Diseases Mediated by Antibodies Against Fixed Cell and Tissue Antigens

As we mentioned earlier, antibodies produced against fixed cellular or tissue antigens are usually autoantibodies. Less frequently, the antibodies may

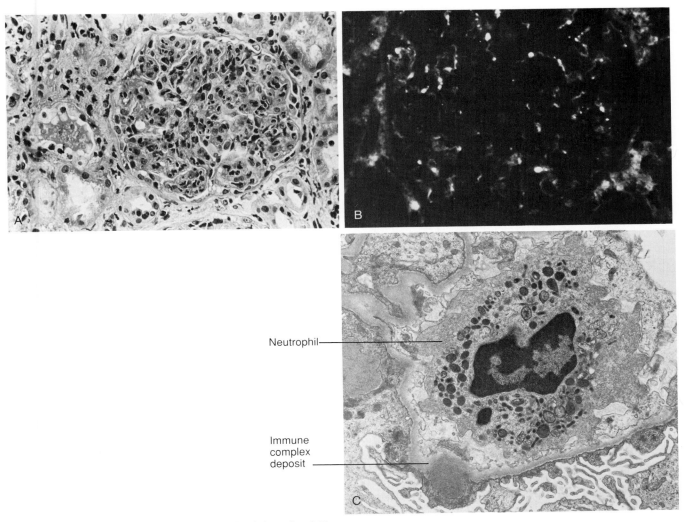

FIGURE 18–4. Histopathology of immune complex–mediated glomerulonephritis.
A. *Light micrograph of a kidney glomerulus, showing hypercellularity caused by infiltration of leukocytes.*
B. *Immunofluorescent stain for IgG showing granular deposits in a glomerulus. (Complement proteins, including C3b, would co-localize with the antibody.)*
C. *Electron micrograph of a glomerular capillary, showing an immune complex deposited in the wall and a neutrophil in the lumen.*
(Courtesy of Dr. Helmut Rennke, Department of Pathology, Brigham and Women's Hospital, Boston; reproduced with permission from Brenner, B. M., F. L. Coe, and F. C. Rector. Clinical Nephrology, Philadelphia, W.B. Saunders Co., 1987.)

be produced against extrinsic antigens but may bind to immunologically similar or cross-reactive antigens present in autologous cells or tissues. Antibodies against self tissues are not always pathogenic. For instance, tissue injury due to ischemia or infection may lead to autoantibody production because of alterations of self antigens or exposure of antigens that are normally sequestered from the immune system. In such situations, the autoantibodies may be the result and not the cause of tissue necrosis. Some patients who suffer myocardial infarctions develop, within a few weeks, antibodies against their own cardiac cells. Obviously, the autoantibodies are not the cause but the result of the infarction.

Many tissue or organ-specific immunologic diseases are associated with the production of, and are thought to be caused by, autoantibodies (Table 18–3). In most of these diseases, specific circulating antibodies can be found in the blood but the mechanisms responsible for autoantibody production are not known. Autoimmune hemolytic anemia and immune thrombocytopenia are due to autoantibodies against erythrocytes and platelets, respectively. The antibodies cause complement-dependent lysis of the circulating cells and opsonize the cells leading to enhanced phagocytosis by mononuclear phagocytes. Autoimmune hemolytic anemia and thrombocytopenia are usually idiopathic and may sometimes be associated with other immunologic abnormalities, e.g., in SLE. Similar diseases occur during idiosyncratic reactions to some drugs and may be due to binding of the drugs to cell surfaces, leading to the creation of neo-antigens which elicit specific antibody responses. **Goodpasture's syndrome** is a disease characterized by lung

TABLE 18–3. Examples of Autoantibodies in Human Diseases

Disease	Principal Clinical Features	Autoantibody Detected: Specificity	Method of Detection
Glomerulonephritis (Goodpasture's syndrome)	Nephritis with proteinuria, renal failure; lung hemorrhages	Type IV collagen in basement membranes of kidney glomeruli and lung alveoli	Immunofluorescence
Autoimmune hemolytic anemia	Hemolysis, anemia	Erythrocyte membrane proteins	Hemagglutination
Autoimmune thrombocytopenic purpura	Platelet deficiency (thrombocytopenia), bleeding disorders	Platelet membrane proteins (e.g., gp IIb/IIIa)	Immunofluorescence
Pemphigus vulgaris	Decreased adhesions between epidermal keratinocytes; skin vesicles (bullae)	Intercellular junctions of epidermal cells	Immunofluorescence
Bullous pemphigoid	Detachment of epidermal cells; skin vesicles	Epidermal basement membrane proteins	Immunofluorescence
Myasthenia gravis	Muscle weakness	Acetylcholine receptor	Immunoprecipitation
Graves' disease (hyperthyroidism)	Hyperthyroidism due to increased production of thyroid hormones	Thyroid-stimulating hormone receptor on thyroid follicular epithelial cells	Bioassay
Insulin-resistant diabetes mellitus	Diabetes, unresponsive to insulin therapy	Insulin receptor	Inhibition of insulin binding to cultured cells
Pernicious anemia	Abnormal erythropoiesis due to vitamin B_{12} deficiency	Intrinsic factor; gastric parietal cells	Bioassay; immunofluorescence

hemorrhages and severe glomerulonephritis. It is caused by an autoantibody that binds to epitopes of type IV collagen found in the basement membranes of pulmonary alveoli and glomerular capillaries and leads to local activation of complement and neutrophils. On microscopic examination, necrosis, leukocytic infiltrates, and linear deposits of antibody and complement along basement membranes can be seen (Fig. 18–5). A number of skin diseases are due to antibodies against epidermal cells or basement membrane antigens.

Autoantibodies against cell surface receptors may lead to functional abnormalities without the involvement of any other effector mechanisms. For instance, some antibodies against cell surface hormone receptors bind to these receptors and lead to aberrations in cellular physiology without inflammation or tissue injury. These functional abnormalities may result from receptor-mediated stimulation of target cells or inhibition due to interference with receptor function (Fig. 18–6).

One example of stimulation by an antibody mimicking a physiologic molecule is **Graves' disease,** an autoimmune disease of the thyroid gland characterized by hyperthyroidism. The clinical syndrome results from excessive production of thyroid hormones such as thyroxine. This disease is usually caused by an autoantibody specific for the receptor for thyroid-stimulating hormone (TSH) on thyroid epithelial cells. TSH is a pituitary hormone whose normal function is to stimulate the production of thyroid hormones by thyroid epithelial cells. Binding of antibody

to the TSH receptor has the same effect as TSH itself, leading to unregulated stimulation of thyroid epithelial cells and excess thyroid hormone production even in the absence of TSH.

An example of anti-receptor antibody-mediated functional inhibition is **myasthenia gravis,** a disease of progressive muscle weakness caused by autoantibodies reactive with acetylcholine receptors in the motor end plates of neuromuscular junctions. Binding of the antibodies interferes with acetylcholine mediated neuromuscular transmission and may lead to a reduction in receptor numbers as a consequence of endocytosis and intracellular degradation ("down-modulation") of the receptors. The result is a failure of muscle to respond to normal neural impulses, leading to progressive muscle weakness. Experimentally, a disease resembling myasthenia gravis can be produced in rats and mice by immunizing them with purified acetylcholine receptors. The experimental disease can be adoptively transferred to normal animals by antibodies against the acetylcholine receptor. Similarly, some patients with diabetes mellitus who are unresponsive to insulin have autoantibodies against insulin receptors that block the binding and the physiologic effects of the hormone.

Autoantibodies against physiologically important circulating molecules, such as hormones, may also lead to functional abnormalities and disease in the absence of cell or tissue destruction. Some cases of **pernicious anemia** are associated with autoantibodies against intrinsic factor, which is a cofactor for the intestinal absorption of vitamin B_{12}. The antibodies are thought to

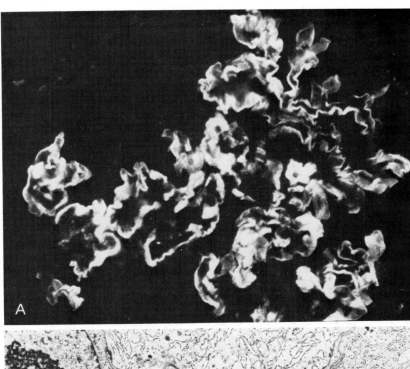

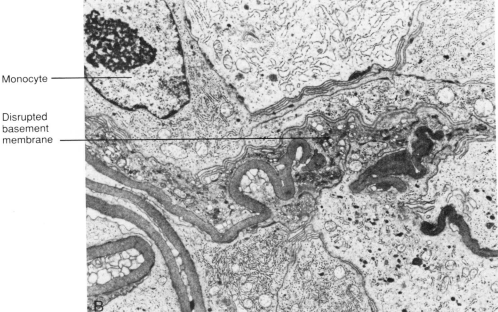

FIGURE 18-5. *Pathology of glomerulone-phritis induced by an antibody against the glomerular basement membrane (Goodpasture's syndrome).*
A. *Immunofluorescent stain for IgG, showing linear deposition of antibody along the capillary basement membrane of a glomerulus. (This pattern is very different from that of immune complex-mediated diseases; see Fig. 18-4B.)*
B. *Electron micrograph of a glomerular capillary, showing destruction of the basement membrane without evidence of immune complex deposition.*
(Courtesy of Dr. Helmut Rennke, Department of Pathology, Brigham and Women's Hospital, Boston; reproduced with permission from Brenner, B. M., F. L. Coe, and F. C. Rector. Clinical Nephrology. Philadelphia, W.B. Saunders Co., 1987.)

Monocyte

Disrupted basement membrane

bind to and inhibit the function of intrinsic factor, resulting in vitamin B_{12} deficiency. This causes abnormal hematopoiesis and megaloblastic anemia.

Some human diseases are also due to antibodies produced against foreign antigens that cross-react with self proteins. Perhaps the best example is **acute rheumatic fever,** which, like post-streptococcal glomerulonephritis, is a late sequela of throat infection caused by streptococci. The bacterial strains associated with rheumatic fever are usually different from those that lead to glomerulonephritis. Rheumatic fever is characterized by arthritis, endocarditis

resulting in lesions of heart valves, myocarditis, and neurologic abnormalities, but no kidney abnormalities. The myocardial injury is thought to be due to an antibody against a streptococcal cell wall protein that binds to a cross-reactive antigen in cardiac muscle cells.

Despite the numerous examples of circulating autoantibodies associated with immunologic diseases, it is important to reiterate that it is often not clear whether a particular antibody is the cause of the disease or is produced as a result of cell or tissue injury. Furthermore, autoantibodies may be present but may

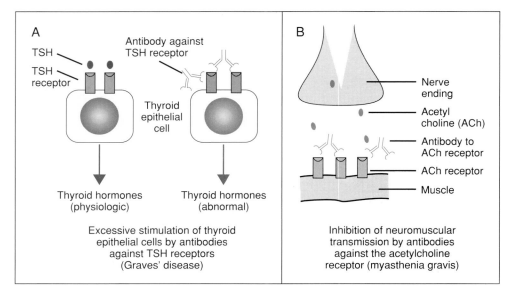

FIGURE 18–6. Effector mechanisms in antibody-mediated diseases: functional abnormalities induced by antibodies against hormone receptors.
A. *Antibodies against thyroid-stimulating hormone (TSH) receptors stimulate thyroid epithelial cells by binding to the receptor and by mimicking the effects of TSH, the physiologic ligand.*
B. *Antibodies against the acetylcholine (ACh) receptor inhibit neuromuscular transmission by binding to the ACh receptor, leading to down-modulation of receptors and competitive inhibition of ACh binding.*

not be responsible for pathologic abnormalities. For instance, patients with **rheumatoid arthritis** (Box 18–2) frequently have a circulating IgM antibody that is specific for their own IgG molecules, usually the Fc portions of these molecules. Such autoantibodies are called rheumatoid factors. Although their presence is a useful diagnostic test for rheumatoid arthritis, there is no evidence that rheumatoid factors are involved in the formation of injurious immune complexes or contribute to the joint lesions in this disease.

DISEASES CAUSED BY T CELLS

The potential importance of T lymphocytes as mediators of human immunologic diseases has been

---

BOX 18–2.   RHEUMATOID ARTHRITIS

Rheumatoid arthritis is a destructive disease involving primarily the joints of the extremities, particularly of the fingers. As the disease progresses, more of the large joints are affected. Rheumatoid arthritis is characterized by destruction of the joint cartilage and inflammation of the synovium, with a morphologic picture suggestive of a local immune response. CD4+ T cells, activated B lymphocytes, and plasma cells are found in the inflamed synovium, and in severe cases, well-formed lymphoid follicles with germinal centers may be present. Numerous cytokines, including interleukin-1 (IL-1), TNF, and IFN-γ, have been detected in the synovial (joint) fluid. It is believed that cytokines activate resident synovial cells to produce hydrolytic enzymes, such as collagenase, that mediate destruction of the cartilage, ligaments, and tendons of the joints. Many of the cytokines thought to play a role in initiating joint destruction are probably produced as a result of local T cell and macrophage activation. The specificity of the T cells that may cause arthritis and the nature of the initiating antigen(s) are not known. Recently, significant numbers of T cells expressing the γδ antigen receptor have been detected in the synovial fluid of patients with rheumatoid arthritis. However, the pathogenic role of this subset of T cells, like their physiologic function, is obscure.

Systemic complications of rheumatoid arthritis include vasculitis, presumably caused by immune complexes, and lung injury. The nature of the antigen or the antibodies in these complexes is not known. Patients with the adult form of rheumatoid arthritis frequently have circulating antibodies, which may be IgM or IgG, reactive with the Fc (and rarely Fab) portions of their own IgG molecules. These autoantibodies are called **rheumatoid factors**, and their presence is used as a diagnostic test for rheumatoid arthritis. Rheumatoid factors seem to play no role in the joint pathology or in the formation of injurious immune complexes. Although activated B cells and plasma cells are often present in the synovia of affected joints, the specificities of the antibodies produced by these cells or their role in causing joint lesions are not known. Susceptibility to rheumatoid arthritis is linked to the HLA-DR4 haplotype and quite specifically to a stretch of amino acid residues in the polymorphic region near the N-terminal of the HLA-DRβ1 chain that is found in HLA-DR4 and some other alleles. (The possible basis of this association is discussed elsewhere in the chapter.)

There are several experimental models of arthritis. MRL/*lpr* mice develop spontaneous arthritis and have high serum levels of rheumatoid factors. The immune mechanisms of joint disease in MRL/*lpr* are not known. T cell–mediated arthritis can be induced in susceptible strains of mice and rats by immunization with type II collagen (the type found in cartilage), and the disease can be adoptively transferred to unimmunized animals with collagen-specific T cells. However, in the human disease there is no convincing evidence for collagen-specific autoimmunity. Experimental arthritis can also be produced by immunization with various bacterial antigens, including mycobacterial and streptococcal cell wall proteins. However, such diseases bear a very superficial resemblance, if any, to human rheumatoid arthritis.

increasingly recognized in the 1980s. This is largely because of two technological advances — the production of monoclonal antibodies that identify phenotypically and functionally distinct subsets of T cells, and methods for isolating and propagating T cells from lymphoid tissues and lesions. As we shall see later in this chapter, the demonstration that T lymphocytes are critical for maintaining self-tolerance to many protein antigens has led to increasing interest in their role in autoimmune disorders.

Mechanisms of T Cell-Mediated Tissue Injury

The T cells that cause tissue injury may be autoreactive, or they may be specific for foreign protein antigens that are present in or bound to one's own cells or tissues. The pathologic lesions vary, depending on the types of T cells that produce these lesions. T cells injure tissues by the same two mechanisms that are responsible for cell-mediated immunity against microbes (see Chapter 12):

1. T cells, usually of the CD4$^+$ subset, secrete cytokines, which activate macrophages, giving rise to **DTH reactions.** Acute tissue injury results from the products of activated macrophages, such as hydrolytic enzymes and toxic oxygen metabolites. Chronic DTH reactions often produce fibrosis as a result of the secretion of cytokines and growth factors by the macrophages (see Chapter 12).

2. CD8$^+$ **cytolytic T lymphocytes** (CTLs) directly lyse target cells bearing class I major histocompatibility complex (MHC)-associated foreign antigens, without the participation of macrophages or any other effector mechanisms.

A role for T cells in causing a particular immunologic disease is suspected largely by the demonstration of T cells in lesions and by the isolation of T cells specific for self antigens from the tissues or blood of patients. Furthermore, cytokines secreted by activated T cells induce alterations in adjacent tissues that are used as indicators of local T cell stimulation. One such cytokine is γ-interferon (IFN-γ), which induces the expression of class II MHC molecules on vascular endothelium as well as on other cells that do not express these molecules constitutively. Abnormal expression of class II MHC molecules in a tissue suggests that T cells have been activated in the immediate environment. Aberrant expression of class II MHC molecules may also lead to excessive T cell activation, because many more cells may acquire the ability to present antigen. However, epithelial and mesenchymal cells that are induced to express class II molecules may not produce costimulators that are necessary for T cell activation and, therefore, may not be efficient at stimulating T cells (Chapter 7).

The presence of activated T cells in the blood or tissues of patients is not always associated with disorders of cell-mediated immunity. For instance, CD4$^+$ T cells function as helper cells in humoral immunity and, therefore, may be abundant in lesions that are mediated by antibodies and not by the T cells themselves. Moreover, as for antibodies, the identification and even isolation of T cells are not, by themselves, proof of their pathogenic role. The most definitive proof is the ability to adoptively transfer the disease to normal recipients, and this is not possible in the clinical situation. However, in experimental models of several immunologic diseases, the lesions have been transferred to normal syngeneic animals by purified T cells or by antigen-specific cloned lines of T cells (Table 18-4). The similarities between these experimentally induced lesions and clinical diseases further support a primary pathogenic role of T cells in the latter. Finally, alterations in the ratio of circulating CD4$^+$ and CD8$^+$ T cells (the normal being about 2:1) have been used as diagnostic indices for T cell-mediated immunologic diseases. Such assays, however, are of limited usefulness because they are not specific for particular immunologic abnormalities.

TABLE 18-4. Identification of Antigen-Specific T Cells in Immunologic Diseases

Disease	Specificity of T Cell Clone/Line	Isolated from Lesions or Blood of		Ability to Transfer Disease in Animal Models
		Patients	*Animal Models*	
Experimental allergic encephalomyelitis	Myelin basic protein	No	Yes	Yes
Experimental allergic neuritis	P2 protein of peripheral nerve myelin	No	Yes	Yes
*Myasthenia gravis**	Acetylcholine receptor	Yes	Yes	Yes
Some cases of Graves' disease, autoimmune thyroiditis*	Thyroid follicular epithelial cells	Yes	Yes	Yes
Viral myocarditis	Viruses (e.g., Coxsackie)	No	Yes†	Yes

* In these cases, the T cells may be helper cells that stimulate local production of autoantibodies, which are responsible for inducing lesions.

† CD8$^+$ cytolytic T lymphocyte (CTL) clones; pathogenic T cells in the other examples listed are CD4$^+$ cells.

Diseases Caused by CD4+ T Cells and Delayed Type Hypersensitivity

A variety of cutaneous diseases that result from topical exposure to foreign antigens or are sequelae of skin infections are due to CD4+ T cell–mediated DTH reactions. These include skin rashes as a result of *contact sensitivity to chemicals,* such as drugs, cosmetics, and environmental antigens. The rashes usually appear hours or even days after exposure to the contact sensitizing agent. The lesions may be due to T cell responses to neo-antigens created by binding of the chemicals to normal cell surface proteins on epidermal keratinocytes or Langerhans cells. Skin biopsy specimens show dermal perivascular infiltrates of lymphocytes and macrophages plus edema and fibrin deposition resulting from leakage of plasma from dermal capillaries and venules (see Chapter 12, Fig. 12–2). Vascular endothelial cells in the lesions may express enhanced levels of cytokine-regulated surface molecules, such as class II MHC molecules. These DTH reactions are quite different mechanistically and morphologically from two other types of immunologic skin lesions, IgE-mediated immediate hypersensitivity and immune complex–mediated Arthus reactions (Table 18–5).

A number of organ-specific autoimmune diseases are thought to be caused by autoreactive T cells. In some patients with **insulin-dependent diabetes mellitus** (IDDM) (Box 18–3), there are infiltrates of lymphocytes and macrophages around islets of Langerhans in the pancreas, with destruction of insulin-producing β cells in the islets and a resultant deficiency in insulin production. Residual islet cells in these lesions express class II MHC molecules, again suggesting local cytokine production. Similar findings have been observed in spontaneous diabetes in rats and mice, in which the lesions have been adoptively transferred to normal animals with CD4+ T cells from diseased animals. CD8+ CTLs may also contribute to insulitis and islet cell destruction in human and experimental diabetes mellitus. The specificity of the T cells that cause insulitis and destroy islet cells, and the nature of the initiating antigen, are unknown. **Experimental allergic encephalomyelitis** (EAE) (Box 18–4) is a neurologic disease that can be induced in experimental animals by immunization with myelin basic protein in adjuvant. Such immunization leads to an autoimmune T cell response against myelin, culminating in activation of macrophages around nerves in the brain and spinal cord, destruction of the myelin, abnormalities in nerve conduction, and neurologic deficits. EAE can be transferred to naive animals with myelin basic protein–specific CD4+ T cells, and the experimental disease can be blocked by antibodies specific for class II MHC or for CD4 molecules, indicating that CD4+ class II MHC–restricted T cells play an obligatory role in this disorder. A role for CTLs in this experimental disease is also suspected but remains unproved. It has

TABLE 18–5. Lesions and Mechanisms of Different Forms of Immunologic Reactions in the Skin

	Immediate Hypersensitivity	Immune Complex–Mediated Injury	Delayed Type Hypersensitivity
Induced by	Antigens that evoke IgE response (genetic predisposition?)	Antigens that induce IgM, IgG antibodies	Protein antigens; chemicals that bind to self proteins
Form of Cutaneous Reaction	Urticaria, wheal	Arthus reaction	Contact sensitivity, tuberculin reaction
Onset After Antigen Challenge	Minutes*	Usually 2–6 hours	Usually 24–48 hours
Pathologic Lesion	Edema, vascular dilatation, local smooth muscle contraction	Necrotizing vasculitis	Perivascular cellular infiltrates and edema
Transferred to Normal Animals by	Serum	Serum	Lymphocytes
Antibody Involved	IgE	IgG (usually complement-fixing subclasses), IgM	None
Effector Cells	Mast cells with IgE bound to Fc receptors	Neutrophils, monocytes (recruited by complement-dependent and complement-independent mechanisms)	CD4+ T cells, macrophages (activated by cytokines)
Secreted Mediators, Effector Molecules	Mast cell–derived mediators: vasoactive amines, lipid mediators	Products of complement activation: membrane attack complex, C3a, C5a	Cytokines, particularly IFN-γ and TNF

* Note that the late phase reaction of immediate hypersensitivity resembles delayed type hypersensitivity.
Abbreviations: Ig, immunuglobulin; IFN, interferon.

BOX 18-3. INSULIN-DEPENDENT DIABETES MELLITUS

Diabetes mellitus is a metabolic disease due to a deficiency of insulin or its inadequate function, leading to abnormalities in glucose metabolism that result in ketoacidosis, thirst, and increased urine production. The late stage of the disease is characterized by progressive atherosclerotic vascular lesions, which can lead to gangrene of the extremities due to arterial obstruction, renal failure due to glomerular and arterial injury, and blindness due to arterial aneurysms and increased fragility of proliferating vessels in the retina. The relationship of abnormal glucose metabolism and vascular lesions is not known. Insulin-dependent diabetes mellitus (IDDM, also called juvenile or type I diabetes) affects about 0.2 per cent of the United States population, with a peak age of onset of 11 to 12 years. These patients have a deficiency of insulin resulting from destruction of the insulin-producing β cells of the islets of Langerhans in the pancreas, and continuous hormone replacement therapy is needed.

Several mechanisms may contribute to β cell destruction, including CTL-mediated lysis of islet cells, local cytokine production, and autoantibodies against islet cells. In the rare cases in which the pancreatic lesions have been examined at the early active stages of the disease, the islets show cellular necrosis and lymphocytic infiltrations. This lesion is also called **insulitis.** The infiltrates consist of both CD8$^+$ and CD4$^+$ T cells. Surviving islet cells often express class II MHC molecules. This aberrant expression of MHC molecules is probably an effect of local production of IFN-γ and other cytokines by the T cells. It has been suggested that abnormally high expression of MHC molecules may amplify T cell responses and worsen islet cell injury, but there is no evidence proving that islet cells can function as antigen-presenting cells (APCs.) Autoantibodies against islet cells and insulin are also detected in the blood of these patients. These antibodies may participate in causing the disease or may be a result of T cell-mediated injury and release of normally sequestered antigens. In fact, in susceptible children who have not developed diabetes (such as relatives of patients) the presence of antibodies against islet cells is predictive of the development of IDDM. This suggests that the anti-islet cell antibodies contribute to injury to the islets. Multiple genes are involved in this disease. Recently, a great deal of attention has been devoted to the role of HLA genes (see text). Non-HLA genes also contribute to the disease, but these are undefined. Furthermore, viral infections, particularly with Coxsackie B-4, may precede the onset of IDDM, perhaps by initiating cell injury, altering self antigens, and triggering an autoimmune response. However, the nature of the antigens which initiate islet-specific immune responses is not known.

Animal models of spontaneous IDDM have been described. The inbred BB rat strain develops a T cell-mediated insulitis that is linked to both MHC and non-MHC genes. The non-obese diabetic (NOD) mouse strain also develops a spontaneous T cell-mediated insulitis. The linkage of this disease with the H-2 complex is remarkably similar to HLA-linked IDDM in humans. Interestingly, certain MHC genes are protective and prevent IDDM. The NOD mouse expresses I-A but not I-E class II MHC molecules, and breeding with I-E-positive strains or the expression of various transgenic I-A or I-E molecules in NOD mice reduces the incidence of the disease.

Finally, two types of transgenic mice have been created that express introduced transgenes in the pancreatic islet cells and develop IDDM. These are interesting experimental models, even though their relation to spontaneous IDDM is not clear. First, it was postulated that if foreign MHC molecules were selectively expressed on pancreatic β cells, these cells would be intrinsic allografts, in effect, and would be rejected by the host, giving rise to IDDM. Based on this hypothesis, several groups of investigators have constructed transgenic inbred mice that express a foreign class I or class II MHC molecule under the control of the insulin promoter and, therefore, preferentially or exclusively in insulin-producing β cells. Such mice do develop IDDM but surprisingly, no insulitis is seen because their T cells are tolerant to the allogeneic MHC (which is seen as "self" by the immune system of the transgenic mice). This induction of T cell tolerance indicates that expression of MHC molecules outside the thymus, i.e., in the pancreas, can induce tolerance. It may be that T cell tolerance to class II molecules expressed by islet cells is not due to clonal deletion, but develops because presentation of the allogeneic MHC antigens by the β cells induces clonal anergy in alloreactive T cells. This may occur because β cells are incompetent APCs that do not produce costimulators necessary for T cell activation. Insulin deficiency in these transgenic mice may be related not to a specific immune response but to excessive synthesis of MHC molecules in the β cells that may interfere with endogenous insulin synthesis or secretion by unknown mechanisms. These are intriguing results but their relation to human IDDM is unclear. Other transgenic mice have been constructed to express cytokines, specifically IFN-γ, under the control of the insulin promoter. These mice develop insulitis and IDDM, probably secondary to local IFN-γ secretion and macrophage activation.

---

been postulated that EAE is an experimental counterpart of a progressive neurologic disease called multiple sclerosis.

Cell-mediated immune responses to microbes and other foreign antigens may also lead to considerable injury of the tissues at the sites of infection or antigen exposure. Intracellular bacteria such as *Mycobacterium tuberculosis* induce strong T cell and macrophage responses, resulting in the formation of granulomas, and fibrosis due to the production of cytokines which stimulate fibroblast proliferation and collagen synthesis (described in Chapter 12). Therefore, mycobacterial infections often result in extensive tissue destruction and scarring that can cause severe functional impairment, for instance in the lungs. Sarcoidosis is a disease of unknown etiology in which granulomas develop in the lungs, lymphoid tissues, liver, and spleen. This disease is probably due to a T cell-mediated immune response to a foreign antigen that has eluded identification.

BOX 18 – 4. EXPERIMENTAL ALLERGIC ENCEPHALOMYELITIS

Experimental allergic encephalomyelitis (EAE) in mice, rats and guinea pigs is probably the best characterized experimental model of an organ-specific autoimmune disease mediated exclusively by T lymphocytes. The disease is induced by immunizing animals with guinea pig, bovine, or mouse myelin basic protein (MBP) with an adjuvant containing pertussis bacteria. About 1 to 2 weeks after immunization, the animals develop encephalomyelitis characterized by perivascular infiltrates composed of lymphocytes and macrophages associated with demyelination in the brain and spinal cord. The neurologic lesions can be mild and self-limited or chronic and relapsing. The chronic form of the experimental disease bears some, albeit superficial, resemblance to multiple sclerosis. This is often quoted as evidence to support the hypothesis that multiple sclerosis is an autoimmune disease.

In mice, EAE is caused by CD4+ T cells specific for MBP. This has been established by many lines of experimental evidence. Mice immunized with MBP contain CD4+ T cells that produce interleukin-2 and proliferate in response to MBP *in vitro*. The disease can be transferred to unimmunized animals by CD4+ T cells from MBP-immune syngeneic mice, or with MBP-specific CD4+ cloned T cell lines. Development of the disease can be prevented by injecting antibodies specific for CD4 or for class II MHC molecules into mice immunized with MBP. More recently, the disease has also been prevented by depleting T cells expressing $V_\beta 8$ and $V_\beta 13$ gene products in their antigen receptors. Therefore, murine EAE is due to MBP-specific, $V_\beta 8$ and/or $V_\beta 13$-expressing CD4+, class II MHC-restricted T cells. It is still not clear why immunization with autologous or heterologous MBP induces specific autoimmunity. It may be that myelin is an anatomically sequestered tissue, so that autologous MBP-reactive T cells are not deleted during thymic maturation. Immunization with this antigen together with an adjuvant leads to a T cell response directed against epitopes of autologous MBP. As the T cells respond to myelin adjacent to blood vessels in the central nervous system, cytokines are released that recruit and activate macrophages. This leads to destruction of the myelin. The role of different cytokines in the disease is not well understood. The observation that MBP-specific cloned T cell lines vary in their ability to induce EAE may allow investigators to define the T cell cytokines

and effector functions that are most important for the development of EAE. Astrocytes in the CNS show an aberrant expression of class II MHC molecules, presumably as a result of local production of IFN-γ. It may be that these astrocytes present MBP to T cells and contribute to persistent and excessive T cell activation.

Much of the recent interest in this disease has focused on the analysis of the fine specificity of MBP-reactive encephalitogenic T cells in different inbred mouse strains. For instance, in mice of the H-2ᵘ strain, the majority of encephalitogenic T cells recognize an MBP peptide consisting of the 9 amino-terminal amino acids in association with the I-Aᵘ molecule. The encephalitogenic T cells in these strains express a limited set of $V\alpha$, $J\alpha$, and $V\beta$ genes. Mutational analysis of various MBP peptides, similar to studies described in Chapter 6, have shown that some amino acid residues are critical for binding to MHC molecules and others for recognition by T cells. For instance, in MBP(1–20), an alanine substitution at position 4 enhances binding to I-Aᵘ whereas an alanine substitution at position 3 abolishes recognition of this peptide by MBP-specific T cells. Based on these findings, the ability of MBP(1–20) Ala 3,4 to inhibit the development of EAE was tested. If the peptide was injected in 10- to 100-fold excess together with MBP at the time of the first immunization, the incidence of EAE was significantly reduced. It is likely that the synthetic peptide binds avidly to I-A molecules and competitively inhibits the binding of the T cell-stimulating processed fragment of native MBP. This antigenic competition blocks activation of MBP-specific T cells and prevents the disease. Such findings provide an elegant *in vivo* demonstration of the phenomenon of antigenic competition at the level of binding to MHC molecules which was described in Chapter 6. These results also raise the exciting possibility that if we can identify self antigens that cause autoimmune diseases, administration of mutated forms of these antigens may be a rational and specific immunotherapy for the diseases. Alternatively, if we can identify MHC molecules that bind and present self antigens, synthetic peptides that bind to these molecules but do not stimulate T cells may inhibit the binding of self antigens and, therefore, the activation of MHC-restricted autoreactive T cells. Such an approach is feasible even without identifying the self antigen that initiates the autoimmune response.

Diseases Caused by Cytolytic T Lymphocytes

The principal physiologic function of CTLs is to eliminate intracellular microbes, primarily viruses. It follows, therefore, that infected cells are lysed during CTL-mediated protective immune responses. Some viruses directly injure infected cells, or are cytopathic, whereas others are not. Since CTLs cannot *a priori* distinguish between cytopathic and non-cytopathic viruses, they will lyse virally infected cells whether or not the infection itself is harmful to the host. *Therefore, CTL responses to viral infections can lead to tissue injury even if the virus itself has no pathologic effects.* Examples of viral infections in which the lesions are due to the host CTL response and not the virus itself include lymphocytic choriomeningitis in mice and viral hepatitis in humans (see Chapter 15).

To date, there are few documented examples of autoimmune diseases mediated by CTLs. In mice infected with the Coxsackie B virus, myocarditis develops, with infiltration of the heart by CD8+ T cells. These animals contain virus-specific, class I MHC-restricted CTLs as well as CTLs that lyse uninfected myocardial cells. It is postulated that the heart lesions are initiated by the virus infection and virus-specific CTLs, but myocardial injury leads to the exposure or alteration of self antigens and the development of autoreactive CTLs. As mentioned above, CTLs may also contribute to tissue injury in many of the disorders that are caused primarily by CD4+ T cells, such as insulitis and EAE. It is likely, however, that extracellular tissue antigens preferentially stimulate CD4+ T cells and that CD8+ CTLs recognize and respond to endogenously synthesized antigens, such as viral proteins. One would, therefore, predict that these two forms of T cell-mediated immunity would be involved in pathologic immunity against distinct types of antigens.

So far in this chapter, we have discussed the various immunologic mechanisms that cause tissue injury and disease. We have also described how immunologic diseases can result from responses to autologous antigens, foreign antigens, or foreign antigens that cross-react with self molecules. In the remainder of this chapter, we discuss the mechanisms that might lead to autoimmunity, which remains the most frequent, the least understood, and the most intensively investigated etiology for human immunologic diseases.

MECHANISMS OF AUTOIMMUNITY

The possibility that an individual's immune system can react against autologous antigens and lead to pathologic tissue injury was appreciated by immunologists from the time that the specificity of the immune system for foreign antigens was recognized. In the early 1900s, Paul Ehrlich coined the rather melodramatic phrase, "horror autotoxicus," for immunity against self. When Macfarlane Burnet proposed the clonal selection hypothesis 50 years later, he added the corollary that clones of autoreactive lymphocytes were deleted during development in order to prevent autoimmune reactions. The ability to discriminate between self and non-self has been emphasized throughout this book as an essential and unique property of the normal immune system. As discussed in Chapters 8 and 10, self-tolerance is due to two principal mechanisms: clonal deletion and clonal anergy.

The most effective mechanism of self-tolerance is the deletion of self-recognizing T and B lymphocytes prior to their maturation to functional competence, because of which normal individuals lack lymphocytes capable of recognizing many autologous antigens. Clonal deletion, however, cannot account for all self tolerance, because autoreactive B cells can be induced to secrete autoantibodies by polyclonal activators and not all self antigens may be present in the thymus to delete developing T cells. The alternative mechanism by which lymphocytes become self-tolerant is clonal anergy, induced by encounter with self antigens so that the self-reactive cells survive but cannot respond to these antigens. Other mechanisms of self-tolerance that have been postulated include suppressor T cells specific for self antigens, but their existence and physiologic role are unproved.

Autoimmunity results from a breakdown or failure of the mechanisms that are normally responsible for maintaining self-tolerance. Failure of self-tolerance can be due to incomplete deletion of self-reactive clones or to aberrant stimulation or regulation of self-reactive lymphocytes that are normally anergic to self antigens. Much of our knowledge of autoimmunity is based on experimental models, in which autoimmune diseases occur spontaneously or are induced by particular immunizations. Several important general

concepts have emerged from the analyses of these models during the last 20 years or so:

1. *Multiple interacting factors contribute to the development of autoimmune disease.* These include immunologic abnormalities, genetic backgrounds that predispose to autoimmunity, and microbial infections that often precede clinical autoimmune diseases and may lead to aberrant lymphocyte stimulation. Because various combinations of these factors may be operative in different disorders, it is not surprising that autoimmune diseases comprise an extraordinarily heterogeneous group of clinical and pathologic abnormalities.

2. *Different types of antigens and immunologic mechanisms may cause systemic and organ-specific autoimmune diseases.* For instance, immune responses to widely disseminated antigens (such as autologous DNA in SLE) and the formation of circulating immune complexes typically produce systemic diseases. In contrast, autoimmune responses against antigens with restricted tissue distributions lead to organ-specific or tissue-specific injury, such as insulitis in diabetes mellitus and motor end-plate lesions in myasthenia gravis. It is also likely that systemic diseases characterized by multiple autoimmune phenomena are due to aberrant regulation or polyclonal activation of numerous clones of lymphocytes. In contrast, organ-specific autoimmune diseases may be due to failure of self-tolerance in lymphocytes specific for one or a few tissue antigens or abnormal activation of lymphocyte clones reactive with a limited number of antigens. The possible mechanisms leading to these two classes of autoimmune reactions are described later in the chapter.

3. *Low levels of autoantibodies are stimulated in normal individuals during immune responses to foreign antigens.* Based largely on the detection of such "natural autoantibodies" in healthy individuals, it has been suggested that the potential for autoreactivity exists normally. Natural autoantibodies are usually low-affinity antibodies of the IgM class that may be generated without T cell help and do not produce tissue injury. Pathologic autoimmunity may develop if larger amounts of high-affinity autoantibodies are produced, presumably as a result of help provided by autoreactive T cells. This concept again emphasizes the importance of T cell tolerance in maintaining unresponsiveness to self antigens.

A major difficulty in defining the mechanisms of human autoimmune diseases has been the inability to identify the antigens that initiate autoimmune responses. As a result, the specific etiologies of most autoimmune diseases are not known. Recent advances in the experimental analysis of self-tolerance, and in techniques for studying the molecular basis of antigen recognition by lymphocytes, are providing new insights into the mechanisms of autoimmunity. In the following sections, we describe the immunologic, genetic, and other factors that contribute to the development of autoimmune responses, keeping in mind that these factors are often interrelated and act in concert to give rise to pathologic autoimmunity.

LYMPHOCYTE ABNORMALITIES IN AUTOIMMUNITY

Autoimmune diseases may result from primary abnormalities of B cells, T cells, or both. Even in disorders mediated by autoantibodies, the defect may lie in helper T lymphocytes, which are necessary for the production of high-affinity antibodies. Experimental myasthenia gravis, for instance, can be adoptively transferred to normal animals with cloned lines of helper T cells specific for acetylcholine receptors, even though the disease is caused by anti-receptor antibodies. Because helper T cells play a central role in the regulation of all immune responses, and because T cell clonal deletion is an effective way of maintaining self-tolerance, much recent attention has focused on the role of T cells in autoimmunity.

Immunologic abnormalities can disrupt self-tolerance in many different ways. First, autoimmunity may develop if self-reactive clones of lymphocytes escape normal deletion mechanisms and are allowed to mature. Since the mechanisms of clonal deletion are not yet known, it is difficult to postulate how self-reactive lymphocytes may evade such deletion. As we shall discuss later, the expression of particular MHC alleles may influence the positive and negative selection of T lymphocytes during thymic maturation. Second, autoreactive lymphocytes that survive but are normally unresponsive to self antigens may be stimulated by cross-reactive antigens or by polyclonal activators that function independently of antigen receptor-mediated stimulation. Third, regulatory mechanisms that normally control the responses of all lymphocytes, including ones that are autoreactive, may be aberrant or nonfunctional. Immunologic studies of autoimmunity have focused on two broad aspects: (1) the stimuli that trigger the proliferation and effector functions of autoreactive lymphocytes, and (2) the nature of autoreactive B and T cells, in particular whether they are normally present cells that escape regulation or abnormal clones that are deleted or absent from healthy individuals.

Immunologic Cross-Reactions of Foreign and Self Antigens

One of the simplest experimental methods for inducing an autoimmune disease is to immunize an animal with a slightly altered form of a self antigen or with the homologous antigen from an animal of a different species. For example, rats and mice immunized with heat-denatured autologous thyroglobulin (a thyroid protein) or with rabbit thyroglobulin in adjuvant develop thyroiditis. Similarly, mice immunized with bovine or guinea pig myelin basic protein in adjuvant develop effector T cells that also recognize the

mouse's own myelin basic protein and cause EAE. Thus, the immune response is induced by a foreign antigen or altered self antigen but the disease develops because the response is also directed against the homologous normal self antigen. Little is known about the mechanisms by which such immunizations with antigens that differ only slightly from self antigens lead to an apparent breakdown of self-tolerance. In the case of experimental autoimmune thyroiditis, it is possible that mice normally contain B cells capable of recognizing some epitope(s) of their own thyroglobulin; however, these B cells do not produce antibody because helper T cells specific for other determinants of the same protein are tolerant or have been deleted. If rabbit thyroglobulin has T cell epitopes that are different from mouse thyroglobulin, the rabbit protein injected into mice will activate helper T cells, which can cooperate with the self thyroglobulin-specific B cells (Fig. 18-7). This leads to stimulation of the B cells and the production of antibodies that bind to the mouse's own thyroglobulin and produce thyroiditis. Such immunologic cross-reactions can explain how autoantibodies might be produced against multideterminant self antigens.

Because autoimmune responses induced by immunologic cross-reactions are likely to generate autoantibodies specific for one or a few related antigens, it is likely that the lesions that develop are organ- or tissue-specific. Infections or inflammation secondary to trauma may lead to alterations in autologous proteins and generate autoimmunity by this mechanism. This may be the basis for the clinical observation that many organ-specific autoimmune diseases follow infectious prodromes or trauma.

Polyclonal Lymphocyte Activation

Autoimmunity can also result from antigen-independent stimulation of self-reactive clones that are not deleted during development. Polyclonal activators stimulate a large number of T or B lymphocytes irrespective of antigenic specificity and often without interacting with antigen receptors. The best example is lipopolysaccharide (LPS), which functions as a polyclonal B cell activator in mice. Mice injected with LPS produce antibodies of many specificities, included among which are autoantibodies. This may be because some self-reactive B cells are not deleted but rendered unresponsive (anergic) to self antigens (see Chapter 10). However, they retain the ability to proliferate and differentiate in response to stimuli such as LPS, which functions even in the absence of antigen receptor expression. *This form of autoimmunity, being a component of a polyclonal response, is usually associated with the production of multiple autoantibodies and therefore gives rise to systemic rather than organ-specific autoimmune diseases.* Systemic lupus erythematosus fits the criterion of a systemic autoimmune disease with multiple autoantibodies (see Box 18-1),

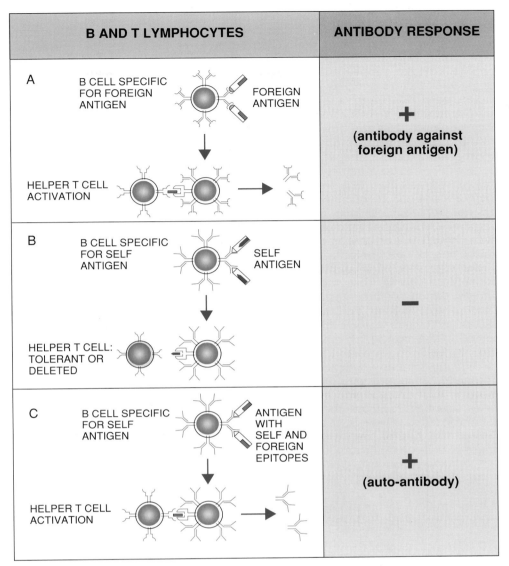

B AND T LYMPHOCYTES	ANTIBODY RESPONSE
A B CELL SPECIFIC FOR FOREIGN ANTIGEN FOREIGN ANTIGEN HELPER T CELL ACTIVATION	**+** (antibody against foreign antigen)
B B CELL SPECIFIC FOR SELF ANTIGEN SELF ANTIGEN HELPER T CELL: TOLERANT OR DELETED	**−**
C B CELL SPECIFIC FOR SELF ANTIGEN ANTIGEN WITH SELF AND FOREIGN EPITOPES HELPER T CELL ACTIVATION	**+** (auto-antibody)

FIGURE 18–7. Role of helper T cells in the production of autoantibodies. In a normal immune response (A), B and T lymphocytes specific for epitopes of a foreign antigen cooperate to stimulate antibody production. B cells specific for a self antigen may not be stimulated if helper T cells specific for the self antigen are absent or tolerant (B). However, these B cells may produce autoantibody if stimulated with an antigen containing foreign epitopes that are recognized by specific helper T cells (C).

but the initiating agent for this disease is unknown. Polyclonal antibody secretion *in vivo* may be induced by microbial cell wall products similar to LPS, and this is another possible link between infections and autoimmunity. Multiple autoimmune phenomena are also associated with graft-versus-host disease (GVHD), which occasionally develops after the transplantation of allogeneic bone marrow (see Chapter 16). In recipients of such transplants, helper T cells may develop from precursors in the transplanted marrow and B cells may be derived from the host. If these two populations are allogeneic, the T cells recognize the host B cells as "foreign" and respond by secreting cytokines. This leads to polyclonal B cell activation and autoantibody production in the absence of specific antigenic stimulation.

Polyclonal T cell activation has also been postulated as a mechanism of autoimmunity. Adjuvants or bacterial "super-antigens" can stimulate large num-

bers of T cells, among which may be clones specific for but normally unresponsive to self antigens.

Abnormalities in Lymphocyte Activation and Regulation

A variety of immunoregulatory abnormalities has been associated with different autoimmune diseases, particularly in animal models. (NZB × NZW)F1 mice develop a disease resembling human SLE (see Box 18–1), and their B lymphocytes produce much higher amounts of antibodies in response to polyclonal activators and exogenous antigens than B cells from other strains that do not develop spontaneous autoimmunity. The biochemical basis of this B cell "hyperresponsiveness" is unknown. In contrast, MRL/*lpr* mice, which develop a SLE–like syndrome associated with

T cell proliferation, have normal B cell responses. It has been postulated that the spontaneously proliferating T cells in these mice constitutively produce a cytokine that stimulates B cell growth and differentiation. This cytokine appears distinct from the known B cell helper factors and has not yet been identified molecularly. It is important to distinguish between autoimmune disorders that may be caused by primary B cell abnormalities and those due to excessive cytokine production, because diagnostic and therapeutic approaches for these categories of diseases would be quite different even if their clinicopathologic manifestations were similar. The search for such immunologic aberrations in human autoimmune disorders has not yielded informative results to date.

It is also striking that many experimental autoimmune diseases, including thyroiditis and EAE, develop only if the antigens are administered with strong adjuvants. Such adjuvants may have two complementary effects. First, they may activate macrophages, which produce costimulators that function normally to overcome T cell anergy (see Chapter 10). Second, adjuvants may contain proteins, possibly resembling super-antigens, that are polyclonal activators of T cells.

Finally, various deficiencies in the numbers and/or function of suppressor T cells have been reported in many experimental and human autoimmune diseases. Attempts to isolate such suppressor cells have generally failed. There is, therefore, little direct evidence for a role of suppressor cells in the maintenance of self-tolerance and, conversely, for suppressor cell defects as a cause of autoimmunity.

The Nature of Autoreactive Lymphocytes: Analysis of Antigen Receptor V Genes in Autoimmunity

It is evident from our discussion so far that we know little about the specificity and development of autoreactive lymphocytes. One can postulate that the expression of particular antigen receptor variable (V) genes may contribute to autoimmunity in different ways. For instance, autoimmunity may be due to the presence in the germline of V genes that encode self antigen-specific receptors and that are absent in normal individuals. Individuals that contain these V genes may have an inherited propensity to develop autoimmunity. If, however, autoimmunity is due to a failure to delete self-reactive lymphocyte clones, then all individuals may contain the same germline V genes but the peripheral lymphocytes of individuals prone to develop these disorders may express antigen receptors that are absent from the normal selected repertoire of mature lymphocytes. It is also possible that autoimmunity is due to aberrant activation and regulation of lymphocytes that are present normally. In this case there may be no difference in V gene expression between autoimmune and normal individuals. Finally,

autoreactive lymphocytes may arise as a consequence of abnormal somatic mutations involving antigen receptors that normally recognize foreign antigens, making these receptors reactive with self antigens.

One approach for evaluating these various possibilities is to compare the Ig and T cell receptor (TCR) V genes in the germlines of inbred strains of mice that do and do not develop spontaneous autoimmunity. In addition, one can determine if self-reactive lymphocytes or antibodies express V genes that are present in normal individuals or in lymphocytes or antibodies specific for foreign antigens. Such analyses are in their infancy and have not yet provided definitive answers to why autoimmunity develops. Nevertheless, the available data have already led to some significant conclusions:

1. *Autoimmunity is not due to a specific Ig or TCR repertoire and is not associated with a specific V gene polymorphism.* Comparisons of restriction fragment length polymorphisms (see Chapter 4, Box 4–1) in humans that do and do not have autoimmune diseases indicate no specific associations of the diseases with Ig gene loci. The Ig germline genes in two strains of mice that develop SLE–like syndromes, (NZB × NZW)F1 and MRL/*lpr* (see Box 18–1), also reveal no consistent differences from other, non-autoimmune strains. Autoantibodies of different specificities do not show similar patterns of V gene usage or somatic mutations. This argues against a common initiating antigen or stimulus for diverse autoimmune disorders. Limited analyses of TCR α and β loci have led to similar conclusions.

2. *Autoreactive B and T lymphocytes express essentially the same antigen receptor genes as do normal lymphocytes specific for foreign antigens.* For instance, anti-DNA antibody producing B cell hybridomas from (NZB × NZW)F1 mice, and rheumatoid factor producing hybridomas from MRL/*lpr* mice, contain Ig V, D, and J gene segments that are also found in various combinations in hybridomas that secrete antibodies specific for foreign antigens. The Ig genes of rheumatoid factor–producing B cells also show somatic mutations in V regions that suggest that these autoantibodies are produced by the same types of antigenic stimulation and lymphocyte selection that are operative in humoral immune responses to foreign antigens. Interestingly, in mice, the small subset of B cells that expresses CD5 accounts for a disproportionately high level of autoantibody production. These cells secrete IgM autoantibodies against a variety of self antigens spontaneously in culture, i.e., without overt antigenic stimulation. The significance of $CD5^+$ B cells in human autoimmune diseases is not clear.

3. *In individual patients or inbred mouse strains with organ-specific autoimmune diseases, the autoreactive lymphocytes may be oligoclonal or may express restricted sets of V genes.* In an oligoclonal population, which is derived from a few precursors, only a small number of antigen receptor genes is expressed. Restricted V gene expression may, however, also be seen in a lymphocyte population that is multiclonal in origin, and this suggests that the population is specific

for one or a few antigenic determinants. For instance, the majority of the T cell clones isolated from the synovium of an individual patient with rheumatoid arthritis express the same germline TCR genes, indicating that they arose from the same T cell. Rheumatoid factor–producing B cells from individual MRL/*lpr* mice are similarly oligoclonal. T cells cloned from the cerebrospinal fluid of individual patients with multiple sclerosis also express only a few V genes. However, different patients or inbred mouse strains with the same disease may express different Ig or TCR V genes in their self-reactive lymphocytes. Therefore, the restricted V gene expression in autoreactive lymphocytes in individuals probably reflects the fact that these cells are specific for one or few antigenic determinants rather than a consistent association between a particular pattern of V gene usage and the development of autoimmunity. Alternatively, if only a few autoreactive cells escape tolerance induction or regulation at any given time, the cells isolated from lesions would be oligoclonal.

The general conclusion of these studies is that *organ-specific autoimmune diseases are usually due to stimulation of lymphocyte clones having a limited repertoire.* The molecular characteristics of many autoreactive antibodies suggest that their production is essentially similar to the generation of antibodies specific for foreign protein antigens. These studies do not tell us whether autoreactive clones are abnormal cells that have escaped the process of self-tolerance or are normally present cells whose aberrant stimulation or regulation leads to pathologic autoimmunity. They also do not indicate whether the primary lesion leading to autoantibody production is in the B cells or in helper T cells or both.

Genetic Factors in Autoimmunity

From the earliest studies of patients with autoimmune disorders, it has been known that some of these diseases run in families and there is a high rate of concordance in monozygotic twins. Much of the interest in the genetic basis of autoimmunity has focused on MHC genes, because of their known role in the selection of T cells and in the induction of immune responses to protein antigens. Although it is not yet clear precisely how MHC genes influence the development of autoimmunity, recent molecular and biochemical studies are providing new insights into mechanisms as well as potential therapeutic approaches.

Role of MHC Genes in Autoimmunity

Human leukocyte antigen (HLA) typing of large groups of patients with various autoimmune diseases has shown that some HLA alleles occur at higher frequencies in patients with particular diseases than in

TABLE 18–6. Examples of Human Leukocyte Antigen (HLA)–Linked Immunologic Diseases

Disease	HLA Allele	Relative Risk*
Rheumatoid arthritis	DR4	6
Insulin-dependent diabetes mellitus	DR3	5
	DR4	6–7
	DR3/DR4	20
	DR3, DQw8	100
	DR2	0.25
Pemphigus vulgaris	DR4	24
Chronic active hepatitis	DR3	14
Sjögren's syndrome	DR3	10
Celiac disease	DR3	12
Ankylosing spondylitis	B27	90

* Relative risk defines the chance of individuals with a particular HLA allele(s) of developing a disease compared with individuals lacking that HLA allele(s).

the general population. From such studies, it is possible to estimate the "relative risk" of developing a disease with every known HLA allele (Table 18–6). The strongest such association is between ankylosing spondylitis, an autoimmune disease of vertebral joints, and the class I MHC allele, HLA–B27. The immunologic basis of this is not well understood. Recently, much more work has been done on the polymorphic class II alleles, HLA–DR and DQ, in autoimmune diseases, because of the realization that class II MHC molecules are crucial for the selection and activation of CD4+ T cells and, therefore, for the regulation of all immune responses to protein antigens.

DNA sequencing of class II MHC genes, combined with analysis of restriction fragment length polymorphisms to identify small genetic differences between patients and controls, have clearly established the association of particular class II MHC sequences with some autoimmune diseases. Two examples are especially illustrative:

1. *Insulin-dependent diabetes mellitus* (Box 18–3) is both positively and negatively associated with HLA genes. Ninety to 95 per cent of Caucasians with this disease have HLA–DR3 or HLA–DR4 or both, in contrast to about 40 per cent of normals, and 40 to 50 per cent of patients are HLA-DR3/DR4 heterozygotes, in contrast to 5 per cent of normals. It is now apparent that the HLA–associated susceptibility to IDDM is more strongly linked to particular HLA–DQ alleles, which are in linkage disequilibrium (i.e., inherited together) with certain HLA–DR alleles. All DQβ chains that are more frequent in Caucasian patients than in controls have one of three amino acids (alanine, valine, or serine) at position 57, whereas the DQβ chains present at lower frequency in patients than in controls have aspartic acid (Asp) at this position. Interestingly, the non-obese diabetic (NOD) mouse, which develops a spontaneous IDDM–like disease, has serine at position 57 of I-Aβ, the murine homolog of DQβ. In contrast, most other mouse strains, including the

closely related non-obese normal, have Asp at this position. These observations led to the hypothesis that Asp 57 in the DQβ chain confers resistance to IDDM and its absence increases susceptibility. This residue forms a part of the antigen-binding cleft of the class II MHC molecule (see Chapter 5), supporting the idea that it influences T cell selection or antigen recognition. There are, however, several exceptions to this association of Asp 57 with IDDM. For instance, Japanese patients with the disease frequently have Asp 57 in their DQβ chains. Moreover, if a transgenic I-A molecule containing serine at position 57 in the β chain is expressed in NOD mice, it too reduces the incidence of IDDM. *It is, therefore, likely that the structure of the peptide-binding cleft of the entire MHC molecule contributes to the development of this autoimmune disease,* and residue 57 may be one of many amino acids that play a role in determining this structure. Furthermore, the HLA linkage of IDDM is unusual, in that it maps as a recessive trait. The likely reason for this is that increased susceptibility is associated with the absence of certain residues in the DQβ chain of both alleles, and these residues in either allele are significantly protective.

2. *Rheumatoid arthritis* (see Box 18-2) is most strongly associated with HLA-DR4 and less so with the DR1 and DRw10 haplotypes. In all these alleles, the amino acid sequences from positions 65 to 75 of the DRβ chain are almost identical. These sequences are located in a polymorphic region of the class II MHC molecule that also participates in the formation of the antigen-binding cleft.

There are several postulated mechanisms to account for the association of autoimmune diseases with class II MHC sequences.

1. The amino acid sequences of MHC molecules in an individual may determine which clones of potentially autoreactive T cells are positively selected or deleted during development. As we discussed in Chapter 8, the expression of particular MHC genes is crucial during thymic education, because T cells recognize peptides attached to the antigen-binding clefts of MHC molecules and this recognition determines the selection of developing T lymphocytes. Thus, if the MHC molecules in the thymus of an individual fail to bind a self protein with high affinity, T cells reactive with this self antigen may escape clonal deletion. Such a mechanism might explain the HLA-DQβ-associated resistance to IDDM. If this MHC molecule is capable of binding and presenting the self antigen(s) responsible for insulitis, the presence of this allele results in deletion or inactivation of T cells specific for this self antigen. In the absence of this MHC allele, the autoreactive T cells might escape negative selection and may later cause insulitis. Presumably, these T cells are restricted to recognizing the relevant self antigen in association with another HLA molecule, which, for unknown reasons, does not negatively select the cells during their maturation.

2. Similarities between MHC molecules and self or microbial antigens may contribute to autoimmunity. For example, if a microbial antigen resembles a self MHC molecule, T cell responses against the microbe may result in cross-reactions against self MHC. This is an example of molecular mimicry. Several bacterial and viral proteins contain stretches of amino acids that are also found in various MHC molecules, but the pathogenic significance of these findings is uncertain.

3. Class II MHC molecules may influence the activation of T cells such as suppressor cells, whose function is to prevent autoimmune reactions. However, as stated above, the role of regulatory T cells in self-tolerance is not clearly established.

4. An older hypothesis was that HLA-disease associations reflected the ability of some but not other MHC molecules to bind self antigens and present these antigens to specific T cells. According to this postulate, autoreactive T cells were neither deleted nor rendered anergic. Instead, they were unable to respond to self antigens because normal individuals could not present these antigens in association with their own MHC molecules. However, we now know that MHC molecules normally bind many, and perhaps all, self peptides and do not discriminate between self and non-self at the stage of antigen presentation (see Chapter 6). Therefore, this hypothesis is unlikely to be correct.

Finally, we should add that disease-associated HLA sequences are found in healthy individuals and, conversely, that alleles commonly present in normal individuals are also found in some patients with autoimmune diseases. *Therefore, the expression of a particular HLA gene is not by itself the cause of any autoimmune disease* but is likely to be one of several factors that contribute to autoimmunity. It is also clear that HLA-disease associations are often weak or partial. In some cases, this may be because an HLA "allele" identified by tissue typing is actually a family of structurally related alleles, some of which have strong disease associations and others that do not.

The concept of HLA-linked autoimmunity does have practical implications. It has some predictive value, the usefulness of which depends on the strength of the disease association. It may also be possible to exploit this concept for specific immunotherapy. For instance, if a polymorphic MHC sequence is associated with a disease in a patient, antibodies against this sequence or peptides that bind to this site in the MHC but do not stimulate T cells may block T cell antigen recognition and alter the course of the disease. This idea has been successfully used to prevent EAE in inbred mice (Box 18-4). Whether or not such approaches will be feasible in the clinical setting remains to be seen.

Association of Other Genes with Autoimmunity

The development of autoimmunity is clearly influenced by multiple genes. Breeding analyses of mouse strains that develop autoimmunity indicate that as many as twenty genes may contribute to different diseases. Even in autoimmune diseases that are associated with class I MHC (HLA–A or HLA–B) alleles, it is thought that the apparent association reflects a linkage disequilibrium with another adjacent gene(s) that is actually responsible for disease susceptibility. Some of these non-MHC genes may influence immune reactions and others may cause disease by non-immune mechanisms. In humans, genes for two complement proteins, C2 and C4, and for two cytokines, tumor necrosis factor (TNF) and lymphotoxin (LT), are located within the MHC locus (see Chapter 5). It is known that C2 and C4 deficiencies lead to impaired phagocytosis of immune complexes and an increased incidence of SLE–like syndromes. In addition, certain alleles of C2 and C4 genes may be in linkage disequilibrium with MHC alleles that predispose to autoimmunity. Recent data suggest that in humans TNF genes are also polymorphic, and some alleles may be associated with autoimmune diseases. Such findings have led to the concept of "extended HLA haplotypes." In some HLA haplotypes, recombination within the locus appears to be suppressed, so that many genes (both HLA genes and other adjacent genes) remain in linkage disequilibrium. We do not know the molecular mechanism or evolutionary advantage of maintaining an extended haplotype in linkage disequilibrium, but some such extended haplotypes are present with increased frequency in patients with certain autoimmune diseases.

In the final analysis, it is clear that genes presently identified do not completely account for the inheritance patterns of autoimmune diseases. However, because of the remarkable progress that has been made in the late 1980s in techniques for identifying disease-producing genes and mapping the human genome, it is likely that the genetic basis of autoimmunity will be understood in increasingly precise terms in the not too distant future.

OTHER FACTORS IN AUTOIMMUNITY

The development of autoimmunity is also related to a number of other factors:

1. *Anatomic alterations* may lead to the exposure of antigens that are normally sequestered and concealed from the immune system. Because of this sequestration, individuals may not be immunologically tolerant to such antigens. Therefore, if such self antigens are released and interact with immunocompetent lymphocytes, specific immune responses may develop. Examples of anatomically sequestered antigens may be intraocular proteins and sperm. Post-traumatic uveitis and orchitis, and orchitis following vasectomy, are thought to be autoimmune responses to self antigens that are released from their normal locations.

2. *Hormonal influences* are also thought to play a role in human and experimental autoimmune dis-

orders. SLE, for instance, affects females about ten times as frequently as males. The lupus-like disease of (NZB × NZW)F1 mice also develops in females and can be retarded by androgen treatment. Many other autoimmune disorders tend to be more frequent in females, although this is clearly not always the case. It is not known whether this is due to the influence of sex hormones or other factors.

3. *Viral and bacterial infections,* as mentioned in the preceding sections, are associated with autoimmunity, and infections often precede the clinical manifestations of autoimmune diseases. In most of these diseases, the infectious microorganism is not present in autoimmune lesions and is not even detectable when autoimmunity develops. Therefore, the lesions are not due to the infectious agent itself but result from host immune responses. The many possible effects of infections include polyclonal lymphocyte activation, alterations of self antigens to create partially cross-reactive neo-antigens, mimicry of self antigens, and tissue injury leading to release of anatomically sequestered antigens.

It is appropriate to conclude by reminding ourselves that "mechanisms of autoimmunity" is a topic in which theories and hypotheses continue to outnumber facts. However, we now know a great deal about the immunologic basis of self/non-self discrimination and the induction and maintenance of self-tolerance, and remarkable technical advances have been made in analyzing genetic polymorphisms and structural variations in Ig, TCR, and MHC genes. There seems little doubt that as these new concepts and methods are applied to human and experimental autoimmune diseases, clearer and more definitive answers to the enigmas of autoimmunity will begin to emerge.

SUMMARY

Diseases in which tissue injury and pathophysiologic abnormalities are due to immunologic mechanisms may be initiated by immune responses to foreign or self (autologous) antigens. Pathogenic mechanisms include antigen-antibody complexes formed during humoral immune responses, autoantibodies against fixed tissue or cell surface antigens, and T lymphocytes. The effector mechanisms by which antibodies and immune complexes induce tissue injury include the complement system and various host inflammatory cells. Antibodies against physiologic agents such as hormones or against cell surface receptors for hormones induce functional abnormalities without the involvement of any other effector systems. CD4+ T lymphocytes recruit and activate macrophages as the principal effectors of tissue injury, and CD8+ cytolytic T lymphocytes themselves lyse antigen-bearing target cells.

Immune responses against foreign antigens may be pathologic either because of immunologic cross-reactivity with self antigens or because the responses are excessive or unregulated (hence the term "hypersensitivity" applied to such reactions). Strong immune responses to self antigens, called autoimmunity, are usually pathologic, because normal individuals are tolerant to self antigens. Autoimmune responses develop as a result of multiple interacting factors. The principal immunologic mechanisms that may contribute to autoimmunity include polyclonal lymphocyte stimulation, the introduction of foreign antigens that are partially cross-reactive with self molecules, and abnormalities in immunoregulation. The strongest genetic association of autoimmunity is with MHC genes, and multiple mechanisms have been proposed to account for such associations. Recent advances in the understanding of self-tolerance and self/non-self discrimination and in techniques for analyzing Ig, TCR, and MHC genes hold great promise for elucidating the mechanisms of autoimmunity and for developing rational therapeutic strategies for this group of diseases.

SELECTED READINGS

Acha-Orbea, H., L. Steinman, and H. O. McDevitt. T cell receptors in murine autoimmune diseases. Annual Review of Immunology 7:371–405, 1989.

Bruijn, J. A., P. J. Hoedemaeker, and G. J. Fleuren. Pathogenesis of anti-basement membrane glomerulopathy and immune complex glomerulonephritis: dichotomy dissolved. Laboratory Investigation 61:480–488, 1989.

Castano, L., and G. S. Eisenbarth. Type 1 diabetes: a chronic autoimmune disease of human, mouse and rat. Annual Review of Immunology 8:647–679, 1990.

Charreire, J. Immune mechanisms in autoimmune thyroiditis. Advances in Immunology 46:263–334, 1989.

Kofler, R., F. J. Dixon, and A. N. Theofilopoulos. The genetic origin of autoantibodies. Immunology Today 8:374–380, 1987.

Kumar, V., D. H. Kono, J. L. Urban, and L. Hood. The T-cell receptor repertoire and autoimmune diseases. Annual Review of Immunology 7:657–682, 1989.

Lindstrom, J. D. Shelton, and Y. Fujii. Myasthenia gravis. Advances in Immunology 42:233–284, 1988.

Samter, M., D. W. Talmage, M. M. Frank, K. Frank Austen, and H. N. Claman (eds.). Immunological Diseases, 4th ed. Boston, Little, Brown & Co., 1989.

Theofilopoulos, A. N., R. Kofler, P. A. Singer, and F. J. Dixon. Molecular genetics of murine lupus models. Advances in Immunology 46:61–110, 1989.

Thompson, G. HLA disease associations: models for insulin-dependent diabetes mellitus and the study of complex human genetic disorders. Annual Review of Genetics 22:31–50, 1988.

Todd, J. A. Genetic control of autoimmunity in type 1 diabetes. Immunology Today 11:122–129, 1990.

Zamvil, S. S., and L. Steinman. The T lymphocyte in experimental allergic encephalomyelitis. Annual Review of Immunology 8:579–621, 1990.

CHAPTER NINETEEN

CONGENITAL

AND ACQUIRED

IMMUNODEFICIENCIES

The integrity of the immune system is essential for defense against infectious organisms and their toxic products and, therefore, for the survival of all individuals. Defects in one or more components of the immune system can lead to serious and often fatal disorders, which are grouped into immunodeficiency diseases. These diseases are broadly classified into two groups. The **congenital** or **primary immunodeficiencies** are genetic defects that result in an increased susceptibility to infections that is frequently manifested early in infancy and childhood but is sometimes clinically detected later in life. It is estimated that in the United States approximately 1 in 500 individuals are born with a defect in some component(s) of the immune system, although only a small proportion are affected severely enough to develop life-threatening complications. **Acquired** or **secondary immunodeficiencies** develop as a consequence of malnutrition, disseminated cancers, treatment with immunosuppressive drugs, or infections of immunocompetent cells, most notably with the human immunodeficiency virus (HIV), the etiologic agent of the acquired immunodeficiency syndrome (AIDS). This chapter describes the major types of congenital and acquired immunodeficiencies, with an emphasis on their pathogenesis and on the components of the immune system that are involved in each.

Before beginning our discussion, it is important to emphasize some general features of immunodeficiencies:

1. *The principal consequence of immunodeficiency is an increased susceptibility to infections.* The nature of the infection in a particular patient depends largely on the component of the immune system that is defective. For instance, deficient humoral immunity usually results in increased susceptibility to infections by pyogenic bacteria, whereas defects in cell-mediated immunity lead to infections by viruses and other intracellular microbes. Specific examples of these will be mentioned later in the chapter.

2. *Patients with immunodeficiencies are also prone to certain types of cancers, particularly those caused by oncogenic viruses.* This is generally seen in T cell immunodeficiencies because, as we discussed in Chapter 17, T cells may play an important role in surveillance against virus-induced tumors. In addition, somewhat paradoxically, certain immunodeficiencies are associated with an increased incidence of autoimmunity.

3. *Clinically and pathologically, immunodeficiency diseases are extremely heterogeneous.* In large part, this is because different diseases involve different components of the immune system. However, such heterogeneity is also seen in various diseases involving the same cells or molecules and even in different patients suffering from the same disorder. The reason for this variability is not well understood.

Deficient immune responses may result from abnormalities in specific or natural immunity. Defective specific immunity is due to abnormal development, activation, or function of specific T or B lymphocytes or both. Among the examples of impaired natural immunity are defects in phagocytes and the complement system. We first describe congenital immunodeficiencies, dividing our discussion into defects in B cells, T cells, and both, and in phagocytes. In each group, the current understanding of the cellular or molecular basis of the immunodeficiency will be illustrated with selected examples. We conclude this chapter with a discussion of AIDS and other acquired immunodeficiencies.

CONGENITAL B CELL DEFICIENCIES

Congenital abnormalities in B lymphocyte development and function result in deficient antibody production. These diseases have been recognized for many years, because assays for measuring serum antibodies have been in routine clinical use since the 1950s. A large number of congenital deficiencies that selectively affect humoral immune responses are now known (Table 19-1). Clinically, these disorders are characterized by recurrent infections with pyogenic

TABLE 19-1. Examples of Congenital B Cell Immunodeficiencies

Disease	Functional Deficiencies	Presumed Mechanism of Defect
X-linked agammaglobulinemia	All Ig isotypes decreased; reduced B cells	Block in pre-B to B cell maturation
Selective IgA deficiency	Decreased serum IgA1 and IgA2; normal B cells	Failure of terminal differentiation of IgA+ B cells
Ig deficiency with increased IgM	Increased IgM; normal or increased IgD; other Ig isotypes decreased	Defect in heavy chain isotype switching
Selective IgG subclass deficiencies	Decrease in one or more IgG subclasses	Defect in isotype switching or terminal B cell differentiation
Ig heavy chain deletions	IgG1, IgG2 or IgG4 absent; sometimes associated with absent IgA or IgE	Chromosomal deletion at 14q 32 (Ig heavy chain locus)
Transient hypogammaglobulinemia of infancy	IgG and IgA decreased; detectable levels of antibacterial antibodies; normal B cells	Unknown; ? delayed maturation of helper T cells in some patients
Common variable immunodeficiency	Variable reductions in multiple Ig isotypes; normal or decreased B cells	Defect in B cell maturation, usually due to intrinsic B cell abnormality

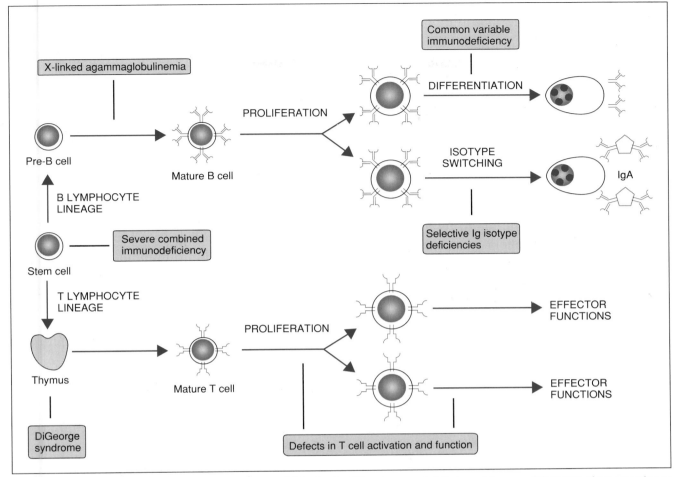

FIGURE 19–1. Sites of cellular abnormalities in congenital immunodeficiencies. *In different congenital (primary) immunodeficiencies, the maturation or activation of B or T lymphocytes may be blocked at different stages.*

organisms, such as pneumococcus, *Haemophilus influenzae,* and streptococcus. In addition, patients are susceptible to certain viral infections, such as polio, and to intestinal parasites such as *Giardia.* Not surprisingly, immunity to these microbes is normally mediated principally by antibodies (see Chapter 15).

In different antibody deficiencies, the primary abnormality may be at different stages of B lymphocyte maturation or in the responses of mature B cells to antigenic stimulation (Fig. 19–1). Abnormal helper T cell function may also result in deficient antibody production. In the following section we describe some examples of antibody immunodeficiencies, emphasizing the mechanisms of B cell defects.

X-linked Agammaglobulinemia

This disease, also called Bruton's agammaglobulinemia, is characterized by the absence of γ globulins in the blood, as the name implies. It is one of the most common congenital immunodeficiencies and the prototype of selective B cell defects. It was also the first immunodeficiency to be recognized, in 1952, and stud-

ies of these patients were useful in proving that plasma cells produced antibodies (both of which are absent in the patients). It is an X chromosome–linked disease, so that females who carry the defective gene on one X chromosome are phenotypically normal because the other X chromosome has a normal gene, but males who inherit the abnormal X chromosome manifest the disease. Thus, X-linked agammaglobulinemia is transmitted from phenotypically normal female carriers to their male offspring. In female carriers of this disease, i.e., the mothers of affected boys, the mutant X chromosome is inactivated in the B cells that survive and mature, whereas the T cells show a normal random pattern of X chromosome inactivation ("lyonization"). Thus, by assessing X chromosome utilization in B cells, it is possible to identify carriers of the disease. Affected boys are susceptible to bacterial and some viral infections, whereas infections by most intracellular microbes and fungi are handled normally. These children suffer from recurrent pyogenic bacterial infections of the conjunctiva, throat, skin, middle ear, bronchi, and lungs. Newborn infants are often normal because maternally derived antibodies provide adequate protection, and the disease is usually recognized late in the first year of life. If untreated the disease is usually fatal.

Patients with X-linked agammaglobulinemia usually have low or undetectable serum immunoglobulin (Ig), reduced or absent B cells in peripheral blood and lymphoid tissues, no germinal centers in lymph nodes, and no plasma cells in tissues. The numbers of pre – B cells in the bone marrow are normal, and these cells synthesize normal μ heavy chains. Thus, the disease is due to a block in the maturation of pre – B cells to surface IgM-positive B cells. Some patients do have mature peripheral B cells and even have elevated levels of serum IgG and IgA. However, in these patients, B cell numbers may be 100-fold lower than normal and antibody responses to immunization are seriously deficient, suggesting that only a very limited repertoire of B cells is present. The maturation, numbers, and functions of T cells are generally normal. Some studies have revealed reduced numbers of activated T cells in patients, which may be a consequence of reduced antigen presentation due to the lack of B cells. Almost 20 per cent of patients develop autoimmune disorders, the mechanisms of which are unknown.

The gene defect in X-linked agammaglobulinemia has been mapped to band q21.3-22 in the long arm of the X chromosome. The protein product of this gene has not yet been identified, nor is the molecular basis of defective B cell development known. In the pre – B cells of these patients, VDJ rearrangement and μ chain production are normal but subsequent light chain gene rearrangements do not occur. It is likely that the primary defect lies not in the light chain genes themselves, but in the mechanisms of rearrangement and expression of light chain genes. There is some evidence that the disease is not due to a single gene defect but that multiple genetic abnormalities located in the X chromosome may lead to agammaglobulinemia. Interestingly, a number of immunologic deficiencies in humans and mice have been mapped to the X chromosome. Some other human diseases are mentioned later in this chapter. A mutant mouse strain called the CBA/N mouse has an X-linked defect in B cell development with impaired antibody responses to polysaccharide antigens. It is thought that a gene locus on the X chromosome regulates lymphocyte maturation, but the nature of this putative regulatory gene(s) or its protein product(s) is unknown.

The infectious complications of X-linked agammaglobulinemia are greatly reduced by periodic (e.g., monthly) intravenous or intramuscular injections of pooled gamma globulin preparations. Such preparations contain pre-formed antibodies against common pathogens and provide effective passive immunity.

Selective Immunoglobulin Isotype Deficiencies

Many immunodeficiencies that selectively involve one or a few Ig isotypes have been described.

The most common is **selective IgA deficiency,** which affects about 1 in 700 individuals of Caucasian descent and is thus the most common primary immunodeficiency. The inheritance pattern of IgA deficiency is variable, different cases being autosomal dominant or recessive. In some patients, the disorder may not be inherited but may occur as a result of embryonic rubella infection or drug exposures. The clinical features are also extremely variable. Many patients are entirely normal, others have occasional respiratory infections and diarrhea, and, rarely, patients have severe, recurrent infections leading to permanent intestinal and airway damage, with associated autoimmune disorders.

IgA deficiency is characterized by abnormally low serum IgA, usually less than $50 \mu g/ml$, with normal or elevated levels of IgM and IgG. The defect in these patients is a block in the differentiation of surface IgA-expressing B cells to antibody-secreting plasma cells. The α heavy chain genes and the expression of membrane-associated IgA are normal. It is not known whether the block in B cell differentiation is due to an intrinsic B cell defect or to an abnormality in T cell help, such as the production of cytokines that enhance IgA secretion (e.g., transforming growth factor – β [TGF – β] and interleukin-5 [IL – 5]), or in B cell responses to these cytokines. No gross abnormalities in the numbers, phenotypes, or functional responses of T cells have been noted in these patients.

Selective IgM deficiency is a rare autosomal recessive disease associated with severe infections, such as bacterial meningitis. As in IgA deficiency, patients with IgM deficiency have normal membrane IgM and IgD expressing B lymphocytes but these cells do not differentiate into antibody-secreting plasma cells. The defect may be in the delivery of T cell help or in the responses of B cells to helper T cell stimuli. **Selective deficiencies of IgG subclasses** have also been described. Most of these are also due to abnormal B cell differentiation. Rarely, the deficiencies are due to homozygous deletions of various constant region (C_γ) genes. Individuals with single C_γ gene deletions are usually normal, which attests to the capacity of the immune system to compensate for selective antibody deficiencies.

IgG and IgA deficiency with increased IgM is usually inherited as an X-linked disorder. Affected male children produce only IgM antibodies and are therefore susceptible to severe bacterial infections. Furthermore, many of the IgM antibodies are autoantibodies reactive with the patient's own red blood cells, leukocytes, and platelets. This leads to secondary deficiencies of these blood cells, further reducing resistance to infections. The C_γ and C_α genes are structurally normal, as are the switch regions located 5' of these genes. However, heavy chain class switching to IgG and IgA does not occur, so that the patients lack B cells with surface IgG or IgA and do not produce these isotypes. Stimulation of B cells with the T cell–independent polyclonal activator, lipopolysaccharide (LPS), or infection with Epstein-Barr virus (EBV) also gives rise to B cells that produce IgM only. Thus, in most cases, the failure of isotype switching is due to an intrinsic B cell defect, the nature of which is not yet known.

Common Variable Immunodeficiency

This antibody deficiency disorder is usually inherited as an autosomal disease. Hypogammaglobulinemia may develop in affected children at different ages, but the increased susceptibility to bacterial infections is usually manifested in late childhood or early adult life. (For this reason, the disease is also called **acquired agammaglobulinemia.**) Patients as well as relatives have a high incidence of autoimmune diseases like rheumatoid arthritis and autoimmune hemolytic anemia.

Common variable immunodeficiency has been attributed to multiple abnormalities, including intrinsic B cell defects, deficient T cell help, and excessive "suppressor cell" activity. It is likely that in the majority of patients the primary abnormality responsible for low antibody production is a defect in the terminal differentiation of B lymphocytes to antibody-secreting cells. In lymphoid tissues, the B cell areas (i.e., lymphoid follicles) are often hyperplastic but plasma cells are absent. These findings suggest that B cells proliferate in response to antigenic stimulation but fail to differentiate normally. It is not known whether this is due to defective reception of helper T cell–derived stimuli or to more distal block(s) in the program of B cell activation. In some patients, IgM production can be induced *in vitro* by transformation with Epstein-Barr virus, which functions as a T cell–independent stimulus. However, even in these individuals, switching to other isotypes, such as IgG and IgA, usually does not occur.

CONGENITAL T CELL DEFICIENCIES

Severe defects in T cell maturation, such as the DiGeorge syndrome (discussed below), have been recognized for many years. More subtle immunodeficiencies attributable to primary T cell abnormalities are being appreciated relatively recently, as our assays for T cell maturation and function are improving. In the previous section of the chapter, we mentioned that some antibody deficiencies may, in fact, be due to abnormal T cell help. We shall now describe immunodeficiencies that primarily influence T lymphocytes and, therefore, lead to impaired cell-mediated immune reactions (Fig. 19–1, Table 19–2).

Cellular immune deficiencies are manifested by increased susceptibility to infections with viruses, fungi, intracellular bacteria, and protozoa. Such microorganisms are often capable of surviving and even replicating inside cells, including phagocytes (which is why their eradication is dependent on T cell immunity, as discussed in Chapter 15). As a result, these infections are usually severe and difficult to control and may be fatal. Patients with T cell deficiencies may also be susceptible to virally induced malignancies.

TABLE 19–2. Examples of Congenital T Cell and Combined Immunodeficiencies

Disease	Functional Deficiencies	Presumed Mechanism of Defect
DiGeorge syndrome	Decreased T cells; normal B cells; normal or decreased serum Ig	Anomalous development of 3rd and 4th branchial pouches, leading to thymic hypoplasia
SCID		
X-linked	Markedly decreased T cells; normal or increased B cells; reduced serum Ig	Defective T cell maturation
Autosomal recessive	Decreased T and B cells; reduced serum Ig	Defective maturation of T and B cells
ADA deficiency	Progressive decrease in T and B cells (mostly T); reduced serum Ig	ADA deficiency leading to accumulation of toxic metabolites
PNP deficiency	Decreased T cells; normal B cells and serum Ig	PNP deficiency leading to accumulation of toxic metabolite in T cells
Class II MHC deficiency	Normal lymphocyte numbers; normal or decreased serum Ig; deficient cell-mediated immunity	Defective transcription of class II MHC genes
Reticular dysgenesis	Markedly decreased T and B cells and other blood cells; reduced serum Ig	Defective maturation of hematopoietic stem cells
Wiskott-Aldrich syndrome	Progressive decrease in T cells; normal B cells; decreased IgM; deficient antibody responses to polysaccharide antigens	Defective glycosylation of membrane proteins, defective maturation of hematopoietic stem cells
Ataxia telangiectasia	Decreased T cells; normal B cells; variable reduction in IgA, IgE, and IgG subclasses	?Defect in DNA repair

Abbreviations: SCID, severe combined immunodeficiency disease; ADA, adenosine deaminase; PNP, purine nucleoside phosphorylase; Ig, immunoglobulin; MHC, major histocompatibility complex.

These aspects are discussed more fully in Chapter 17 and later in this chapter when we discuss the clinical features of AIDS, the prototypical acquired T cell immunodeficiency. T cell immunodeficiencies are diagnosed by reduced numbers of peripheral blood T cells, abnormally low proliferative responses to polyclonal T cell activators, e.g., phytohemagglutinin (PHA), and deficient cutaneous delayed type hypersensitivity (DTH) reactions to ubiquitous microbial antigens, such as *Candida* antigens.

The DiGeorge Syndrome (Thymic Hypoplasia)

This selective T cell deficiency is due to a congenital malformation that results in defective development of the third and fourth pharyngeal pouches. These structures give rise to the thymus and the parathyroid glands at weeks 6 to 8 of gestation and to the aortic arch and portions of the lips and ears at 12 weeks of fetal life. Developmental anomalies induced at this stage of gestation lead to partial or complete DiGeorge syndrome, manifested by hypoplasia or agenesis of the thymus (leading to deficient cell-mediated immunity), absent parathyroid glands (causing abnormal calcium homeostasis and muscle twitching, or tetany), abnormal development of the great vessels, and facial deformities. Different patients may show varying degrees of these abnormalities. Furthermore, the nature of the developmental insult is usually not known. Some cases are associated with maternal alcohol consumption, and rare cases show autosomal dominant patterns of inheritance or are associated with translocations involving chromosome 22.

The hypoplasia of the thymus leads to defective maturation of all T lymphocytes, because of which peripheral blood T lymphocytes are absent or greatly reduced in number. Sometimes the total peripheral blood lymphocyte count is near normal, but most of the cells are B lymphocytes (which make up only 10 to 20 per cent of the blood lymphocytes in normal individuals). Peripheral blood lymphocytes do not respond to polyclonal T cell activators or in mixed leukocyte reactions (MLRs). Antibody levels are usually normal but may be reduced in severely affected patients. In the peripheral lymphoid tissues, the B cells appear normal. As in other severe T cell deficiencies, patients are susceptible to mycobacterial, viral, and fungal infections.

The disease can be corrected by fetal thymic transplant. This is usually not necessary, however, because T cell function tends to improve with age and is often normal by 5 years. This is probably because extrathymic sites assume the function of T cell maturation. The existence of extrathymic sites of T cell development has been suspected, but no such tissue has been defined anatomically. It is also possible that as these patients grow older, typical thymus tissue develops at ectopic sites (i.e., other than the normal loca-

tion). Similarly, ectopic parathyroids develop with age, with consequent improvement of tetany.

An example of T cell immunodeficiency in animals is the **nude (athymic) mouse.** These mice have an inherited defect of epithelial cells in the skin, leading to hairlessness, and in the lining of the third and fourth pharyngeal pouches, causing thymic hypoplasia. The disorder is due to a recessive gene on chromosome 11 and is therefore manifested in homozygotes (called nu/nu). Affected mice have rudimentary thymuses in which T cell maturation cannot occur normally. As a result, there are few or no mature T cells in peripheral lymphoid tissues and a failure of all cell-mediated immune reactions, including allograft rejection, DTH, and antibody responses to T cell–dependent protein antigens. As the mice age to about 1 year, some mature T cells do develop but the site of T cell maturation is not defined. Nu/nu mice are susceptible to many infections, but somewhat surprisingly they are able to eradicate some intracellular bacteria. It is thought that this is because of normal or even increased numbers of natural killer (NK) cells, which produce γ-interferon (IFN-γ), which activates macrophages and serves to eliminate the microbes. NK cells may also account for the lack of susceptibility of nu/nu mice to spontaneous tumors (see Chapter 17). A similar inherited abnormality has been observed in rats, but nu/nu rats have not been analyzed in as much detail.

Defects in T Cell Activation and Function

In the late 1980s, isolated case reports of abnormalities in T cell responses to antigenic or mitogenic stimulation began to appear. These defects are associated with T cell immunodeficiencies of varying clinical severity. They may be due to multiple mechanisms, including (1) defective surface expression of the T cell receptor (TCR):CD3 complex; (2) abnormal signal transduction by the TCR:CD3 complex; (3) defective production of cytokines such as IL-2 and IFN-γ; and (4) defective expression of receptors for IL-2 or IL-1. These patients may have selective T cell or mixed T and B cell immunodeficiencies despite normal or even elevated numbers of blood lymphocytes. It is likely that such abnormalities will be recognized more frequently in coming years and their molecular basis as well as clinical significance understood in much more detail.

COMBINED IMMUNODEFICIENCIES (MIXED B AND T CELL DEFECTS)

Combined immunodeficiencies affecting both the B and T cell compartments may arise as a result of primary lymphoid abnormalities or in association with other congenital diseases. In both situations, the immunodeficiencies are clinically and mechanistically heterogeneous (Table 19–2).

Severe Combined Immunodeficiencies

The term severe combined immunodeficiency disease (SCID) is given to a heterogeneous group of disorders characterized by defective development of B and T lymphocytes, profound lymphopenia, and deficient humoral and cell-mediated immunity. The first example of the disease was discovered in Switzerland in the 1950s (because of which this disorder was originally called Swiss type agammaglobulinemia). The transmission of the disease may be autosomal recessive or X-linked recessive; many cases of the former are due to known enzyme deficiencies, described below.

SCID is usually due to an abnormal development of B and T lymphocytes from bone marrow stem cells. In most cases, the mechanisms of abnormal lymphocyte development are not known. The thymus as well as the peripheral lymphoid organs contain few or no lymphocytes. Infants show markedly reduced blood lymphocyte counts and antibody titers, and are deficient in all immune functions. Unless treated, they usually succumb to infections during the first year of life.

About 50 per cent of the autosomal recessive form of SCID (and about 20 per cent of all cases) are due to deficiency of an enzyme called **adenosine deaminase** (ADA). ADA catalyzes the irreversible deamination of adenosine and deoxyadenosine to inosine and 2'deoxyinosine, respectively (Fig. 19–2). The ADA gene is located on chromosome 2, and deficiency of the enzyme can be due to deletions or mutations in the gene. The enzyme is widely distributed but is particularly abundant and active in lymphocytes. Its deficiency leads to the accumulation of deoxyadenosine and deoxy ATP (adenosine triphosphate) in cells, particularly in developing T lymphocytes. These metabolites are toxic to lymphocytes because they block DNA synthesis by inhibiting ribonucleotide reductase activity and by causing the accumulation of compounds that inhibit transmethylation reactions. Thus, ADA deficiency leads to reduced numbers of lymphocytes, especially mature T cells, and a resultant immunodeficiency. Some patients may have near normal numbers of T cells but defective responses of these cells to antigenic stimulation. ADA deficiency is a prime candidate for treatment by specific gene transfer. The ADA gene has been cloned, and it is constitutively expressed. The disease is manifested in bone marrow–derived cells and may thus be treatable by transfection of a functional gene into autologous self-renewing marrow cells and transplantation of these cells back into the patient.

A rarer autosomal recessive form of SCID is due to the deficiency of another enzyme, called **purine nucleoside phosphorylase** (PNP), that is involved in purine catabolism. PNP catalyzes the conversion of inosine to hypoxanthine and guanosine to guanine. Deficiency of PNP leads to accumulation of deoxyguanosine and deoxy GTP (guanosine triphosphate), with toxic effects similar to ADA deficiency (Fig. 19–2). The gene for PNP is located on chromosome 14. Enzyme deficiency due to deletions or mutations in this gene usually result in deficient T cell immunity of

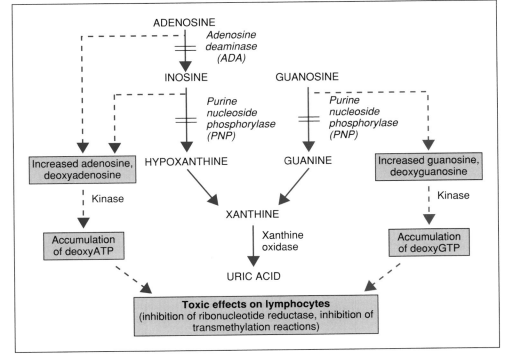

FIGURE 19–2. Congenital abnormalities in purine metabolism. *The major pathways for metabolism of purines (adenosine and guanosine) are shown in solid lines. Deficiencies of the enzymes adenosine deaminase (ADA) and purine nucleoside phosphorylase (PNP) block these metabolic pathways at different steps. This leads to shunting into secondary metabolic pathways, indicated by dashed lines, and the accumulation of toxic metabolites (in boxes).*

variable severity, with normal B cell function. Patients present with variable susceptibility to infections.

Recently, an autosomal recessive form of SCID with deficiency in class II major histocompatibility complex (MHC) gene expression has been recognized, and is called the **bare lymphocyte syndrome.** These patient express little or no human leukocyte antigen (HLA) – DP, DQ, or DR on B lymphocytes, macrophages, and dendritic cells and fail to express class II MHC molecules in response to IFN – γ. They express normal or only slightly reduced levels of class I MHC molecules and β_2-microglobulin and do synthesize the invariant (γ) chain upon stimulation with IFN – γ. The defect is due to an abnormality in a DNA – binding protein that normally stimulates transcription of class II genes by binding to the "X box" regulatory element located 5' of the class II locus (see Chapter 5). In the bare lymphocyte syndrome, either the production of this *trans*-acting DNA – binding protein is reduced, or it is structurally abnormal and, therefore, inactive. This results in reduced transcription of class II MHC genes. The consequence of deficient class II expression is a failure of antigen presentation to CD4$^+$ T cells. As a result, affected individuals are deficient in DTH responses and in antibody responses to T-dependent protein antigens, and they are susceptible to infections, particularly viral infections. In some patients, the numbers of mature CD4$^+$ T cells in peripheral blood and tissues are reduced. This may be because in the absence of class II MHC expression in the thymus, positive selection of CD4$^+$ T cells cannot occur (see Chapter 8).

Apart from the specific disease entities mentioned above, the cellular and molecular bases of all other forms of SCID are not known. It is suspected that many of these cases may be due to defects in the rearrangement and expression of antigen receptor genes, but such defects have not been identified in humans. An instructive experimental model is the **SCID mouse,** which arose as a spontaneous mutant of an inbred strain called CB – 17. In the SCID mutant strain, both B and T cells are absent because of an early block in maturation from bone marrow precursors. The defect in SCID mice is an abnormality in the recombinase that mediates rearrangement of TCRs and Ig genes. In cell lines derived from immature B and T cells of SCID mice, the J_H exons of Ig genes and J_β exons of TCR genes are often deleted because of an aberrant recombination of the D segment directly to one of the constant (C) region genes. As a result, VDJ rearrangements do not occur and antigen receptors are not expressed. Developing lymphocytes that fail to produce antigen receptors are eliminated *in vivo*. It is not known whether the SCID mouse lacks the normal recombinase gene itself or another gene that regulates the activity of the recombinase. The *scid* mutation has been localized to chromosome 16, but the protein product of this gene is not identified yet. Recently, two other genes called RAG – 1 and RAG – 2 (for "recombination activating genes") have been identified that trigger VDJ recombination when transfected into cells that normally lack recombinase activity. The RAG – 1 and RAG – 2 genes are not present on chromo-

some 16, and their relationship with the defective recombinase activity of SCID mice is not clear. About 15 per cent of inbred SCID mice are "leaky," in that they produce reduced but readily detectable numbers of mature B and T cells. The lymphocytes in these mice express limited repertoires of antigen receptor genes, suggesting that normal Ig or TCR rearrangements can occur in some developing clones.

Immunodeficiency Associated with Other Defects

Variable degrees of B and T cell immunodeficiency occur in certain congenital diseases in which there is a wide spectrum of abnormalities involving multiple organ systems. One such disorder is called the **Wiskott-Aldrich syndrome,** an X-linked disease characterized by eczema, thrombocytopenia (reduced blood platelets), and susceptibility to bacterial infections. In the initial stages of the disease, lymphocyte numbers are normal and the principal defect is an inability to produce antibodies in response to polysaccharide antigens, which are typical "type 2 thymus-independent (TI – 2)" antigens (see Chapter 9). These patients are especially susceptible to infections with encapsulated pyogenic bacteria. The lymphocytes (and platelets) are smaller than normal. With increasing age, the patients show reduced numbers of lymphocytes and more severe immunodeficiency. The gene (or genes) responsible for the Wiskott-Aldrich syndrome has been mapped to band p11.1 in the short arm of the X chromosome. The protein product of this gene is not defined. In patients with this disease, there is a defect in the glycosylation of membrane proteins, resulting in reduced expression of many cell surface glycoproteins. One such protein is a sialic acid – rich 115 kD glycoprotein called CD43 (or sialophorin), which is normally expressed on lymphocytes (both B and T), macrophages, neutrophils, and platelets. The role of CD43 deficiency in the abnormal lymphocyte function associated with this disease is not clear. It is unlikely to be the primary defect, because CD43 is encoded by a gene on chromosome 16.

Another disease associated with immunodeficiency is **ataxia telangiectasia,** an autosomal recessive disorder characterized by abnormal gait (ataxia), vascular malformations (telangiectasias), various neurologic deficits, increased incidence of tumors, and immunodeficiency. The immunologic defects are of variable severity and may affect both B and T cells, the latter usually being more impaired. Patients experience infections, multiple autoimmune phenomena, and increasingly frequent cancers with advancing age. Multiple genetic defects may give rise to this constellation of clinical and pathologic abnormalities. The cells, including lymphocytes, of some patients contain numerous chromosomal deletions and translocations that may involve Ig or TCR loci. DNA repair mechanisms in all cells may be defective, as suggested by an increased susceptibility of patients' cells to ionizing radiation. Such defects may contribute to abnormal lymphocyte development as well as abnormal proliferative responses to antigenic stimulation.

CONGENITAL DISORDERS OF PHAGOCYTES AND OTHER CELLS OF NATURAL IMMUNITY

Natural immunity is mediated principally by phagocytes and complement, and it constitutes the first line of defense against infectious organisms. In addition, phagocytes and complement participate in the effector phases of specific immunity. Therefore, congenital disorders of phagocytes and the complement system result in recurrent infections of varying severity. Complement deficiencies have been described in Chapter 13. In this section of the chapter, we discuss some examples of congenital phagocytic disorders.

Chronic Granulomatous Disease

Chronic granulomatous disease (CGD) is rare, estimated to affect about 1 in 1 million individuals in the United States. About two thirds of the cases show an X-linked recessive pattern of inheritance, and the remainder are autosomal recessive. The disease is characterized by recurrent bacterial infections, usually from early childhood. The infections are usually not controlled by neutrophilic inflammation and may result in the formation of granulomas composed of activated macrophages. The disease is often fatal, even with aggressive antibiotic therapy.

CGD is due to a defect in the production of superoxide anion, which constitutes a major microbicidal mechanism of phagocytes. In response to an encounter with bacteria, neutrophils and macrophages rapidly consume oxygen and liberate superoxide, which is a precursor of the active oxygen species that serve to kill bacteria. Superoxide generation is mediated by an enzyme called nicotinamide adenine dinucleotide phosphate (NADPH)–oxidase, which upon activation catalyzes the one-electron reduction of oxygen (O_2) to superoxide (O_2^-). A neutrophil-specific protein, called neutrophil cytochrome b, is part of the enzyme complex that catalyzes this reaction. The neutrophils of patients with X-linked CGD are defective in this b type cytochrome and, therefore, fail to produce superoxide. It is now known that cytochrome b is a heterodimer composed of a 91 kD and a 22 kD chain. In the majority of X-linked CGD patients, the defect involves the gene encoding the 91 kD chain, which is located in band p21 of the X chromosome. The gene may be absent, truncated, or mutated so that it is either not transcribed or the RNA is unstable. Failure to produce the 91 kD protein often leads to diminished synthesis of the coordinately regulated 22 kD chain as well. The defect in most cases of the autosomal recessive form of CGD does not involve the genes encoding the cytochrome b protein. Recent evidence indicates that two other components of the NADPH–oxidase system, a 47 kD and a 67 kD cytosolic protein, are affected in the autosomal recessive form. In both the X-linked and autosomal recessive forms, the end result is severe impairment of neutrophil superoxide generation.

Recently, it has been found that IFN–γ stimulates the production of superoxide by normal neutrophils as well as CGD neutrophils, especially in cases where the cytochrome b genes are present but their transcription is reduced. IFN–γ enhances transcription of the cytochrome b genes and also stimulates other components of the enzyme system that catalyzes superoxide generation. Once neutrophil superoxide production is enhanced to within 10 to 12 per cent of normal, there is greatly improved resistance to infection. The results of clinical trials of IFN–γ treatment of X-linked CGD are promising, showing both increased neutrophil microbicidal function and resistance to infection. The granulomatous reactions to infections seen during the natural history of the disease may reflect the body's attempt to mount a T cell response, with increased IFN–γ production and macrophage activation, to compensate for the neutrophil defect.

Leukocyte Adhesion Deficiency

Leukocyte adhesion deficiency is a rare autosomal recessive disorder characterized by recurrent bacterial and fungal infections and impaired wound healing. In these patients, most adhesion-dependent functions of leukocytes are abnormal. These functions include adherence to endothelium; neutrophil aggregation and chemotaxis; phagocytosis; and cytotoxicity mediated by neutrophils, NK cells, and T lymphocytes. The molecular basis of the defect is absent or deficient expression of the $\beta2$ integrins, or the CD11CD18 family of glycoproteins, which includes leukocyte function–associated antigen–1 (LFA–1 or CD11aCD18), Mac-1 (CD11bCD18) and p150,95 (CD11cCD18). These proteins participate in the adhesion of leukocytes to other cells (see Box 7–4, Chapter 7) and in the phagocytosis of complement-coated particles (see Chapter 13). In all patients studied so far, the defect has been mapped to the 95 kD β chain (CD18). The gene encoding this chain may be mutated, producing an aberrant transcript, or its transcription may be reduced. In fact, even in the limited number of cases analyzed, the reduced biosynthesis of the β chain has been shown to result from different molecular abnormalities.

To date, fewer than 100 patients with this disorder have been described. Like other genetic defects affecting leukocytes, leukocyte adhesion deficiency is a candidate for bone marrow transplantation and ultimately specific gene therapy.

Chédiak-Higashi Syndrome

This rare autosomal recessive disorder is characterized by recurrent infections by pyogenic bacteria, partial oculocutaneous albinism, and infiltration of various organs by non-neoplastic lymphocytes. Early studies showed that the neutrophils, monocytes, and lymphocytes of these patients contained giant cytoplasmic granules. It is now thought that this disease is due to a more generalized cellular abnormality leading to increased fusion of cytoplasmic granules. This affects the lysosomes of neutrophils and monocytes (causing reduced resistance to infections), melanocytes (causing albinism), cells of the nervous system (causing nerve defects), and platelets (leading to bleeding disorders). The molecular basis of the defect is not known. It may be due to abnormal membrane fluidity, which causes uncontrolled granule fusion and also defects in cell motility and microtubule function.

The giant lysosomes found in neutrophils form during the maturation of these cells from myeloid precursors. Some of these neutrophil precursors die prematurely, resulting in moderate leukopenia. Surviving neutrophils may contain reduced levels of lysosomal enzymes, which function in microbial killing. These cells are also defective in chemotaxis and phagocytosis, further contributing to their deficient microbicidal activity. NK cell function in these patients is impaired, probably because of an abnormality in the cytoplasmic granules that store proteins that mediate cytolysis (see Chapter 12). Interestingly, cytolytic T lymphocyte (CTL)–mediated killing is normal. A mutant mouse strain, called the **beige mouse,** is an animal model for the Chédiak-Higashi syndrome. This strain is characterized by deficient NK cell function and giant lysosomes in leukocytes. The beige mouse can be cured by transplantation of bone marrow from normal syngeneic animals, raising the possibility of using this treatment in the clinical situation.

THERAPEUTIC APPROACHES FOR CONGENITAL IMMUNODEFICIENCIES

In theory, the therapy of choice for congenital disorders of lymphocytes is to replace the defective gene in self-renewing precursor cells. This remains a distant goal for most human immunodeficiencies at present, despite considerable effort. Thus, current treatment for immunodeficiencies has two aims — to minimize and control infections and to replace the defective or absent components of the immune system by adoptive transfer and/or transplantation. Among the agents that have proved useful as replacement therapy are the following:

1. Pooled gamma globulins are enormously valuable for agammaglobulinemic patients and have been life-saving for many boys with X-linked agammaglobulinemia.

2. Bone marrow transplantation is currently the treatment of choice for SCID, with careful T cell depletion from the marrow and full or partial HLA matching to prevent graft-versus-host disease (GVHD) (see Chapter 16). If a child with SCID is given a transplant of semi-syngeneic marrow cells from a parent (also

called a "haploidentical" transplant because it is identical to the recipient at one of the two HLA haplotypes), the T cells that arise from the marrow must now develop in the partly foreign host. These T cells become restricted to recognizing foreign antigens in association with HLA molecules of the host, which are the HLA molecules that the donor T cells encounter during their maturation in the thymus. This, of course, is analogous to mouse bone marrow chimeras, which provided the initial evidence for the role of MHC molecules in the thymus in determining the selection of the T cell repertoire (see Chapter 8).

HUMAN IMMUNODEFICIENCY VIRUS AND THE ACQUIRED IMMUNODEFICIENCY SYNDROME

Acquired immunodeficiency syndrome is a disease first described in the early 1980s, characterized by profound immunosuppression with diverse clinical features, including opportunistic infections, malignancies, and central nervous system (CNS) degeneration. AIDS is one of a group of clinical syndromes caused by a retrovirus called human immunodeficiency virus. *HIV primarily infects CD4 expressing T cells, including helper T cells, and macrophages.* The degree of morbidity and mortality caused by HIV and the global impact of HIV infection on health care resources and economics are already enormous and continue to grow. In the United States alone, more than 1.5 million people have been infected; in central Africa the number of infected individuals is far greater and the risk groups are difficult to define. Currently, there is no prophylactic immunization or cure for AIDS. More than 30,000 people in the United States have already died of AIDS, and the disease will probably be fatal to at least half of, and perhaps most, infected individuals. In this section of the chapter we describe the molecular and biologic properties of HIV, the nature and possible causes of HIV–induced immunosuppression, and the clinical and epidemiologic features of HIV–related diseases.

Molecular and Biologic Features of HIV

HIV is considered to be a member of the lentevirus family of animal retroviruses, on the basis of genomic sequence homologies, morphology, and life cycle. Lenteviruses, including the visna virus of sheep, and the bovine, feline, and simian immunodeficiency viruses, are all capable of long-term latent infection of cells or short-term cytopathic effects, and they all produce slowly progressive, fatal diseases. Two closely related types of HIV, designated HIV–1 and HIV–2, have been identified. Although these viruses have distinct differences in genomic structure

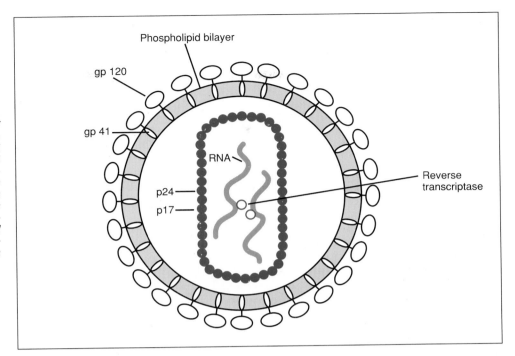

FIGURE 19–3. Structure of human immunodeficiency virus–1 (HIV–1). HIV–1 consists of two identical strands of RNA (the viral genome) with associated reverse transcriptase and core polypeptides (p18, p24), all enclosed in a phospholipid membrane envelope derived from the host cell. Virally encoded proteins (gp120 and gp41) are bound to the envelope. (Modified with permission from Rosenberg, Z. F., and A. S. Fauci. The immunopathogenesis of HIV infection. Advances in Immunology 47:377–431, 1989.)

and antigenicity, both types cause indistinguishable clinical syndromes. HIV–1 is a far more common cause of AIDS than HIV–2 in the United States.

An infectious HIV particle consists of two identical strands of RNA, each approximately 9.2 to 9.7 kilobases (kb) long, packaged within a core of viral proteins, surrounded by a phospholipid bilayer envelope derived from the host cell membrane but including virally encoded membrane proteins (Fig. 19–3). The HIV genome shares the basic structure of all known retroviruses, including nucleotide sequences called *gag* that encode core structural proteins; *env* sequences encoding envelope glycoproteins; and *pol* sequences encoding reverse transcriptase, endonuclease, and viral protease enzymes required for viral replication. In addition to these typical retrovirus genes, HIV also includes at least six other genes, including *vpr, vif, tat, rev, nef*, and *vpu* genes, whose

products regulate viral reproduction in various ways, to be discussed below (Fig. 19–4, Table 19–3).

HIV infection occurs when viral particles or infected cells in blood, semen, or other body fluids from one individual bind to cells of another individual. *Two HIV envelope glycoproteins, gp120 and gp41, are critical for HIV infection.* (Conventional notation of viral and cellular proteins includes a "p" for protein, or "gp" for glycoprotein, followed by a number designating the molecular weight in kilodaltons.) The first step is the *high-affinity binding of gp120 to CD4 molecules* on the surface of a primate T cell or mononuclear phagocyte. HIV does not bind to CD4 molecules in non-primate species. There are two ways in which this first binding step and subsequent HIV infection can occur. Free HIV particles released from one infected cell can bind to an uninfected cell. Alternatively, gp120, which is expressed on the plasma membrane of infected cells

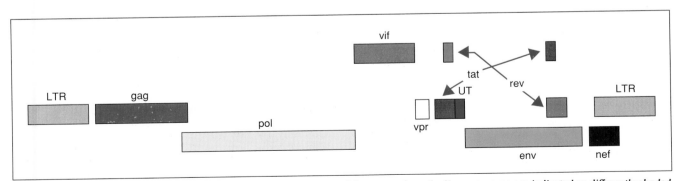

FIGURE 19–4. Human immunodeficiency virus–1 (HIV–1) genes. The positions of the genes along the linear genome are indicated as differently shaded blocks. Similarly shaded blocks separated by arrows indicate genes whose coding sequences are separated in the genome and require RNA splicing to produce functional messenger RNA (mRNA). The products and/or functions of each gene are described in Table 19–3. UT, untranslated segment; LTR, long terminal repeat. (Courtesy of Dr. Anthony S. Fauci, National Institutes of Health.)

TABLE 19–3. Genes of Human Immunodeficiency Virus

Name of Gene	Protein Products	Functions of Gene Products
gag	p55 precursor p17, p24, p15, mature proteins	Structural core proteins
pol	protease	Protease cleaves *gag* precursors;
	reverse transcriptase (64 kD+51 kD) integrase (34 kD)	Reverse transcriptase makes proviral DNA from RNA; Integrase required for proviral insertion
env	gp160 precursor gp120, gp41 mature proteins	gp 120 binds CD4 for infection; gp 41 required for viral fusion with cell
vpr	?	Unknown, not required for infection or cytopathicity
vif	23 kD	Involved in infection by free virus; not required for cell to cell infection
tat	p14	Binds to viral LTR sequence and activates transcription of all viral genes
rev	20 kD	Required for post-transcriptional expression of *gag* and *env* genes
nef	27 kD	Inhibits HIV transcription and retards viral replication
vpu	16 kD	?Required for optimal assembly/packaging of new virions

before virus is released, can bind to CD4 on another cell, initiating a membrane fusion event, and HIV genomes can be passed between the fused cells directly. The role of gp41 is discussed below.

Detailed molecular mapping studies are under way to define which regions of the CD4 and gp120 molecules are involved in binding to one another. This information will be potentially useful in the design of therapeutic strategies aimed at blocking virus interaction with CD4 expressing cells. Three well-conserved, noncontiguous regions in the carboxy terminus of gp120 of HIV–1 and HIV–2 are required for CD4 binding. Interestingly, these regions are separated by sequences that are extremely variable from one HIV isolate to another; this is significant to the way HIV may evade the host immune system, which we will discuss later. Such studies have already determined that various residues in the amino terminal domain of human CD4 are critical for binding. Genetically engineered soluble CD4 molecules can block HIV infection of cells, and this phenomenon has been applied to experimental treatment protocols for AIDS.

HIV particles that bind to CD4 may enter cells by receptor-mediated endocytosis. However, this may not be necessary, because HIV can efficiently infect cells expressing mutant CD4 molecules that are incapable of being internalized. It is likely that HIV can enter cells after binding to the cell surface, by direct fusion of the virus membrane with the host cell membrane. In a current model of HIV infection, gp120 binding to CD4 permits the associated viral gp41 molecule to insert its hydrophobic amino terminal head into the adjacent cell membrane, initiating fusion of the virus envelope with the cell. Other cellular factors may be critical for infection besides the CD4 molecule, as is suggested by the fact that murine cells expressing transfected human CD4 genes cannot be infected by HIV.

Once an HIV virion enters a cell, the enzymes within the nucleoprotein complex become active and begin the viral reproductive cycle (Fig. 19–5). The RNA genome of HIV is transcribed into a double-stranded DNA form by viral reverse transcriptase, and then viral integrase protein catalyzes the integration of the viral DNA into the host cell genome. The integrated DNA form of HIV is called the **provirus.** The provirus may remain transcriptionally inactive for months or years, with little or no production of new viral proteins or virions, and in this way HIV infection can be latent. In addition to the integrated provirus, many T cells may contain viral RNA genomes that do not become reverse transcribed into DNA as well as large amounts of reverse transcribed double-stranded viral DNA that do not become integrated. These pools of unintegrated viral nucleic acids probably contribute to the cytopathic effect of the virus, and if they do not kill the cell, they may also represent another form of latent infection.

Transcription of the genes of the integrated DNA provirus is regulated by long terminal repeat (LTR) sequences, which flank either side of the viral structural genes. The LTRs contain polyadenylation signal sequences, TATA box promoter sequence, and *cis*-acting regulators of transcription of the viral genes. These *cis*-acting sequences include tandemly repeated enhancer sequences that are known to bind at least two nuclear regulatory factors NFκ-B and Sp1. NFκ-B-like nuclear regulatory proteins, which bind to sequences in the regulatory regions of IL–2 and IL–2 receptor genes, can also bind to similar sequences in HIV LTRs and activate HIV transcription.

Initiation of HIV gene transcription in T cells is probably linked to physiologic activation of the T cell by antigen or cytokine stimulation. The LTRs of HIV are influenced by TCR and cytokine stimulation of the host cells. For example, TCR–binding lectins, tumor necrosis factor (TNF) and IL–6, all stimulate HIV LTR directed expression of linked genes and increase HIV virion production. TCR and cytokine stimulation of HIV gene transcription probably involves the induction of nuclear factors that bind to the NF-κB binding sequences in the viral LTR. This phenomenon may be significant to the pathogenesis of AIDS in two ways. First, physiologic activation of a latently infected T cell may be the way in which latency is ended and virus production begins. Second, the multiple infections that AIDS patients acquire lead to elevated TNF production; this, in turn, may stimulate HIV production and infection of additional cells. *Thus HIV replication is stimulated by the same mechanisms that promote growth of the host T cell.* In addition to the enhancer

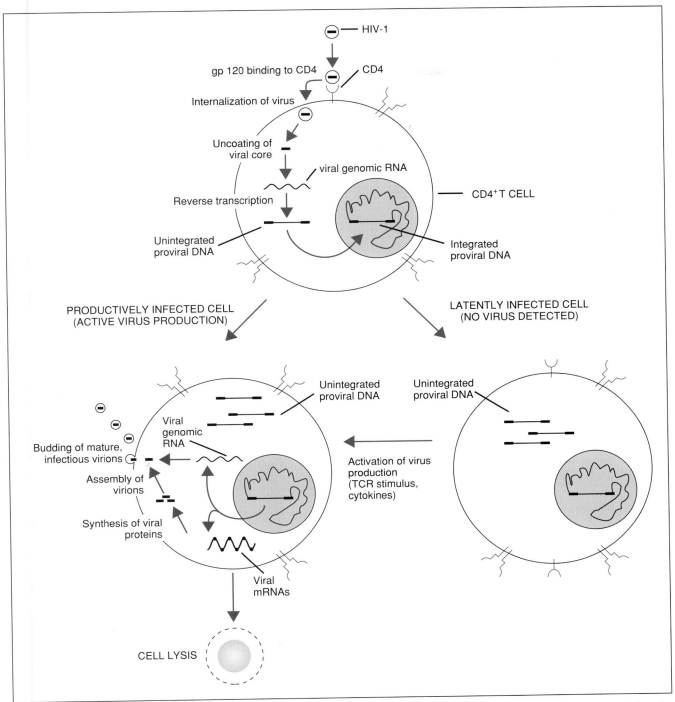

FIGURE 19 – 5. Life cycle of human immunodeficiency virus – 1 (HIV – 1). *HIV – 1 infection of a CD4 – expressing T cell is schematically depicted, including the* relationship between latent infection and productive, lytic infection.

elements, there are also silencer sequences in the HIV LTR that are involved in negative regulation of transcription. The activation state of the T cell probably determines which nuclear binding proteins are available for binding to these enhancer or silencer sequences, which in turn influences the transcriptional activity of the proviral genome and new viral production. It is interesting that when the regulatory sequences of the HIV LTR are linked to other genes and transfected into various cell types, they work efficiently. Therefore, the tissue specificity of productive HIV infection is not a function of these regulators but, rather, reflects the specificity of virus binding to and internalization by CD4+ cell types.

Synthesis of mature, infectious viral particles begins after the various viral genes are expressed as proteins, and full-length genomic viral RNA transcripts are produced. The *pol* gene product is a precursor protein that is sequentially cleaved to form reverse transcriptase, protease, and integrase enzymes. As mentioned above, the reverse transcriptase and integrase proteins are required for establishment of the integrated DNA proviral form of HIV. The *gag* gene encodes a 55 kD protein that is then proteolytically cleaved into p24, p17, and p15 polypeptides by the action of the viral protease encoded by the *pol* gene. These polypeptides are the mature core proteins that are required for assembly of infectious viral particles. The primary product of the *env* gene is a

160 kD glycoprotein (gp160) which is cleaved by cellular proteases within the endoplasmic reticulum into the CD4 binding protein, gp120, expressed on the external surface of the envelope, and the gp41 transmembrane glycoprotein. Gp120 does not contain a transmembrane domain, but it remains bound to the cell surface by non-covalent interactions with gp41. As mentioned above, both these molecules are crucial for viral infectivity. In addition, a soluble (virus-free) form of gp120 may be responsible for some of the immunopathology caused by HIV (see next page).

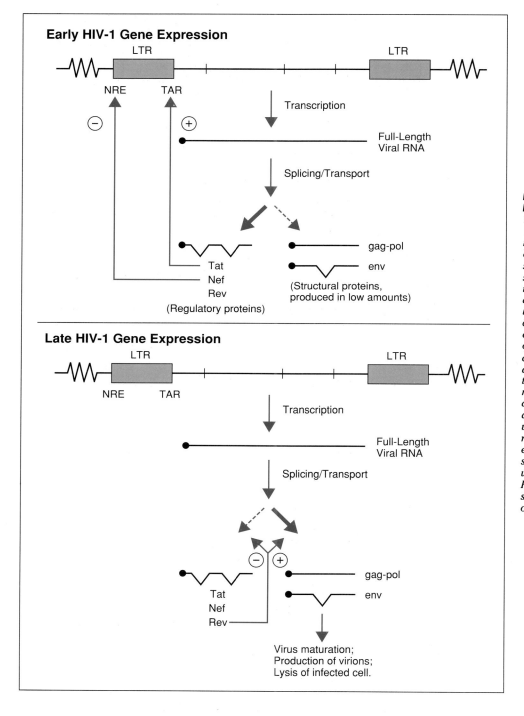

FIGURE 19–6. Early and late phases of human immunodeficiency virus–1 (HIV–1) gene expression. *During early HIV–1 gene expression, the predominant type of transcripts transported out of the nucleus are multiply spliced messenger RNA (mRNA) species encoding regulatory proteins Tat, Nef, and Rev. Tat and Nef act on genomic sequences to regulate further transcription. Rev causes a change to late phase gene expression by altering the balance of mRNA transport out of the nucleus. Specifically, Rev causes a relative increase in the transport and translation of singly or unspliced mRNAs encoding viral structural and enzymatic proteins that are required for production of mature viral particles. LTR, long terminal repeat; NRE, negative regulatory element; TAR, trans-acting responsive sequences. (Modified with permission from Greene, W. C. Regulation of HIV–1 gene expression. Annual Review of Immunology 8:453–475, 1990.)*

In addition to the conventional retroviral genes described above, namely *gag, pol,* and *env,* at least two other HIV genes are essential for viral replication. First, the *tat* gene encodes a 14 kD protein that is reported to have transcriptional, post-transcriptional, and translational effects. This protein binds to sequences present in the LTR called the *trans*-activating response element, resulting in stimulation of expression of all HIV genes. Second, the *rev* gene encodes a 20 kD protein that acts post-transcriptionally to ensure proper transport and processing of viral messenger RNA (mRNA) transcripts of the *gag, pol,* and *env* genes. At the same time, the *rev* product down-regulates expression of the HIV regulatory genes, including *tat, nef,* and *rev* itself. HIV gene expression may be divided into an early stage, during which the regulatory genes are expressed, and a late stage, during which structural genes are expressed (Fig. 19–6). The Rev protein is apparently critical for the transition from the early to late stage. This two-stage sequence of viral gene transcription probably serves to limit the duration of the expression of viral structural proteins, thereby diminishing the chance that the host immune system will recognize these proteins and destroy the virally infected cells in which they are expressed.

The *nef* gene encodes a 27 kD myristolated protein found predominantly in the cytoplasm of infected cells. The *nef*-encoded protein is not essential for viral replication or cytopathic effects. This protein may serve a negative regulatory function, slowing down viral replication, but its mode of action is unknown.

Three other HIV genes, which are not essential to the viral life cycle and whose functions are still poorly characterized, have been identified. The *vif* gene encodes a 23 kD protein that is involved in controlling the infectivity of HIV by an unknown mechanism. A functional *vif* gene is required for efficient infection of cells by viral particles, but it may not be involved in infection occurring by direct cell-cell contact. The *vpu* gene encodes a 16 kD protein that may be involved in assembly of new virions. The *vpr* gene has been identified by DNA sequence analysis only and no protein product has been definitively demonstrated.

In addition to their functions in the viral life cycle, the protein products of the various HIV genes are also significant because they stimulate immune responses in the host that may be either beneficial or detrimental (discussed below).

After transcription of these various viral genes, viral proteins are synthesized in the cytoplasm. Assembly of infectious viral particles then begins by packaging full-length RNA transcripts of the proviral genome within a nucleoprotein complex that includes the *gag* core proteins and the *pol*-encoded enzymes required for the next cycle of integration. This nucleoprotein complex is then enclosed within a membrane envelope and released from the cell by a process of budding from the plasma membrane. Production of mature virus is associated with lysis of the cell.

HIV–2 has basically the same molecular organization and reproductive biology as HIV–1. There are, however, several molecular differences. First, HIV–2 contains a gene called *vpx,* not present in the HIV–1 genome, which encodes a 14 kD protein of unknown function. Second, HIV–2 does not contain the *vpu* gene, which is present in the HIV–1 genome. Third, there is a large insertion in HIV–2 *rev* gene. Fourth, distinct differences in the *env* genes between the two types of HIV result in the fact that antibodies against one type will not react with the other. This is important, since most diagnostic tests for HIV in the United States rely on antibodies that recognize only HIV–1 and not HIV–2.

Immunology of HIV Infection

The clinical course of HIV infection reflects a complex interplay between the effects of the virus on the function of immunocompetent cells and the host's immune response to the virus. We next describe what is known or hypothesized to be the basis for HIV-induced immunosuppression and discuss the role of the host's immune response in both aggravating and limiting the pathologic effects of the virus (Table 19–4).

TABLE 19–4. Mechanisms of Human Immunodeficiency Virus (HIV)–Induced Pathogenesis

Pathologic Effect	Mechanism
Immunodeficiency	
Depletion of CD4$^+$ T cells: direct effects on infected cells	Lysis of CD4$^+$ T cells caused by viral budding and/or *env* glycoprotein insertion
	Cytopathic effect of unintegrated viral RNA and DNA
	Cytopathic effect of intracellular binding of gp120 to newly synthesized or recycled CD4
Depletion of CD4$^+$ T cells: indirect effects	Inhibition of CD4$^+$ T cell maturation
	Syncytia formation due to gp120 on infected cells binding to CD4 on uninfected cells
	Autoimmune destruction of uninfected CD4$^+$ T cells due to presence of normal T cell surface molecules that cross react with viral proteins
	Lysis of class II MHC expressing, infected T cells by class II-MHC restricted, gp120–specific CTLs
Functional impairment of immune system	Soluble gp120 blocks interaction of CD4$^+$ T cells with class II MHC on APCs
	Soluble gp120-induced down-regulation of CD3 and CD4 on T cells
	Impaired macrophage and NK cell function, unknown mechanism
Central Nervous System (CNS) Damage	Release of inflammatory cytokines from HIV-infected CNS macrophages; soluble gp120 may interfere with neurotransmitter action on neurons

Abbreviations: MHC, major histocompatibility complex; APC, antigen-presenting cell; CTL, cytolytic T lymphocyte.

NATURE AND MECHANISMS OF IMMUNOSUPPRESSION

The effects of HIV infection on the immune system are largely due to the specific tropism of HIV gp120 for the CD4 molecule. CD4 is expressed on helper T cells, and these cells play a central role in the induction of most immune responses. HIV infection can lead to lysis of CD4$^+$ T cells or functional inactivation of these cells without cytolysis. In either case, the diminished helper T cell activity results in impairment of all types of immune responses.

The cytolytic effects of HIV on CD4$^+$ T cells are reflected by the marked reduction of these cells in AIDS patients. The ratio of CD4$^+$ T cells to CD8$^+$ T cells in the peripheral blood is approximately 2:1 in normal individuals but is often reduced to as low as 0.5 in AIDS patients. CD4$^+$ T cells are also reduced in lymphoid tissues and at sites of inflammation. This profound depletion of helper T cells occurs despite the fact that in these patients probably less than 1 per cent of CD4$^+$ T cells are directly infected with HIV and more than 99 per cent of these infected cells are latently infected without detectable viral RNA transcripts. Furthermore, various immunologic abnormalities are present in HIV–infected individuals even before their CD4$^+$ T cells are reduced in numbers. Therefore, in order to understand HIV–induced immunosuppression, it is crucial to elucidate why the number of CD4$^+$ T cells destroyed is far greater than the number infected, and why those immune cells that are not killed still do not function properly.

Although the answer is not yet known, it is likely that the depletion of CD4$^+$ T cells is due to a combination of both direct lysis of infected cells, and indirect mechanisms involving both infected and uninfected cells. *At least three mechanisms of direct HIV–induced cytolysis of infected CD4$^+$ T cells have been described:*

1. The process of virus production leads to lysis of infected T cells because of increased plasma membrane permeability resulting from *env* glycoprotein insertion and/or virion budding. The increased permeability results in influx of ions and water, leading to osmotic lysis or an influx of a lethal amount of calcium.

2. A large amount of cytoplasmic viral DNA remains in the cytoplasm, as we mentioned previously, and is not incorporated into the cellular genome in HIV–infected cells. This may be toxic to infected cells. Similarly, high levels of nonfunctional viral mRNA transcripts in the cytoplasm may also interfere with normal cellular functions.

3. *Env* gene products, such as gp120, may bind newly synthesized or recycled CD4 molecules within the cytoplasm, and this intracellular interaction may be lethal to the cell.

Although HIV can infect macrophages, these cells are relatively resistant to the cytolytic effects of the virus. This may reflect the fact that high levels of CD4 expression are required not only for viral entry into cells but also for virus-induced cytotoxicity. The lower expression of CD4 on macrophages in comparison with helper T cells may protect the former from virus-induced killing. Many macrophages, in fact, may become infected by a CD4 independent route, such as phagocytosis of other infected cells or Fc receptor–mediated endocytosis of antibody-coated HIV. *Since macrophages can be infected but generally not killed by the virus, they are probably a major reservoir for the virus during the long clinical course of HIV–related disease.* In fact, the quantity of macrophage-associated HIV far exceeds T cell–associated virus in most tissues from AIDS patients, including brain, lung, and lymph node.

At least three mechanisms are hypothesized to account for indirect HIV–induced depletion of uninfected CD4$^+$ T cells:

1. HIV may block maturation of CD4$^+$ T cells by infecting cells that produce cytokines required for T cell maturation.

2. HIV–infected cells, expressing cell surface gp120, can bind to and fuse with uninfected CD4$^+$ T cells; this can lead to the formation of fused cells, multinucleated giant cells, or syncytia, *in vitro*. The life span of these giant cells is short. It is possible that this phenomenon may contribute to CD4$^+$ T cell depletion *in vivo*, although there is no direct evidence for this.

3. HIV infection of some CD4$^+$ T cells may lead to autoimmune destruction of both infected and uninfected CD4$^+$ T cells. Soluble gp120 released from infected cells can bind to CD4 on the surface of uninfected cells. Many patients have circulating anti-gp120 antibodies that could mediate destruction of these gp-120 coated T cells, by antibody-dependent cell-mediated cytotoxicity (ADCC) or by complement fixation. It is also possible that antibodies specific for viral proteins may cross-react with normal T cell surface proteins, leading to their destruction. For example, the viral envelope gp41 molecule has a region of homology with the β1 domain of class II MHC molecules. Since activated human T cells express class II MHC, antibodies against gp41 may cross react with and mediate killing of these T cells. Similarly, gp120 and IL–2 share regions of homology and anti-gp120 antibodies in AIDS patients may bind to IL–2 and interfere with IL–2 dependent growth of T cells. Alternatively, gp120 binding to uninfected CD4$^+$ T cells can render them susceptible to lysis by gp120-specific CTLs. This has been demonstrated *in vitro* and occurs when uninfected CD4$^+$ T cells internalize and process the gp120 protein and present a peptide derivative in association with class II MHC molecules. Class II–restricted, gp120-specific CTLs have been isolated and cloned from the peripheral blood of HIV–infected patients, and these CTLs can lyse other CD4$^+$ T cells that have processed and presented the gp120 molecule.

In addition to depletion of CD4$^+$ T cells, which becomes most significant late in the course of HIV infection, *the virus also causes functional impairment of CD4$^+$ T cells in ways not directly related to cytotoxic* *effects or T cell depletion.* Uninfected T cells in HIV–infected patients have a decreased expression of IL–2 receptors and diminished secretion of IL–2 in response to soluble antigens both *in vivo* and *in vitro.* Humoral responses to soluble antigens and CTL responses to certain viruses are also impaired, probably as a consequence of the failure of CD4+ helper T cells to secrete adequate amounts of the appropriate cytokines required for functional differentiation of B cells and CTLs.

As with the cytolytic effects, these functional abnormalities of CD4+ T cells are most likely due to the binding of HIV or free gp120 to CD4 molecules on helper T cells. Such binding could have numerous consequences. CD4 that has bound gp120 may not be available to interact with class II MHC molecules on antigen-presenting cells (APCs), and thus T cell responses to soluble antigens would be inhibited. Alternatively, gp120 binding to CD4 may down-regulate surface expression of a variety of molecules required for T cell activation, including CD3 and CD4 itself. This down-regulation may be due to gp120-induced modulation of CD4 and, perhaps, associated CD3, as well as inhibition of transcription of CD4 and CD3 genes. In addition, the HIV Tat protein can also block antigen induced responses of T cells, presumably by interfering with intracellular T cell activation pathways.

The immunosuppressive effects of HIV may also be partly related to effects the virus has on cells other than CD4+ T cells. Abnormalities in B lymphocyte activation are frequently observed in HIV–infected individuals. Paradoxically, these patients typically have elevated serum Ig levels resulting from polyclonal activation of B cells. This may be a result of a polyclonal activating effect of HIV or gp120 itself. Polyclonal activation of B cells may also be caused by EBV infection, which can be largely uncontrolled in HIV–infected individuals as a result of poor T cell immune responses. Despite this generalized B cell hyperactivity, humoral immune responses to newly introduced antigens are greatly impaired. Diminished T cell help, as well as refractoriness of the B cells themselves, may both play a role in this deficit.

Macrophages are frequently infected with the virus, and there are reports that various macrophage functions are impaired in HIV–infected patients. These impairments include decreased chemotaxis, IL–1 production, and oxygen metabolite-dependent killing of microbes. In addition, antigen-presenting capabilities of monocytes and macrophages are reduced in AIDS patients. One possible mechanism for this effect is the down-regulation of class II MHC expression, which is reported to occur in HIV infected macrophages.

NK cells from AIDS patients are also reported to be functionally impaired by an unknown mechanism, and this may be a reason for inadequate anti-viral immunity in these individuals.

It is apparent from the discussion above that many abnormalities in the cells of the immune system have been shown to result from HIV infection. It is, however, not yet clear which defects contribute most significantly to the immunodeficiency.

Immune Responses to HIV

Both humoral and cell-mediated immune responses specific for a wide variety of HIV gene products have been demonstrated in HIV–infected patients. Given the extremely high fatality rate among HIV–infected individuals, it is clear that these immune responses to the virus do not confer adequate protection. This is, of course, partly due to the fact that the CD4+ T cells required to initiate protective immune responses against the virus are killed or inactivated by the virus, and thus the immune responses may be too compromised to eliminate the virus. In addition, the HIV genome displays a remarkable degree of genetic variability, as a result of high rates of mutations, insertions and deletions, and recombinations between different viral strains. This results in antigenic variations that may serve to evade the host immune system. Despite the poor effectiveness of immune responses to the virus, it is important to characterize them for two reasons. First, the immune responses may be detrimental to the host, as we have alluded to previously; they result in autoimmune killing of uninfected T cells, or they may stimulate uptake of opsonized virus into uninfected cells by Fc receptor–mediated endocytosis. Second, the design of effective vaccines for immunization against HIV requires knowledge of the viral epitopes that are most likely to stimulate protective immune responses.

The most immunogenic molecules on HIV appear to be the envelope glycoproteins, and high titers of anti-gp120 and anti-gp41 antibodies are present in most HIV–infected individuals. Other immunoglobulins found frequently in patients' sera include antibodies to p24, reverse transcriptase, and *gag* and *pol* products. The effect of these antibodies on the clinical course of HIV–related diseases is probably minimal. Interestingly, the anti-envelope antibodies are generally poor inhibitors of viral infectivity or cytopathic effects, supporting the hypothesis that the most immunogenic epitopes of the envelope glycoproteins are least important for the functions of these molecules. Furthermore, the antibodies are usually virus strain–specific, so that antibodies from one infected individual often do not recognize HIV isolated from other infected individuals. This implies that the immunogenic portions of HIV not only are functionally unimportant but also are encoded by variable genes. It is possible that the host immune response may work as a selective pressure that promotes survival of the most genetically variable viruses. Low titers of neutralizing antibodies that can inactivate HIV are present in HIV–infected patients, as are antibodies that can mediate ADCC. These antibodies are usually specific for gp120. Whether there is a correlation between the titer of these antibodies and the clinical course remains controversial.

Experimentally produced neutralizing antibodies, made by immunizing animals with HIV− or purified HIV−encoded proteins, are potentially useful for treating infected individuals. Since HIV can spread by cell-cell fusion, antibodies that block fusion as well as neutralize free virus particles would be needed. Furthermore, such antibodies would need to recognize nonvariable parts of the virus.

The role of T cell-mediated immune responses to HIV infection is also incompletely understood. MHC−restricted CTLs specific for *env, gag,* and *pol* gene products have been detected in HIV−infected individuals. In addition, NK cell activity against HIV infected targets is present in these patients. These effector mechanisms are clearly important in the immunologic control of other types of viral infections, and their role in HIV infection requires more research.

Clinical Features of HIV Infection

Because of the complex biology of HIV, the clinical manifestations of infection are quite variable. Initial infection is either asymptomatic or is accompanied by a flu-like illness with fever, muscle aches, sore throat, and rash. The virus is replicating abundantly during this period and is present within the blood and cerebrospinal fluid. After this initial phase, extracellular virus practically disappears but latent infection of CD4+ T cells, macrophages, and microglial cells in the CNS continues. The appearance of serum antibodies against HIV usually occurs between 3 and 20 weeks after initial exposure to the virus. The duration of the latent phase may be anywhere from 2 to 10 years, and perhaps longer. Generalized lymphadenopathy develops in many patients during this latent phase, but the immune system is functioning normally. In some patients, a syndrome called **AIDS−related complex** (ARC) develops and is characterized by fevers, weight loss, and diarrhea. ARC patients produce virions, and have immunologic abnormalities, including depletion of CD4+ T cells, but they do not suffer from frequent infections or neoplasms, which typify AIDS. Many patients with ARC proceed to develop AIDS, but it is not clear whether all ARC patients will, nor is it clear whether ARC is a necessary precursor to AIDS.

As we described earlier, AIDS is characterized by profound global immunosuppression with depletion of CD4+ T cells. AIDS patients continue to have lymphadenopathy and weight loss characteristic of ARC. They also acquire numerous infections that can be life-threatening, often with organisms which are not normally pathogenic for immunocompetent individuals. These infections are a result of the lack of either humoral or cell-mediated immune responses to the organisms. Pneumonia caused by the protozoan *Pneumocystis carinii* is the most commonly acquired infection in AIDS patients, occurring in more than 50 per cent of patients; *Pneumocystis* pneumonia is perhaps the most frequent cause of death in AIDS. Other protozoal and helminthic organisms that frequently infect AIDS patients include *Cryptosporidium, Toxoplasma,* and *Strongyloides.* Bacteria that often cause

infections in AIDS patients include *Mycobacterium avium−intracellulare, Mycobacterium tuberculosis, Nocardia,* and *Salmonella.* Fungal infections with *Candida, Cryptococcus neoformans, Coccidioides immitis,* and *Histoplasma capsulatum* are common, as are viral infections with cytomegalovirus, herpes simplex, and varicella-zoster. The inflammatory responses to these various organisms are often unlike those seen in immunocompetent individuals; this probably reflects the lack of T cells that would normally secrete cytokines, which promote acute and chronic inflammation. For example, well-formed granulomas with activated macrophages are not seen in mycobacterial or fungally infected tissues in AIDS patients.

Various malignant neoplasms are frequently found in AIDS patients, and these represent another major cause of AIDS−related morbidity and mortality. Up to 30 per cent of AIDS patients develop Kaposi's sarcoma, a mesenchymal tumor histologically characterized by vascular spaces and malignant spindle cells. AIDS−related Kaposi's tumors, unlike sporadic forms of this neoplasm, are highly aggressive and disseminated, involving skin, mucosa, lymph nodes, and multiple visceral organs. The cause of this tumor in the setting of AIDS remains obscure. AIDS patients also develop malignant lymphomas at a much higher rate than immunocompetent individuals. Burkitt's lymphoma and other B cell tumors are most frequent, and they are often positive for EBV. The development of these tumors may result from immunologically unchecked EBV infections leading to polyclonal B cell proliferation and subsequent malignant transformation (see Box 17−2, Chapter 17). Primary lymphomas of the CNS are also common in AIDS patients.

The brain is a major site of HIV infection, and up to 66 per cent of AIDS patients suffer from a form of dementia called AIDS−encephalopathy or AIDS−dementia complex, characterized by memory loss and various other nonspecific neuropsychiatric disturbances. Macrophages are the cells most likely to be infected in the brain, although some evidence suggests direct infection of cerebrovascular endothelium and neurons. Neuronal damage is seen on pathologic examination of brains from AIDS autopsies, but the causes are not clear. It is possible that HIV−infected macrophages secrete cytokines that are toxic to neurons or that HIV interferes with neurotropic peptide factors or neurotransmitters.

Transmission of HIV and Epidemiology of AIDS

The modes of transmission of HIV from one individual to another are the major determinants of the epidemiologic features of AIDS. The virus is transmitted by three major routes:

1. Intimate sexual contact is the most frequent mode of transmission, most often involving homosexual male partners. The virus is present in semen and gains access to the previously uninfected partner ei-

ther through traumatized rectal mucosa or vaginal mucosa. Transmission from infected females to males may also occur.

2. Inoculation of a recipient with infected blood or blood products is the second most frequent mode of HIV transmission. Needles shared by intravenous drug abusers account for most cases of this form of transmission, and transfusion of blood or blood products, in a clinical setting, accounts for a small portion of HIV infections. Patients infected in this way may then infect other individuals by sexual contact.

3. Mother to child transmission of HIV accounts for the majority of pediatric cases of AIDS. This occurs most frequently *in utero* or during childbirth, although transmission through breast milk is also possible.

Epidemiologists, e.g., at the Center for Disease Control (CDC), have identified six major groups at risk for developing AIDS in the United States, including:

1. Homosexual or bisexual males (approximately 70 per cent of cases).
2. Intravenous drug abusers (approximately 18 per cent of cases).
3. Recipients of unscreened blood, plasma, or blood cell transfusions (approximately 2.5 per cent of cases).
4. Hemophiliacs who were transfused with pooled, concentrated coagulation factors (approximately 1 per cent of cases).
5. Heterosexual partners of members of the above risk groups (approximately 4 per cent).
6. Babies born from infected mothers.

In Africa, the vast majority of HIV infections occur by sexual transmission from one heterosexual partner to another, with no other identifiable risk factors, making African AIDS a particularly ominous epidemic.

Treatment of HIV infection and AIDS remains largely experimental and no satisfactorily effective intervention has been developed. The drug 3'-azido-3'-deoxythymidine (AZT) is an inhibitor of reverse transcriptase and has some efficacy in prolonging asymptomatic periods in HIV–infected individuals. Unfortunately, the drug does not eliminate latent virus and ultimately fails to stem the progression of immunodeficiency. As we mentioned earlier, AIDS patients have been treated with soluble CD4 molecules, in an attempt to interfere with spread of the virus. This approach has had limited success. The individual infections experienced by AIDS patients are treated with the appropriate antibiotics and support measures. More aggressive antibiotic therapy is often required than for similar infections in less compromised hosts.

The development of an effective vaccine for immunoprophylaxis against HIV has become a major priority for biomedical research institutions worldwide. The task has been complicated by the genetic potential of the virus for great antigenic variability. Furthermore, although we know many of the viral gene products that induce naturally occurring humoral re-

sponses, these responses are ineffective in preventing disease. Perhaps vaccine development will require identification of viral epitopes that stimulate effective cell-mediated immune responses. Vaccines effective in preventing simian immunodeficiency virus (SIV) infection of macaques have already been developed. This is encouraging because SIV is molecularly closely related to HIV and causes a disease similar to AIDS in macaques. Given the tremendous amount we have already learned about HIV even though the existence of the virus was not even known 10 years ago, it is not unrealistic to assume that the HIV epidemic will be controlled in the near future.

OTHER ACQUIRED IMMUNODEFICIENCIES

Overall, acquired immunodeficiencies caused by other factors besides HIV infection are still more common than AIDS. These immunodeficiency states fall into two general etiologic categories. First, there is immunosuppression, as a biologic complication of another disease process. Second, there are immunodeficiencies that are complications of the therapy for other diseases, so-called iatrogenic immunodeficiency.

Diseases in which immunodeficiency is a common complicating element include malnutrition, neoplasias, and infections. Protein-calorie malnutrition is extremely common in developing countries and is associated with impaired cellular and humoral immunity to microorganisms. Much of the morbidity and mortality that afflicts malnourished people is due to infections. The basis for the immunodeficiency is not well defined, but it is reasonable to assume that the global metabolic disturbances in these individuals, caused by deficient intake of protein, fat, vitamins, and minerals, will adversely affect the maturation and function of the cells of the immune system.

Patients with advanced widespread cancers are often susceptible to infections because of impaired cell-mediated and humoral immune responses to a variety of organisms. Bone marrow tumors, including cancers metastatic to marrow and leukemias that arise in the marrow, may interfere with the growth and development of normal lymphocytes. Alternatively, tumors may produce substances that interfere with lymphocyte development or function, such as transforming growth factor-β (TGF-β). An example of malignancy associated immunodeficiency is the impairment of T cell function commonly observed in patients with a type of malignant lymphoma called Hodgkin's disease. This defect was first characterized as an inability to mount a DTH reaction upon dermal injection of various common antigens to which the patients were previously exposed, such as *Candida* or tetanus toxoid. Other *in vitro* measures of T cell function, such as proliferative responses to polyclonal activators, are also impaired in Hodgkin's disease. Such a generalized deficiency in DTH responses is called

anergy. The basis for these T cell abnormalities is currently unknown.

Various types of infections lead to immunosuppression. Viruses other than HIV are known to impair immune responses and lead to complicating infections by other organisms. Examples include the measles virus and human T lymphotropic virus–1 (HTLV–1). Both viruses can infect lymphocytes, and this may be a basis for their immunosuppressive effects. Like HIV, HTLV–1 is a retrovirus with tropism for CD4+ T cells; however, instead of killing helper T cells, it transforms them, producing an aggressive T cell malignancy called adult T cell leukemia/lymphoma (ATL). In ATL patients, typically there is severe immunosuppression with multiple opportunistic infections. Chronic infections with *Mycobacterium tuberculosis* and various fungi frequently result in anergy to many antigens. Chronic parasitic infections may also lead to immunosuppression. For example, African children with chronic malarial infections have depressed T cell function and this may be important in the pathogenesis of EBV–associated malignancies (see Box 17–2, Chapter 17).

Iatrogenic immunosuppression is most often due to drug therapies which either kill or functionally inactivate lymphocytes. Some drugs are given intentionally to immunosuppress patients, either for treatment of inflammatory diseases or to prevent rejection of tissue allografts. The most commonly used immunosuppressive drugs are corticosteroids and cyclosporin A, discussed in Chapter 16. Various chemotherapeutic drugs are administered to cancer patients, and these drugs are usually cytotoxic to both mature and developing lymphocytes as well as to granulocyte and monocyte precursors. Thus, cancer chemotherapy is almost always accompanied by a period of immunosuppression and risk of infections. Radiation treatment of cancer carries the same risks.

One final form of acquired immunosuppression that should be mentioned results from the absence of a spleen, caused by surgical removal of the organ after trauma or for the treatment of certain hematologic diseases or as a result of infarction in sickle cell disease. Patients without spleens are more susceptible to infections by some organisms, particularly encapsulated bacteria such as *Streptococcus pneumoniae.* The spleen is apparently required for the induction of protective humoral immune responses to such organisms.

Summary

Immunodeficiency diseases are caused by congenital or acquired defects in lymphocytes, phagocytes, or other mediators of specific and natural immunity. These diseases are associated with an increased susceptibility to infections, the nature and severity of which depend largely on which component of the immune system is abnormal and the extent of the abnormality. In addition, patients with immunodeficiencies often show an increased incidence of cancers and autoimmune diseases.

Congenital (or primary) immunodeficiencies may be due to defects in B or T lymphocytes or both. An example of a selective B cell deficiency is X-linked agammaglobulinemia, an inherited block in the maturation of pre–B cells to B lymphocytes that results in an absence of mature B cells and antibodies. Congenital disorders selectively affecting the production of one or a few Ig isotypes, including IgA, IgM, and various IgG subclasses, are usually due to a failure of mature B cells to switch to particular Ig heavy chain isotypes. Common variable immunodeficiency is most often due to an intrinsic defect in the Ig secretory responses of mature B cells to antigenic stimulation.

The best-defined congenital T cell immunodeficiency is the DiGeorge syndrome, caused by a genetic abnormality in the development of the thymus. This results in a failure of T cell maturation. Diverse abnormalities in the functional responses of mature T lymphocytes to receptor-mediated stimulation have been described, but their underlying mechanisms are not known yet.

Severe combined immunodeficiencies constitute a group of disorders with defects in the development of both B and T lymphocytes. Some cases are due to inherited deficiencies of enzymes, such as adenosine deaminase, that are involved in purine metabolism. Other cases are attributable to poorly understood blocks in the development of antigen receptor expressing lymphocytes from precursors in the bone marrow. Deficiencies of B and T lymphocytes are also associated with diseases that affect multiple organ systems, such as the Wiskott-Aldrich syndrome and ataxia telangiectasia.

Acquired immunodeficiency syndrome (AIDS) is a severe T cell immunodeficiency caused by infection with the human immunodeficiency virus (HIV). This virus selectively infects CD4+ T lymphocytes, causing depletion of these cells by direct lysis as well as several indirect mechanisms that lead to death, defective maturation, and abnormal function of uninfected T cells. The depletion of T cells results in greatly increased susceptibility to infection by a number of opportunistic microorganisms, including *Pneumocystis carinii,* mycobacteria, and various fungi and viruses. In addition, patients have a propensity to tumors, particularly Kaposi's sarcoma and Epstein-Barr virus–associated B cell lymphomas, and frequently develop an encephalopathy, the mechanism of which is not fully understood. Despite enormous effort, an effective cure or prophylactic vaccine for this disease is not available.

Acquired immunodeficiencies are also associated with malnutrition, disseminated cancers, and immunosuppressive therapy for transplant rejection or autoimmune diseases.

Selected Readings

Anderson, D. C., and T. A. Springer. Leukocyte adhesion deficiency: an inherited defect in the Mac-1, LFA–1, and p150,95 glycoproteins. Annual Review of Medicine 38:175–194, 1987.

Green, W. C. Regulation of HIV–1 gene expression. Annual Review of Immunology 8:453–476, 1990.

Kantoff, P. W., S. M. Freeman, and W. F. Anderson. Prospects for gene therapy for immunodeficiency diseases. Annual Review of Immunology 6:581–594, 1988.

Ochs, H. D., and R. J. Wedgwood. IgG subclass deficiencies. Annual Review of Medicine 38:325–340, 1987.

Orkin, S. H. Molecular genetics of chronic granulomatous disease. Annual Review of Immunology 7:277–307, 1989.

Primary immunodeficiency diseases: report of a WHO sponsored meeting. Immunodeficiency Reviews 1:173–205, 1989.

Rosen, F. S., M. D. Cooper, and R. J. P. Wedgwood. The primary immunodeficiencies. New England Journal of Medicine 311:235–242, 300–310, 1984.

Rosenberg Z. F., and A. S. Fauci. The immunopathogenesis of HIV infection. Advances in Immunology 47:377–431, 1989.

Rosenberg Z. F., and A. S. Fauci. Immunopathogenic mechanisms of HIV infection: cytokine induction of HIV expression. Immunology Today 11:176–180, 1990.

Rotrosen, D., and J. I. Gallin. Disorders of phagocyte function. Annual Review of Immunology 5:127–150, 1987.

Shultz, L. D., and C. L. Sidman. Genetically determined murine models for immunodeficiency. Annual Review of Immunology 5:367–403, 1987.

Stiehm, E. R. (ed.). Immunologic Disorders in Infants and Children, 3rd ed. Philadelphia, W. B. Saunders Co., 1989.

APPENDIX: PRINCIPAL FEATURES OF KNOWN CD MOLECULES

The following table is based on a workshop held in February 1989 to update the list of human CD molecules. More detailed descriptions of individual CD molecules, with relevant references, can be found in the workshop report, which was published as a book: *Leukocyte Typing IV. White Cell Differentiation Antigens,* by Knapp W., B. Dorken, W.R. Gilks, et al. (eds.). Oxford, Oxford University Press, 1989.

CD Designation	Common Synonym(s)	Molecular Structure	Main Cellular Expression	Known or Proposed Function(s)
CD1a*†	T6	49 kD; β_2 microglobulin-associated	Thymocytes, dendritic cells (incl. Langerhans cells)	? Ligand for some $\gamma\delta$ T cells
CD1b	–	45 kD; β_2 microglobulin-associated	Same as CD1a	Same as CD1a
CD1c	–	43 kD; β_2 microglobulin-associated	Same as CD1a	Same as CD1a
CD2	T11; LFA-2; sheep red blood cell receptor	50 kD	T cells, NK cells	Adhesion molecule (binds LFA-3); T cell activation
CD3	T3; Leu-4	Composed of five chains (see Chapter 7)	T cells	Signal transduction as a result of antigen recognition by T cells
CD4	T4; Leu-3; L3T4 (mice)	55 kD	Class II MHC–restricted T cells	Adhesion molecule (binds to class II MHC); signal transduction
CD5	T1; Lyt1	67 kD	T cells; B cell subset	?
CD6	T12	100 kD	Subset of T cells; some B cells	?
CD7	–	40 kD	Subset of T cells	?
CD8	T8; Leu-2; Lyt2	Composed of two 34 kD chains; expressed as $\alpha\alpha$ or $\alpha\beta$ dimer	Class I MHC–restricted T cells	Adhesion (binds to class I MHC); signal transduction
CD9	–	24 kD	Pre-B and immature B cells; monocytes, platelets	? Role in platelet activation
CD10	CALLA	100 kD	Immature and some mature B cells; lymphoid progenitors, granulocytes	Structurally identical to neural endopeptidase (enkephalinase)
CD11a‡	LFA-1 α chain	180 kD; associates with CD18 to form LFA-1 integrin	Leukocytes	Adhesion (binds to ICAM-1)
CD11b	Mac-1; CR3 (iC3B receptor) α chain	165 kD; associates with CD18 to form Mac-1 integrin	Granulocytes, monocytes, NK cells	Adhesion; phagocytosis of iC3b-coated (opsonized) particles
CD11c	p150,95; CR4 α chain	150 kD; associates with CD18 to form p150,95 integrin	Monocytes, granulocytes, NK cells	Adhesion; ? phagocytosis of iC3b-coated (opsonized) particles
CDw12§	–	? 90–120 kD	Monocytes, granulocytes	Nature and properties of "CDw12" need to be re-evaluated
CD13	–	150 kD	Monocytes, granulocytes	Aminopeptidase; ? role in oxidative burst
CD14	Mo2	55 kD; PI-linked	Monocytes	? Role in oxidative burst
CD15	–	Carbohydrate epitope	Granulocytes	?
CD16	FcRIII	50–70 kD; PI-linked and transmembrane	NK cells, granulocytes, macrophages	Low-affinity Fcγ receptor: ADCC, activation of NK cells
CDw17	–	Carbohydrate epitope (lactosylceramide)	Granulocytes, macrophages, platelets	?
CD18	β chain of LFA-1 family ($\beta2$ integrins)	95 kD; noncovalently linked to CD11a, CD11b, or CD11c	Leukocytes	See CD11a, CD11b, CD11c
CD19	B4	90 kD	Most B cells	? Role in B cell activation or regulation
CD20	B1	Heterodimer: 35 and 37 kD chains	Most or all B cells	? Role in B cell activation or regulation
CD21	CR2; C3d receptor	145 kD	Mature B cells	Receptor for C3d, Epstein-Barr virus; ? role in B cell activation

CD Designation	Common Synonym(s)	Molecular Structure	Main Cellular Expression	Known or Proposed Function(s)
CD22	–	135 kD	B cells	?
CD23	FcεRIIb	45–50 kD	Activated B cells, macrophages	Low-affinity Fcε receptor, induced by IL–4; function unknown
CD24	–	Heterodimer of 38 and 41 kD chains	B cells, granulocytes	?
CD25	TAC; p55; low-affinity IL–2 receptor	55 kD	Activated T and B cells; activated macrophages	Complexes with p70 to form high-affinity IL–2 receptor; T cell growth
CD26	–	120 kD	Activated T and B cells; macrophages	Serine peptidase, function unknown
CD27	–	Homodimer of 55 kD chains	Most T cells; ? some plasma cells	? Role in B cell growth
CD28	Tp44	Homodimer of 44 kD chains	T cells (most CD4+, some CD8+ cells)	? T cell receptor for costimulator molecule(s)
CD29	β chain of VLA antigens (β1 integrins)	130 kD; noncovalently associated with VLA α chains (CDw49)	Broad	Adhesion to extracellular matrix proteins, cell-cell adhesion (see CDw49)
CD30	Ki-1	105 kD	Activated T and B cells; Reed-Sternberg cells in Hodgkin's disease	?
CD31	Platelet gpIIa	140 kD	Platelets; monocytes, granulocytes, B cells, endothelial cells	?
CDw32	FcRII	~40 kD	Macrophages, granulocytes, B cells, eosinophils	Fc receptor for aggregated IgG; role in phagocytosis, ADCC
CD33	–	67 kD	Monocytes, myeloid progenitor cells	?
CD34	–	105–120 kD	Precursors of hematopoietic cells	?
CD35	CR1; C3b receptor	Polymorphic; four forms are 190–280 kD	Granulocytes, monocytes, erythrocytes, B cells	Binding and phagocytosis of C3b-coated particles and immune complexes
CD36	Platelet gpIIIb	90 kD	Monocytes, platelets	? Platelet adhesion
CD37	–	Composed of 2 or 3 40–52 kD chains	B cells, some T cells	?
CD38	T10	45 kD	Plasma cells, thymocytes, activated T cells	?
CD39	–	70–100 kD	Mature B cells	?
CD40	–	Heterodimer of 44 and 48 kD chains	B cells	? Role in B cell growth, memory cell generation
CD41	gpIIb/IIIa complex (gpIIIa is CD61)	Complex of gpIIb heterodimer (120 and 23 kD) and gpIIIa (CD61)	Platelets	Platelet aggregation and activation: receptor for fibrinogen, fibronectin (binds to R-G-D sequence)
CD42a	Platelet gpIX	23 kD; forms complex with CD42b	Platelets, megakaryocytes	Platelet adhesion, binding to von Willebrand factor
CD42b	Platelet gpIb	Dimer of 135 and 25 kD chains, forms complex with CD42a	See CD42a	See CD42a
CD43	Sialophorin	95 kD, highly sialylated	Leukocytes (except circulating B cells)	? Role in T cell activation
CD44	Pgp-1; Hermes	80–>100 kD, highly glycosylated	Leukocytes, erythrocytes	May function as homing receptor; receptor for matrix components (e.g., hyaluronate)
CD45	T200; leukocyte common antigen	Four isoforms, 180–220 kD	Leukocytes	? Role in signal transduction (tyrosine phosphatase)
CD45R	Restricted forms of CD45	CD45RO: 180 kD CD45RA: 220 kD CD45RB: 190, 205 and 220 kD isoforms	CD45RO: memory T cells CD45RA: naive T cells CD45RB: B cells; subset of T cells	See CD45
CD46	Membrane cofactor protein (MCP)	45–70 kD	Leukocytes; epithelial cells, fibroblasts	Regulation of complement activation

CD Designation	Common Synonym(s)	Molecular Structure	Main Cellular Expression	Known or Proposed Function(s)
CD47	–	47 – 52 kD	Broad	?
CD48	–	41 kD; PI – linked	Leukocytes	?
CDw49a‖	VLA α1 chain	210 kD; associates with CD29 to form VLA – 1 (β1 integrin)	T cells, monocytes	Adhesion to collagen, laminin
CDw49b	VLA α2 chain; platelet gpIa	170 kD; associates with CD29 to form VLA – 2 (β1 integrin)	Platelets, activated T cells, monocytes, some B cells	Adhesion to extracellular matrix: receptor for collagen
CDw49c	VLA α3 chain	Dimer of 130 and 25 kD; associates with CD29 to form VLA – 3 (β1 integrin)	T cells; some B cells, monocytes	Adhesion to fibronectin, laminin
CDw49d	VLA α4 chain	150 kD; associates with CD29 to form VLA – 4 (β1 integrin)	T cells, monocytes, B cells	Peyer's patch homing receptor, binds to VCAM – 1; adhesion to fibronectin
CDw49e	VLA α5 chain	Dimer of 135 and 25 kD; associates with CD29 to form VLA – 5 (β1 integrin)	T cells; few B cells and monocytes	Adhesion to fibronectin
CDw49f	VLA α6 chain	150 kD; associates with CD29 to form VLA – 6 (β1 integrin)	Platelets, megakaryocytes; activated T cells	Adhesion to extracellular matrix: receptor for laminin
CDw50	–	108 – 140 kD; ?PI – linked	Leukocytes	?
CD51	α chain of vitronectin receptor	140 kD heterodimer, associates with CD61	Platelets	Adhesion: receptor for vitronectin, fibrinogen, von Willebrand factor (binds R-G-D sequence)
CDw52	–	? 21 – 28 kD	Leukocytes	?
CD53	–	32 – 40 kD	Leukocytes, plasma cells	?
CD54	ICAM – 1	80 – 114 kD	Broad; many activated cells (cytokine-inducible)	Adhesion: ligand for LFA – 1
CD55	Decay accelerating factor (DAF)	70 kD; PI – linked	Broad	Regulation of complement activation
CD56	Leu-19	Heterodimer of 135 and 220 kD chains	NK cells	Homotypic adhesion; isoform of neural cell adhesion molecule (N – CAM)
CD57	HNK – 1, Leu-7	110 kD	NK cells, subset of T cells	?
CD58	LFA – 3	55 – 70 kD; PI – linked	Broad	Adhesion: ligand for CD2
CD59	Membrane inhibitor of reactive lysis (MIRL)	18 – 20 kD; PI – linked	Broad	Regulation of complement (MAC) action
CDw60	–	Carbohydrate epitope	Subset of T cells, platelets	?
CD61	β chain of vitronectin receptor (β3 integrin); gpIIIa	110 kD; associates with CD51 (α chain of vitronectin receptor)	Platelets, megakaryocytes	See CD51
CD62	GMP – 140	140 kD; platelet granule protein that is translocated to cell surface upon activation	Platelets, endothelial cells	Neutrophil and monocyte adhesion to endothelium, platelets
CD63	–	53 kD; present in platelet lysosomes, translocated to cell surface upon activation	Activated platelets; monocytes, macrophages	?
CD64	FcRI	75 kD	Monocytes, macrophages	High-affinity Fcγ receptor: role in phagocytosis, ADCC, macrophage activation
CDw65	–	Carbohydrate epitope	Granulocytes	? Role in neutrophil activation
CD66	–	180 – 200 kD phosphorylated glycoprotein	Granulocytes	?
CD67	–	100 kD; PI – linked	Granulocytes	?
CD68	–	110 kD, intracellular protein, weak surface expression	Monocytes, macrophages	?
CD69	–	Homodimer of 28 – 34 kD chains, phosphorylated glycoprotein	Activated B and T cells, macrophages, NK cells	?
CDw70	–	?	Activated T and B cells	?
CD71	T9; transferrin receptor	95 kD homodimer	Activated T and B cells, macrophages, proliferating cells	Receptor for transferrin: role in iron metabolism, cell growth

CD Designation	Common Synonym(s)	Molecular Structure	Main Cellular Expression	Known or Proposed Function(s)
CD72	–	Heterodimer of 39 and 43 kD chains	B cells	?
CD73	–	69 kD; PI–linked	Subsets of T and B cells	Ecto-5'-nucleotidase, regulates nucleotide metabolism
CD74	Class II MHC invariant (γ) chain; I$_i$	Three protein species: 35, 41, and 53 kD	B cells, monocytes, macrophages; other class II$^+$ cells	Associates with newly synthesized class II MHC molecules
CDw75	–	53 kD	Mature B cells	?
CD76	–	Heterodimer of 67 and 85 kD chains	Mature B cells, subset of T cells	?
CD77	–	Carbohydrate epitope	Follicular center B cells	?
CDw78	Ba	?	B cells	?

* CD molecules to which reference has been made in the text of this book are indicated in boldface.

† The small letters affixed to some CD numbers refer to complex CD molecules that are encoded by multiple genes or that belong to families of structurally related proteins. For instance, CD1a, CD1b, and CD1c are structurally related but distinct forms of a β_2 microglobulin–associated nonpolymorphic protein.

‡ CD11a, CD11b, and CD11c are three α chains that can noncovalently associate with the same β chain (CD18) to form three different integrins, all of which are members of the "CD11CD18" family (also called the "LFA–1 family" or the "$\beta 2$ integrins").

§ Antibodies that have been submitted recently, or whose reactivity has not been fully confirmed, are said to identify putative CD molecules, indicated with a "w" (for "workshop") designation.

‖ CD49a, CD49c, and CD49e are tentative names because not enough antibodies reactive with these molecules are available yet to permit the designation of "clusters of differentiation."

Abbreviations: LFA, leukocyte function–associated antigen; MHC, major histocompatibility complex; kD, kilodalton; ICAM, intercellular adhesion molecule; NK, natural killer; VLA, very late antigen; IL, interleukin; MAC, membrane attack complex; Ig, immunoglobulin; ADCC, antibody-dependent cell-mediated cytotoxicity; VCAM, vascular cell adhesion molecule; GP, glycoprotein; GMP, granule membrane protein; PI, phosphatidylinositol; TAC, T cell activation antigen.

INDEX

Note: Numbers in *italics* refer to illustrations. Numbers followed by
(t) indicate tables; numbers followed by (b) indicate boxed material.